HUMAN HEALTH AND DISEASE

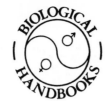

II

HUMAN HEALTH
AND DISEASE

COMPILED AND EDITED BY

Philip L. Altman and Dorothy Dittmer Katz

Federation of American Societies for Experimental Biology

BETHESDA, MARYLAND

Library of Congress Catalog Card Number: 76-53166

International Standard Book Number: 0-913822-11-6

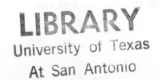

FOREWORD

The new series of Biological Handbooks is designed to provide as reliable biological data as there exists to investigators in biomedical research. The first volume, *Cell Biology,* was oriented mainly toward those engaged in laboratory research, and this second volume is oriented more toward those in clinical investigation. Nonetheless, we hope that these volumes, and all subsequent volumes, will be of broad use to the biomedical community.

In designing and implementing this series, the Editorial Board is constantly aware that it must steer a perilous course between Scylla and Charybdis: the availability of "hard" biological data is limited, and conflict with standard textbooks of medicine and pathology must be avoided. We have addressed the first problem by restricting the contents of this volume to man, with substantiating data for animals only where necessary, by requesting quantitative data wherever possible, and by rigorous peer review of all the data. The second issue was handled by omitting discussion of the treatment of disease and by using drug data only when it was of fundamental biological interest.

The Editorial Board realizes that the publication of a series of Biological Handbooks is an ambitious and difficult enterprise. However, we feel very strongly that the prime responsibility of a learned society is to provide reliable data to the scientific community that it serves. The progress of science depends upon the systematic accumulation of facts—preferably in quantitative terms—upon which all investigators can build. The process of cataloging such information is often tedious and fraught with the passions and prejudices of the moment. Hopefully, the collective efforts of the biomedical scientific community under the aegis of the Federation will provide this vital collection of information in a dispassionate and reliable manner and present it in a systematic and useful format.

The Editorial Board wishes to acknowledge the support provided from several sources to the preparation of this volume. The National Institutes of Health awarded a grant to support the peer review process which assures maximal reliability of the data. The Burroughs Welcome Fund, the Commonwealth Fund, the International Business Machines Corporation, the Johnson and Johnson Associated Industries Fund, the Henry J. Kaiser Family Foundation, the Kroc Foundation, Eli Lilly and Company, and the Foundation for Microbiology provided support for the preparation and distribution of this book.

18 January 1977
Pittsburgh, Pennsylvania

Thomas J. Gill III, M.D., *Chairman*
Biological Handbooks Editorial Board

BIOLOGICAL HANDBOOKS EDITORIAL BOARD

HUMAN HEALTH AND DISEASE ADVISORY COMMITTEE

FASEB PUBLICATIONS COMMITTEE

OFFICE OF BIOLOGICAL HANDBOOKS STAFF

CONTRIBUTORS AND REVIEWERS

AAMODT, ROGER L.
NIH, Clinical Center, Nuclear Medicine
Department
Bethesda, Maryland 20014

ABRAHAMSON, SEYMOUR
University of Wisconsin
Madison, Wisconsin 53706

ADKINSON, N. FRANKLIN, JR.
Johns Hopkins University School of
Medicine
Baltimore, Maryland 21205

ALFORD, CHARLES A.
University of Alabama Medical Center
Birmingham, Alabama 35294

ALFORD, ROBERT H.
Veterans Administration Hospital
Nashville, Tennessee 37203

ALPER, CHESTER A.
Center for Blood Research
Boston, Massachusetts 02115

AMMANN, ARTHUR J.
University of California
San Francisco, California 94143

ANDREWS, J. ROBERT
4428 Volta Place, N.W.
Washington, D.C. 20007

AOKI, THOMAS T.
Elliott P. Joslin Research Laboratory
Boston, Massachusetts 02215

ARBUS, G. S.
Hospital for Sick Children
Toronto, Ontario, M5G 1X8, Canada

ARNASON, BARRY G.
University of Chicago
Chicago, Illinois 60637

ARONSON, STANLEY M.
Brown University
Providence, Rhode Island 02912

AUSTEN, K. FRANK
Robert B. Brigham Hospital
Boston, Massachusetts 02120

AXELROD, LLOYD
Harvard Medical School
Boston, Massachusetts 02115

AYOUB, ELIA M.
University of Florida College of
Medicine
Gainesville, Florida 32610

BAEHNER, ROBERT L.
Indiana University School of Medicine
Indianapolis, Indiana 46202

BALOWS, ALBERT
DHEW, Center for Disease Control
Atlanta, Georgia 30333

BANKER, BETTY Q.
Case Western Reserve University School
of Medicine
Cleveland, Ohio 44109

BARINGER, J. RICHARD
Veterans Administration Hospital
San Francisco, California 94121

BARRY, ARTHUR L.
University of California School of
Medicine
Sacramento, California 95817

BARTELS, HEINZ
Medizinische Hochschule Hannover
3 Hannover, German Federal Republic

BARTLETT, JOHN G.
Veterans Administration Hospital
Boston, Massachusetts 02130

BATES, DAVID V.
University of British Columbia
Vancouver, British Columbia,
V6T 1W5, Canada

BEARN, ALEXANDER G.
New York Hospital-Cornell Medical
Center
New York, New York 10021

BEITINS, INESE Z.
295 Harvard Street
Cambridge, Massachusetts 02139

BELL, WILLIAM R.
Johns Hopkins Medical Institutions
Baltimore, Maryland 21205

BELZER, FOLKERT O.
University of Wisconsin Hospitals
Madison, Wisconsin 53706

BERK, PAUL D.
NIH, National Institute of Arthritis,
Metabolism, and Digestive Diseases
Bethesda, Maryland 20014

BEUTLER, ERNEST
City of Hope National Medical Center
Duarte, California 91010

BICKFORD, REGINALD G.
University of California School of
Medicine
La Jolla, California 92093

BINFORD, CHAPMAN H.
Armed Forces Institute of Pathology
Washington, D.C. 20305

BISSONETTE, DAVID J.
University of Pittsburgh School of
Medicine
Pittsburgh, Pennsylvania 15213

BISTRIAN, BRUCE R.
New England Deaconess Hospital
Boston, Massachusetts 02115

BLACK, F. OWEN
Eye and Ear Hospital of Pittsburgh
Pittsburgh, Pennsylvania 15213

BLACKBURN, GEORGE L.
New England Deaconess Hospital
Boston, Massachusetts 02215

BLAESE, R. MICHAEL
NIH, National Cancer Institute,
Metabolism Branch
Bethesda, Maryland 20014

BLOOMER, JOSEPH R.
Yale University School of Medicine
New Haven, Connecticut 06510

BLUME, K. -G.
City of Hope National Medical Center
Duarte, California 91010

BOND, V. P.
Brookhaven National Laboratory
Upton, Long Island, New York 11973

BONDAREFF, WILLIAM
Northwestern University Medical
School
Chicago, Illinois 60611

BORZY, MICHAEL
University of Wisconsin Hospitals
Madison, Wisconsin 53706

BOWMAN, BARBARA H.
University of Texas Medical Branch
Galveston, Texas 77550

BOXER, LAURENCE A.
Indiana University School of Medicine
Indianapolis, Indiana 46202

BRANDTZAEG, PER
University of Oslo
Oslo 1, Norway

BRINKHOUS, K. M.
University of North Carolina School
of Medicine
Chapel Hill, North Carolina 27514

BRISCOE, WILLIAM A.
New York Hospital-Cornell Medical
Center
New York, New York 10021

BRODER, JOHN R.
State University of New York
Buffalo, New York 14215

BROOKS, FRANK P.
Hospital of the University of
Pennsylvania
Philadelphia, Pennsylvania 19104

BROSEUS, ROGER W.
NIH, Division of Research Services,
Radiation Safety Branch
Bethesda, Maryland 20014

BROWN, AUDREY K.
State University of New York
Brooklyn, New York 11203
BROWN, RICHARD B.
Peter Bent Brigham Hospital
Boston, Massachusetts 02115
BUCKLEY, REBECCA H.
Duke University Medical Center
Durham, North Carolina 27710
BUIST, NEIL R. M.
University of Oregon Health Sciences
Center
Portland, Oregon 97201
BULGER, ROGER J.
University of Massachusetts Medical
School
Worcester, Massachusetts 01605
BULLOCK, WARD E.
Yale University School of Medicine
New Haven, Connecticut 06510
BURKHOLDER, PETER
University of Wisconsin Medical
School
Madison, Wisconsin 53706

CAHILL, GEORGE F., JR.
Elliott P. Joslin Research Laboratory
Boston, Massachusetts 02215
CANFIELD, CRAIG J.
NIH, National Institute of Allergy and
Infectious Diseases
Bethesda, Maryland 20014
CAREY, W. D.
Mayo Clinic
Rochester, Minnesota 55901
CARRUTHERS, MARY M.
Northwestern University Medical
School
Chicago, Illinois 60611
CASARETT, GEORGE W.
University of Rochester School of
Medicine
Rochester, New York 14620
CASTOR, C. WILLIAM
University of Michigan School of
Medicine
Ann Arbor, Michigan 48104
CERDA, JAMES J.
University of Florida College of
Medicine
Gainesville, Florida 32610
CHARACHE, SAMUEL
Johns Hopkins Medical Institutions
Baltimore, Maryland 21205
CHERRY, JAMES D.
University of California School of
Medicine
Los Angeles, California 90024

CHRISTIAN, CHARLES L.
Cornell University Medical College
New York, New York 10021
CHOW, ANTHONY W.
Harbor General Hospital
Torrance, California 90509
CLEVE, HARTWIG
Institute for Anthropology and Human
Genetics
8 Munich, German Federal Republic
CLINE, MARTIN J.
University of California School of
Medicine
Los Angeles, California 90024
CLOWES, GEORGE H. A., JR.
Boston City Hospital
Boston, Massachusetts 02118
CLYDE, DAVID F.
Louisiana State University Medical
Center
New Orleans, Louisiana 70112
COBBS, C. GLENN
University of Alabama Medical Center
Birmingham, Alabama 35294
COGAN, DAVID G.
NIH, National Eye Institute
Bethesda, Maryland 20014
COGGINS, CECIL H.
Harvard Medical School
Boston, Massachusetts 02115
COHEN, ALAN S.
Boston University School of Medicine
Boston, Massachusetts 02118
CONLEY, C. LOCKARD
Johns Hopkins Medical Institutions
Baltimore, Maryland 21205
CONRAD, MARCEL E.
University of Alabama
Birmingham, Alabama 35294
COOPER, MAX D.
University of Alabama Medical Center
Birmingham, Alabama 35294
COUNTS, GEORGE W.
Harborview Medical Center
Seattle, Washington 98104
COX, KAYE B.
Lenox Hill Hospital
New York, New York 10021
CRAIG, WILLIAM A.
Veterans Administration Hospital
Madison, Wisconsin 53705
CRANE, LAWRENCE R.
Wayne State University School of
Medicine
Detroit, Michigan 48201
CROSBY, WILLIAM H.
Scripps Clinic and Research Founda-
tion
La Jolla, California 92037

CROWLEY, WILLIAM F., JR.
Massachusetts General Hospital
Boston, Massachusetts 02114
CUSHING, RALPH D.
Detroit General Hospital
Detroit, Michigan 48226

DANIELS, GILBERT H.
Massachusetts General Hospital
Boston, Massachusetts 02114
DAVENPORT, FRED M.
University of Michigan
Ann Arbor, Michigan 48109
DAVIS, RICHARD L.
University of Southern California
School of Medicine
Los Angeles, California 90033
DeMARIA, ANTHONY N.
University of California School of
Medicine
Davis, California 95616
D'ESOPO, NICHOLAS
Veterans Administration Hospital
West Haven, Connecticut 06516
DILLON, HUGH C.
University of Alabama Medical Center
Birmingham, Alabama 35294
DOHERTY, R. L.
Queensland Institute of Medical
Research
Brisbane, Queensland 4006, Australia
DONALDSON, ROBERT M., JR.
Veterans Administration Hospital
San Francisco, California 94121
DOOLITTLE, RUSSELL F.
University of California
La Jolla, California 92037
DOWDLE, WALTER R.
DHEW, Center for Disease Control
Atlanta, Georgia 30333
DREILING, DAVID A.
Mount Sinai School of Medicine
New York, New York 10029
DREYFUS, PIERRE M.
University of California School of
Medicine
Davis, California 95616
DRUTZ, DAVID J.
University of Texas Health Science
Center
San Antonio, Texas 78284
DULL, H. BRUCE
DHEW, Center for Disease Control
Atlanta, Georgia 30333

EASTERDAY, B. C.
University of Wisconsin
Madison, Wisconsin 53706

EDSALL, GEOFFREY
  5 Ellerdale Road, Hampstead
  London, NW3 6BA, England
ERBE, RICHARD W.
  Massachusetts General Hospital
  Boston, Massachusetts 02114
ERSLEV, ALLAN J.
  Jefferson Medical College
  Philadelphia, Pennsylvania 19107
EXTON, JOHN H.
  Vanderbilt University School of
  Medicine
  Nashville, Tennessee 37232

FAIRBANKS, VIRGIL F.
  Mayo Clinic
  Rochester, Minnesota 55901
FALKNER, FRANK
  Fels Research Institute
  Yellow Springs, Ohio 45387
FASS, ROBERT J.
  Ohio State University Hospital
  Columbus, Ohio 43210
FEIGENBAUM, HARVEY
  Indiana University School of Medicine
  Indianapolis, Indiana 46202
FELIG, PHILIP
  Yale University School of Medicine
  New Haven, Connecticut 06510
FENNER, FRANK
  Australian National University
  Canberra, A.C.T. 2600, Australia
FIELDS, JAMES P.
  U.S. Public Health Service Hospital
  Staten Island, New York 10304
FINEGOLD, SYDNEY M.
  Wadsworth Hospital Center
  Los Angeles, California 90073
FISHER, EVELYN J.
  Henry Ford Hospital
  Detroit, Michigan 48202
FITCH, COY D.
  Saint Louis University School of
  Medicine
  St. Louis, Missouri 63104
FITZPATRICK, THOMAS B.
  Massachusetts General Hospital
  Boston, Massachusetts 02114

GAMBINO, S. RAYMOND
  College of Physicians and Surgeons of
  Columbia University
  New York, New York 10032
GANGAROSA, EUGENE J.
  DHEW, Center for Disease Control
  Atlanta, Georgia 30333
GARCIA, JULIO H.
  University of Maryland Hospital
  Baltimore, Maryland 21201

GARDNER, PIERCE
  Pritzker School of Medicine
  Chicago, Illinois 60637
GARDNER, REED M.
  Latter Day Saints Hospital
  Salt Lake City, Utah 84143
GEIGER, KLAUS K.
  Harvard Medical School
  Boston, Massachusetts 02115
GEWURZ, HENRY
  Rush Medical College
  Chicago, Illinois 60612
GIBBS, ERNA L.
  720 North Michigan Avenue
  Chicago, Illinois 60611
GIBBS, FREDERIC A.
  720 North Michigan Avenue
  Chicago, Illinois 60611
GIBLETT, ELOISE R.
  Puget Sound Blood Center
  Seattle, Washington 98104
GILDEN, DONALD
  University of Pennsylvania Hospital
  Philadelphia, Pennsylvania 19104
GOLDMAN, ARMOND S.
  University of Texas Medical Branch
  Galveston, Texas 77550
GOLDSTEIN, JOSEPH L.
  University of Texas Southwestern
  Medical School
  Dallas, Texas 75235
GOTTO, ANTONIO M., JR.
  Baylor College of Medicine
  Houston, Texas 77030
GRAY, GARY M.
  Stanford University Medical Center
  Stanford, California 94305
GREEN, RALPH
  Scripps Clinic and Research Founda-
  tion
  La Jolla, California 92037
GREGG, MICHAEL B.
  DHEW, Center for Disease Control
  Atlanta, Georgia 30333
GREAVES, M. F.
  University College London
  London, WC1E 6BT, England
GUMP, FRANK E.
  College of Physicians and Surgeons of
  Columbia University
  New York, New York 10032
GUREWICH, VICTOR
  St. Elizabeth's Hospital
  Brighton, Massachusetts 02135

HAGAN, A. D.
  Naval Regional Medical Center
  San Diego, California 92134

HANAHAN, DONALD J.
  University of Texas Health Science
  Center
  San Antonio, Texas 78284
HARRIS, H. WILLIAM
  New York University Medical Center
  New York, New York 10016
HAUSLER, W. J., JR.
  University of Iowa
  Iowa City, Iowa 52242
HAYWARD, ANTHONY R.
  University of Alabama Medical Center
  Birmingham, Alabama 35294
HEDLEY-WHYTE, JOHN
  Harvard Medical School
  Boston, Massachusetts 02115
HILLEMAN, MAURICE R.
  Merck Institute for Therapeutic
  Research
  West Point, Pennsylvania 19486
HOBBY, GLADYS L.
  Veterans Administration Hospital
  East Orange, New Jersey 07019
HOEPRICH, PAUL D.
  University of California School of
  Medicine
  Davis, California 95615
HOLLAND, PAUL B.
  NIH, Clinical Center, Blood Bank
  Bethesda, Maryland 20014
HONG, RICHARD
  University of Wisconsin Hospitals
  Madison, Wisconsin 53706
HOROWITZ, SHELDON
  University of Wisconsin Hospitals
  Madison, Wisconsin 53706
HOWELL, DAVID S.
  University of Miami School of
  Medicine
  Miami, Florida 33152
HUISMAN, TITUS H. J.
  Medical College of Georgia
  Augusta, Georgia 30902
HURSH, JOHN B.
  34 Woodland Road
  Pittsford, New York 14534
HYATT, R. E.
  Mayo Clinic
  Rochester, Minnesota 55901
HYDE, RICHARD W.
  University of Rochester School of
  Medicine and Dentistry
  Rochester, New York 14642

JACKSON, DUDLEY P.
  Georgetown University Hospital
  Washington, D.C. 20007

JACOBSON, ROBERT R.
U.S. Public Health Service Hospital
Carville, Louisiana 70721

JANNETTA, PETER J.
University of Pittsburgh School of
Medicine
Pittsburgh, Pennsylvania 15213

JANOWITZ, HENRY D.
Mount Sinai School of Medicine
New York, New York 10029

JENSEN, WALLACE N.
Albany Medical College
Albany, New York 12208

JOHNSON, KARL M.
DHEW, Center for Disease Control
Atlanta, Georgia 30333

JOHNSON, KENNETH P.
Veterans Administration Hospital
San Francisco, California 94121

JOHNSON, THOMAS W.
Meharry Medical College
Nashville, Tennessee 37208

JONES, E. ANTHONY
NIH, National Institute of Arthritis,
Metabolism, and Digestive Diseases
Bethesda, Maryland 20014

KANSU, EMIN
Jefferson Medical College
Philadelphia, Pennsylvania 19107

KAPLAN, EDWARD L.
University of Minnesota
Minneapolis, Minnesota 55455

KARPATKIN, SIMON
New York University Medical Center
New York, New York 10016

KARZON, DAVID T.
Vanderbilt University School of
Medicine
Nashville, Tennessee 37232

KATZ, MICHAEL
College of Physicians & Surgeons of
Columbia University
New York, New York 10032

KATZ, SAMUEL L.
Duke University Medical Center
Durham, North Carolina 27710

KAUFMAN, HERBERT E.
University of Florida College of
Medicine
Gainesville, Florida 32610

KENDALL, WILLIAM F.
William Beaumont Army Medical
Center
El Paso, Texas 79920

KERBER, RICHARD E.
University of Iowa College of
Medicine
Iowa City, Iowa 52242

KERSEY, JOHN H.
University of Minnesota Medical
School
Minneapolis, Minnesota 55455

KESSLER, GERALD
Jewish Hospital of St. Louis
St. Louis, Missouri 63178

KEUTMANN, HENRY T.
Massachusetts General Hospital
Boston, Massachusetts 02114

KHURANA, RAMESH K.
University of Maryland School of
Medicine
Baltimore, Maryland 21201

KIBRICK, SIDNEY
Boston University School of Medicine
Boston, Massachusetts 02118

KILBOURNE, EDWIN D.
Mount Sinai School of Medicine
New York, New York 10029

KLIMAN, BERNARD
Harvard Medical School
Boston, Massachusetts 02115

KNIGHT, VERNON
Baylor College of Medicine
Houston, Texas 77025

KOFF, RAYMOND S.
Boston University School of Medicine
Boston, Massachusetts 02115

KOLTS, BYRON E.
University of Florida College of
Medicine
Gainesville, Florida 32610

KORNGOLD, LEONHARD
Hospital for Special Surgery
New York, New York 10021

KOTCHER, EMIL
Louisiana State University Medical
Center
Shreveport, Louisiana 71130

KRAUSE, RICHARD M.
NIH, National Institute of Allergy and
Infectious Diseases
Bethesda, Maryland 20014

KRIGMAN, MARTIN R.
University of North Carolina School of
Medicine
Chapel Hill, North Carolina 27514

KUEPPERS, FRIEDRICH
Mayo Clinic
Rochester, Minnesota 55901

LAASBERG, L. H.
Harvard Medical School
Boston, Massachusetts 02115

LAUTER, CARL B.
Wayne State University School of
Medicine
Detroit, Michigan 48201

LEHRICH, JAMES R.
Massachusetts General Hospital
Boston, Massachusetts 02114

LEMANN, JACOB, JR.
Medical College of Wisconsin
Milwaukee, Wisconsin 53226

LESSELL, SIMMONS
Boston University School of Medicine
Boston, Massachusetts 02118

LEVY, HARVEY L.
Massachusetts General Hospital
Boston, Massachusetts 02114

LEWIS, C.
Harvard Medical School
Boston, Massachusetts 02115

LICHTENSTEIN, LAWRENCE M.
Johns Hopkins University School of
Medicine
Baltimore, Maryland 21205

LITWIN, STEPHEN D.
New York Hospital-Cornell Medical
Center
New York, New York 10021

LOEWENSTEIN, MATTHEW S.
Boston City Hospital
Boston, Massachusetts 02118

LUBY, JAMES P.
University of Texas Health Science
Center
Dallas, Texas 75235

MALOOF, FARAHE
Massachusetts General Hospital
Boston, Massachusetts 02114

MANN, DEAN L.
NIH, National Cancer Institute,
Immunology Branch
Bethesda, Maryland 20014

MARTIN, WILLIAM J.
University of California
Los Angeles, California 90024

MAYS, CHARLES W.
University of Utah
Salt Lake City, Utah 84132

McCOLLUM, ROBERT W.
Yale University School of Medicine
New Haven, Connecticut 06510

McCRORY, W. W.
New York Hospital-Cornell Medical
Center
New York, New York 10021

McCURDY, PAUL R.
American Red Cross
Washington, D.C. 20006

McDUFFIE, FREDERIC C.
Mayo Clinic
Rochester, Minnesota 55901

McGUIRE, JOSEPH
Yale University School of Medicine
New Haven, Connecticut 06510

McMICHAEL, ANDREW J.
Stanford University Medical Center
Stanford, California 94305
MELVIN, MAE
DHEW, Center for Disease Control
Atlanta, Georgia 30333
MENA, H.
University of Maryland Hospital
Baltimore, Maryland 21201
MERIGAN, THOMAS C.
Stanford University Medical Center
Stanford, California 94305
MERSON, MICHAEL H.
195 David Avenue
Brookline, Massachusetts 02146
MERZ, TIMOTHY
Medical College of Virginia
Richmond, Virginia 23298
MEUWISSEN, HILAIRE J.
Birth Defects Institute
Albany, New York 12237
MILLER, LOUIS H.
NIH, National Institute of Allergy and
Infectious Diseases
Bethesda, Maryland 20014
MOORE, FRANCIS D.
Peter Bent Brigham Hospital
Boston, Massachusetts 02115
MOORE-EDE, M. C.
Harvard Medical School
Boston, Massachusetts 02115
MOOSSY, JOHN
University of Pittsburgh School of
Medicine
Pittsburgh, Pennsylvania 15261
MORGAN, KARL Z.
Georgia Institute of Technology
Atlanta, Georgia 30332
MORRIS, JAMES F.
Veterans Administration Hospital
Portland, Oregon 97207
MOSLEY, JAMES W.
University of Southern California
School of Medicine
Los Angeles, California 90007

NEEL, JAMES V.
University of Michigan Medical School
Ann Arbor, Michigan 48104
NELSON, ERLAND R.
University of Maryland School of
Medicine
Baltimore, Maryland 21201
NELSON, JAMES S.
Washington University School of
Medicine
St. Louis, Missouri 63110
NEWCOMBE, HOWARD B.
Atomic Energy of Canada Limited
Chalk River, Ontario, K0J 1J0, Canada

NIEWIAROWSKI, STEFAN
Temple University School of Medicine
Philadelphia, Pennsylvania 19140
NORTHERN, JERRY L.
University of Colorado Medical Center
Denver, Colorado 80220
NUTTER, DONALD O.
Emory University School of Medicine
Atlanta, Georgia 30303

O'BRIEN, DONOUGH
University of Colorado Medical Center
Denver, Colorado 80220
OGRA, PEARAY L.
State University of New York School
of Medicine
Buffalo, New York 14222
O'REILLY, RICHARD J.
Memorial Sloan-Kettering Cancer
Center
New York, New York 10021
ORENSTEIN, WALTER
DHEW, Center for Disease Control
Atlanta, Georgia 30333
OSTROW, J. DONALD
Veterans Administration Hospital
Philadelphia, Pennsylvania 19104
OWEN, OLIVER E.
Temple University Medical School
Philadelphia, Pennsylvania 19140

PARKER, M. T.
Central Public Health Laboratory
London, NW9 5HT, England
PATERSON, PHILIP Y.
Northwestern University Medical
School
Chicago, Illinois 60611
PECHET, LIBERTO
University of Massachusetts Medical
Center
Worcester, Massachusetts 01605
PERPER, JOSHUA A.
Allegheny County Coroner's Office
Pittsburgh, Pennsylvania 15219
PETERSDORF, ROBERT G.
University of Washington
Seattle, Washington 98195
PIERRE, R. V.
Mayo Clinic
Rochester, Minnesota 55901
PLAUT, MARSHALL
Johns Hopkins University School of
Medicine
Baltimore, Maryland 21205
POLK, HIRAM C., JR.
University of Louisville School of
Medicine
Louisville, Kentucky 40201

PRINEAS, J. W.
Veterans Administration Hospital
East Orange, New Jersey 07019
PRITHAM, GORDON H.
8415 Spring Valley Road
Raytown, Missouri 64138
PURCELL, ROBERT H.
NIH, National Institute of Allergy and
Infectious Diseases
Bethesda, Maryland 20014

QUEVEDO, WALTER C., JR.
Brown University
Providence, Rhode Island 02912
QUIE, PAUL G.
University of Minnesota Medical
School
Minneapolis, Minnesota 55455

RAINE, CEDRIC S.
Albert Einstein College of Medicine
Bronx, New York 10461
RALEIGH, JAMES W.
Harris County Hospital District
Houston, Texas 77019
RAMMELKAMP, CHARLES H.
Case Western Reserve University
Cleveland, Ohio 44106
RE, RICHARD
Harvard Medical School
Boston, Massachusetts 02115
REEVES, JOHN T.
University of Colorado Medical Center
Denver, Colorado 80220
REYES, MILAGROS P.
Wayne State University School of
Medicine
Detroit, Michigan 48201
RIDGWAY, E. CHESTER
Massachusetts General Hospital
Boston, Massachusetts 02114
ROBINS, STEPHEN M.
NIH, National Eye Institute
Bethesda, Maryland 20014
ROBSON, ALAN M.
St. Louis Children's Hospital
St. Louis, Missouri 63110
ROCKLIN, ROSS E.
Robert B. Brigham Hospital
Boston, Massachusetts 02120
ROGERS, ARVEY I.
Veterans Administration Hospital
Miami, Florida 33125
ROOT, RICHARD K.
Yale University School of Medicine
New Haven, Connecticut 06510
RORKE, LUCY B.
Philadelphia General Hospital
Philadelphia, Pennsylvania 19104

ROSE, NOEL R.
Wayne State University School of
Medicine
Detroit, Michigan 48201
ROSENBERG, GARY L.
Johns Hopkins University School of
Medicine
Baltimore, Maryland 21205
ROSENBERG, LEON E.
Yale University School of Medicine
New Haven, Connecticut 06510
ROTHFIELD, NAOMI F.
University of Connecticut School of
Medicine
Farmington, Connecticut 06032
ROUHE, STANLEY A.
Loma Linda University School of
Medicine
Loma Linda, California 92354
ROWELL, LORING B.
University of Washington
Seattle, Washington 98195
RUBIN, ROBET H.
Massachusetts General Hospital
Boston, Massachusetts 02114
RUDDY, SHAUN
Medical College of Virginia
Richmond, Virginia 23298
RUDERMAN, NEIL B.
Elliott P. Joslin Research Laboratory
Boston, Massachusetts 02215
RYTEL, MICHAEL W.
Medical College of Wisconsin
Milwaukee, Wisconsin 53226

SANFORD, JAY P.
Uniformed Services University of the
Health Sciences
Bethesda, Maryland 20014
SCHALLER, JANE
University of Washington School of
Medicine
Seattle, Washington 98195
SCHLANT, ROBERT C.
Emory University School of Medicine
Atlanta, Georgia 30303
SCHRIER, ROBERT W.
University of Colorado Medical Center
Denver, Colorado 80220
SCHWARTZ, MORTON K.
Memorial Sloan-Kettering Cancer
Center
New York, New York 10021
SCHWARTZ, WILLIAM B.
Tufts University School of Medicine
Boston, Massachusetts 02111
SCRIVER, CHARLES R.
McGill University
Montreal, Quebec, H3H 1P3, Canada

SELKURT, EWALD E.
Indiana University School of Medicine
Indianapolis, Indiana 46202
SEVERINGHAUS, JOHN W.
University of California School of
Medicine
San Francisco, California 94143
SHEAGREN, JOHN N.
George Washington University Medical
Center
Washington, D.C. 20037
SHEPHERD, JOHN T.
Mayo Clinic
Rochester, Minnesota 55901
SHIH, VIVIAN E.
Massachusetts General Hospital
Boston, Massachusetts 02114
SILVA, JOSEPH, JR.
University Hospital
Ann Arbor, Michigan 48104
SIMMONS, RICHARD L.
University of Minnesota Hospitals
Minneapolis, Minnesota 55455
SLAVIN, RICHARD E.
Baltimore City Hospitals
Baltimore, Maryland 21224
SLEISENGER, MARVIN H.
Veterans Administration Hospital
San Francisco, California 94121
SOBER, ARTHUR J.
Massachusetts General Hospital
Boston, Massachusetts 02114
SOUTH, MARY A.
University of Pennsylvania School of
Medicine
Philadelphia, Pennsylvania 19174
STANNARD, J. NEWELL
University of Rochester School of
Medicine and Dentistry
Rochester, New York 14642
STEVENSON, STUART S.
2 Fifth Avenue
New York, New York 10011
STOLLERMAN, GENE H.
University of Tennessee
Memphis, Tennessee 38163
STORB, RAINER
Fred Hutchinson Cancer Research
Center
Seattle, Washington 98104
STOSSEL, THOMAS P.
Children's Hospital Medical Center
Boston, Massachusetts 02115
SUTTER, VERA L.
Wadsworth Hospital Center
Los Angeles, California 90073
SWAIN, ROBERT W.
NIH, National Cancer Institute,
Radiation Branch
Bethesda, Maryland 20014

TAN, ENG M.
Scripps Clinic and Research Founda-
tion
La Jolla, California 92037
TAYLOR, ANDREW, JR.
Veterans Administration Hospital
San Diego, California 92161
THOMPSON, JOHN H., JR.
Mayo Clinic
Rochester, Minnesota 55901
THORUP, OSCAR A., JR.
University of Virginia College of
Medicine
Charlottesville, Virginia 22901
TILLOTSON, JAMES R.
Albany Medical College
Albany, New York 12208
TRERICE, MARY S.
New England Deaconess Hospital
Boston, Massachusetts 02215
TUCKER, ALAN
Wright State University
Dayton, Ohio 45431

VALENTINE, WILLIAM N.
University of California School of
Medicine
Los Angeles, California 90024
VAN PILSUM, JOHN
University of Minnesota Medical
School
Minneapolis, Minnesota 55455
VAUGHAN, VICTOR C., III
St. Christopher's Hospital for Children
Philadelphia, Pennsylvania 19133
VERITY, M. ANTHONY
University of California School of
Medicine
Los Angeles, California 90024

WAGNER, WILLIAM M.
NIH, Division of Research Services,
Radiation Safety Branch
Bethesda, Maryland 20014
WALDMAN, ROBERT H.
West Virginia University School of
Medicine
Morgantown, West Virginia 26506
WANNAMAKER, LEWIS W.
University of Minnesota Hospitals
Minneapolis, Minnesota 55455
WASHINGTON, JOHN A., II
Mayo Clinic
Rochester, Minnesota 55901
WEATHERALL, D. J.
University of Oxford
Oxford, OX2 6HE, England
WEHRLE, PAUL F.
University of Southern California
Medical Center
Los Angeles, California 90033

WEINSTEIN, LOUIS
Peter Bent Brigham Hospital
Boston, Massachusetts 02115
WEIR, GORDON
Harvard Medical School
Boston, Massachusetts 02115
WEISSLER, ARNOLD M.
Wayne State University School of
Medicine
Detroit, Michigan 48201
WHITE, DAVID O.
University of Melbourne
Melbourne, Victoria 3052, Australia
WIESNER, PAUL J.
DHEW, Center for Disease Control
Atlanta, Georgia 30333
WILLIAMS, WILLIAM J.
State University Hospital
Syracuse, New York 13210

WILMORE, DOUGLAS W.
Brooke Army Medical Center
Fort Sam Houston, Texas 78234
WILSON, FRANCIS M.
Wayne State University School of
Medicine
Detroit, Michigan 48201
WITTE, JOHN J.
DHEW, Center for Disease Control
Atlanta, Georgia 30333
WOLINSKY, EMANUEL
Metropolitan General Hospital
Cleveland, Ohio 44109
WOODWARD, THEODORE E.
University of Maryland School of
Medicine
Baltimore, Maryland 21201

WRAY, SHIRLEY H.
Massachusetts Eye and Ear Infirmary
Boston, Massachusetts 02114

YOUNG, DONALD S.
NIH, Clinical Pathology Department
Bethesda, Maryland 20014

ZEE, DAVID S.
Johns Hopkins Hospital
Baltimore, Maryland 21205
ZELIS, ROBERT
Milton S. Hershey Medical Center
Hershey, Pennsylvania 17033
ZORUB, DAVID S.
University of Pittsburgh School of
Medicine
Pittsburgh, Pennsylvania 15213

CONTENTS

II. IMMUNOLOGICAL FACTORS

III. METABOLIC DISORDERS

V. NEUROLOGIC DISEASES

INTRODUCTION

HUMAN HEALTH AND DISEASE is volume II in a new series of Biological Handbooks. Each volume is devoted to the presentation of reference data on a discrete subject of vital importance to investigators, teachers, and students. Present plans are for the production of one such volume per year.

Contents and Review
HUMAN HEALTH AND DISEASE is arranged in seven sections with the material organized in the form of 186 tables of quantitative and descriptive data. With few exceptions, which are clearly indicated, coverage throughout the book is for man. Contents of this volume were authenticated by 326 outstanding experts in the fields of biology and medicine. The review process to which the data were subjected was designed to eliminate, insofar as possible, material of questionable validity and errors of transcription.

Headnote
An explanatory headnote, serving as an introduction to the subject matter, may precede a table. More frequently, tables are prefaced by a short headnote containing such important information as units of measurement, abbreviations, definitions, and estimate of the range of variation. To interpret the data, it is essential to read the related headnote.

Exceptions
Occasionally, differences in values for the same specifications, certain inconsistencies in nomenclature, and some overlapping of coverage may occur among tables. These result, not from oversight or failure to choose between alternatives, but from a deliberate intent to respect the judgment and preferences of the individual contributors.

Conventions and Terminology
The main conventions used throughout this volume were adapted from the third edition of the *CBE Style Manual,* published in 1972 for the Council of Biology Editors by the American Institute of Biological Sciences. Terminology was checked against *Webster's Third New International Dictionary,* published in 1961 by G. & C. Merriam Company.

Contributors and References
Appended to the tables are the names of the contributors, and a list of the literature citations arranged in alphabetical sequence. The reference abbreviations conform to those in the *Bibliographic Guide for Editors and Authors,* published by The American Chemical Society in 1974.

Enzyme Nomenclature
Enzyme names and Enzyme Commission numbers were verified in *Enzyme Nomenclature,* the 1972 recommendations of the Commission on Biochemical Nomenclature, published by Elsevier Scientific Publishing Company for the International Union of Pure and Applied Chemistry and the International Union of Biochemistry.

Range of Variation
Values are generally presented as either the mean plus and minus the standard deviation, or the mean and the lower and upper limit of the range of individual values about the mean (either observed or statistical). Usually, it is of greater importance that the range be given rather than the mean. The several methods used to estimate the range—depending on the information available—are designated by the letters "a, b, c, or d" to identify the type of range in descending order of accuracy.

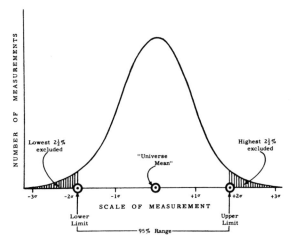

"a"—When the group of values is relatively large, a 95% range is derived by curve fitting. A recognized type of normal frequency curve is fitted to a group of measured values, and the extreme 2.5% of the area under the curve at each end is excluded (*see* illustration).

"b"—When the group of values is too small for curve fitting, as is usually the case, a 95% range is estimated by a simple statistical calculation. Assuming a normal symmetrical distribution, the standard deviation is multiplied by a factor of 2, then subtracted from and added to the mean to give the lower and upper range limits.

"c"—A less dependable, but commonly applied, procedure takes as range limits the lowest value and the highest value of the reported sample group of measurements. It underestimates the 95% range for small samples and overestimates for larger sample sizes, but where there is marked asymmetry in the position of the mean within the sample range, this method may be used in preference to the preceding one.

"d"—Another estimate of the lower and upper limits of the range of variation is based on the judgment of an individual experienced in measuring the quantity in question.

ABBREVIATIONS AND SYMBOLS

Only those abbreviations and symbols not generally defined in the
headnote, body, or footnotes of a table are included in this list.

Measurements

yr = year

mo = month

wk = week

d = day

h = hour

min = minute

s = second

ms = millisecond (10^{-3} second)

A.M. = *ante meridiem* (before noon)

P.M. = *post meridiem* (after noon)

m = meter; milli (prefix, 10^{-3})

km = kilometer (10^{-3} meters)

cm = centimeter (10^{-2} meter)

mm = millimeter (10^{-3} meter)

μm = micrometer (10^{-6} meter)

nm = nanometer (10^{-9} meter)

Å = angstrom (10^{-1} nanometer)

wt = weight

g = gram

kg = kilogram (10^{3} grams)

mg = milligram (10^{-3} gram)

μg = microgram (10^{-6} gram)

ng = nanogram (10^{-9} gram)

pg = picogram (10^{-12} gram)

mmole = millimole (10^{-3} mole)

μmole = micromole (10^{-6} mole)

nmole = nanomole (10^{-9} mole)

meq = milliequivalent

μeq = microequivalent

neq = nanoequivalent

mol wt = molecular weight

mM = millimolar (10^{-3} molar)

μM = micromolar (10^{-6} molar)

dl = deciliter (10^{-1} liter)

ml = milliliter (10^{-3} liter)

μl = microliter (10^{-6} liter)

% = percent (parts per hundred)

IU = international unit

μU = microunit

pH = negative logarithm of hydrogen ion concentration

pK' = first apparent dissociation constant

temp = temperature

°C = degrees Celsius

kcal = kilocalorie (10^{3} calories)

kPa = kilopascal

cm H_2O = centimeters of water

mm H_2O = millimeters of water

mm Hg = millimeters of mercury

mosmole = milliosmole

P_{O_2} = oxygen pressure

P_{CO_2} = carbon dioxide pressure

dB = decibel

Hz = hertz

mA = milliampere

Ω = ohm

kV = kilovolt

μV = microvolt

KeV = kiloelectron-volt

R = roentgen

mrem = millirem

mCi = millicurie

μCi = microcurie

no. = number

+ = plus; positive

− = minus; negative

± = plus or minus

X = times; by; crossed with

/ = per; divided by

$\sim$ = approximately

$\approx$ = approximately equal to

< = less than

> = greater than

<< = much less than

>> = much greater than

$\leqslant$ = less than or equal to

$\geqslant$ = greater than or equal to

$\lesssim$ = approximately less than or equal to

° = degree (angular)

Biological and Chemical Specifications

♂ = male

♀ = female

♂♀ = male and female

sp. = species (singular)

spp. = species (plural)

var. = variety

C2 (C3, C4) = second (third, fourth) cervical vertebra or spinal root

L1 = first lumbar vertebra or spinal root

T1 = (T12) first (twelfth) thoracic vertebra or spinal root

Hb = hemoglobin

RBC = red blood cell (erythrocyte)

WBC = white blood cell (leukocyte)

CNS = central nervous system

GI = gastrointestinal

ECG = electrocardiogram

IQ = intelligence quotient

K_m = Michaelis constant

SV40 = simian vacuolating virus

i.m. = intramuscular (ly)

i.p. = intraperitoneal (ly)

i.v. = intravenous (ly)

s.c. = subcutaneous (ly)

nat = naturally-occurring

ACTH = adrenocorticotropic hormone

DPT = diphtheria-pertussis-tetanus

EDTA = ethylenediaminetetracetic acid

C1r, C1s, etc. = complement factors

HLA = human histocompatibility leukocyte antigen

IgA, IgD, IgE, IgG, IgM = immunoglobulin A, D, E, G, and M, respectively

DNA = deoxyribonucleic acid

RNA = ribonucleic acid

Tyr = tyrosine

ADP = adenosine 5'-diphosphate

AMP = adenosine 5'-monophosphate

cAMP = cyclic adenosine 3',5'-monophosphate

ATP = adenosine 5'-triphosphate

ATPase = adenosinetriphosphatase

DPNH = diphosphopyridine nucleotide, reduced form

FAD = flavin adenine dinucleotide

NAD = nicotinamide adenine dinucleotide

NAD^+ = nicotinamide adenine dinucleotide, oxidized form

NADH = nicotinamide adenine dinucleotide, reduced form

$NADP^+$ = nicotinamide adenine dinucleotide phosphate, oxidized form

NADPH = nicotinamide adenine dinucleotide phosphate, reduced form

UDP = uridine diphosphate

CoA = coenzyme A

dl = racemic mixture

l = levorotatory

D = dextro (configuration)

L = levo (configuration)

n = normal (configuration)

N = normal (concentration); *nitro*

O = *oxy*

S = *sulfo*

m = *meta*

o = *ortho*

p = *para*

s = symmetrical (ring compounds)

tert = tertiary

Δ^n = position of double bond

Miscellaneous

Fn = footnote

ref. = reference

vs. = versus

e.g. = *exempli gratia* (for example)

i.e. = *id est* (that is)

et al. = *et alii* (and others)

etc. = *et cetera* (and so forth)

HUMAN HEALTH AND DISEASE

I. INFECTIOUS DISEASES

1. PROPERTIES OF MICROORGANISMS AND VIRUSES

Symbols: + indicates "yes" or "present"; − indicates "no" or "not present."

	Organisms	DNA & RNA	Ribo-somes	Binary Fission	Growth on Non-living Media	Sensitivity to Antibiotics	Sensitivity to Interferon
1	Viruses	−	−	−	−	−	+
2	Chlamydiae	+	+	+	−	+	+
3	Rickettsiae	+	+	+	−	+	−
4	Mycoplasmas	+	+	+	+	+	−
5	Bacteria	+	+	+	+	+	−

Contributors: Fenner, Frank, and White, David O.

Reference: Fenner, F., and D. O. White. 1976. Medical Virology. Ed. 2. Academic Press, New York. p. 4.

2. COMPONENTS OF A COMPLETE VIRUS PARTICLE (VIRION)

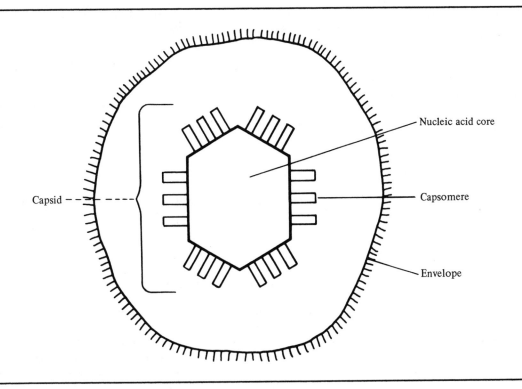

Contributor: Reyes, Milagros P.

Reference: Wintrobe, M. M., et al., ed. 1974. Harrison's Principles of Internal Medicine. Ed. 7. McGraw-Hill, New York. v. 1, p. 924.

3. MAJOR GROUPS OF VIRUSES INFECTING MAN

The viruses causing hepatitis A (infectious hepatitis) or hepatitis B (serum hepatitis) in man are at present unclassified.

	Group	Representative Virus ⟨Synonym⟩	Size nm	Symmetry	Presence of Envelope	Diethyl Ether Sensitivity
		DNA Viruses				
1	Parvovirus	Norwalk agent	18-22	Cubic	No	No
2	Papovavirus	Papilloma (warts), simian vacuolating virus ⟨SV40⟩	40-55	Cubic	No	No
3	Adenovirus	....	65-85	Cubic	No	No
4	Herpesvirus	*Herpesvirus hominis*, B virus ⟨monkey B⟩, varicella-herpes zoster, cytomegalovirus, Epstein-Barr	120-180	Cubic	Yes	Yes
5	Poxvirus	Variola, vaccinia, orf, milker's nodes, molluscum contagiosum	150-300	Complex[1]	Yes	Yes/No
		RNA Viruses				
6	Picornavirus	Enteroviruses: Coxsackieviruses, groups A and B, echoviruses, polioviruses; rhinoviruses	17-30	Cubic	No	No
7	Reovirus	Colorado tick fever; rotaviruses; orbiviruses	74	Cubic	No	No
8	Togaviruses	Rubella; most alphaviruses[2]: equine encephalitis, Semliki Forest; most flaviviruses[3]: dengue, Japanese B, Russian tick-borne, yellow fever	50	Cubic[1]	Yes	Yes
9	Myxovirus	Orthomyxoviruses: influenzas A, B, & C; paramyxoviruses: parainfluenza, mumps, measles[4]; metamyxoviruses: respiratory syncytial	80-200	Helical	Yes	Yes
10	Rhabdovirus	Rabies	65-180	Helical[1]	Yes	Yes
11	Arenavirus	Lymphocytic choriomeningitis ⟨LCM⟩; Tacaribe complex: Junin & Machupo (South American hemorrhagic fevers)	50-300	....	Yes	Yes
12	Coronavirus	....	70-120[1]	....	Yes	Yes
13	Arboviruses not yet classified in other groups	Group C: Marituba, Oriboca; Ungrouped: phlebotomus fever ⟨sand-fly fever⟩, Rift Valley fever	20-100	....	?	Yes

[1] From Melnick, J. L. 1972. Prog. Med. Virol. 14:321-332. [2] Formerly arboviruses group A. [3] Formerly arboviruses group B. [4] Synonym: Rubeola.

Contributor: Reyes, Milagros P.

Reference: Wintrobe, M. M., et al., ed. 1974. Harrison's Principles of Internal Medicine. Ed. 7. McGraw-Hill, New York. v. 1, p. 925.

4. HEMAGGLUTINATION BY VIRUSES

Herpetoviridae, Iridoviridae, and Arenaviridae do not produce hemagglutination.

	Virus		Erythrocytes Agglutinated	pH & Temperature
	Family	Genus or Common Name		
1	Parvoviridae	Adeno-associated virus type 4	Man, guinea pig	Temp, 4°C
2	Papovaviridae	Polyoma virus	Guinea pig	Temp, 4°C
3	Adenoviridae	Most types	Monkey, rat	Not critical
4	Poxviridae	Variola (smallpox), vaccinia	Fowl (some birds only)	Temp, 37°C

continued

4. HEMAGGLUTINATION BY VIRUSES

	Virus		Erythrocytes Agglutinated	pH & Temperature
	Family	**Genus or Common Name**		
5	Picornaviridae	Coxsackievirus (some serotypes)	Man	Vary with serotype
6		Echovirus (some serotypes)	Man	Vary with serotype
7		*Rhinovirus* (some serotypes)	Sheep	Temp, 4°C
8	Togaviridae	*Alphavirus, Flavivirus,* Rubella	Goose, pigeon	pH & temp critical
9	Orthomyxoviridae	Influenza types A & B	Fowl, man, guinea pig	Temp, 4°C or 22°C
10	Paramyxoviridae	Parainfluenza, mumps	Fowl, man, guinea pig	Temp, 4°C or 22°C
11		Measles	Monkey	Temp, 37°C
12	Rhabdoviridae	Rabies	Goose	Temp, 4°C
13	Coronaviridae	Human strains	Rat, mouse, fowl	Temp, 37°C
14	Bunyaviridae	*Bunyavirus*	Goose	pH critical
15	Reoviridae	*Reovirus*	Man	Not critical

Contributors: Fenner, Frank, and White, David O.

Reference: Fenner, F., and D. O. White. 1976. Medical Virology. Ed. 2. Academic Press, New York. p. 43.

5. MODES OF TRANSMISSION OF HUMAN VIRUSES

Virus: EB virus = Epstein-Barr virus.

	Mode of Transmission	Specification	Family	Virus
1	Respiratory	Local symptoms	Adenoviridae	Many serotypes
2			Picornaviridae	*Rhinovirus:* Many serotypes; *Enterovirus:* A few serotypes
3			Orthomyxoviridae	Influenza types A & B
4			Paramyxoviridae	Parainfluenza; respiratory syncytial virus
5			Coronaviridae	Many serotypes
6		General symptoms	Herpetoviridae	Varicella-zoster; EB virus
7			Poxviridae	Variola (smallpox)
8			Togaviridae	Rubella
9			Paramyxoviridae	Mumps, measles
10			Arenaviridae	Lymphocytic choriomeningitis; Lassa virus
11	Alimentary	Local symptoms	Adenoviridae	A few serotypes
12			Picornaviridae	A few enteroviruses
13			Reoviridae	Including rotavirus
14		General symptoms	Picornaviridae	Many enteroviruses, including polioviruses
15			Unclassified	Hepatitis viruses, especially A
16	Contact (skin)	....	Papovaviridae	Papilloma (warts)
17			Herpetoviridae	Herpes simplex types 1 (oral) and 2 (genital); EB virus
18			Poxviridae	Molluscum contagiosum; cowpox; orf; milker's nodes
19	Arthropod bite	Mechanical	Poxviridae	Tanapox virus
20		Propagative	Togaviridae	Alphaviruses, various; flaviviruses, various
21			Bunyaviridae	Bunyaviruses, various
22			Reoviridae	Orbiviruses, various
23	Animal bite	....	Herpetoviridae	B virus
24			Rhabdoviridae	Rabies virus
25	Injection	....	Unclassified	Hepatitis B
26		By transfusion	Herpetoviridae	Cytomegalovirus, EB virus (infectious mononucleosis)
27	Transplacental	....	Herpetoviridae	Cytomegalovirus
28			Togaviridae	Rubella

Contributors: Fenner, Frank, and White, David O.

Reference: Fenner, F., and D. O. White. 1970. Medical Virology. Academic Press, New York. p. 143.

6. EPIDEMIOLOGICAL FEATURES OF SOME COMMON HUMAN VIRAL DISEASES

Incubation Period indicates time from exposure until first appearance of prodromal symptoms; diagnostic signs, e.g., rash or paralysis, may not appear until 2-4 days later. **Period of Communicability:** Most viral diseases are highly transmissible for a few days before symptoms appear; short = <4 days; moderate = 4-10 days; long = >10 days; very long = years. **Incidence of Subclinical Infections:** high = >90%; moderate = 10-90%; low = <10%.

	Disease	Common Mode of Transmission	Incubation Period, d	Period of Communicability	Incidence of Subclinical Infections
1	Acute respiratory disease (A.R.D.) [1]	Respiratory	5-7	Short	Moderate
2	Bronchiolitis; croup	Respiratory	3-5	Short	Moderate
3	Chicken pox	Respiratory	13-17	Moderate	Moderate
4	Common cold	Respiratory	1-3	Short	Moderate
5	Dengue	Mosquito bite	5-8	Short	Moderate
6	Enteroviral diseases	Alimentary	6-12	Long	High
7	Hepatitis A	Alimentary	15-40	Long	High
8	Hepatitis B	Inoculation	50-150	Very long	High
9	Herpes simplex	Contact	5-8	Long	Moderate
10	Infectious mononucleosis	Contact	30-50	? Long	High
11	Influenza	Respiratory	1-2	Short	Moderate
12	Measles	Respiratory	9-12	Moderate	Low
13	Mumps	Respiratory	16-20	Moderate	Moderate
14	Poliomyelitis	Alimentary	5-20	Long	High
15	Rabies	Animal bite	30-100	Nil	Nil
16	Rubella	Respiratory	17-20	Moderate	Moderate
17	Smallpox	Respiratory	12-14	Moderate	Low
18	Warts	Contact	50-150	Long	Low

[1] Caused by adenoviruses.

Contributors: Fenner, Frank, and White D. O.

Reference: Fenner, F., and D. O. White. 1976. Medical Virology. Ed. 2. Academic Press, New York. p. 199.

7. PATTERNS OF ILLNESS WITH RESPIRATORY VIRUSES IN OLDER CHILDREN AND ADULTS

Manifestation: Constitutional—CNS = central nervous system. *Symbols:* ++ = severe; + = moderately severe; ± = mild; ? = unknown or uncommon.

	Agent	Relative Frequency of Occurrence	Rhinitis	Pharyngitis	Tracheo-bronchitis	Pneumonia	Constitutional
1	Rhinovirus	40	++	±	+	Rare	±; usually afebrile
2	Herpesvirus	10	+	++	Rare	Rare	+
3	Influenza A & B viruses	10	+	+	++	Severe when present	++; high fever common
4	Parainfluenza viruses	8	+	++	++ [1]	Rare	+; low or no fever
5	Coronaviruses	8	+	+	+	?	+
6	Respiratory syncytial virus	6	++	+	+ [2]	?	+; usually afebrile
7	Adenoviruses	2	+	++	++	Severe when present	++; high fever
8	Coxsackieviruses & echo-viruses	<1	±	+	+	?	++; fever; visceral & CNS complications
9	Other	13	?	?	?	?	?

[1] Laryngeal involvement common. [2] Especially in older patients.

Contributor: Knight, Vernon

Reference: Thorn, G., et al., ed. 1977. Harrison's Principles of Internal Medicine. Ed. 8. McGraw-Hill, New York.

8. CLASSIFICATION OF HUMAN RESPIRATORY VIRUSES

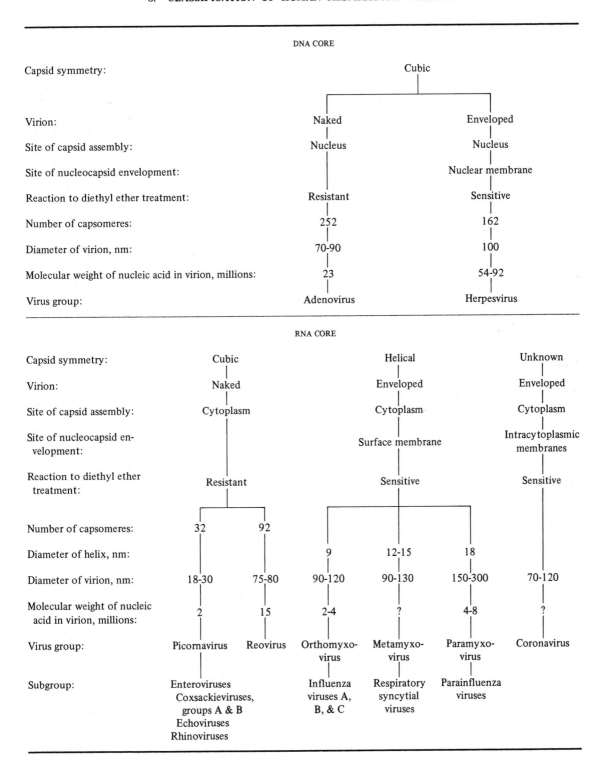

DNA CORE

Capsid symmetry:		Cubic
Virion:	Naked	Enveloped
Site of capsid assembly:	Nucleus	Nucleus
Site of nucleocapsid envelopment:		Nuclear membrane
Reaction to diethyl ether treatment:	Resistant	Sensitive
Number of capsomeres:	252	162
Diameter of virion, nm:	70-90	100
Molecular weight of nucleic acid in virion, millions:	23	54-92
Virus group:	Adenovirus	Herpesvirus

RNA CORE

Capsid symmetry:	Cubic		Helical			Unknown
Virion:	Naked		Enveloped			Enveloped
Site of capsid assembly:	Cytoplasm		Cytoplasm			Cytoplasm
Site of nucleocapsid envelopment:			Surface membrane			Intracytoplasmic membranes
Reaction to diethyl ether treatment:	Resistant		Sensitive			Sensitive
Number of capsomeres:	32	92				
Diameter of helix, nm:			9	12-15	18	
Diameter of virion, nm:	18-30	75-80	90-120	90-130	150-300	70-120
Molecular weight of nucleic acid in virion, millions:	2	15	2-4	?	4-8	?
Virus group:	Picornavirus	Reovirus	Orthomyxovirus	Metamyxovirus	Paramyxovirus	Coronavirus
Subgroup:	Enteroviruses Coxsackieviruses, groups A & B Echoviruses Rhinoviruses		Influenza viruses A, B, & C	Respiratory syncytial viruses	Parainfluenza viruses	

Contributor: Knight, Vernon

Reference: Thorn, G., et al., ed. 1977. Harrison's Principles of Internal Medicine. Ed. 8. McGraw-Hill, New York.

9. INFLUENZA VIRUSES AND THEIR MAJOR SUBTYPES

Influenza viruses belong to the genus *Orthomyxovirus*. **Subtype:** Each is a major antigenic variant with respect to hemagglutinin (H) and/or neuraminidase (N) external virion antigens. Chronologic transition from one subtype to another constitutes antigenic "shift," and is usually associated with pandemic disease. **Antigenic Variants:** Each is a minor antigenic variant within a subtype, probably resulting from a series of point mutations and selection. These changes constitute antigenic "drift" and may effectively challenge subtype-specific immunity within an interpandemic period. Data were adapted from reference 2.

	Type	Subtype	Former Name	Prevalence	Antigenic Variants
	A	Human			
1		H0N1	Influenza A	? 1929-1947	Several
2		H1N1	Influenza A'	1947-1957	Several
3		H2N2	Asian	1957-1968	Several
4		H3N2	Hong Kong	1968-	A/Hong Kong/1/68 [1]
5					A/England/42/72
6					A/Port Chalmers/73
7					A/Victoria/3/75, etc.
		Animal			Only minor intrasubtype variation has
8		Swine: HswN1 [2]	....	? 1918-1929; 1976-	been observed
		Horse	....	....	
9		Heq1Neq1			
10		Heq2Neq2			
11		Avian: Hav1Nav3, etc. [3]	....	....	
12	B	No true subtypes, but antigenic variation is equivalent to that within an influenza A subtype	....	....	....
13	C	None	....	....	Significant variation has not been defined

[1] Strain designation is A/Hong Kong/1/68 (H3N2) [ref. 1]. [2] Probable human prototype strain of 1918-1929; recent appearance in humans in New Jersey in January 1976.

[3] 9 subtypes based on nature of hemagglutinin. All 10 of the known neuraminidase antigens have been found among the viruses recovered from avian species.

Contributor: Kilbourne, Edwin D.

References
1. Chanock, R. M., et al. 1971. Bull. WHO 45:119-124.

2. Kilbourne, E. D. 1975. The Influenza Viruses and Influenza. Academic Press, New York. p. 4.

10. ILLNESSES OR SYNDROMES ASSOCIATED WITH COXSACKIEVIRUS OR ECHOVIRUS INFECTIONS

Virus Types: The listing is not inclusive. Data were adapted from reference 20.

	Illness or Syndrome	Virus Types			Reference
		Coxsackievirus		Echovirus	
		Group A	Group B		
1	No illness [1]	1-24	1-6	1-9, 11-34	12,19
2	Mild or moderate illness Undifferentiated mild febrile illness (non-specific)	1-24	1-6	1-8, 11-34	14,18
3	Upper respiratory syndromes: rhinitis, pharyngitis (including herpangina & lymphonodular pharyngitis), conjunctivitis	1-10, 16, 21 [2], 22, 24	1-5	1, 3, 6, 9, 16, 19, 20, 28	18

[1] In probably 75% of cases. [2] Also known as Coe virus.

continued

10. ILLNESSES OR SYNDROMES ASSOCIATED WITH COXSACKIEVIRUS OR ECHOVIRUS INFECTIONS

	Illness or Syndrome	Virus Types			Reference
		Coxsackievirus		Echovirus	
		Group A	Group B		
4	Laryngotracheitis	9	5	11	7,18
5	Exanthems (various)	2, 4, 5, 7, 9, 10, 16	1-5	1-7, 9, 11, 13, 14, 16-19, 22, 25, 30, 32, 33	7,18,22,35
6	Lymphadenitis, with or without splenomegaly	5, 6, 9	5	4, 9, 16, 20	18
7	Pleurodynia, sometimes with pleural effusion	4, 6, 10	1-5	1, 6, 9	2,18
8	Orchitis	....	1-5	9	8,9,30
9	Gastroenteritis	....	3, 4	2, 3, 6-9, 11-14, 18, 19, 22-24	18
	Severe or life-threatening illness				
10	Hepatitis	4, 9	5	4, 9	17,24,28, 31,32
11	Hemolytic-uremic syndrome	4	4	....	1,13
12	Pneumonia	9	1, 4	3, 8, 9, 19, 20	18
13	Diabetes mellitus[3/]	....	4	....	10,11
	Cardiac				
14	Myocarditis/pericarditis	1, 2, 4, 5, 8, 9, 16	1-5	1, 4, 6, 8, 9, 14, 19, 22, 25, 30	16,21
15	Chronic myocardiopathy	....	2, 4, 5	....	29
16	Subendocardial fibroelastosis[3/]	....	3	....	21
17	Endocardial deformities	....	4	....	5,6
18	Constrictive pericarditis	....	1, 2	....	15,23,26, 27
19	Congenital malformations[3/]	9	3, 4	....	3,4
	Neurologic				
20	Aseptic meningitis/encephalitis, including variants b-f	7, 9, 16	1-5	1-9, 11-23, 25, 30-32	18
21	Acute cerebellar ataxia	4, 9	......	9	18
22	Benign intracranial hypertension	....	4	....	36
23	Post-encephalitic parkinsonism	....	2	....	25,34
24	Guillain-Barré syndrome[3/]	2, 5, 6, 9	......	6, 22	18
25	Chronic myopathy	9	......	....	33

[3/] Suggested (and probable) relationship, but cause not established.

Contributor: Reyes, Milagros P.

References

1. Austin, T., and C. Ray. 1973. J. Infect. Dis. 127:698-701.
2. Bain, H. W., et al. 1961. Pediatrics 27:889-903.
3. Brown, G. C., and T. N. Evans. 1967. J. Am. Med. Assoc. 199:151-155.
4. Brown, G. C., and R. S. Karunas. 1972. Am. J. Epidemiol. 95:207-217.
5. Burch, G. E., and H. L. Colcolough. 1969. Ann. Intern. Med. 71:963-970.
6. Burch, G. E., et al. 1967. Am. Heart J. 74:13-23.
7. Cherry, J. D. 1969. Adv. Pediatr. 16:233-286.
8. Craighead, J. E., et al. 1962. N. Engl. J. Med. 267:498-500.
9. Dalldorf, G. 1955. Annu. Rev. Microbiol. 9:277-296.
10. Gamble, D. R., and K. W. Taylor. 1969. Br. Med. J. 3:631-633.
11. Gamble, D. R., et al. 1969. Ibid. 3:627-630.
12. Gelfand, H. M. 1961. Prog. Med. Virol. 3:193-244.
13. Glasgow, L. A., and P. Balduzzi. 1964. N. Engl. J. Med. 273:754-756.
14. Horstmann, D. M. 1965. Am. J. Med. 38:738-750.
15. Howard, E., and H. Maier. 1968. Am. Heart J. 75:247-250.
16. Johnson, R. T., et al. 1961. Arch. Intern. Med. 108:823-832.
17. Karzon, D. T., et al. 1961. Am. J. Dis. Child. 101:610-622.
18. Kibrick, S. 1964. Prog. Med. Virol. 6:27-70.
19. Kogon, A., et al. 1969. Am. J. Epidemiol. 89:51-61.
20. Lerner, A. M. 1974. In M. M. Wintrobe, et al., ed. Harrison's Principles of Internal Medicine. Ed. 7. McGraw-Hill, New York. v. 1, p. 944.
21. Lerner, A. M., and F. M. Wilson. 1973. Prog. Med. Virol. 15:63-91.
22. Lerner, A. M., et al. 1960. N. Engl. J. Med. 263:1265-1272.

continued

23. Matthews, J. D., et al. 1970. Thorax 25:624-626.
24. Morris, J. A., et al. 1962. N. Engl. J. Med. 267:1230-1233.
25. Poser, C. M., et al. 1969. Acta Neurol. Scand. 45:199-215.
26. Rabiner, S. F., et al. 1954. N. Engl. J. Med. 251:425-428.
27. Ruffy, R., et al. 1973. Rocky Mt. Med. J. 70:37-39.
28. Sabin, A. B., et al. 1958. Am. J. Dis. Child. 96:197-219.

29. Sainani, G. S., et al. 1968. Medicine (Baltimore) 47:133-147.
30. Sanford, J. P., and S. E. Sulkin. 1959. N. Engl. J. Med. 261:1113-1122.
31. Siegel, W., et al. 1963. Ibid. 268:1210-1216.
32. Solomon, P., et al. 1959. J. Pediatr. 55:609-619.
33. Tang, T., et al. 1975. N. Engl. J. Med. 292:608-611.
34. Walters, J. H. 1960. Ibid. 263:744-747.
35. Wenner, H. A. 1973. Prog. Med. Virol. 16:269-336.
36. Wooley, C. F. 1960. Neurology 10:572-574.

11. NON-BACTERIAL PNEUMONIAS IN OLDER CHILDREN AND ADULTS

Clinical Findings include results of X rays. Figures in heavy brackets are reference numbers.

	Causative Organism	Characteristics of Susceptible Patients	Pathogenesis	Clinical Findings	Laboratory Diagnosis	Therapy
1	Influenza virus	Valvular heart disease, chronic lung disease [7]; near-term pregnancy [5]	Exogenous aspiration [4]	High fever, cough, dyspnea, cyanosis. Generalized wheezing and rales. Diffuse bilateral nodular infiltrates. [1]	Virus isolation from throat into embryonated chicken egg or monkey kidney tissue culture. Rise in complement fixation ⟨CF⟩ antibody [9]	Amantadine, vaccine for prevention [9]
2	Varicella-zoster virus	Non-immune over age 20 [15]	Exogenous aspiration [6]	Fever, cough, pleurisy, hemoptysis, dyspnea of variable degree. Generalized rhonchi or wheezing. Nodular peribronchial infiltrate. [15]	Multinucleated giant cells on Tzanck smear of skin lesion [15]. Isolation of virus from vesicle into human embryo tissue culture [6].	Supportive [15]
3	Cytomegalovirus	Immunosuppressed host [12]	Reactivation; exogenous aspiration [12]	Fever, cyanosis, dyspnea, non-productive cough. Bilateral interstitial infiltrates [11]	Lung biopsy: virus isolation into human fibroblast cell culture. Intranuclear inclusions on tissue stain with hematoxylin and eosin. [3]	Supportive [11]
4	*Chlamydia psittaci* [1]	Exposure to birds, especially parakeets [14]	Exogenous aspiration [16]	Cough and/or sputum, fever, malaise, sore throat. Rales or consolidation. Patchy infiltrate. [14] May have epidemics [16].	4 × rise or fall of CF antibody [14]. Isolation of agent from sputum into chicken egg yolk sack, or mice [16].	Tetracycline [14]
5	*Mycoplasma pneumoniae*	Older children, & adults in 2nd & 3rd decades [10]	Exogenous aspiration	Fever, chills, cough, general malaise. Localized rhonchi & rales. Variable X-ray appearance. Characteristically unilateral, segmental bronchopneumonia in a lower lobe. [10]	Isolation of organism in broth & 1% solid agar. 4 × rise or fall of CF antibody. Cold hemagglutinins suggestive. [10]	Tetracycline or erythromycin [10]
6	*Pneumocystis carinii* [2]	Immunosuppressed host [2]	Exogenous aspiration; reactivation [2]	Cough, dyspnea, cyanosis, fever. Either insidious or acute onset. Clear chest or scattered rales. Perihilar haziness with progressive spread to periphery. [2]	Lung biopsy: Gram-Weigert stain of imprint, methenamine silver stain of tissue [13]	Pentamidine isethionate [13]; trimethoprim-sulfamethoxazole [8]

[1] Causative agent of psittacosis. [2] Taxonomic position uncertain.

Contributor: Wilson, Francis M.

continued

11. NON-BACTERIAL PNEUMONIAS IN OLDER CHILDREN AND ADULTS

References

1. Beeson, P. B., and W. McDermott, ed. 1975. Textbook of Medicine. Ed. 14. W. B. Saunders, Philadelphia.
2. Burke, B. A., and R. A. Good. 1973. Medicine (Baltimore) 52:23-51.
3. Craighead, J. E. 1971. Am. J. Pathol. 63:487-504.
4. Davenport, F. M. 1961. Bacteriol. Rev. 25:294-300.
5. Freeman, D. W., and A. Barno. 1959. Am. J. Obstet. Gynecol. 78:1172-1175.
6. Gordon, J. E. 1962. Am. J. Med. Sci. 244:362-389.
7. Harford, C. G. 1960. Am. J. Med. 29:907-909.
8. Hughes, W. T., et al. 1975. Can. Med. Assoc. J. 112 (Spec. No. 13):47-50.
9. Jackson, G. G., and R. L. Muldoon. 1975. J. Infect. Dis. 131:308-357.
10. Murray, H. W. 1975. Am. J. Med. 58:229.
11. Neiman, P., et al. 1973. Transplantation 15:478-485.
12. Plummer, G. 1973. Prog. Med. Virol. 15:92-125.
13. Rosen, P. P., et al. 1975. Am. J. Med. 58:794-802.
14. Schaffner, W., et al. 1967. Arch. Intern. Med. 119: 433-443.
15. Triebwasser, J. H., et al. 1967. Medicine (Baltimore) 46:409-423.
16. Wilson, G. S., and A. A. Miles, ed. 1964. Topley and Wilson's Principles of Bacteriology and Immunity. Ed. 6. Williams and Wilkins, Baltimore.

12. ANTIRABIES POST-EXPOSURE PROPHYLAXIS GUIDE

The recommendations given below are only intended as a guide. They should be used in conjunction with knowledge of the animal species involved, circumstances of the bite or other exposure, vaccination record of the animal, and presence of rabies in the region. In municipal areas that have been deemed "rabies-free," post-exposure therapy is not recommended for wounds inflicted by domestic animals.

Animals not listed below should be considered individually, according to the status of the animal and the epidemiology of rabies for the particular species in the specific geographic locale. Relevant information can and should be obtained from local or state public health authorities, or from the Viral Diseases Branch, Epidemiology Program, Center for Disease Control, Atlanta, Georgia.

SPECIFIC TREATMENT

Thoroughly flush and cleanse wounds with either a soap solution or a quaternary ammonium compound.

B = begin antiserum (S) and vaccine (V_1) at first signs of rabies in attacking animal during period of observation (10 days).

S = antirabies antiserum
of equine origin: give in dose of 40 I.U./kg.
of human origin: give in dose of 20 I.U./kg.
Use up to 50% of antiserum to infiltrate wound; give the remainder intramuscularly.

V_1 = antirabies vaccine, 21 doses of 1 ml each. Give subcutaneously over period of 14 days—
1st 7 days: 2 doses/day.
2nd 7 days: 1 dose/day.
Give booster injections 10 and 20 days after completion of primary course.

V_2 = duck embryo antirabies vaccine, 14 doses of 1 ml each. Give subcutaneously over period of 14 days.

D = discontinue vaccine if fluorescent studies of brain of animal killed at time of attack are negative.

| | Animal | Condition at Time of Attack | Specific Treatment | |
			Bite	Non-Bite
1	Domestic: dog or cat	Healthy	None, B	None, B
2		Escaped (unknown)	S, V_1	V_2
3		Rabid	S, V_1, D	S, V_1, D
4	Wild: skunk	Regard as rabid	S, V_1, D	S, V_1, D
5	raccoon	Regard as rabid	S, V_1, D	S, V_1, D
6	fox	Regard as rabid	S, V_1, D	S, V_1, D
7	bat	Regard as rabid	S, V_1, D	S, V_1, D

Contributor: Rubin, Robert H.

Reference: Public Health Service Advisory Committee on Immunization Practices. 1972. U.S. Public Health Serv. Publ. HSM 72-8154:20.

Serology: CF = complement fixation; CRN = complement requiring neutralization; CRN/N ≥4/1 ratio indicates recent antigenic stimulation; CSF = cerebrospinal fluid; HI = hemagglutination inhibition; HpI = hemadsorption inhibition; IFA = indirect fluorescence; N = neutralization; Pha = passive hemagglutination; RIA = radioimmunoassay; S antigen = "soluble" antigen; V antigen = "viral" antigen. Data in brackets refer to the column heading in brackets.

	Virus	Subjects Infected [Non-Human Hosts]	Seasonal Prevalence [Epidemic]	Paralysis, Seizures, or Coma [Mortality [1]]	Diagnosis & Virus Isolation	Serology	Prophylaxis or Therapy	Reference
1	Herpesvirus ⟨Herpes simplex⟩ Type 1	All ages; ♀ > ♂ [None]	None [No]	Common [40-80%[2]]	Autopsy or biopsy for isolation to tissue culture; direct immunofluorescence	CF, N, CRN, RIA, IFA, CRN/N, Pha; antibodies in sera, CSF	None of proven value; antiviral drugs being tested	1,7,9, 25,27-29,34, 35
2	Type 2[3]	All ages; ♀ = ♂	None [No]	Rare [Very rare in adults, 75% in newborn]	Virus isolation from CSF or blood leukocytes		None	
3	Coxsackie, Group A or B[4]	Children > adults; ♀ = ♂	Summer [Yes]	Rare [Rare]	Isolation from nose, throat, stool, CSF	Not practical; CF, HI, N	None	3,18,23, 37,42
4	Polio, types 1, 2, or 3	50% under 5 yr, 80% under 10 yr; ♂ > ♂ [None]	Summer [No]	Paralysis in ∿50% [Greater after age 25; bulbar, 20-60%; overall, 4-15%]	Isolation from stool, nasopharynx, tonsil, very rarely CSF	CF, N	Vaccines: (i) inactivated, (ii) live attenuated oral	4,37-39, 45,48
5	Mumps[5]	Especially at 5-15 yr; rare under 4 yr or over 40 yr; ♂ < ♀ [None]	Winter [Yes, no]	Rare [Rare]	Isolation from saliva, CSF, blood, urine	HI, N, RIA, HpI, IFA, CF with "V" & "S" antigens	Vaccine: live attenuated	11,12, 21,24, 26,30
6	Measles[6]	Usually under 10 yr; ♀ = ♂ [None]	Winter, spring [Occasional]	Rare [0.1-1%[7]]	Clinical picture; isolation from nasopharynx, blood, urine	CF, N, HI, IFA	Vaccine: live attenuated	6,31,32, 43,44, 47
7	Lymphocytic choriomeningitis	Especially at 10-40 yr; ♂ > ♀ [Monkeys, mice[8], hamsters]	Fall, winter, spring [Yes, no]	Rare [Rare]	Isolation from blood, CSF	CF, N	None	2,15,46
8	Western equine encephalitis	Especially infants & after age 50; ♀ < ♂ [Horses & birds, via mosquitoes[9]]	Early summer[10] [Yes]	Common in infants, rare in adults [Overall, 10%]	Isolation very difficult from blood or CSF; occasionally isolated from brain	CF, HI, N	Mosquito vector control	13,14, 33,40
9	Eastern equine encephalitis	50-70% under 10 yr; ♂ = ♀	Summer[11] [Yes]	Frequent [Nearly 70%]	Very difficult to isolate from blood or CSF, or brain at autopsy	CF, HI, N	Mosquito vector control	14,16, 17,19, 40

[1] Case fatality rate of patients with overt central nervous system disease. [2] Most common fatal non-epidemic encephalitis. [3] Often associated with genital infections. [4] On rare occasions may mimic poliovirus infection. [5] Occasionally may mimic poliovirus infection. [6] Synonym: Rubeola. [7] Variant CNS slow virus infection = subacute sclerosing panencephalitis; usually fatal. [8] Endemic in house mouse. [9] *Culex* spp. [10] Incubation period, 5-10 days. [11] Incubation period, 7-10 days.

continued

10

	Virus	Subjects Infected [Non-Human Hosts]	Seasonal Prevalence [Epidemic]	Paralysis, Seizures, or Coma [Mortality [1]]	Diagnosis & Virus Isolation	Serology	Prophylaxis or Therapy	Reference
10	Venezuelan equine encephalitis	All ages, but mostly under 10 yr; ♂ = ♀ [Horses, small rodents, via mosquitoes [9]]	Summer [12] [Yes]	Rare [Mostly under 5 yr]	Isolation from blood, throat swab	CF, HI, N	Vaccines: (i) formalin-inactivated for horses, (ii) experimental live attenuated for humans	8,19,20, 40
11	St. Louis encephalitis	All ages; ♀ = ♂ [Birds, via mosquitoes [9]]	Late summer, early fall [13] [Yes]	Rare [Greater, after age 50 (30%); overall, ∿2-20%]	No isolations reported from CSF or blood of humans; occasionally from brain	CF, HI, N	Mosquito vector control	14,22, 40,41, 49
12	California encephalitis	Mostly under 16 yr; ♀ < ♂ [Small mammals, via mosquitoes [14]]	Summer [10] [Yes]	Common in infants, rare in adults [Probably <5%]	No isolation reported from CSF or blood of humans	CF, HI, N	Protective clothing, nets, repellents	5,10,14, 36,40, 50

[1] Case fatality rate of patients with overt central nervous system disease. [9] *Culex* spp. [10] Incubation period, 5-10 days. [12] Infectious by respiratory route, and may resemble influenza. [13] Incubation period, up to 2 weeks (?). [14] *Aedes* spp.

Contributor: Lauter, Carl B.

References
1. Adams, H., and D. Miller. 1973. Postgrad. Med. J. 49: 393-397.
2. Armstrong, D., et al. 1969. J. Am. Med. Assoc. 209: 265-266.
3. Artenstein, M. S., et al. 1965. Ann. Intern. Med. 63: 597-603.
4. Aycock, W. L., and J. F. Kessel. 1943. Am. J. Med. Sci. 205:454-465.
5. Balfour, H. H., et al. 1973. Pediatrics 52:680-691.
6. Black, F. L. 1974. In E. H. Lennette, et al., ed. Manual of Clinical Microbiology. Ed. 2. American Society for Microbiology, Washington, D.C. pp. 709-715.
7. Boston Interhospital Virus Study Group, et al. 1975. N. Engl. J. Med. 292:599-603.
8. Briceño Rossi, A. L. 1967. Prog. Med. Virol. 9:176-203.
9. Craig, C. P., and A. J. Nahmias. 1973. J. Infect. Dis. 127:365-372.
10. Cramblett, H. G., et al. 1966. J. Am. Med. Assoc. 198: 108-112.
11. Cushing, R. D., and A. M. Lerner. 1976. In T. C. Eickhoff, ed. Practice of Medicine. Harper and Row, Hagerstown, MD. v. 4, ch. 7 (sect. 2), pp. 5-7.
12. Deinhardt, F. W., and G. J. Shramek. 1974. (Loc. cit. ref. 6). pp. 703-708.
13. Eklund, C. M. 1946. Am. J. Hyg. 43:171-193.
14. Eklund, C. M. 1972. In F. H. Top, Sr., and P. F. Wehrle, ed. Communicable and Infectious Diseases. Ed. 7. C. V. Mosby, St. Louis. pp. 208-220.
15. Farmer, T. W., and C. A. Janeway. 1942. Medicine (Baltimore) 21:1-63.
16. Feemster, R. F. 1957. N. Engl. J. Med. 257:701-704.
17. Hart, K. L., et al. 1964. Am. J. Trop. Med. Hyg. 13: 331-334.
18. Herrmann, E. C., Jr., et al. 1972. Mayo Clin. Proc. 47: 577-586.
19. Johnson, K. M. 1975. In P. B. Beeson and W. McDermott, ed. Textbook of Medicine. Ed. 14. W. B. Saunders, Philadelphia. pp. 229-238.
20. Johnson, K. M., and D. H. Martin. 1974. Adv. Vet. Sci. Comp. Med. 18:79-116.
21. Johnstone, J. A., et al. 1972. Arch. Dis. Child. 47: 647-651.
22. Jones, A. B. 1934. J. Am. Med. Assoc. 103:825.
23. Kibrick, S. 1964. Prog. Med. Virol. 6:27-70.
24. Kilham, L. 1949. Am. J. Dis. Child. 78:324-333.
25. Lauter, C. B., et al. 1975. Proc. Soc. Exp. Biol. Med. 150:23-27.
26. Lerner, A. M. 1970. J. Infect. Dis. 122:116-121.
27. Lerner, A. M., and C. B. Lauter. 1973. In F. Tice, ed. Practice of Medicine. Harper and Row, Hagerstown, MD. v. 4, ch. 7, pp. 1-4.
28. Lerner, A. M., et al. 1972. Proc. Soc. Exp. Biol. Med. 140:1460-1466.
29. Lerner, A. M., et al. 1976. Scand. J. Infect. Dis. 8: 37-44.
30. Levitt, L. P., et al. 1970. Neurology 20:829-834.
31. Linnemann, C. C., Jr. 1973. Am. J. Epidemiol. 97: 365-371.
32. Meulen, V. ter, et al. 1972. Lancet 2:1172-1175.
33. Meyer, K. F., et al. 1931. Science 74:227-228.
34. Nahmias, A. J., et al. 1970. Adv. Pediatr. 17:185-226.

continued

35. Nolan, D. C., et al. 1973. Ann. Intern. Med. 78:243-246.
36. Parkin, W. E., et al. 1972. Am. J. Trop. Med. Hyg. 21:964-978.
37. Philips, C. A. 1974. (Loc. cit. ref. 6). pp. 723-727.
38. Sabin, A. B. 1960. Arch. Intern. Med. 106:5-9.
39. Salk, J. E. 1959. J. Am. Med. Assoc. 169:1829-1838.
40. Shope, R. E. 1974. (Loc. cit. ref. 6). pp. 740-775.
41. Southern, P. M., Jr., et al. 1969. Ann. Intern. Med. 71:681-689.
42. Stern, H. 1961. Br. Med. J. 1:1061-1066.
43. Tidstrøm, B. 1968. Acta Med. Scand. 184:411-415.
44. Top, F. H., Sr. 1938. Am. J. Public Health 28:935-943.
45. Top, F. H., Sr., and H. F. Vaughan. 1941. Ibid. 31:777-790.
46. Top, F. H., Sr., and P. F. Wehrle. 1972. (Loc. cit. ref. 14). pp. 372-377.
47. Top, F. H., Sr., and P. F. Wehrle. 1972. (Loc. cit. ref. 14). pp. 389-400.
48. Top, F. H., Sr., et al 1972. (Loc. cit. ref. 14). pp. 231-252.
49. White, M. G., et al. 1969. Ann. Intern. Med. 71:691-702.
50. Young, D. J. 1966. Ibid. 65:419-428.

14. COMPARISON OF EPIDEMIOLOGIC FEATURES OF HEPATITIS A AND B

Hepatitis A is also called infectious hepatitis ⟨IH⟩, MS-1, or short-incubation hepatitis. **Hepatitis B** is also called serum hepatitis ⟨SH⟩, MS-2, or long-incubation hepatitis.

	Feature	Hepatitis A	Hepatitis B
1	Age predominance	Children, young adults	All ages
2	Seasonal peak	Autumn, winter	None
	Epidemiologic patterns		
3	Sporadic cases	Yes	Yes
4	Post-transfusion [1]	Yes	Yes
5	Needle-associated	Yes	Yes
6	Common-source outbreaks	Yes	No [2]
	Route of infection		
7	Fecal-oral	Yes	No
8	Parenteral	Yes	Yes
9	Venereal	?	?
10	Respiratory	?	?
11	Incubation period	15-50 d	30-180 d
12	Onset	Acute	Often insidious
13	Prodromal "serum-sickness"-like syndrome	No	Common
14	Hepatitis B surface antigen ⟨HB_sAg⟩	No	Yes
	Viremia		
15	Incubation period & acute phase	Yes (2 wk before onset of illness)	Yes (2 wk-3 mo before onset of illness)
16	Convalescence	No	5-10% (persistent circulating HB_sAg)
	Virus in feces		
17	Incubation period & acute phase	Yes	No
18	Convalescence	Rare, if ever	No
19	Carrier state	Rare, if ever	(0.1-1%) [3]
	Immunity		
20	Homologous	Yes	Yes [4]
21	Heterologous	No	No
22	Immune serum globulin prophylaxis	Modifies illness if given early after exposure	May modify illness if given early after exposure; more effective if very high titer antibody to HB_sAg ⟨anti-HB_s⟩ is given

[1] Most post-transfusion hepatitis (in the United States) is due to neither hepatitis A nor B. [2] Except for vaccine- or blood-product-associated epidemics, outbreaks in oncology or hemodialysis centers, and outbreaks among parenteral drug abusers sharing equipment. [3] In the United States. [4] The existence of multiple subtypes is now recognized, but antibody to "a," a common antigenic determinant, is believed to provide broad immunity.

continued

14. COMPARISON OF EPIDEMIOLOGIC FEATURES OF HEPATITIS A AND B

Contributor: Koff, Raymond S.

General References

1. Koff, R. S. 1970. Crit. Rev. Environ. Control 1:383-442.
2. Mosley, J. W., and J. Galambos. 1975. In L. Schiff, ed. Diseases of the Liver. Ed. 4. J. B. Lippincott, Philadelphia. pp. 500-593.
3. National Research Council, Committee on Viral Hepatitis. 1975. Am. J. Med. Sci. 270(1,2):1-412.
4. Tygstrup, N., ed. 1974. Clin. Gastroenterol. 3:239-474.
5. Vyas, G. N., et al., ed. 1972. Hepatitis and Blood Transfusion. Grune and Stratton, New York.
6. Zuckerman, A. J. 1975. Human Viral Hepatitis. Ed. 2. North-Holland, Amsterdam.

15. HAZARD OF HEPATITIS FROM BLOOD PRODUCTS

	Product	Specification	Risk
1	Whole blood	Single donor	Average
	Erythrocytes (Red cells)		
2	Packed	Single donor	Average
3	Frozen-glycerolized	Single donor	Average[1]
4	Granulocyte concentrates	Single donor	Average
5	Platelet concentrates	Single donor	Average
6		Multiple donors, pooled	High
7	Plasma, fresh-frozen or aged	Single donor	Average
8	Plasma protein fraction	Multiple donors, adequately treated[2]	None
9	Albumin, human	Multiple donors, adequately treated[2]	None
10	Serum globulin, immune & hyperimmune	Multiple donors, adequately treated[2]	None
11	Fibrinogen	Multiple donors	High
12	Prothrombin complex (Coagulation factors II, VII, IX, & X) concentrates	Multiple donors	High
	Coagulation factor VIII (Antihemophilic factor)		
13	Concentrates	Single donor	Average
14		Multiple donors	High
15	Cryoprecipitates	Multiple donors	High

[1] Preliminary data suggest a reduced risk for this product. [2] Blood product heated at 60°C for 10 h, or cold ethanol fractionated (method of Cohn).

Contributor: Koff, Raymond S.

General References

1. Cronberg, S., et al. 1963. Lancet 1:967-969.
2. Gellis, S. S., et al. 1948. J. Clin. Invest. 27:239-244.
3. Grady, G. F., and A. J. Bennett. 1972. J. Am. Med. Assoc. 220:692-701.
4. Mainwaring, R. L., and G. G. Brueckner. 1966. Ibid. 195:437-441.
5. Maycock, W.d'A. 1972. Br. Med. Bull. 28:163-168.
6. Meyers, J. D., et al. 1974. Ann. Intern. Med. 81:145-151.
7. Mosley, J. W., and H. B. Dull. 1966. Anesthesiology 27:409-416.
8. Sandler, S. G., et al. 1973. Ann. Intern. Med. 79:485-491.
9. Tullis, J. L., et al. 1970. J. Am. Med. Assoc. 214:719-723.
10. World Health Organization. 1973. WHO Tech. Rep. Ser. 512:1-52.
11. Zuckerman, A. J. 1975. Human Viral Hepatitis. Ed. 2. North-Holland, Amsterdam. pp. 207-223.

16. PRESUMPTIVE DIAGNOSIS IN PATIENTS WITH INFECTIOUS BACTERIAL DISEASES

Tables 16 and 17 should be used together. Prior to therapy, a complete history and physical examination must be made of any patient with an infection. The results of cultures and sensitivity studies determine definitive therapy. Most patients with bacterial infections have elevated leukocyte (white blood cell) counts; the sickest patients may have normal or subnormal counts. Fever is a non-specific sign of inflammation. Data in brackets refer to the column heading in brackets.

	Site	Physical Findings	Historic Points	Laboratory Tests		Diagnosis	Reference
				Special Test	X ray [Serology]		
1	Head or neck	Meningism (Meningismus); confusion	Headache	Lumbar tap	....	Meningitis	12
2		Proptosis; ophthalmoplegia	Facial lesion; bacteremia	? Lumbar tap	? Orbits	Cavernous sinus thrombosis	17,26
3		Focal neurologic	Ear, nose, throat, lung, or heart disease	Brain scan	Skull	Brain abscess	6
4		Red throat, with or without exudate	Previous viral illness	....	[Antistreptolysin O or streptozyme]	Tonsillitis	20
5		"Hot potato" voice; swollen epiglottis	Painful throat; dysphagia	....	Neck, lateral	Epiglottiditis (Epiglottitis)	23
6	Chest	Diffuse rales; rhonchi	Chronic lung disease	Gram stain of sputum	Chest	Bronchopneumonia	10
7		Lobar consolidation	Upper respiratory infection	Gram stain of sputum	Chest	Lobar pneumonia	10
8		Amphoric breathing	Aspiration; periodontal disease; putrid sputum	Gram stain of sputum	Chest	Lung abscess	5
9	Heart	New or changing murmur; embolic lesions	Congenital or valvular disease	Blood cultures	....	Subacute endocarditis	11
10		Sepsis; needle tracks	Intravenous drug use	Blood cultures	Chest	Acute endocarditis	19
11	Abdomen	Diffuse tenderness	Watery or bloody diarrhea	Stool stain & culture	Abdomen	Bacterial diarrhea	4
12		Bradycardia; rose spots; splenomegaly	Fever; cough; travel with no immunization	Stool culture	Chest [Febrile agglutination]	Typhoid fever	8
13		Tenderness, rebound, guarding	Nausea; vomiting; pain	Paracentesis	Abdomen: flat & up	Peritonitis	3
14		Localized signs	Vomiting; pain	....	Abdomen: flat & up	Abscess; disease requiring surgery	3
15	Urogenital	Tender cervix	Sexual history	Cervical, rectal, & throat cultures	....	Pelvic inflammatory disease	2,22
16		Pelvic discharge & tenderness	Post-surgery or post-abortion	Culture of cervix	Abdomen; chest	Endometritis	2
17		Sepsis; foul lochia	Difficult delivery	Culture of lochia & blood	Chest; abdomen	Puerperal sepsis	2
18		Flank tenderness	Dysuria; fever	Urinalysis & urine culture	Abdomen	Pyelonephritis	9
19		Suprapubic tenderness	Frequency of urination; dysuria	Urinalysis & urine culture	....	Cystitis	9
20		Pelvic & prostate tenderness	Dysuria; fever	Culture & stain of urine after prostatic massage	....	Prostatitis	9,13
21		Urethral discharge	Sexual contact	Gram stain & culture of urethral discharge	....	Urethritis	22
22	Lymph	Fluctuant nodes	Flea bite	Giemsa stain of aspirate	Chest	Plague	15,18
23	Skin & soft	Ulcer on finger; fluctuant nodes	Rabbit exposure	Foshay's test	Chest [Agglutination]	Tularemia	16
24	tissues	Ulcer, with eschar on extremity	Wool or hide exposure	Gram stain & culture	....	Anthrax	1

continued

16. PRESUMPTIVE DIAGNOSIS IN PATIENTS WITH INFECTIOUS BACTERIAL DISEASES

	Site	Physical Findings	Historic Points	Laboratory Tests		Diagnosis	Reference
				Special Test	X ray [Serology]		
25		Redness; fluctuance	Injury	Gram stain & culture of pus	....	Abscess	26
26		Redness; heat; no pus	Injury	Gram stain & culture of aspirate	[Streptozyme]	Cellulitis	21,25, 26
27		Redness; crepitation	Injury	Gram stain & culture	Extremity	Gas gangrene	7
28	Joint	Hot joint; effusion	Injury; bacteremia	Gram stain & culture of aspirate	....	Septic arthritis	14,26
29	Bone	Swelling; drainage	Injury; bacteremia	Culture	Extremity	Osteomyelitis	24

Contributor: Cushing, Ralph D.

References
1. Borts, I. H. 1972. In F. H. Top, Sr., and P. F. Wehrle, ed. Communicable and Infectious Diseases. Ed. 7. C. V. Mosby, St. Louis. pp. 108-111.
2. Charles, D., and M. Finland. 1973. Obstetric and Perinatal Infections. Lea and Febiger, Philadelphia. pp. 247-253.
3. Cope, Z. 1972. Early Diagnosis of the Acute Abdomen. Oxford Univ. Press, London.
4. DuPont, H., and R. Hornick. 1973. Medicine (Baltimore) 52:265-270.
5. Finegold, S., et al. 1975. Ann. Intern. Med. 83:357-389.
6. Garfield, J. 1969. Br. Med. J. 2:7-11.
7. Holland, J. A., et al. 1975. Surgery 77:75-85.
8. Hornick, R. B., et al. 1970. N. Engl. J. Med. 283:686-691.
9. Kunin, C. M. 1974. Detection, Prevention and Management of Urinary Tract Infections. Lea and Febiger, Philadelphia.
10. Lerner, A. M., and K. Jankauskas. 1975. Dis. Mon. (Feb.).
11. Lerner, P. I., and L. Weinstein. 1966. N. Engl. J. Med. 274:199-206, 323-331, 388-393.
12. Meade, R. H. 1963. J. Am. Med. Assoc. 185:1023-1030.
13. Meares, W. M., and T. A. Stamey. 1972. Br. J. Urol. 44:175-179.
14. Nelsen, J. 1971. N. Engl. J. Med. 284:349-353.
15. Poland, J. D., and F. H. Top, Sr. 1972. (Loc. cit. ref. 1). pp. 450-456.
16. Poland, J. D., and F. H. Top, Sr. 1972. (Loc. cit. ref. 1). pp. 743-749.
17. Price, C. D., et al. 1971. South. Med. J. 64:1243-1247.
18. Reed, W., et al. 1970. Medicine (Baltimore) 49:465-486.
19. Reyes, M., et al. 1973. Ibid. 53:173-194.
20. Rosenstein, B. J., et al. 1968. J. Pediatr. 73:513-520.
21. Uman, S., and C. Kunin. 1975. Arch. Intern. Med. 135:959-961.
22. U.S. Public Health Service, Center for Disease Control. 1974. U.S. Public Health Serv. Publ. 96-552.
23. Vetto, R. R. 1960. J. Am. Med. Assoc. 173:990-994.
24. Waldvogel, F. A., et al. 1970. N. Engl. J. Med. 282:198-206.
25. Wannamaker, L. 1970. Ibid. 282:78-85.
26. Wise, R. 1973. Medicine (Baltimore) 52:295-304.

17. THERAPY OF BACTERIAL INFECTIONS BASED ON PRESUMPTIVE DIAGNOSIS

The therapy suggested is for adults with infectious diseases. Definitive therapy must be based upon results of culture and sensitivity reports. Patients should be monitored for signs of antibiotic toxicity. All doses stated below assume normal liver and kidney functioning. Duration of therapy is frequently guided by clinical response. Second and third **Antibiotics** listed are alternates to the first drug, unless otherwise indicated. **Dose & Route:** i.v. = intravenous infusion over 15-30 minutes, unless otherwise specified; p.o. = orally; i.m. = intramuscularly. **Interval:** Const = constant infusion. **References** are discussions of the disease entity; sometimes the dose listed is based on the contributor's interpretation of more than one source.

	Diagnosis	Organism (Synonym)	Special Procedure	Antibiotic	Dose & Route	Interval h [1]	Duration	Reference
1	Meningitis	Neisseria meningitidis	Gram stain of spinal fluid	Penicillin G, aqueous	1×10^6 units, i.v.	2	7-14 d	11,
2				Chloramphenicol	1 g, i.v.	6-8	7-14 d	14
3		Streptococcus pneumoniae	Gram stain of spinal fluid	Penicillin G, aqueous	1×10^6 units, i.v.	2	7-14 d	11,
4				Chloramphenicol	1 g, i.v.	6-8	7-14 d	14

[1] Unless otherwise specified.

continued

	Diagnosis	Organism (Synonym)	Special Procedure	Antibiotic	Dose & Route	Interval h [1]	Duration	Reference
5	Cavernous sinus	*Staphylococcus au-*	Blood culture	Methicillin sodium [2]	(1-2) g, i.v.	4	14-21 d	19,
6	thrombosis	*reus*		Penicillin G, aqueous [2]	(1-2) × 10^6 units, i.v.			30
7	Brain abscess	Mixed anaerobes	Surgical drain-	Penicillin G, aqueous [2]	(1-2) × 10^6 units, i.v.	2-4	14-21 d	7
8			age	Chloramphenicol [2]	1 g, i.v.	6-8		
9	Tonsillitis	*Streptococcus pyo-*	Throat culture	Penicillin V [3]	500 mg, p.o.	6	10 d	22
10		*genes*		Benzathine penicillin G	1.2 × 10^6 units, i.m.	Once only	....	
11				Erythromycin	500 mg, p.o.	6	10 d	
12	Epiglottiditis [4]	*Haemophilus influ-*	Relief of airway	Ampicillin	1 g, i.v.	4	7 d	25
13		*enzae*	obstruction	Chloramphenicol	1 g, i.v.	8	7 d	
14	Pneumonia	*Streptococcus pneu-*	Blood culture	Penicillin G, aqueous	6 × 10^5 units, i.m. or i.v.	4	5-10 d	12
15		*moniae*		Lincomycin	3 g, i.v.	Const	5-10 d	
16		*Klebsiella penumo-*	....	Gentamicin [2]	80 mg, i.m.	8	14-21 d	12
17		*niae*		Chloramphenicol [2]	1 g, i.v.	8		
18				Cephalothin	2 g, i.v.	4	14-21 d	
19	Aspiration	Mixed anaerobes	....	Penicillin G, aqueous	(1-2) × 10^6 units, i.v.	4	1-2 mo	5
20				Clindamycin	600 mg, i.v.	8	1-2 mo	
21	Lung abscess	Mixed anaerobes	Bronchoscopy	Penicillin G, aqueous	(1-2) × 10^6 units, i.v.	4	1-2 mo	5
22				Clindamycin	600 mg, i.v.	8	1-2 mo	
	Endocarditis	*Streptococcus*						
23		⟨*S. viridans*⟩	Serum bacteri-	Penicillin G, aqueous	1 × 10^6 units, i.v.	3	28 d	2
24			cidal level	Penicillin V [2,3]	750 mg, p.o.	4	14 d	23
25				Streptomycin [2]	1 g, i.m.	12		
26		⟨*Enterococcus*⟩	Serum bacteri-	Penicillin G, aqueous [2]	(20-30) × 10^6 units, i.v.	Const	42 d	29
27			cidal level	Gentamicin [2]	(60-100) mg, i.m.	8		
		Staphylococcus aureus						
28		Penicillinase +	Serum bacteri- cidal level	Methicillin sodium or other semisynthetic penicillin	(1-2) g, i.v.	4	42 d	28
29		Penicillinase −	Serum bacteri- cidal level	Penicillin G, aqueous	(10-20) × 10^6 units, i.v.	Const	42 d	28
30		*Pseudomonas aerugi-*	Serum bacteri-	Carbenicillin [2]	5 g, i.v.	4	42 d	21
31		*nosa*	cidal level	Gentamicin [2]	100 mg, i.m.	8		
32	Shigellosis	*Shigella* sp.	Methylene blue	Ampicillin	1 g, p.o.	8	3 d	2
33			stain of stool	Tetracycline	2.5 g, p.o.	Once only	....	
34	Typhoid fever	*Salmonella typhi* ⟨*S. typhosa*⟩	....	Chloramphenicol	1 g, p.o.	8	14 d	9
35	Peritonitis	Mixed flora	Surgical drain-	Penicillin G, aqueous [2]	1 × 10^6 units, i.v.	4-8	7-14 d	6
36			age	Tetracycline [2]	1 g, i.v.	12		
37				Gentamicin	(80-100) mg, i.m. or i.v.	8	7-14 d	
38				Clindamycin	300-600 mg, i.v.	8	7-14 d	
39	Pelvic abscess	Mixed anaerobic flora	Surgical drain- age	Chloramphenicol	0.5 g, i.v.	6	7-10 d	3
40	Pelvic inflam- matory dis- ease	*Neisseria gonorrhoeae*	Endocervical culture on Thayer-Martin media	Penicillin G, aqueous	20 × 10^6 units, i.v.	Const	10 d	24
41	Puerperal sepsis	Mixed flora	Consider surgi-	Penicillin G, aqueous [2]	1 × 10^6 units, i.v.	4	10-14 d	3
42	& endometri- tis		cal drainage	Gentamicin [2]	80 mg, i.m.	8		
43	Pyelonephritis	*Escherichia coli*	Intravenous py-	Ampicillin	500 mg, i.m.	6	10-14 d	10
44			elogram	Sulfisoxazole	(2-4) g, p.o.	6-8	10-14 d	
45	Prostatitis	....	3-glass urinaly- sis	Trimethoprim, 80 mg, & sulfamethoxazole, 400 mg	2 tablets, p.o.	12	2-6 wk	10, 15

[1] Unless otherwise specified. [2] Both used together. [3] Synonym: Phenoxymethylpenicillin. [4] Synonym: Epiglottitis.

16

continued

17. THERAPY OF BACTERIAL INFECTIONS BASED ON PRESUMPTIVE DIAGNOSIS

	Diagnosis	Organism ⟨Synonym⟩	Special Procedure	Antibiotic	Dose & Route	Interval h[1]	Duration	Reference
46	Urethritis	Neisseria gonorrhoeae	Culture on Thayer-Martin media	Procaine penicillin G[2]	4.8 × 10⁶ units, i.m.	Once only	....	24
47				Probenacid[2]	1 g, p.o.			
48				Tetracycline	1.5 g, p.o., once, then 0.5 g, p.o.	6	4 d	
49	Plague	Yersinia pestis	....	Tetracycline[2]	3 g, p.o., once, then 1 g, p.o.	6	14 d	17, 20
50				Streptomycin[2]	0.5 g, i.m.	4		
51	Tularemia	Francisella tularensis	Foshay's test	Streptomycin[2]	0.5 g, i.m.	6	5 d	18
52				Tetracycline[2]	0.5 g, p.o.	6	10 d	
53	Anthrax	Bacillus anthracis	....	Tetracycline	0.5 g, p.o.	6	7-21 d	1
54	Septic shock	Gram-negative rods	Search for source; consider steroids & vasopressors	Gentamicin	(80-120) mg, i.v.	8	7-14 d	4,13
55	Abscess in soft tissue	Staphylococcus aureus, penicillinase +	....	Cloxacillin or other semisynthetic penicillin	(250-500) mg, p.o.	6	7-10 d	16
56	Cellulitis in soft tissue	Streptococcus pyogenes	....	Benzathine penicillin G	1.2 × 10⁶ units, i.m.	Once only	....	27
57	Gas gangrene	Clostridium sp.	Amputation	Penicillin G aqueous	(20-30) × 10⁶ units, i.v.	Const	10-14 d	8
58	Septic arthritis	Neisseria gonorrhoeae	Aspirate of joint	Penicillin G aqueous	10 × 10⁶ units	Const	10 d	24
59		Staphylococcus aureus, penicillinase +	Aspirate of joint	Methicillin sodium or other semisynthetic penicillin	(1-2) g, i.v. or i.m.	4-6	2-4 wk	30
60	Osteomyelitis, acute	Staphylococcus aureus, penicillinase +	....	Methicillin sodium or other semisynthetic penicillin	(1-2) g, i.v. or i.m.	4-6	4-6 wk	26

[1] Unless otherwise specified. [2] Both used together.

Contributor: Cushing, Ralph D.

References
1. Borts, I. H. 1972. In F. H. Top, Sr., and P. F. Wehrle, ed. Communicable and Infectious Diseases. Ed. 7. C. V. Mosby, St. Louis. pp. 108-111.
2. Braude, A. 1976. Antimicrobial Drug Therapy. W. B. Saunders, Philadelphia.
3. Charles, D., and M. Finland. 1973. Obstetric and Perinatal Infections. Lea and Febiger, Philadelphia. pp. 247-253.
4. Davies, D. G., et al. 1974. Postgrad. Med. J. 50(Suppl. 7):9-16.
5. Finegold, S., et al. 1975. Ann. Intern. Med. 83:357-389.
6. Fullen, W. D., et al. 1972. J. Trauma 12:282-289.
7. Garfield, J. 1969. Br. Med. J. 2:7-11.
8. Holland, J. A., et al. 1975. Surgery 77:75-85.
9. Hornick, R. B., et al. 1970. N. Engl. J. Med. 283:686-691.
10. Kunin, C. M. 1974. Detection, Prevention and Management of Urinary Tract Infections. Lea and Febiger, Philadelphia.
11. Lepper, M. H., and H. F. Dowling. 1951. Arch. Intern. Med. 88:489-494.
12. Lerner, A. M., and K. Jankauskas. 1975. Dis. Mon. (Feb.).
13. Martin, C., et al. 1969. J. Infect. Dis. 119:506-517.
14. Meade, R. H. 1963. J. Am. Med. Assoc. 185:1023-1030.
15. Meares, W. M., and T. A. Stamey. 1972. Br. J. Urol. 44:175-179.
16. Medical Letter, Inc. 1973. Med. Lett. Drugs Ther. 15(23):93-94.
17. Poland, J. D., and F. H. Top, Sr. 1972. (Loc. cit. ref. 1). pp. 450-456.
18. Poland, J. D., and F. H. Top, Sr. 1972. (Loc. cit. ref. 1). pp. 743-749.
19. Price, C. D., et al. 1971. South. Med. J. 64:1243-1247.
20. Reed, W., et al. 1970. Medicine (Baltimore) 49:465-486.
21. Reyes, M., et al. 1973. Ibid. 53:173-194.
22. Rosenstein, B. J., et al. 1968. J. Pediatr. 73:513-520.
23. Tan, J. S., et al. 1971. Lancet 2:1340-1343.
24. U.S. Public Health Service, Center for Disease Control. 1974. U.S. Public Health Serv. Publ. 96-552.
25. Vetto, R. R. 1960. J. Am. Med. Assoc. 173:990-994.
26. Waldvogel, F. A., et al. 1970. N. Engl. J. Med. 282:198-206.
27. Wannamaker, L. 1970. Ibid. 282:78-85.
28. Watanakunakorn, C., et al. 1973. Am. J. Med. 54:473-481.
29. Weinstein, A., and R. Moellering. 1973. J. Am. Med. Assoc. 233:1030-1032.
30. Wise, R. 1973. Medicine (Baltimore) 52:295-304.

18. CLINICAL AND LABORATORY MANIFESTATIONS OF ACUTE RHEUMATIC FEVER

The Jones criteria (revised) have been employed as a guide in the diagnosis of rheumatic fever. The presence of two major manifestations, or of one major and two minor manifestations, indicates a high probability of the presence of rheumatic fever *if supported by evidence of a preceding streptococcal infection.* The absence of the latter should make the diagnosis doubtful, except in situations in which rheumatic fever is first discovered after a long latent period from the antecedent infection, e.g., Sydenham's chorea or low-grade carditis. Items under **Laboratory** manifestations are not intended to be matched with those items on the same line in the **Clinical** column.

	Clinical	Laboratory
	Major Manifestations	
1	Carditis	....
2	Polyarthritis	
3	Chorea	
4	Erythema marginatum	
5	Subcutaneous nodules	
	Minor Manifestations	
6	Previous rheumatic fever or rheumatic heart disease	Acute phase reactions: elevated erythrocyte sedimentation rate;
7	Arthralgia	C-reactive protein; leukocytosis
8	Fever	Electrocardiogram: prolonged P-R interval
	Supporting Evidence of Preceding Streptococcal Infection	
9	Recent scarlet fever	Increased antistreptolysin O antibody (ASO) or other streptococcal antibodies
10		Positive throat culture for group A *Streptococcus*

Contributor: Krause, Richard M.

Reference: American Heart Association Committee. 1965. Circulation 32:664-668.

19. CHARACTERISTIC FEATURES OF CLASSICAL BACTERIAL PNEUMONIAS

Antibiotic Therapy: [r] indicates that resistant strains have been reported. Figures in heavy brackets are reference numbers.

	Pathogen	Usual Route of Infection	Contagion	Pneumonic Infiltrate	Complications		Antibiotic Therapy
					Intrathoracic	**Other**	
1	*Klebsiella pneumoniae* (Friedlander's bacillus)	Endogenous aspiration [4]	Rare [4]	Lobar consolidation, abscess, atelectasis, ipsilateral tracheal shift, convex bowing of interlobar fissure [6]	Occasional meta- or post-pneumonic empyema [7]	Chronic alcoholism [6]	Two of the following[1]: gentamicin, chloramphenicol [r], tetracycline [r], cephalothin [r], kanamycin [r] [7]
2	*Staphylococcus aureus*	Endogenous or exogenous aspiration; occasionally bacteremic [7]	Common [7]	Bronchopneumonia with multiple small abscesses and pneumatoceles [8]	Infants: early empyema with pneumothorax; adults: postpneumonic empyema [7]	Otitis media, purulent rhinitis, acute adenitis, suppurative parotitis, furunculosis, bacteremia; epidemic with influenza outbreak [7]	Penicillin G, or penicillinase-resistant semisynthetic penicillin (methicillin [r]), cephalosporin [r], vancomycin, lincomycin [r] [7]

[1] Combination of gentamicin and cephalothin may be nephrotoxic [7].

continued

19. CHARACTERISTIC FEATURES OF CLASSICAL BACTERIAL PNEUMONIAS

	Pathogen	Usual Route of Infection	Contagion	Pneumonic Infiltrate	Complications — Intrathoracic	Complications — Other	Antibiotic Therapy
3	*Streptococcus pneumoniae* (pneumococcus)	Endogenous aspiration [7] or exogenous aspiration [5]	Uncommon, but may occur in families [5]	Lobar consolidation [3]; patchy in emphysema [10]	Abscess (type III), atelectasis, metapneumonic empyema, sterile pleural effusion, pericarditis [7]	Otitis media, upper respiratory infection, meningitis, arthritis, peritonitis, endocarditis [7]	Penicillin G [r] [7]; erythromycin [r] [9]; lincomycin [r] [1]
4	*S. pyogenes* (Group A beta-hemolytic streptococci)	Exogenous aspiration via airborne droplets or their nuclei [2]	Usual [2]	Interstitial with large prepneumonic empyema [7]	Suppurative; residual pleural thickening; rarely mediastinitis, pericarditis [7]	Epidemic in closed populations [2]	Penicillin G, erythromycin [r], lincomycin [r] [7]

Contributor: Wilson, Francis M.

References

1. Anderson, R. 1968. Am. Rev. Respir. Dis. 97:914-918.
2. Basiliere, J. L., et al. 1968. Am. J. Med. 44:580-589.
3. Cecil, R. L., et al. 1927. Arch. Intern. Med. 40:253-280.
4. Erasmus, L. D. 1956. Q. J. Med. 25:507-521.
5. Finland, M. 1942. Medicine (Baltimore) 21:307-344.
6. Lampe, W. T., II. 1964. Dis. Chest 46:599-606.
7. Lerner, A. M. 1975. The Classic Bacterial Pneumonias. Year Book, Chicago.
8. Rebhan, A. W., and H. E. Edwards. 1960. Can. Med. Assoc. J. 82:513-517.
9. Witt, R. L., and M. Hamburger. 1963. Med. Clin. North Am. 47:1257-1270.
10. Ziskind, M. M., et al. 1970. Ann. Intern. Med. 72:835-839.

20. CLINICAL FINDINGS IN ADULTS WITH PNEUMONIAS CAUSED BY GRAM-NEGATIVE BACTERIA

	Bacteria	Subjects	Predisposing Conditions or Chronic Diseases	Pathogenesis	Clinical Findings	Therapy of Choice in 1976	Reference
1	*Pseudomonas aeruginosa*	♂, elderly	Chronic lung disease, leukemia, neoplastic diseases, granulocytopenia, sometimes heart disease	Bacteremia, endogenous or exogenous aspiration	Diffuse or nodular lower lobe bronchopneumonias with coalescing microabscesses (confusion, bradycardia, cyanosis, reversal diurnal temp, abnormal liver function, azotemia)	Carbenicillin plus one of the following: gentamicin, tobramycin or amikacin	3,6
2	*Escherichia coli*	♂♀, middle-aged	Pyelonephritis, diabetes mellitus, surgery, gastrointestinal infection, sometimes heart disease	Bacteremia (or endogenous aspiration)	Lower lobe bronchopneumonias with metapneumonic empyemas	Two of the following recommended: kanamycin or gentamicin, tetracycline, ampicillin, cephalothin, chloramphenicol	4
3	*Klebsiella pneumoniae*	♂, middle-aged	Lung disease, heart disease, sometimes pyelonephritis, diabetes mellitus, alcoholism, neoplastic diseases	Endogenous aspiration	Lobar pneumonia with abscess, convex bowing of interlobar fissure, ipsilateral tracheal shift, occasional meta- or post-pneumonic empyema	Gentamicin or kanamycin, plus tetracycline, cephalothin or chloramphenicol	2

continued

	Bacteria	Subjects	Predisposing Conditions or Chronic Diseases	Pathogenesis	Clinical Findings	Therapy of Choice in 1976	Reference
4	*Proteus* spp.	Usually ♂, middle-aged to elderly	Lung disease, alcoholism, sometimes heart disease or diabetes mellitus	Endogenous aspiration	Dense cavitary lobar pneumonias, ipsilateral tracheal shift	Gentamicin (*see* entry 2); ampicillin for strains of *P. mirabilis*	5
5	*Haemophilus influenzae*	Infants, occasionally children, rarely adults	Infection with type b in persons lacking circulating bactericidal antibodies	Endogenous aspiration	Lobar pneumonia which is difficult to differentiate from pneumococcal pneumonia	Ampicillin [1], tetracycline [2] or chloramphenicol	8
6		Usually ♂, middle-aged	Chronic lung diseases, usually non-typable	Endogenous aspiration	Diffuse bronchopneumonia, miliary pattern		
7	*Bacteroides fragilis*	♀	Acute or subacute pelvic infections	Bacteremia	Acute illnesses. Lower lobe bronchopneumonia with empyema, sometimes abscess formation.	Tube thoracotomy, correction of pelvic condition (often surgical), clindamycin or chloramphenicol	7
8	Oral strains of *Bacteroides;* other oral anaerobic bacteria	Middle-aged men or women	Chronic lung disease, sometimes heart disease, alcoholism, carcinoma of the colon, stroke, epilepsy, general anesthesia, heroin addiction	Endogenous aspiration	Subacute illnesses. Lower lobe bronchopneumonia with large recurring empyemas, often abscess formation.	Tube thoracotomy, penicillin, clindamycin	1,7

[1] Drug of first choice unless ampicillin-resistant stains of *Haemophilus* present in community.   [2] Tetracycline relatively contraindicated in pediatric age group.

Contributor: Crane, Lawrence R.

References

1. Bartlett, J. G., et al. 1974. Am. J. Med. 56:202-207.
2. Edmondson, E. B., and J. P. Sanford. 1967. Medicine (Baltimore) 46:323-340.
3. Pennington, J. E., et al. 1973. Am. J. Med. 55:155-160.
4. Tillotson, J. R., and A. M. Lerner. 1967. N. Engl. J. Med. 277:115-122.
5. Tillotson, J. R., and A. M. Lerner. 1968. Ann. Intern. Med. 68:287-294.
6. Tillotson, J. R., and A. M. Lerner. 1968. Ibid. 68:295-307.
7. Tillotson, J. R., and A. M. Lerner. 1968. Ibid. 68:308-317.
8. Tillotson, J. R., and A. M. Lerner. 1968. Arch. Intern. Med. 121:428-432.

21. SOME PARASITES OF WILD ANIMALS WHICH ALSO CAUSE INFECTIOUS DISEASE IN MAN

Diseases listed represent the range of reactions observed. Data in brackets refer to the column heading in brackets.

	Parasite	Primary Hosts [Vector]	Manifestation	
			Non-human Hosts	Human Hosts
		Viruses		
1	Colorado tick fever virus	Squirrels, chipmunks, mice, porcupines [Ticks]	No apparent disease	Fever, malaise, leukopenia

continued

21. SOME PARASITES OF WILD ANIMALS WHICH ALSO CAUSE INFECTIOUS DISEASE IN MAN

	Parasite	Primary Hosts [Vector]	Manifestation Non-human Hosts	Human Hosts
	Arboencephaloviruses			
2	Eastern equine encephalitis	Small birds, ducks, horses [Mosquitoes]	No apparent disease; horses die	Encephalomyelitis
3	Western equine encephalitis	Birds, squirrels, snakes, horses [Mosquitoes]	No apparent disease; horses die	Encephalomyelitis
4	Venezuelan equine encephalitis	Rodents, horses [Mosquitoes]	No apparent disease; horses die	Encephalitis
5	Japanese B encephalitis	Birds, swine, horses, cattle [Mosquitoes]	No apparent disease; domestic animals may die	Encephalitis
6	Murray Valley encephalitis	Birds [Mosquitoes]	No apparent disease	Encephalomyelitis
7	St. Louis encephalitis	Birds [Mosquitoes]	No apparent disease	Encephalomyelitis
8	Tick-borne encephalitis	Rodents, birds [Ticks]	No known apparent disease	Encephalitis
9	Russian spring-summer encephalitis	Small mammals, birds [Ticks]	No known apparent disease	Encephalitis
10	California encephalitis	Rabbits, hares, squirrels, deer, horses, cattle [Mosquitoes]	No apparent disease	Encephalitis
11	Yellow fever virus	Non-human primates [Mosquitoes]	No apparent disease; death	Yellow fever
12	Rabies virus	Weasel-skunk, civet-ferret families, with bats, foxes, skunks most important; dogs, cats, cattle	No apparent disease; death with paralysis	Excitation, paralysis, death
13	Arenaviruses	Rodents, non-human primates [Ticks, mites, mosquitoes]	No apparent disease; death	No clinical disease; malaise, fever, shock, meningitis, encephalitis, hemorrhagic fever
		Chlamydias		
14	Ornithosis chlamydias	Psittacine birds, pigeons, poultry	No apparent disease; death	Fever, cough, pneumonia
		Rickettsias		
15	*Rickettsia akari*	Mice [Mites]	No apparent disease	Rickettsialpox
16	*R. rickettsii*	Rabbits, squirrels, rats, mice, groundhogs [Ticks]	No apparent disease	Rocky Mountain spotted fever
17	*R. typhi* [1]	Rats [Fleas]	No apparent disease	Murine typhus
18	*Coxiella burnetii*	Wild ungulates	No apparent disease	Q fever
		Bacteria		
19	*Borrelia* spp.	Rodents, porcupines, opossums, armadillos [Soft ticks]	No apparent disease; death	Relapsing fever, hemorrhage
20	*Leptospira* spp.	Rats, mice, opossums, skunks, raccoons, wildcats, foxes, dogs, shrews, bandicoots, cattle, swine—almost all mammals	No apparent disease; abortion, hemorrhage, nephritis	Weil's disease, nephritis, hepatitis, conjunctivitis
21	*Spirillum minor* [2]	Rats, mice, cats	No apparent disease	Fever, rash
22	*Pseudomonas pseudomallei*	Rats, mice, rabbits, ruminants, dogs, cats, non-human primates	No apparent disease; death	Pulmonary abscesses, septicemia
23	*Brucella* spp.	Wild ungulates	No apparent disease; abortion	Brucellosis
24	*Francisella tularensis*	Rabbits, squirrels, rats, skunks, bears, muskrats, coyotes, cats, dogs, swine, sheep, cattle [Ticks, deerflies, mosquitoes]	No apparent disease; lymphadenitis, septicemia	Tularemia
25	*Yersinia pestis*	Rats, mice, prairie dogs, squirrels, marmots, rabbits, gerbils [Fleas]	No apparent disease; death	Bubonic, pneumonic, septicemic plague
26	*Streptobacillus moniliformis*	Rats, squirrels, weasels, turkeys	No apparent disease	Fever, rash

[1] Synonym: *R. mooseri*. [2] Synonym: *S. minus.*

continued

21. SOME PARASITES OF WILD ANIMALS WHICH ALSO CAUSE INFECTIOUS DISEASE IN MAN

	Parasite	Primary Hosts [Vector]	Manifestation Non-human Hosts	Manifestation Human Hosts
27	*Listeria monocytogenes*	Wild mammals, birds; domestic mammals	No apparent disease; death	Meningitis, abortion
		Protozoans		
28	*Leishmania* spp.	Rodents, carnivores [Sandflies]	No apparent disease; skin ulcers	Chronic skin ulcerations, mucocutaneous lesions, kala-azar syndrome
29	*Trypanosoma cruzi*	Armadillos, bats, rodents, opossums, non-human primates, dogs, cats [Triatomids]	No known apparent disease	Skin rash, myocarditis, conjunctivitis, myositis, neurologic dysfunctions
30	*T. gambiense; T. rhodesiense*	Wild ungulates [Tsetse flies]	No apparent disease; death in coma	Meningoencephalitis
31	*Pneumocystis carinii* [3]	Rodents, non-human primates, sheep, goats, dogs	No known apparent disease	Plasma cell pneumonia
		Helminths		
32	*Fasciola hepatica*	Snails, fish, cattle, sheep	No apparent disease; death	Acute hepatitis, cholecystitis, cirrhosis
33	*Schistosoma* spp.	Snails, rodents	No apparent disease; death	Colitis, hepatitis, cystitis
34	*Diphyllobothrium latum*	Freshwater fish, bears, dogs, cats	No known apparent disease	Tapeworm infection
35	*Hymenolepis diminuta; H. nana*	Mice, rats	Tapeworm infection	Tapeworm infection
36	*Brugia* spp.	Non-human primates, wild carnivores, rodents [Mosquitoes]	No known apparent disease	Lymphadenopathy, lymphedema
37	*Dracunculus medinensis*	Wild carnivores, non-human primates [Water fleas]	No known apparent disease	Skin ulcers
38	*Trichinella spiralis*	Wild carnivores	No known apparent disease	No apparent disease; death

[3] Taxonomic position uncertain.

Contributor: Hoeprich, Paul D.

Reference: Hoeprich, P. D., ed. 1977. Infectious Diseases. Ed. 2. Harper and Row, Hagerstown, MD.

22. INTRADERMAL (MANTOUX) TUBERCULIN SKIN TEST

Units: TU = international tuberculin unit. **PPD:** Biological activity equivalent to that produced by listed quantities of PPD-S (Purified Protein Derivative-Standard). **Old Tuberculin: Dry Weight** assumes 1000 mg/ml of concentrated old tuberculin.

	Test Strength	Units TU	PPD mg/0.1 ml	Old Tuberculin Dilution	Old Tuberculin Dry Weight mg/0.1 ml dose
1	First	1	0.00002	1:10,000	0.01
2	Intermediate (usual test dose)	5	0.00010	1:2,000	0.05
3	Second	250	0.00500	1:100	1.0

Contributor: Hoeprich, Paul D.

Reference: Hoeprich, P. D., ed. 1977. Infectious Diseases. Ed. 2. Harper and Row, Hagerstown, MD.

23. SOME CHARACTERISTICS OF A FEW MYCOBACTERIUM SPECIES

Part I. General

Growth Temperature: 0 = no growth; + = growth; Few = few strains (<50%); Most = most strains (>50%).

Runyon Group		Species	Colony Appearance			Growth Temperature, °C				Rate of Growth
			Type	Pigment		22-24	32-33	35-39	41-43	
				In Dark	After Light					
1	Tuberculosis	*Mycobacterium tuberculosis*	Rough	None	None	0	+	+	0	Slow
2	complex	*M. bovis*	Rough	None	None	0	+	+	0	Slow
3	I	*M. kansasii*	Usually rough	None	Yellow	+	+	+	0	Slow
4		*M. marinum*	Usually smooth	None	Yellow	+	+	0	0	Slow
5	II	*M. scrofulaceum*	Smooth	Yellow or orange	Yellow or orange	+	+	+	0	Slow
6	III	*M. xenopi*	Smooth	Yellow or orange	Yellow or orange	0	Few	+	+	Slow
7		*M. avium/intracellulare*	Smooth	None	None	Few	+	+	Few	Slow
8		*M. ulcerans*	Rough	None	None	Most	+	0	0	Slow
9	IV	*M. fortuitum* complex	Rough or smooth	None	None	+	+	+	Most	Rapid

Contributor: Harris, H. William

Reference: Harris, H. W. 1977. In P. D. Hoeprich, ed. Infectious Diseases. Ed. 2. Harper and Row, Hagerstown, MD.

Part II. Biochemical and Clinical

Resistant to TCH: TCH = 2-thiophenecarboxylic acid hydrazide. **Clinical Significance** indicates pathogenicity of isolates from clinical specimens (sputum, etc.). **Symbols:** + = reacts, or yes; 0 = does not react, or no; Few = few strains (<50%); Many = many strains (>50%).

Runyon Group		Species	Niacin Test	Catalase		Tween Hydrolysis 5 d	Nitrate Reduction	Resistant to TCH 10 µg/ml	Clinical Significance
				Semi-quantitative >45 mm	68°C for 20 min				
1	Tuberculosis	*Mycobacterium tuberculosis*	+	0	0	Few	+	+	Always pathogenic
2	complex	*M. bovis*	0	0	0	0	0	0	Always pathogenic
3	I	*M. kansasii*	0	+	+	+	+	+	Usually pathogenic
4		*M. marinum*	Few	0	Few	+	0	+	Usually pathogenic
5	II	*M. scrofulaceum*	0	+	+	0	0	+	May be pathogenic or non-pathogenic
6	III	*M. xenopi*	0	0	+	0	0	+	May be pathogenic or non-pathogenic
7		*M. avium/intracellulare*	0	0	+	0	0	+	Usually pathogenic; may be non-pathogenic
8		*M. ulcerans*	0	+	+	0	0	+	Always pathogenic
9	IV	*M. fortuitum* complex	0	+	+	Many	+	+	Usually non-pathogenic

Contributor: Harris, H. William

Reference: Harris, H. W. 1977. In P. D. Hoeprich, ed. Infectious Diseases. Ed. 2. Harper and Row, Hagerstown, MD.

24. ANTITUBERCULOUS DRUGS

Usual Daily Dose is for adults. **Major Toxic Manifestations:** GI = gastrointestinal; CNS = central nervous system.

	Drug ⟨Abbreviation⟩	Contribution to Antituberculous Regimen	Route of Administration	Usual Daily Dose	Major Toxic Manifestations	Relative Frequency of Toxicity	Relative Efficacy
				Initial Treatment			
1	Isoniazid ⟨INH⟩	Major	Oral	300 mg once daily	Hepatic; neurologic	Uncommon	Highly effective
2	Rifampin ⟨RMP⟩	Major	Oral	600 mg once daily	Hepatic; hematologic	Uncommon	Highly effective
3	Streptomycin ⟨SM⟩	Major	Intramuscular	0.5-1 g once daily	Cranial nerve VIII; renal	Common	Highly effective
4	Ethambutol ⟨EMB⟩	"Companion"	Oral	15-25 mg/kg once daily	Optic neuritis	Uncommon	Limited effectiveness; good "companion" drug
5	p-Aminosalicylic acid ⟨PAS⟩	"Companion"	Oral	12-14 g in divided doses	GI intolerance	Common	Limited effectiveness; poor patient tolerance
				Retreatment			
6	Pyrazinamide ⟨PZA⟩	"Companion"	Oral	1.5-3.0 g in divided doses	Hepatic; hyperuricemia	Common	Effective "companion" drug; hepatitis may be severe
7	Ethionamide ⟨ETA⟩	"Companion"	Oral	0.5-1.0 g in divided doses	GI intolerance; hepatic	Common	Moderately effective; poor patient tolerance
8	Cycloserine ⟨CS⟩	"Companion"	Oral	0.5-1.0 g in divided doses	CNS (psychosis, seizures)	Common	Limited effectiveness; rarely indicated
9	Viomycin ⟨VM⟩	Major	Intramuscular	1 g once daily	Cranial nerve VIII; renal	Common	Moderately effective
10	Kanamycin ⟨KM⟩	Major	Intramuscular	1 g once daily	Cranial nerve VIII; renal	Common	Moderately effective
11	Capreomycin ⟨CM⟩	Major	Intramuscular	1 g once daily	Cranial nerve VIII; renal	Common	Moderately effective

Contributor: Harris, H. William

Reference: Harris, H. W. 1977. In P. D. Hoeprich, ed. Infectious Diseases. Ed. 2. Harper and Row, Hagerstown, MD.

25. NEPHRITOGENIC SEROTYPES OF RECOGNIZED IMPORTANCE

Group A streptococci are serotyped by two methods: a slide agglutination method [ref. 6] which uses trypsinized suspensions and identifies the T-antigens, and a precipitin method [ref. 11] which identifies the M-antigens. Usually one streptococcal strain has only one M-antigen, and this is the antigen that plays an important part in the virulence of the streptococcus.

	Streptococcal Antigens		Usual Site of Antecedent Infection		Reference
	Type T	Type M	Skin	Throat	
1	1	1	.....	+	13
2	2 [1/]	2 [1/]	.....	+	1

[1/] Limited number of cases reported to date.

continued

25. NEPHRITOGENIC SEROTYPES OF RECOGNIZED IMPORTANCE

	Streptococcal Antigens		Usual Site of Antecedent Infection		Reference
	Type T	Type M	Skin	Throat	
3	4	4	.....	+	13
4	4	60[2,3]	+	+	2,4,9
5	6[1]	6[1]	.....	+	13
6	12	12[3]	.....	+	10
7	14/49	49[2,3]	+	+	3,5,7,12,14
8	8/25/Imp. 19	2[2,3]; 55[2,3]; 57[2,3]	+	.....	3-5,7,8

[1] Limited number of cases reported to date. [2] Predominantly associated with pyoderma. [3] Strains of major and/or epidemic importance.

Contributor: Dillon, Hugh C.

References

1. Anthony, B. F., et al. 1974. J. Infect. Dis. 129:336-340.
2. Dillon, H. C., and M. S. A. Dillon. 1974. Infect. Immun. 9:1070-1078.
3. Dillon, H. C., et al. 1968. Lancet 1:543-545.
4. Dillon, H. C., et al. 1974. J. Infect. Dis. 130:257-267.
5. Dillon, H. C., Jr. 1970. Postgrad. Med. J. 46:641-652.
6. Griffith, F. 1934. J. Hyg. 34:542-584.
7. Parker, M. T. 1969. Br. J. Dermatol. 81(Suppl. 1):37-46.
8. Potter, E. V., et al. 1968. J. Lab. Clin. Med. 71:126-137.
9. Potter, E. V., et al. 1971. J. Clin. Invest. 50:1197-1205.
10. Rammelkamp, C. H., Jr., and R. S. Weaver. 1953. Ibid. 32:345-358.
11. Swift, H. F., et al. 1943. J. Exp. Med. 78:127-133.
12. Updyke, E. L., et al. 1955. Science 121:171-172.
13. Wannamaker, L. W. 1967. Acute Glomeronephritis Proc. 17th Annu. Symp. Kidney, pp. 39-67.
14. Wannamaker, L. W. 1970. N. Engl. J. Med. 282:23-31, 78-85.

26. RELATIVE VALUE OF STREPTOCOCCAL ANTIBODY TESTS IN ACUTE GLOMERULO-NEPHRITIS IN RELATION TO ANTECEDENT SITE OF INFECTION

Average Frequency of Elevated Titers: **Pharyngitis-AGN**—antecedent site of infection was throat; **Pyoderma-AGN**—antecedent site of infection was skin. *Abbreviation:* AGN = acute glomerulonephritis.

	Antibody	Average Frequency of Elevated Titers, %		Reference
		Pharyngitis-AGN	Pyoderma-AGN	
1	Anti-streptolysin O	80-85	50	1-5
2	Anti-DNase B	80	90	1,2,5
3	Anti-hyaluronidase	.....	>80	4
4	Anti-NADase	>80	<25	1,2,5

Contributor: Dillon, Hugh C.

References

1. Ayoub, E. M., and L. W. Wannamaker. 1962. Pediatrics 29:527-538.
2. Dillon, H. C., Jr., and M. S. Reeves. 1974. Am. J. Med. 56:333-346.
3. Kaplan, E. L. 1970. J. Clin. Invest. 49:1405-1414.
4. Potter, E. V., et al. 1968. J. Pediatr. 72:871-884.
5. Wannamaker, L. W. 1970. N. Engl. J. Med. 282:23-31, 78-85.

Laboratory Findings: AFB = acid-fast-staining bacilli; VDRL = Venereal Disease Research Laboratories; C1q = a subcomponent of complement component one. **Fre**quency = occurrence in percent of cases. Data in brackets refer to the column heading in brackets.

	Organ Site	Clinical Manifestations	Laboratory Findings [Frequency]
1	Skin	Macules or papules: multiple, bilaterally symmetrical, usually erythematous	Infiltrates of foamy macrophages; lymphocytes scanty; absence of giant cells & epithelioid cells; masses of AFB; dermal basement membrane deposition of IgM
2		Diffuse infiltration	
3		Erythema nodosum (50-75% of cases), often accompanied by fever & arthralgias[1]	
4		Brawny edema of hands & feet; thickening of facial & ear skin; loss of eyebrows	
5	Nerves	Mononeuritis multiplex; anesthesia; atrophic changes; nerve thickening	Slowed conduction velocity; Schwann cell invasion by AFB; perineural proliferation; demyelination; axonal degeneration
6	Eyes	"Beading" of corneal nerve; granulomatous conjunctivitis; punctate keratitis; iridocyclitis; blindness	Granulomatous infiltrates
7	Nose: mucous membranes	Epistaxis; nasal congestion; nasal septum perforation	Masses of AFB
8	Blood	....	Chronic bacteremia [>75%]
9			Reversal of B:T lymphocyte ratio in peripheral blood[2] (*see* entry 11)
10	Serology	Clinical manifestations of amyloid deposition; erythema nodosum[3]; vasculitis (Lucio phenomenon)[3]; glomerulonephritis[3]	Amyloid-related serum component protein [>50%]; cryoproteinemia [>30%]; rheumatoid factor [5-50%]; polyclonal hypergammaglobulinemia; anti-nuclear factor [1-30%]; false positive VDRL test [>10%]; serum C1q precipitin activity[2] (*see* entry 3)
11	Lymphoid organs	Specific skin test anergy to *Mycobacterium leprae*; non-specific anergy to other skin test antigens	Macrophage infiltration of lymph node paracortical areas and splenic white pulp; granulomata in liver & bone marrow
12	Urogenital organs	....	Amyloid deposition
13			Abnormal urinary sediment; proteinuria[4]
14			Proliferative glomerulonephritis (*see* entry 10)
15		Epididymo-orchitis; testicular atrophy; gynecomastia	Increase in total urinary gonadotropins; decrease in plasma testosterone; granulomatous inflammation with fibrotic changes

[1] Also may rarely be associated with leukemoid reaction (*see* entry 10). [2] Frequency not established. [3] This clinical manifestation may or may not be related to the accompanying laboratory findings. [4] Associated with erythema nodosum (entry 3).

Contributor: Bullock, Ward E.

General References

1. Bullock, W. E. 1971. In M. Samter, ed. Immunological Diseases. Ed. 2. Little, Brown; Boston. pp. 630-643.
2. Cochrane, R. G., and T. F. Davey, ed. 1964. Leprosy in Theory and Practice. Ed. 2. Williams and Wilkins, Baltimore.
3. Drutz, D. J., et al. 1972. N. Engl. J. Med. 287:159-164.
4. Ridley, D. S., and W. H. Jopling. 1966. Int. J. Lepr. 34:255-273.

28. KINDS AND SOURCES OF FOODS KNOWN TO HAVE LED TO BOTULISM IN THE UNITED STATES

The data below are derived from 735 outbreaks between 1899 and 1975 [ref. 3]. For additional information, consult references 1 and 2.

Food	Outbreaks %
Kinds	
1 Vegetables	54
2 Fish & fish products	9
3 Meats	7
4 Fruit (including pimientos)	5
5 Miscellaneous products (including pickles, olives, & milk products)	5

Food	Outbreaks %
6 Unknown	20
Sources	
7 Home preserved	71
8 Commercially preserved	9
9 Unknown	20

Contributor: Gangarosa, Eugene J.

References

1. Meyer, K. F., and B. Eddie. 1965. 65 Years of Human Botulism in the United States and Canada. Univ. California Press, Berkeley.

2. U.S. Public Health Service, Center for Disease Control. 1974. U.S. Dep. Health Educ. Welfare Publ. 74-8279.
3. U.S. Public Health Service, Center for Disease Control. Unpublished. CDC Surveillance Data. Atlanta, GA.

29. RICKETTSIAL DISEASES

Data in brackets refer to the column heading in brackets.

Disease [Agent]	Geographic Distribution	Arthropod Host [Mammalian Host]	Transmission to Man	Serologic Diagnosis	
				Weil-Felix Reaction	Complement Fixation
Spotted Fever Group					
1 Rocky Mountain spotted fever [*Rickettsia rickettsii*]	Western hemisphere	Ticks [Wild rodents, dogs]	Tick bite	Positive OX-19, OX-2	Positive group- and type-specific
2 Boutonneuse fever [*R. conorii*]	Africa, Europe, Middle East, India	Ticks [Wild rodents, dogs]	Tick bite	Positive OX-19, OX-2	Positive group- and type-specific
3 Queensland tick typhus [*R. australis*]	Australia	Ticks [Marsupials, wild rodents]	Tick bite	Positive OX-19, OX-2	Positive group- and type-specific
4 North Asian tick-borne rickettsiosis [*R. sibirica*]	Siberia, Mongolia	Ticks [Wild rodents]	Tick bite	Positive OX-19, OX-2	Positive group- and type-specific
5 Rickettsialpox [*R. akari*]	United States, Russia, ? Africa	Blood-sucking mite [House mouse, other rodents]	Mite bite	Negative	Positive group- and type-specific
Typhus Group					
6 Endemic (murine) typhus [*R. typhi* [1]]	Worldwide	Flea [Small rodents]	Infected flea feces into broken skin	Positive OX-19	Positive group- and type-specific
7 Epidemic typhus [*R. prowazekii*]	Worldwide	Body louse [Man]	Infected louse feces into broken skin	Positive OX-19	Positive group- and type-specific

[1] Synonym: *R. mooseri.*

continued

29. RICKETTSIAL DISEASES

Disease [Agent]	Geographic Distribution	Arthropod Host [Mammalian Host]	Transmission to Man	Serologic Diagnosis	
				Weil-Felix Reaction	Complement Fixation
8 Brill-Zinsser disease [*R. prowazekii*]	Worldwide	Recurrence years after original attack of epidemic typhus		Usually negative	Positive group- and type-specific
9 Scrub typhus [*R. tsutsugamushi*]	Asia, Australia, Pacific islands	Trombiculid mites [Wild rodents]	Mite bite	Positive OX-K	Positive in ∿50% of patients
Other					
10 Q fever [*Coxiella burnetii* 2/]	Worldwide	Ticks [Small mammals, cattle, sheep, goats]	Inhalation of dried infected material	Negative	Positive
11 Trench fever [*Rochalimaea quintana* 3/]	Europe, Africa, North America	Body louse [Man]	Infected louse feces into broken skin	Negative	None available

2/ Synonym: *Rickettsia burnetii.*   3/ Synonym: *Rickettsia quintana.*

Contributor: Woodward, Theodore E.

Reference: Wintrobe, M. M., et al., ed. 1974. Harrison's Principles of Internal Medicine. Ed. 7. McGraw-Hill, New York.
p. 910.

30. SEROLOGIC DIAGNOSIS OF RICKETTSIAL DISEASES OF THE UNITED STATES

Group	Disease	Testing Agent	Illustrative Titer			Cases with Diagnostic Titer
			Day 10	Day 20	Day 30	
Weil-Felix Reaction						
1 Spotted fever	Rocky Mountain spotted fever	*Proteus* OX-19	40	320	......	Most
2		OX-2	20	160	......	
3	Rickettsialpox	*Proteus* OX-19	0	0	......	None
4		OX-2	0	0	......	
5 Typhus	Endemic (murine) typhus	*Proteus* OX-19	160	640	......	Most
6		OX-2	10	40	......	
7	Brill-Zinsser disease	*Proteus* OX-19	160	20	......	Infrequent
8		OX-2	0	0	......	
9 Other	Q fever	*Proteus* OX-19	0	0	......	None
10		OX-2	0	0	......	
Complement-Fixation Tests with Type-specific Antigen						
11 Spotted fever	Rocky Mountain spotted fever	*Rickettsia rickettsii*	20	160	80	Most
12	Rickettsialpox	*R. akari*	0	64	128	Most
13 Typhus	Endemic (murine) typhus	*R. typhi* 1/	0	160	160	Most
14	Brill-Zinsser disease	*R. prowazekii*	1280	640	320	Most
15 Other	Q fever	*Coxiella burnetii* 2/	10	80	160	Most

1/ Synonym: *R. mooseri.*   2/ Synonym: *Rickettsia burnetii.*

Contributor: Woodward, Theodore E.

Reference: Wintrobe, M. M., et al., ed. 1974. Harrison's Principles of Internal Medicine. Ed. 7. McGraw-Hill, New York.
p. 912.

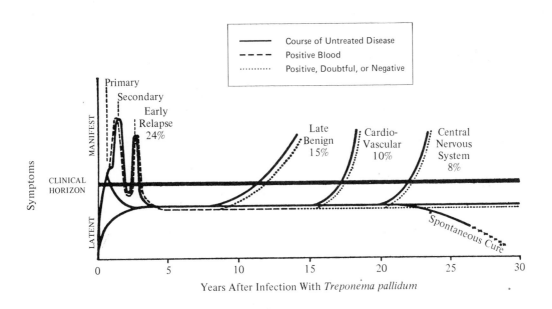

Contributor: Johnson, Thomas W.

Reference: Johnson, T. W. 1972. In P. D. Hoeprich, ed. Infectious Diseases. Harper and Row, Hagerstown, MD. p. 543.

32. HUMORAL ANTIBODIES CHARACTERISTIC OF SYPHILIS AND THEIR RELATION TO SEROLOGIC TESTS FOR SYPHILIS

	Antibody	Antigen	Test
	Reagin: Non-specific anti-	Lipid extracts of normal human	Complement fixation
1	bodies that appear as a	or non-human tissues suffice;	Wassermann
2	consequence of syphilis	cardiolipin as now in use is a	Eagle
3	and many other diseases	highly purified lipid extract	Kolmer
		of beef heart combined with	Flocculation
4		lecithin & cholesterol	Venereal Disease Research Laboratory ⟨VDRL⟩
5			Hinton
6			Kahn
7			Kline
8			Eagle
	Specifically anti-trepone-	*Treponema pallidum*	
9	mal	Reiter strain (avirulent)	Reiter protein complement fixation ⟨RPCF⟩
10		Nichols strain (virulent)	*Treponema pallidum* immobilization ⟨TPI⟩
11			Fluorescent treponemal antibody ⟨FTA⟩
12			Fluorescent treponemal antibody absorption ⟨FTA-ABS⟩

Contributor: Johnson, Thomas W.

Reference: Johnson, T. W. 1972. In P. D. Hoeprich, ed. Infectious Diseases. Harper and Row, Hagerstown, MD. p. 551.

33. TREATMENT OF SYPHILIS

Penicillin dosages for pregnant women are the same as for the non-pregnant. For pregnant women allergic to penicillin, erythromycin is recommended in the same dosages as for the non-pregnant. Tetracycline therapy is *not* recommended during pregnancy.

	Type of Syphilis	Antibiotic	Dose
	Without Penicillin Allergy		
1	Early: primary; secondary; latent syphilis of <1-yr duration; exposed contacts	Benzathine penicillin G	2.4 million units total by i.m. injection at a single visit
2		Procaine penicillin G, aqueous	4.8 million units total: 600,000 units by i.m. injection daily for 8 d
3	Syphilis of >1-yr duration: latent syphilis of indeterminate or >1-yr duration; cardiovascular; late benign; neurosyphilis[1]	Benzathine penicillin G	7.2 million units total: 2.4 million units by i.m. injection weekly for three successive weeks
4		Procaine penicillin G, aqueous	9.0 million units total: 600,000 units by i.m. injection daily for 15 d
5	Congenital With abnormal cerebrospinal fluid	Procaine penicillin G, aqueous	50,000 units/kg by i.m. injection daily, for a minimum of 10 d
6		Penicillin G, aqueous	50,000 units/kg by i.m. or i.v. injection daily in 2 divided doses, for a minimum of 10 d
7	With normal cerebrospinal fluid	Benzathine penicillin G	50,000 units/kg by i.m. injection in a single dose
	With Penicillin Allergy		
8	Early: primary; secondary; latent syphilis of <1-yr duration; exposed contacts	Erythromycin (base, or ethyl succinate, or stearate)	500 mg by mouth, 4 times/d for 15 d
9		Tetracycline HCl	500 mg by mouth, 4 times/d for 15 d
10	Syphilis of >1-yr duration: latent syphilis of indeterminate or >1-yr duration; cardiovascular; late benign; neurosyphilis	Erythromycin (base, or ethyl succinate, or stearate)	500 mg by mouth, 4 times/d for 30 d
11		Tetracycline HCl	500 mg by mouth, 4 times/d for 30 d
12	Congenital (with or without abnormal cerebrospinal fluid)	Erythromycin (base, or ethyl succinate, or stearate), or tetracycline HCl	After neonatal period, dosage of erythromycin, or tetracycline, for congenital syphilitics who are allergic to penicillin should be individualized, but need not exceed dosages used in adult syphilis of >1-yr duration. Tetracycline should *not* be given to children <8-yr old.

[1] Some clinicians prefer to treat symptomatic neurosyphilis with aqueous penicillin G, 2-4 million units, i.v., every 4 h for 10 d.

Contributor: Wiesner, Paul J.

Reference: U.S. Public Health Service, Center for Disease Control. 1976. Syphilis, CDC Recommended Treatment Schedules. Atlanta, GA.

34. SOME PROPERTIES OF ANTIMALARIAL DRUGS

Data were adapted from reference 5. **Class of Agent:** Blood schizonticides eliminate asexual erythrocytic parasites; hepatic schizonticides eliminate exoerythrocytic (hepatic) schizonts, and therefore prevent relapses (radical cure); sporonticides prevent development of sexual forms in the mosquito. **Drug Resistance: Type**—RI = clearance of

continued

asexual parasitemia followed by recrudescence; RII = marked reduction of asexual parasitemia but no clearance; RIII = no marked reduction of asexual parasitemia. Data in brackets refer to the column heading in brackets.

Class of Agent	Drug	Drug Action		Drug Resistance		Toxicity	Reference
		Site of Action	Therapeutic Use	Resistant Species [Geographic Distribution]	Mechanism [Type]		
Blood schizonticide							
1 Rapid-acting	4-Aminoquinolines: chloroquine, amodiaquin	Food vacuole; DNA	Acute attack; chemoprophylaxis	*Plasmodium falciparum* [Asia, Latin America]	Reduced accumulation of drug by erythrocytes [RI, RII, RIII]	Minimal in suppressive doses	3,4, 7,9
2	Quinine	Food vacuole; DNA	Acute attack caused by chloroquine-resistant *Plasmodium falciparum*	*P. falciparum* [Asia, Latin America]	? [RI]	Cinchonism; immune hemolysis	7
3	Mefloquine [1]	?	Acute attack caused by chloroquine-resistant *P. falciparum*; chemoprophylaxis	None known	....	Not determined (limited experience)	7,8
4 Combination use	Pyrimethamine [2]	Block of tetrahydrofolate dehydrogenase [3]	Used in combination with sulfonamides (*see* entry 7)	*P. falciparum* [Worldwide]	Decreased binding to tetrahydrofolate dehydrogenase [3] [RI, RII, RIII]	Minimal; thrombocytopenia	2,7
5				*P. vivax; P. malariae* [Worldwide]	Decreased binding to tetrahydrofolate dehydrogenase [3]		
6	Sulfonamides	Block utilization of *p*-aminobenzoic acid	Used in combination with pyrimethamine (*see* entry 7)	*P. falciparum*	?	Minimal; agranulocytosis; Stevens-Johnson syndrome	7
7	Pyrimethamine + sulfonamides	Synergistic (*see* entries 4-6)	Acute attack; chemoprophylaxis against chloroquine-resistant *P. falciparum*	*P. falciparum* [Asia]	? [RI, RII, RIII]	(*See* entries 4-6)	7
8 Slow-acting	Antibiotics: tetracycline	Inhibition of protein synthesis	Acute attack caused by chloroquine-resistant *P. falciparum*, in combination with rapid-acting schizonticidal agent (e.g., quinine)	None known	....	Dental staining of fetuses & children; diarrhea	1,7
9 Hepatic schizonticide; sporonticide	8-Aminoquinolines: primaquine	?	Radical cure in infections with *P. vivax & P. ovale*	*P. vivax* [New Guinea, 30%; Vietnam, 10%; Central America, 5%]	?	Hemolysis in glucose-6-phosphate dehydrogenase deficiency; methemoglobinemia	6,7

[1] Experimental. [2] Also a primary hepatic schizonticide when asexual parasite is pyrimethamine-sensitive. [3] Synonym: Dihydrofolate reductase.

Contributors: Miller, Louis H., and Canfield, Craig J.

References
1. Colwell, E. J., et al. 1972. Am. J. Trop. Med. Hyg. 21:144-149.
2. Ferone, R., et al. 1970. Science 167:1263-1264.
3. Fitch, C. D. 1972. Proc. Helminthol. Soc. Wash. Spec. Issue 39:265-271.

continued

4. Hahn, F. E. 1975. In J. W. Corcoran and F. E. Hahn, ed. Antibiotics. Springer Verlag, New York. v. 3, pp. 58-78.

5. Miller, L. H. 1972. In P. D. Hoeprich, ed. Infectious Diseases. Harper and Row, Hagerstown, MD. pp. 1113-1125.

6. Miller, L. H., et al. 1974. Am. J. Trop. Med. Hyg. 23: 309-310.

7. Peters, W. 1970. Chemotherapy and Drug Resistance in Malaria. Academic Press, London and New York.

8. Trenholme, G. M., et al. 1975. Science 190:792-794.

9. Warhurst, D. C. 1973. Chemother. Agents Study Parasites Symp. Br. Soc. Parasitol. 11:1-28.

35. OVA OF INTESTINAL HELMINTHS

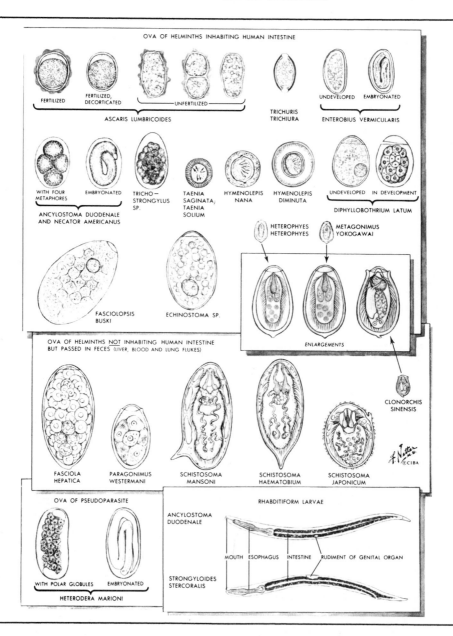

Contributor: Cox, Kaye B.

Reference: Netter, F. H. 1962. The CIBA Collection of Medical Illustrations. CIBA Pharmaceutical Company, Summit, NJ. v. 3, pt. 2, p. 184.

36. IMPORTANT CHARACTERISTICS OF INTESTINAL HELMINTHS

Data were adapted from reference 3. Data in brackets refer to the column heading in brackets.

| | Class[1] & Species | Adults | | Eggs | | |
		Average Size, mm[1] [Extreme Range mm[1]]	Significant Characteristics	Average Size, μm [Extreme Range μm]	Embryonal Contents	Significant Characteristics
			Helminths Inhabiting Intestinal Tract			
1	Nematoda[2] *Ancylostoma duodenale*	♂, 10 × 0.45 [(6-11) × (0.4-0.5)]; ♀, 12 × 0.6 [(9-16) × (0.35-0.60)]	Buccal capsule has 2 ventral pairs of teeth. ♂ has copulatory bursa; ♀ has vulva in posterior half of body. Gray-white.	58 × 38 [(56-60) × (36-40)]	2- to 8-cell stage	Thin, transparent shell; hyaline
2	*Ascaris lumbricoides*	♂, 240 × 3 [(150-310) × (2-4)]; ♀, 300 × 5 [(200-350) × (3-6)]	Large, glistening worms. Mouth with 3 oval papillate lips. ♂ has curved posterior extremity with 2 spicules. White.	Fertile: 60 × 45 [(45-75) × (35-50)]	Undeveloped embryo	Mamillated external coating, usually present; golden brown
3				Infertile: 90 × 42 [(88-94) × (39-44)]	Amorphous, granular	Irregular mamillated external coating; bizarre shapes; golden brown
4	*Capillaria philippinensis*	♂, 2.7 × 0.025 [(2.3-3.2) × 0.025]; ♀, 3.9 × 0.038 [(2.5-4.3) × 0.038]	♂ has long copulatory spicule & very long aspinous sheath; ♀ has vulva immediately behind esophagus, double reflex of oviduct	40 × 21 [(36-45) × (20-22)]	Undeveloped embryo, or larva	Thick shell (shell may be absent); translucent flattened polar plugs
5	*Enterobius vermicularis*	♂, 4 × 0.15 [(2-5) × (0.1-0.2)]; ♀, 10 × 0.4 [(6-13) × (0.3-0.5)]	♂ is seldom seen, has coiled posterior extremity; ♀ has anterior cuticular alae & long, pointed tail. White.	55 × 26 [(50-60) × (20-32)]	Developed embryo	One side convex, one side flattened; hyaline
6	*Necator americanus*	♂, 7 × 0.3 [(5-11) × (0.30-0.45)]; ♀, 10 × 0.35 [(9-13) × (0.35-0.60)]	Buccal capsule has 2 semilunar cutting plates. ♂ has copulatory bursa; ♀ has vulva in anterior half of body. Gray-white.	66 × 38 [(64-76) × (36-40)]	2- to 8-cell stage	Thin, transparent shell; hyaline
7	*Strongyloides stercoralis*	♂, 0.7 × 0.04 [(0.6-0.8) × (0.03-0.05)]; ♀, 2.2 × 0.04 [(2-3) × (0.04-0.10)]	♂ is seldom seen; filariform, parasitic ♀ has single file of eggs in uterus. Colorless, transparent.	54 × 32 [(50-60) × (30-35)]	Undeveloped embryo, or larva	Thin, transparent shell; hyaline. Rarely seen in feces.
8	*Trichuris trichiura*	♂, 38 × 1.3 [(30-45) × (1.2-1.5)]; ♀, 42 × 1.7 [(35-50) × (1.6-1.8)]	Narrow whiplike anterior 3/5, more robust posterior 2/5 of body. ♂ has coiled posterior extremity with copulatory spicule. Gray-white.	52 × 23 [(50-54) × (22-24)]	Undeveloped embryo	Thick shell; translucent polar plugs. Bile-stained.
9	Cestoda *Diphyllobothrium latum*	(3-10) m × 12 mm [(3-18) m × (10-20) mm]	Scolex has 2 elongate sucking grooves. 3000-4000 proglottids; mature proglottid has coiled, rosette-like uterus, diffuse testes & ovaries, median genital & uterine pores. Ivory-white.	65 × 45 [(55-76) × (37-56)]	Undeveloped embryo	Inconspicuous operculum; small abopercular thickening. Light yellow.

[1] Unless otherwise indicated. [2] Phylum.

continued

33

	Class & Species	Adults		Eggs		
		Average Size, mm[1] [Extreme Range mm[1]]	Significant Characteristics	Average Size, μm [Extreme Range μm]	Embryonal Contents	Significant Characteristics
10	*Dipylidium caninum*	300 × 2.5 [(100-800) × (2.5-4.0)]	Scolex has 4 suckers, hooklets, retractile rostellum. 60-175 proglottids; mature proglottid has diffuse testes, uterus with nest-like compartments, bilateral genital pore. Pink-red.	35 [25-60]	Hexacanth embryo	No operculum. Packets of 10-25 eggs. Brick red.
11	*Hymenolepis diminuta*	45 × 4 [(40-640) × (3-5)]	Scolex has 4 suckers, rostellum. 800-1000 proglottids; mature proglottid has 3 round testes, discrete bilobed ovary, unilateral genital pore. Ivory-white.	78 × 65 [(70-86) × (50-79)]	Hexacanth embryo	No operculum; double membrane, no filaments. Light yellow.
12	*H. nana*	20 × 0.7 [(20-45) × (0.5-0.9)]	Scolex has 4 suckers, hooklets, retractile rostellum. Up to 200 proglottids; mature proglottid has 3 round testes, discrete bilobed ovary, unilateral genital pore. Ivory-white.	47 × 35 [(44-50) × (30-37)]	Hexacanth embryo	No operculum; double membrane, 4-8 polar filaments; hyaline
13	*Taenia saginata*	(4-10) m × (12-20) mm [(4-25) m × (7-20) mm]	Scolex has 4 suckers. 1000-2000 proglottids; mature proglottid has diffuse testes, discrete bilobed ovary, irregularly alternate genital pore, gravid proglottid has 15-25 main branches on each side of uterus. Ivory-white.	35 × 25 [(30-40) × (20-30)]	Hexacanth embryo	No operculum; radially striated shell. Yellow-brown.
14	*T. solium*	(2-4) m × (8-12) mm [(2-8) m × (3-12) mm]	Scolex has 4 suckers, hooklets. 800-1000 proglottids; mature proglottid has diffuse testes, discrete trilobed ovary, irregularly alternate genital pore; gravid proglottid has 7-13 main branches on each side of uterus. Ivory-white.	35 [30-43]	Hexacanth embryo	Indistinguishable from *T. saginata*
15	Trematoda *Fasciolopsis buski*	50 × 14 [(20-80) × (8-20)]	Thick, ovate; small spines. Oral sucker much smaller than ventral. Flesh-colored gray.	135 × 82 [(130-140) × (80-85)]	Undeveloped embryo	Indistinct operculum. Uniformly granular contents. Yellow-brown.
16	*Gastrodiscoides hominis*	11 × 6 [(5-14) × (3-8)]	Bluntly pyriform with conical anterior, rounded posterior; aspinous. Small oral sucker, vary large posterior sucking disk. Pink.	160 × 65 [(150-170) × (60-72)]	Undeveloped embryo	Indistinct operculum. Uniformly granular contents. Green-brown.
17	*Heterophyes heterophyes*	1.4 × 0.5 [(1.0-1.7) × (0.3-0.7)]	Elongate, pyriform; scale-like spines. Ventral sucker much larger than oral; genital sucker. Gray.	29 × 16 [(28-30) × (15-17)]	Developed embryo	Distinct operculum, slight opercular shoulder. Thick shell. Usually small abopercular knob. Blunt ends. Yellow-brown.
18	*Metagonimus yokogawai*	1.5 × 0.6 [(1.0-2.5) × (0.4-0.8)]	Pyriform with rounded posterior; small scale-like spines. Oral sucker smaller than ventral; ventral sucker to right of midline. Gray.	28 × 16 [(27-29) × (16-17)]	Developed embryo	Distinct operculum; slight opercular shoulders. Thin shell. Usually no abopercular knob. Blunt ends. Yellow-brown.

[1] Unless otherwise indicated.

continued

34

	Adults		Eggs		
Class & Species	Average Size, mm [Extreme Range mm]	Significant Characteristics	Average Size, μm [Extreme Range μm]	Embryonal Contents	Significant Characteristics
Enteric-associated Helminths					
Trematoda 19 Clonorchis sinensis	18 X 4 [(10-25) X (3-5)]	Flat, elongate, tapering anteriorly; aspinous. Ventral sucker smaller than oral. Gray (brown when bile-stained).	30 X 16 [(27-35) X (12-20)]	Developed embryo	Distinct operculum; prominent abopercular knob. Yellow-brown.
20 Fasciola hepatica	25 X 10 [(20-30) X (8-13)]	Flat, leaf-like, conical anterior; scale-like spines. Suckers of equal size. Brown.	140 X 76 [(130-150) X (63-90)]	Undeveloped embryo	Indistinct operculum. Uniformly granular contents. Yellow-brown.
21 Opisthorchis felineus & O. viverrini	10 X 2.3 [(7-12) X (1.5-3.0)]	Flat, elongate, tapering anteriorly; aspinous. Ventral sucker smaller than oral. Yellow-red.	28 X 12 [(26-31) X (11-13)]	Developed embryo	Distinct operculum; prominent opercular shoulders; prominent abopercular knob. Yellow-brown.
22 Paragonimus westermani	12 X 6 [(7-16) X (4-8)]	Flat, spoon-shaped to spherical; scale-like, simple, or toothed spines. Suckers of equal size. Red-brown.	85 X 55 [(73-118) X (46-67)]	Undeveloped embryo	Distinct operculum; prominent opercular shoulders; thickened abopercular shell. Yellow-brown.
23 Schistosoma haematobium	♂, 13 X 0.9 [(10-15) X (0.8-1.0)]; ♀, 22 X 0.25 [(20-25) X (0.24-0.26)]	Elongate, cylindrical. Oral & ventral suckers of equal size. ♂ has fine cuticular tubercles; ♀ uterus is long with 20-30 eggs, ovary in posterior half of body. Gray-white.	143 X 60 [(112-170) X (40-73)]	Undeveloped embryo, or miracidium	No operculum; large terminal spine. Light yellow-brown.
24 S. japonicum	♂, 15 X 0.7 [(9-22) X (0.5-0.9)]; ♀, 19 X 0.30 [(12-26) X (0.25-0.30)]	Elongate, cylindrical. Oral & ventral suckers of equal size. ♂ has smooth cuticle; ♀ uterus is long with 50-100 eggs, ovary in middle of body. Gray-white.	88 X 65 [(70-106) X (50-80)]	Undeveloped embryo, or miracidium	No operculum; inconspicuous lateral projection. Usually debris-covered. Light yellow-brown.
25 S. mansoni	♂, 10 X 1.2 [(6-14) X (1.0-2.0)]; ♀, 14 X 0.16 [(7-17) X (0.10-0.20)]	Elongate, cylindrical. Oral & ventral suckers of equal size. ♂ has gross cuticular tubercles; ♀ uterus is short with 1-4 eggs, ovary in anterior half of body. Gray-white.	155 X 66 [(114-182) X (45-73)]	Undeveloped embryo, or miracidium	No operculum; large lateral spine. Light yellow-brown.

Contributor: Cox, Kaye B.

References

1. Belding, D. L. 1965. Textbook of Parasitology. Ed. 3. Appleton-Century-Crofts, New York. pp. 397-481, 581-625, 671-681, 701-708, 735-736.

2. Brown, H. W. 1975. Basic Clinical Parasitology. Ed. 4. Appleton-Century-Crofts, New York. pp. 4-9, 112-138, 168, 178-193, 217-225.

3. Cahill, K. M., and K. B. Cox. 1972. In P. D. Hoeprich. ed. Infectious Diseases. Harper and Row, Hagerstown, MD. pp. 627-637, 673-681.

4. Faust, E. C., et al. 1970. Craig and Faust's Clinical Parasitology. Ed. 8. Lea and Febiger, Philadelphia. pp. 272-279, 284-317, 330-343, 460, 465-469, 492-494, 508-514, 522-538.

5. Spencer, F. M., and L. S. Monroe. 1975. The Color Atlas of Intestinal Parasites. Rev. ed. 1. C. C. Thomas, Springfield, IL. pp. 90-99, 102-105, 108-111, 114-115, 118-132, 137-138.

37. RECOMMENDED DOSAGES OF ANTIMICROBIALS IN OLIGURIC PATIENTS

Oliguric patients are here defined as patients whose creatinine clearance is less than 10% of normal. **Dosage Significantly Affected by Dialysis:** Even if significant amounts of a drug are removed by dialysis, this does not necessarily mean that the dosage is affected. **Additional Medication Required: Hemodialysis**—Dosages listed are for parenteral administration unless otherwise indicated. **Peritoneal Dialysis**—When antibiotic blood levels are significantly affected by peritoneal dialysis, the agents should be added to the dialysate at the desired serum concentration while continuing the usual intravenous or intramuscular administration; figures in brackets represent suitable concentrations when adding to peritoneal dialysis fluid. Data in brackets refer to the column heading in brackets.

	Agent	Dosage Off Dialysis	Dosage Significantly Affected by Dialysis [Additional Medication Required]	
			Hemodialysis	Peritoneal Dialysis
	Aminoglycosides			
1	Gentamicin	1-2 mg/kg body wt every 3 half-lives[1]	Yes [1 mg/kg after each dialysis]	....
2	Kanamycin	7 mg/kg body wt every 3 half-lives[2] or 0.5 g every 3-4 d	Yes [250 mg after each dialysis]	Yes [20 μg/ml]
3	Streptomycin[3]	1 g; then 0.5 g every 2-3 d	No	No
4	Amphotericin B	Modest reductions in advanced renal failure	No	No
	Cephalosporins			
5	Cephaloridine[4]	1 g every 24 h	Yes [0.5 g every 4 h]	Yes [20 μg/ml]
6	Cephalothin	2-3 g loading dose; then 1 g every 12-24 h	Yes [1 g after each dialysis]	Yes [20 μg/ml]
7	Chloramphenicol	0.5 g every 6 h	No	No
8	Erythromycin	0.5 g every 6 h	No	No
9	5-Fluorocytosine[5]	6-8 mg/kg body wt every half-life[6]	Effectively dialyzed	....
10	Lincomycin	250 mg every 12 h	No	No
	Penicillins			
11	Ampicillin	1 g; then 0.5 g every 8 h	Yes [0.5-1.0 g every 6 h][7]	No
12	Carbenicillin	2 g every 6-24 h	Yes [2 g after each dialysis]	Yes [100 μg/ml]
13	Dicloxacillin	0.5 g every 8 h	No	Yes [25 μg/ml]
14	Methicillin	1 g every 8-12 h	No	No
15	Oxacillin	1 g every 8-12 h	No	No
16	Penicillin G	0.5-2 million units every 6-8 h	No	No
	Polymyxins			
17	Colistin[8]	200-300 mg; then 100-150 mg every 2-4 d	No	No
18	Polymyxin B	100-150 mg; then 50-100 mg every 2-4 d	No	No
	Tuberculostatic agents			
19	Ethambutol	7-15 mg/kg body wt each day	Readily dialyzable	....
20	Isoniazid	Same as in patients with normal renal function	No	No
21	Rifampin	Same as in patients with normal renal function	No	No
22	Vancomycin	1 g every 10-14 d	No	....

[1] Half-life ⟨T½⟩ in hours = serum creatinine concentration in mg/100 ml X 4. [2] Half-life ⟨T½⟩ in hours = serum creatinine concentration in mg/100 ml X 3. [3] Seldom indicated in renal failure because of the threat to the eighth cranial nerve, and because less toxic alternatives are usually available. [4] Not used because of nephrotoxicity; may prove useful in patients on chronic dialysis programs to whom nephrotoxicity is of no significance. [5] Synonym: Flucytosine. [6] Half-life ⟨T½⟩ in hours = serum creatinine concentration in mg/100 ml X 6. [7] Dosage for oral or parenteral administration. [8] Synonym: Polymyxin E.

Contributor: Bulger, Roger J.

Reference: Anderson, R. J., et al. 1976. In B. M. Brenner and F. C. Rector, Jr., ed. The Kidney. W. B. Saunders, Philadelphia. v. 2, pp. 1911-1948.

	Disease, Condition, or Medical Procedure	Efficacy of Prophylaxis	Drug
1	Aspiration of gastric contents	Ineffective	....
2	Bacterial endocarditis (valvular heart disease), associated with: dental operations; ear, nose, & throat operations; or gastrointestinal & urogenital tract operations	Usually effective	Gentamicin plus one of the following: penicillin, erythromycin, or vancomycin
3	Bronchitis, chronic	Sometimes effective	Ampicillin; tetracycline
4	Burns (streptococcal infection)	Sometimes effective	Penicillin
5	Catheterization: arterial, urethral, or venous	Ineffective	....
6	Coma	Ineffective	....
7	Congestive heart failure	Ineffective	....
8	*Escherichia coli* diarrheal disease in infants	Usually effective	Neomycin; kanamycin
9	Gonococcal infection exposure	Sometimes effective	Penicillin
10	Gonococcal ophthalmia	Usually effective	Silver nitrate; penicillin
11	Impaired host defenses	Ineffective	....
12	Injury, grossly contaminated	Sometimes effective	Oxacillin; tetracycline
13	Labor, prolonged	Sometimes effective	Ampicillin
14	Malaria	Usually effective	Chloroquine
15	Meningococcal infection	Usually effective	Sulfonamides; rifampin
16	Operations, "clean"	Ineffective	....
17	With prostheses: cardiac or orthopedic	Usually effective	Oxacillin plus gentamicin
18	Post-operative wound infection Abdominal operations, "contaminated"	Usually effective	Cephalosporins; or penicillin plus gentamicin plus clindamycin (or chloramphenicol)
19	Gynecologic operations	Sometimes effective	Ampicillin; cephalosporins
20	Oropharyngeal operations, "contaminated"	Sometimes effective	Ampicillin; cephalosporins
21	Prematurity	Ineffective	....
22	Rheumatic fever (*Streptococcus* Group A infection)	Usually effective	Penicillin; sulfonamides
23	Steroid therapy, high dose	Ineffective	....
24	Syphilis exposure	Usually effective	Penicillin
25	Tuberculosis	Usually effective	Isoniazid
26	Viral exanthems	Ineffective	....
27	Viral pharyngitis	Ineffective	....
28	Viral respiratory disease	Ineffective	....

Contributor: Counts, George W.

Reference: Wintrobe, M. M., et al., ed. 1974. Harrison's Principles of Internal Medicine. Ed. 7. McGraw-Hill, New York. v. 1, p. 752.

39. SUSCEPTIBILITY OF ANAEROBES TO ANTIMICROBIAL AGENTS

Aminoglycosides, such as gentamicin and kanamycin, are generally quite inactive against the majority of anaerobes. The activity of **Erythromycin** varies significantly according to the testing procedure. **Metronidazole** is not yet approved by the Food and Drug Administration for anaerobic infections. **Penicillin G**: Other penicillins and cephalosporins are frequently less active. Ampicillin, carbenicillin, and cephaloridine are roughly comparable to penicillin G on a weight basis, but the high blood levels safely achieved with carbenicillin make it effective against 95% of the strains of *Bacteroides fragilis*. Cefoxitin, a compound resistant to penicillinase ⟨β-lactamase I⟩ and cephalosporinase ⟨β-lactamase II⟩, also appears promising, but is still in the experimental stage. **Tetracycline**: Doxycycline and minocycline are more active than other tetracyclines, but susceptibility testing is indicated to ensure activity. *Symbols:* ++++ = drug of choice;

continued

39. SUSCEPTIBILITY OF ANAEROBES TO ANTIMICROBIAL AGENTS

+++ = good activity; ++ = moderate activity; + = poor or inconsistent activity. There is no difference in activity between drugs rated +++ and those rated ++++; the symbol ++++ indicates a drug with good activity, good pharmacologic characteristics, and low toxicity.

	Bacterium	Chloram-phenicol	Clinda-mycin	Erythro-mycin	Linco-mycin	Metronid-azole	Penicillin G	Tetra-cycline	Vanco-mycin
1	Microaerophilic & anaerobic cocci	+++	++ to +++	++ to +++	+++	++	+++ to ++++	++	+++
2	*Bacteroides fragilis*	+++	+++	+ to ++	+ to ++	+++	+	+ to ++	+
3	*B. melaninogenicus*	+++	+++	+++	+++	+++	+++[1]	++ to +++	+
4	*Fusobacterium varium*	+++	+ to ++	+	+ to ++	+++	+++[1]	++	+
5	Other *Fusobacterium* spp.	+++	+++	+	+++	+++	++++	+++	+
6	*Clostridium perfringens*	+++	+++[2]	+++	++ to +++	+++	++++[1]	++ to +++	+++
7	Other *Clostridium* spp.	+++	++	++ to +++	+	++ to +++	+++	++	++ to +++
8	*Eubacterium* & *Actinomyces*	+++	++ to +++	+++	++ to +++	+ to ++	++++	++ to +++	++ to +++

[1] A few strains are resistant. [2] Rare strains are resistant.

Contributors: Sutter, Vera L. and Finegold, Sydney M.

General References

1. Sutter, V. L., and S. M. Finegold. 1976. Antimicrob. Agents Chemother. (in press).

2. Sutter, V. L., and S. M. Finegold. Unpublished. Veterans Administration, Wadsworth Hospital Center, Los Angeles, CA, 1976.

40. ZONE DIAMETER INTERPRETIVE STANDARDS AND APPROXIMATE MINIMUM INHIBITORY CONCENTRATION CORRELATES FOR ANTIMICROBIAL AGENTS

Zone Diameter: Values have been rounded to the nearest whole millimeter. **MIC** = minimum inhibitory concentration.

	Antimicrobial Agent	Disk Content μg	Zone Diameter, mm			Approximate MIC Correlates, μg/ml[1]	
			Resis-tant	Inter-mediate	Suscep-tible	Resistant	Suscep-tible
	Aminoglycosides						
1	Gentamicin	10	≤12	....	≥13	≥6	≤6
2	Kanamycin	30	≤13	14-17	≥18	≥25	≤6
3	Neomycin	30	≤12	13-16	≥17	....	≤10
4	Streptomycin	10	≤11	12-14	≥15	≥15	≤6
5	Tobramycin	10	≤11	12-13	≥14	....	≤6
6	Cephalothin[2]	30	≤14	15-17	≥18	≥32	≤10
7	Chloramphenicol	30	≤12	13-17	≥18	≥25	≤12.5
8	Clindamycin	2	≤14	15-16	≥17	≥2	≤1
9	Erythromycin	15	≤13	14-17	≥18	≥8	≤2
	Penicillins						
10	Ampicillin[3]—when testing gram-negative enteric organisms & enterococci	10	≤11	12-13	≥14	≥32	≤8

[1] Unless otherwise indicated. [2] Class disk for cephalothin, cephaloridine and cephalexin, cephazolin, and cephapirin.
[3] Class disk for ampicillin, hetacillin, and amoxicillin.

continued

40. ZONE DIAMETER INTERPRETIVE STANDARDS AND APPROXIMATE MINIMUM INHIBITORY CONCENTRATION CORRELATES FOR ANTIMICROBIAL AGENTS

	Antimicrobial Agent	Disk Content μg	Zone Diameter, mm			Approximate MIC Correlates, μg/ml[1]	
			Resistant	Intermediate	Susceptible	Resistant	Susceptible
11	Ampicillin[3]—when testing staphylococci & penicillin G-susceptible microorganisms	10	≤20	21-28	≥29	≥32[4]	≤0.2
12	Ampicillin[3]—when testing *Haemophilus* species	10	≤19	....	≥20	....	≤2
13	Carbenicillin—when testing *Proteus* species & *Escherichia coli*	100	≤17	18-22	≥23	≥32	≤16
14	Carbenicillin—when testing *Pseudomonas aeruginosa*	100	≤13	14-16	≥17	≥250	≤125
15	Methicillin[5]—when testing staphylococci	5	≤9	10-13	≥14	....	≤3
16	Oxacillin or nafcillin	1	≤10	11-12	≥13	....	≤1
17	Penicillin G[6]—when testing staphylococci	10	≤20	21-28	≥29	Fn[4]	≤0.1
18	Penicillin G[6]—when testing other microorganisms	10	≤11	12-21[7]	≥22	≥32	≤1.5
	Polymyxins						
19	Colistin	10	≤8	9-10	≥11	Fn[8]	....
20	Polymyxin B	300	≤8	9-11	≥12	≥50 units/ ml[8]	....
21	Tetracycline[9]	30	≤14	15-18	≥19	≥12	≤4
	Urinary tract antimicrobics[10]						
22	Nalidixic acid	30	≤13	14-18	≥19	≥32	≤12
23	Nitrofurantoin	300	≤14	15-16	≥17	≥100	≤25
24	Sulfonamides	250 or 300	≤12	13-16	≥17	≥350	≤100
25	Trimethoprim-sulfamethoxazole	25[11]	≤10	11-15	≥16	≥200	≤35

[1] Unless otherwise indicated. [3] Class disk for ampicillin, hetacillin, and amoxicillin. [4] Resistant strains of *Staphylococcus aureus* produce penicillinase; their MIC's with penicillin and ampicillin will be extremely variable and method-dependent, usually 0.5 μg/ml or greater. [5] Class disk for penicillinase-resistant penicillins. [6] Class disk for penicillin G ⟨benzyl penicillin⟩, penicillin V ⟨phenoxymethyl penicillin⟩, and phenethicillin. [7] Intermediate category includes some microorganisms, such as enterococci and certain gram-negative bacilli, that may cause systemic infections treat-able with high dosages of penicillin G, but not penicillin V or phenethicillin. [8] Colistin and polymyxin B diffuse poorly in agar; thus the accuracy of diffusion tests is less than that found with other antimicrobics, and MIC correlates cannot be calculated reliably from regression analysis. [9] Class disk for tetracyclines. [10] Used only for testing isolates from urinary tract infections. [11] The disks used for testing the combination of trimethoprim-sulfamethoxazole contain 1.25 μg trimethoprim and 23.75 μg sulfamethoxazole.

Contributor: Barry, Arthur L.

Reference: Barry, A. L. 1977. In P. D. Hoeprich, ed. Infectious Diseases. Ed. 2. Harper and Row, Hagerstown, MD. (In press).

41. ROUTES OF ELIMINATION AND HALF-LIVES OF ANTIMICROBIAL AGENTS

Route of Excretion or Inactivation: Minor routes of drug disposition are indicated in parentheses. **Maintenance Dose Intervals,** based on typical dosage schedules, should be considered only as representative. Other dosage schedules for an individual agent can be adjusted in proportion to the changes shown. Loading doses are not influenced by alterations of drug disposition. $Cc_{>80}$ indicates creatinine clearance >80 ml/min; Cc_{50-80} indicates creatinine clearance of 50-80 ml/min; Cc_{10-50} indicates creatinine clearance of 10-50 ml/min; $Cc_{>10}$ indicates creatinine clearance of <10 ml/min. NR = not recommended. **Dosage Significantly Affected by Dialysis** indicates whether additional medication following dialysis is required; **H** = hemodialysis; **P** = peritoneal dialysis; (+) = significant; (−) = insignificant; (±) = may

continued

or may not be significant. A lack of requirement for additional medication after dialysis does not necessarily indicate a lack of utility of dialysis for the treatment of intoxication by the drug. Data in brackets refer to the column heading in brackets.

	Drug	Route of Excretion or Inactivation [Normal Half-Life, h]	Maintenance Dose Intervals, h				Dosage Significantly Affected by Dialysis	
			$Cc_{>80}$	Cc_{50-80}	Cc_{10-50}	$Cc_{<10}$	H	P
	Aminoglycosides							
1	Gentamicin	Renal [2]	8	12	12-36	48-72	+	−
2	Kanamycin	Renal [3-4]	8	24	24-72	72-96	+	+
3	Streptomycin	Renal [2.5]	12	24	24-72	72-96	+	+
4	Amphotericin B	Non-renal [18-24]	24	24	24	24-36	−	...
	Cephalosporins							
5	Cephazolin	Renal (hepatic) [1.5]	6	12	12[1]	24[2]	−	−
6	Cephalexin	Renal (non-renal) [0.6-1]	6	6	6-12	18-24	+	+
7	Cephaloridine	Renal [1.5]	6	NR	NR	NR	+	+
8	Cephalothin	Renal, hepatic [0.5-0.8]	6	6	8	8-12	+	+
9	Chloramphenicol	Hepatic (renal) [2.5]	6	6	6	6	−	−
10	Clindamycin	Hepatic (renal) [2]	6	6	6	6	−	−
11	Colistimethate	Renal [2]	12	24	36-60	60-90	±	±
12	Erythromycin	Hepatic [1.5]	6	6	6	6	−	−
13	5-Fluorocytosine[3]	Renal [3-4]	6	12	12-24	NR	+	+
14	Lincomycin	Hepatic (renal) [5]	6	6	6	8-12	−	−
	Penicillins							
15	Amoxicillin	Renal [1]	8	8	12	16	+	...
16	Ampicillin	Renal, hepatic [1.5]	6	6	9	12	+	−
17	Carbenicillin	Renal, hepatic [1.5]	4	4	6-12	12-16	+	−
18	Cloxacillin; dicloxacillin	Hepatic, renal [0.5]	6	6	6	6	−	...
19	Methicillin	Renal, hepatic [0.5]	4	4	4	8-12	−	−
20	Nafcillin	Hepatic (renal) [0.5]	6	6	8	12	−	...
21	Oxacillin	Renal, hepatic [0.5]	6	6	6	8-12	−	−
22	Penicillin G	Renal, hepatic [0.5]	8	8	8	12	−	−
23	Sulfisoxazole	Renal [5]	6	6	8-12	12-24	+	+
	Tetracyclines							
24	Chlortetracycline; oxytetracycline; tetracycline	Renal, hepatic [6-9]	6	NR	NR	NR	−	−
25	Demethylchlortetracycline[4]; methacycline	Renal, hepatic [15-17]	12	NR	NR	NR	−	−
26	Doxycycline	Hepatic, renal [20]	12-24	12-24	12-24	12-24	−	−
27	Minocycline	Hepatic, renal [18]	12-24	NR	NR	NR	−	−
	Tuberculostatic agents							
28	Ethambutol	Renal [6-8]	24	24	24-36	48	+	+
29	Isoniazid	Renal, hepatic[5] [2-4]	8	8	8	8	+	+
30	Rifampin	Hepatic [3]	24	24	24	24	?	?
	Urinary tract antiseptics							
31	Methenamine mandelate	Renal [4]	6	6	NR	NR	?	?
32	Nalidixic acid[6]	Renal [1.5-2]	6	6	6	6	?	?
33	Nitrofurantoin	Renal [0.3]	8	8	8	NR	+	...
34	Vancomycin	Renal [6]	6	24-72	72-240	240	−	−

[1] Reduce dose to 7 mg/kg every 12 h. [2] Reduce dose to 5 mg/kg every 24 h. [3] Synonym: Flucytosine. [4] Synonym: Demeclocycline. [5] There is genetic variation in the hepatic disposition of isoniazid. Slow acetylators of the drug who have reduced renal function may require prolongation of the dose interval. [6] Inactive, non-toxic metabolite accumulates.

continued

41. ROUTES OF ELIMINATION AND HALF-LIVES OF ANTIMICROBIAL AGENTS

Contributors: Weinstein, Louis, and Brown, Richard B.

Reference: Goodman, L. S., and A. Gilman, ed. 1975. The Pharmacological Basis of Therapeutics. Ed. 5. Macmillan, New York. pp. 1108-1109.

42. PLASMA LEVEL AND RENAL EXCRETION OF PENICILLIN G

This schematic chart was constructed from various reported data on the plasma concentration and the renal elimination of penicillin G in adults with good renal function. As shown below, an intramuscular injection of 300,000 units of an aqueous solution of penicillin G sodium was made at zero time. Observe that the peak plasma level of 8 units/ml was reached between 15 and 30 minutes after injection, and that the concentration then fell quickly to 0.1 unit/ml by the end of 5 hours. This decline is the result of the rapid renal excretion of penicillin G, which is due primarily to tubular secretion. Within the 5-hour period depicted in the chart, nearly 60% (180,000 units) of the administered dose was eliminated in the urine. At the height of the excretory process, nearly 3000 units were being excreted each minute and about 500 ml of plasma were being cleared of penicillin during the same time span.

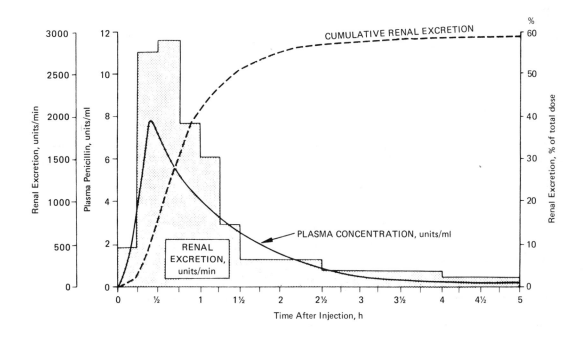

Contributors: Weinstein, Louis, and Brown, Richard B.

Reference: Goodman, L. S., and A. Gilman, ed. 1975. The Pharmacological Basis of Therapeutics. Ed. 5. Macmillan, New York. p. 1137.

43. SOME PROBLEMS ENCOUNTERED DURING DEVELOPMENT AND USE OF VIRAL VACCINES

SV40 = a simian polyomavirus.

	Classification	Vaccine	Problems
1	Live vaccines	Smallpox	Inadequate attenuation leading to complications
2			Overattenuation leading to lack of protection
3		Poliovirus (Sabin)	Contaminating viruses (e.g., SV40)
4			Interference by endemic enteroviruses
5		Type III	Back-mutation to virulence
6		Measles (Edmonston)	Inadequate attenuation leading to fever and rash
7		Rubella (HPV-77) Dog-kidney-cell grown	Inadequate attenuation leading to arthritis in adult females
8		Duck-cell modified	No problems
9		Yellow fever (pre-war)	Contaminating hepatitis B in human serum contained in "stabilizing" medium
10	Inactivated vaccines	Poliovirus (Salk)	Residual live virulent virus
11			Contaminating virus (SV40) resisting formaldehyde
12		Influenza	Pyrogenicity; toxicity
13		Measles; respiratory syncytial	Hypersensitivity reactions on subsequent natural infection or live vaccine booster
14		Rabies (Semple)	Allergic encephalomyelitis

Contributors: Fenner, Frank, and White, D. O.

Reference: Fenner, F., and D. O. White. 1976. Medical Virology. Ed. 2. Academic Press, New York. p. 229.

44. COMPARISON OF ADVANTAGES AND DISADVANTAGES OF LIVE AND INACTIVATED VACCINES

	Type	Advantages	Disadvantages
1	Live vaccines	Single dose, given ideally by natural	Reversion to virulence [1]
2		route, invokes full range of immu-	Natural spread to contacts
3		nological responses, including local	Contaminating viruses [1]
4		IgA as well as systemic IgG produc-	"Human cancer viruses" [2]
5		tion, leading to possibility of local	Viral interference
6		eradication of wild-type viruses	Inactivation by heat in the tropics
7	Inactivated vaccines	Stability	Multiple doses & boosters needed, given by injection
8			High concentration of antigen needed: economic problems in production with some viruses

[1] With care, these difficulties have been largely overcome.
[2] Theoretical objection that has been raised against use of human diploid cell strains as substrate for vaccine production, but vaccines prepared in such cells are now licensed in several countries, including Great Britain and the United States.

Contributors: Fenner, Frank, and White, D. O.

Reference: Fenner, F., and D. O. White. 1976. Medical Virology. Ed. 2. Academic Press, New York. p. 230.

45. COMPARISON OF RESPONSES TO LIVE ORAL AND INACTIVATED PARENTERAL POLIOVIRUS VACCINES

Graphs show the detailed sequence of Immunoglobulin G ⟨IgG⟩, immunoglobulin M ⟨IgM⟩, and immunoglobulin A ⟨IgA⟩ poliovirus antibody formation in serum and secre-tions after immunization. The serum neutralizing-antibody response ⟨Neut, serum⟩ has been recorded for comparison.

Immunization with three doses of trivalent inactivated virus at monthly intervals, beginning at 2 months of age. Arrows indicate time of dose.

Immunization with live attenuated virus: Type 1 monovalent poliovaccine given at 2 months, and types 3 and 2 at monthly intervals thereafter. Arrows indicate time of dose.

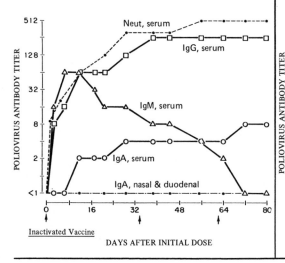 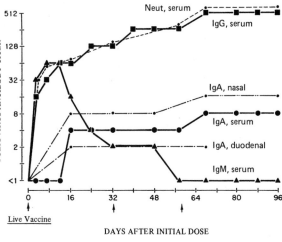

Contributor: Karzon, David T.

Reference: Ogra, P. L., et al. 1968. N. Engl. J. Med. 279:898.

46. SCHEDULES FOR ACTIVE IMMUNIZATION AGAINST VIRAL DISEASES

Prior to the administration of any vaccine, the manufac-turer's product information sheet should be consulted for specific dosage, route, and contraindications. **Type**: I = in-activated; A = attenuated. Data in brackets refer to the col-umn heading in brackets.

	Disease	Vaccine		Indications & Applicable Age Groups	Dosage		Adverse Reactions	Contra-indications
		Name [Type]	Preparation & Components		Primary	Booster		
1	Smallpox	Smallpox vaccine [A]	Vaccinia virus re-covered from calf lymph or chorio-allantoic mem-brane of chicken eggs	Individuals travel-ing in smallpox endemic areas; laboratory person-nel working with smallpox & other poxviruses	One vac-cination resulting in a typ-ical Jen-nerian vesicle	Every 3 yr	Neurologic complica-tions; eczema vaccina-tum, generalized vaccin-ia, progressive vaccinia, autoinoculation; gener-alized exanthems	Altered immune states; preg-nancy; skin disorders in the prospective vaccinee or in family contacts
2	Poliomye-litis	Poliovi-rus vac-cine, live, oral, tri-valent [A]	Attenuated poliovi-rus types I, II, & III grown in mon-key kidney or hu-man WI-38 tissue cultures	All children >2 mo old; selected un-immunized adults who are likely to be exposed	3 doses 6-8 wk apart	At 1½ yr & 5 yr of age; fur-ther boos-ters at times of exposure	Rarely neuro-logic compli-cations; these are more common in previously unimmunized adults	Altered immune states

continued

	Disease	Vaccine Name [Type]	Vaccine Preparation & Components	Indications & Applicable Age Groups	Dosage Primary	Dosage Booster	Adverse Reactions	Contra-indications
3		Poliovirus vaccine [I]	Poliovirus types, 1, 2, & 3 grown in monkey kidney tissue culture	Previously unimmunized adults followed by 2 doses attenuated vaccine	3 doses 4 wk apart,	Further boosters with attenuated vaccine at times of exposure	None	None
4	Rubella	Rubella virus vaccine, live [A]	Attenuated rubella virus grown in rabbit kidney or duck embryo tissue culture	All children between 1 yr & puberty; all seronegative adolescent girls & adult women of child-bearing age	1 dose	None	Arthralgias & arthritis, especially in post-pubertal females	Altered immune states; should not be given within 3 mo prior to pregnancy or during pregnancy [1]
5	Yellow fever	Yellow fever vaccine [A]	Attenuated yellow fever virus grown in chicken embryo	Individuals 6 mo or older who live or travel in areas where yellow fever infection is prevalent	1 dose	Every 10 yr	Mild headache, myalgia, low-grade fever; rarely neurologic complications	Altered immune states; pregnancy
6	Influenza	Influenza virus vaccine, bivalent [I]	Current strains of influenza viral types A & B grown in chicken embryos	Individuals of all ages with chronic debilitating conditions; individuals providing essential community services	2 doses[2] 4-8 wk apart	1 dose annually	Allergic reaction to vaccine components; sore arm, myalgia, fever, chills, sweats	Egg allergy; reaction following previous influenza immunization
7		Influenza virus vaccine, bivalent type A[3] [I]	Influenza viral types A/Victoria & A/Swine					
8		Influenza virus vaccine, monovalent [I]	Current strain of influenza A virus, which is significantly different from previous strains, grown in chicken embryos	All ages	2 doses[2] 4-8 wk apart	1 dose annually	Allergic reaction to vaccine components	
9	Mumps	Mumps virus vaccine, live [A]	Attenuated mumps virus grown in chicken embryo tissue culture	All >1 yr old who have not had mumps	1 dose	None	None	Altered immune states; pregnancy
10	Measles	Measles virus vaccine, live [A]	Attenuated measles virus, grown in chicken embryo tissue culture	All >1 yr old who have not had measles[4]; children who have previously received killed vaccine	1 dose	None	Mild fever & rash; rarely neurologic complications	Altered immune states; pregnancy

[1] The risk of congenital rubella syndrome appears to be lower in patients inadvertently vaccinated in pregnancy compared to those who develop rubella in pregnancy.
[2] One dose may be adequate for primary immunization.
[3] All persons receiving bivalent type A vaccine should also receive monovalent influenza B vaccine; preferably bivalent type A and monovalent B vaccines should be administered at least one week apart. [4] In areas of high measles prevalence, vaccination at 6-12 months old is indicated; these children should be reimmunized later.

continued

46. SCHEDULES FOR ACTIVE IMMUNIZATION AGAINST VIRAL DISEASES

	Disease	Vaccine		Indications & Applicable Age Groups	Dosage		Adverse Reactions	Contra-indications
		Name [Type]	Preparation & Components		Primary	Booster		
11	Rabies	Rabies vaccine [I]	Rabies virus grown in duck embryo	Individuals likely to be exposed (veterinarians, animal handlers, etc.)	2 doses, 4 wk apart	1 dose 6 mo after primary, and every 2-3 yr thereafter	Allergic reactions to vaccine components; local soreness; very rarely neurologic complications	Any life-threatening reaction to duck embryo vaccine is indication for use of vaccine currently under investigation made from human WI-38 tissue culture[5/]
12				All individuals with bite wounds from rabid or possibly rabid animals; individuals with scratches, abrasions, or open wounds which have been exposed to rabies virus	21 daily doses plus human rabies immune globulin	2 doses, 10 & 20 days after primary series		

[5/] Available from Center for Disease Control, Atlanta, Georgia.

Contributor: Cherry, James D.

General References

1. Benenson, A. S., ed. 1975. Control of Communicable Diseases in Man. Ed. 12. American Public Health Association, Washington, D.C.
2. Public Health Service Advisory Committee on Immunization Practices. 1972. Morb. Mortal. Rep. Suppl. 21(25).
3. Public Health Service Advisory Committee on Immunization Practices. 1975. Ibid. 24(12).
4. Steigman, A. J., ed. 1974. Report of the Committee on Infectious Diseases. Ed. 17. American Academy of Pediatrics, Evanston, IL.

47. ANTIVIRAL AGENTS CURRENTLY USEFUL

Mechanism of Action: Ara-AMP = arabinosyladenine monophosphate; Ara-ATP = arabinosyladenine triphosphate. **Disease, Recommended Dosage, & Duration of Therapy:**

DMSO = dimethyl sulfoxide, which is not yet licensed in the United States.

	Agent ⟨Synonym⟩	Antiviral Spectrum	Mechanism of Action	Disease, Recommended Dosage, & Duration of Therapy	Remarks	Reference
1	Amantadine HCl ⟨1-Adamantanamine HCl; Symmetrel⟩	Influenza A_2	Blocks penetration of virus into cell and/or inhibits uncoating of virus particle	Influenza A: prophylaxis—200 mg/d in adults, up to 90 d; questionable role in therapy of established infection	Also anti-Parkinson's disease action. Rimantidine HCl = similar agent chemically	14,19, 20,22, 36,41, 43,45, 50
2	Arabinosyladenine ⟨Adenine arabinoside; Ara-A; 9-β-D-arabinofuranosyladenine; Vidarabine⟩	Herpesvirus ⟨herpes simplex virus⟩; ? B virus ⟨herpes B⟩; ? cytomegalovirus; varicella-zoster; vaccinia	Selective depression of viral DNA synthesis; metabolized to Ara-AMP or Ara-ATP; either causes preferential inhibition of viral DNA nucleotidyltransferase, ribonucleotide reductase, or other virus-specific enzymes	Herpetic keratitis: 3% Ara-A ointment 5 times/d for 7-10 d[1/] Herpetic kerato-uveitis, or serious herpes simplex or herpes zoster infections: 10-20 mg Ara-A per kg per day i.v. infusion over 8-12 h, for 7-10 d[1/]	Arabinosylhypoxanthine and phosphorylated derivatives of Ara-A are also being tested	1,8,9, 21,23, 29,42, 44,49, 52

[1/] Under investigation at the present time.

continued

45

	Agent ⟨Synonym⟩	Antiviral Spectrum	Mechanism of Action	Disease, Recommended Dosage, & Duration of Therapy	Remarks	Reference
3	Idoxuridine ⟨Io-dodeoxyuri-dine; 5-iodo-2'-deoxyuridine; IUdR; IDU; Herplex; Stoxil⟩	Herpesvirus ⟨herpes simplex virus⟩; B virus ⟨herpes B⟩; varicella-zoster; vaccinia	Direct inhibition or feedback of enzymes involved in pathway of incorporation of thymidine into DNA, and/or formation of IUdR-DNA that is functionally deficient	Herpetic keratitis: 0.5% solution or 0.1% ointment for 3-5 d after healing Cutaneous herpes simplex or cutaneous herpes zoster: 5-40% in DMSO	Studies in encephalitis show toxicity of drug; no evidence of efficacy	4,16, 18,26-28,30, 31,34, 37,39, 40,47, 48
4	Interferon, human	Almost (?) all viruses in vitro; herpesviruses; rhinoviruses	Binds to cells and induces them to become resistant to a number of viruses (?) through an induced antiviral protein that requires RNA, protein synthesis	Rhinovirus; prevention of recurrent herpes simplex; prevention of dissemination of herpes zoster	Interferon inducers of various types not yet clinically useful	2,10, 12,13, 15,24, 25,33, 35,38, 46
5	Methisazone ⟨N-Methylisatin-β-thiosemicarbazone; IBT; Marboran⟩	Vaccinia; variola (smallpox)	? Defect in viral nucleic acid synthesis. ? Binds to metal atoms in DNA & RNA nucleotidyltransferase molecules.	Vaccinia (also eczema vaccinatum & vaccinia gangrenosa) therapy: Loading dose, 200 mg/kg; then 400 mg/kg/d in divided doses over 48 h Smallpox prophylaxis[2/]: 1.5 g 2 times/d for 4 d; 3.0 g 2 times/d for 4 d	Related agents are isoquinoline-1-thiosemicarbazone ⟨IQ-TSC⟩ & kethoxal bis(thiosemicarbazone) ⟨KTS⟩	3,5-7, 11,17, 32,51

[2/] Two treatment regimens were tested in the same study and were equally effective [ref. 3].

Contributor: Lauter Carl B.

References

1. Abel, R., Jr., et al. 1975. In D. Pavan-Langston, et al., ed. Adenine Arabinoside: An Antiviral Agent. Raven Press, New York. pp. 393-400.
2. Anonymous. 1974. Lancet 2:761-762.
3. Bauer, D. 1965. Ann. N.Y. Acad. Sci. 130:110-117.
4. Boston Interhospital Virus Study Group, et al. 1975. N. Engl. J. Med. 292:599-603.
5. Brainerd, H. D., et al. 1967. Ibid. 276:620-621.
6. Brockman, R. W., et al. 1970. Proc. Soc. Exp. Biol. Med. 133:609-614.
7. Burns, G. R. 1968. Inorg. Chem. 7:277-283.
8. Ch'ien, L. T., et al. 1973. In W. A. Carter, ed. Selective Inhibitors of Viral Function. CRC Press, Cleveland, pp. 227-256.
9. Ch'ien, L. T., et al. 1975. Intersci. Conf. Antimicrob. Agents Chemother. 15th, Abstr. 360.
10. DeClerq, E., and W. E. Steward, II. 1973. (Loc. cit. ref. 8). pp. 81-106.
11. Easterbrook, K. B. 1962. Virology 17:245-251.
12. Field, A. K. 1973. (Loc. cit. ref. 8). pp. 149-176.
13. Field, A. K., et al. 1967. Proc. Natl. Acad. Sci. USA 58:1004-1010.
14. Galbraith, A. W., et al. 1971. Lancet 2:113-121.
15. Gatmaitan, B. G., et al. 1973. J. Infect. Dis. 127:401-407.
16. Goz, B., and W. H. Prusoff. 1970. Annu. Rev. Pharmacol. 10:143-170.

17. Hamre, D., et al. 1951. J. Immunol. 67:305-312.
18. Herrmann, E. C., Jr. 1961. Proc. Soc. Exp. Biol. Med. 107:142-145.
19. Hoffmann, C. E. 1973. (Loc. cit. ref. 8). pp. 199-211.
20. Hoffmann, C. E., et al. 1965. J. Bacteriol. 90:623-628.
21. Hyndiuk, R. A., et al. 1975. (Loc. cit. ref. 1). pp. 331-335.
22. Jackson, G. G. 1971. Hosp. Pract. 6:75-87.
23. Jones, D. B. 1975. (Loc. cit. ref. 1). pp. 371-379.
24. Jordan, G. W., et al. 1974. J. Infect. Dis. 130:56-62.
25. Jordan, W. S., Jr., et al. 1973. Ibid. 128:261-264.
26. Juel-Jensen, B. E. 1970. Ann. N.Y. Acad. Sci. 173:74-82.
27. Kaufman, H. E. 1963. Invest. Ophthalmol. 2:504-518.
28. Kaufmann, H. E. 1965. Prog. Med. Virol. 7:116-159.
29. Laibson, P. R., and J. H. Krachmer. 1975. (Loc. cit. ref. 1). pp. 323-330.
30. Lerner, A. M. 1974. In F. G. McMahon, ed. Principles and Techniques of Human Research and Therapeutics. Futura, New York. v. 7, pp. 71-80.
31. Lerner, A. M., and E. J. Bailey. 1972. J. Clin. Invest. 51:45-49.
32. Levinson, W. 1973. (Loc. cit. ref. 8). pp. 213-226.
33. Lockart, R. Z., Jr. 1964. Biochem. Biophys. Res. Commun. 15:513-518.

continued

34. MacCallum, F. O., and B. E. Juel-Jensen. 1966. Br. Med. J. 2:805-807.

35. Merigan, T. C., et al. 1973. Lancet 1:563-567.

36. Neumayer, E. M., et al. 1965. Proc. Soc. Exp. Biol. Med. 119:393-396.

37. Nolan, D. C., et al. 1973. Ann. Intern. Med. 78:243-246.

38. Panusarn, C., et al. 1974. N. Engl. J. Med. 291:57-61.

39. Rawls, W. E., et al. 1964. Proc. Soc. Exp. Biol. Med. 115:123-127.

40. Roizman, B., et al. 1963. Virology 21:482-498.

41. Sabin, A. B. 1967. J. Am. Med. Assoc. 200:943-950.

42. Schabel, F. M., Jr. 1968. Chemotherapy 13:321-338.

43. Schwab, R. S., et al. 1969. J. Am. Med. Assoc. 208:1168-1170.

44. Shipman, C., Jr., and J. C. Drach. 1974. Abstr. Annu. Meet. Am. Soc. Microbiol., p. 97(M-187).

45. Smorodintsev, A. A., et al. 1970. J. Am. Med. Assoc. 213:1448-1454.

46. Stewart, W. E., II, et al. 1972. J. Virol. 10:707-712.

47. Umeda, M., and C. Heidelberger. 1969. Proc. Soc. Exp. Biol. Med. 130:24-29.

48. Weinstein, L. 1975. In L. S. Goodman and A. Gilman, ed. The Pharmacological Basis of Therapeutics. Ed. 5. Macmillan, New York. pp. 1224-1227.

49. Whitley, R. J., et al. 1975. Intersci. Conf. Antimicrob. Agents Chemother. 15th, Abstr. 359.

50. Wingfield, W. L., et al. 1969. N. Engl. J. Med. 281:579-584.

51. Woodson, B., and W. K. Joklik. 1965. Proc. Natl. Acad. Sci. USA 54:946-953.

52. York, J. L., and G. A. LePage. 1966. Can. J. Biochem. 44:19-26.

48. PASSIVE IMMUNOPROPHYLAXIS

	Disease	Antibody Source & Preparation	Dose & Route of Injection	Value	Adverse Reactions
			Viral Diseases		
1	Varicella	Human serum globulins	0.6 ml/kg body wt, i.m.	Slight	Local pain, tenderness, induration
2		Human zoster serum globulins	1.25-5.0 ml, i.m.	Definite	None
3	Smallpox & vaccinia	Human hyperimmune serum globulins	0.3 ml/kg body wt, i.m.	Definite	None
4	Poliomyelitis	Human serum globulins	0.35 ml/kg body wt, i.m.	Definite	None
5	Rubella	Human serum globulins	20-50 ml, i.m.	Doubtful	Local pain, tenderness, induration
6	Mumps	Human hyperimmune serum globulins	5-10 ml, i.m.	Doubtful	Local pain, tenderness, induration
7	Measles	Human serum globulins	0.22 ml/kg body wt, i.m., to prevent; 0.04 ml/kg body wt, i.m., to modify	Definite	None
8	Rabies	Horse serum, refined & concentrated	40 units/kg body wt, part infiltrated in region of bite, the rest i.m.	Definite	Hypersensitivity; serum sickness
9		Human immune serum globulins	20 units/kg body wt	Definite	Local pain, tenderness
10	Hepatitis A	Human serum globulins	0.02-0.06 ml/kg body wt, i.m.	Definite	None
11	Hepatitis B	Human serum globulins	10 ml, i.m., repeated after 4 wk	Unproved	Local pain, tenderness
12		Human hyperimmune serum globulins	3-5 ml, i.m., repeated after 4 wk	Definite	Local pain, tenderness
			Bacterial Diseases		
13	Pertussis	Human hyperimmune serum	20 ml, i.m.	Definite	None
14		Human hyperimmune serum globulins	2.5 ml, i.m.	Definite	None
15	Botulism	Horse serum, refined & concentrated, trivalent (A, B, E)	Therapeutic A: 60,000 units B: 44,000 units E: 68,000 units i.v. injection, plus same dose i.m.	Definite	Hypersensitivity; serum sickness

continued

	Disease	Antibody Source & Preparation	Dose & Route of Injection	Value	Adverse Reactions
16	Gas gangrene	Horse serum, refined & concentrated, pentavalent	26,000-104,000 units, i.v.	None	Hypersensitivity; serum sickness
17	Tetanus	Horse serum, refined & concentrated	1,500-10,000 units, i.m.	Definite	Hypersensitivity; serum sickness
18		Human serum globulins	250 units, i.m.	Definite	None
19	Diphtheria	Horse serum, refined & concentrated	30,000-40,000 units, i.m., if mildly to moderately ill	Definite	Hypersensitivity; serum sickness

Contributor: Hoeprich, Paul D.

Reference: Hoeprich, P. D., ed. 1977. Infectious Diseases. Ed. 2. Harper and Row, Hagerstown, MD.

49. ACTIVE IMMUNOPROPHYLAXIS

Agent: $TCID_{50}$ = median tissue culture infectious dose; L_f = flocculation unit; BCG = bacille Calmette-Guérin. Dose—Basic: CCA = chicken cell agglutinating unit.

	Disease	Agent	Age Applicable	Dose Basic	Dose Booster	Route	Value	Adverse Reactions
				Viral Diseases				
1	Variola	Live vaccinia virus, from calf lymph or chick embryos, 10^3 pockforming units/ml	>6 mo	1 drop	1 drop every 3 yr; annually if in endemic area	Multiple-pressure acupuncture	>90%	Fever, malaise, lymphadenopathy; local scarring
2	Poliomyelitis	Live, attenuated polio virus: type 1—800,000 $TCID_{50}$; type 2—100,000 $TCID_{50}$, type 3—500,000 $TCID_{50}$	>2 mo	1 dose, trivalent, at 8 wk intervals for 2 doses, and a 3rd dose 8-12 mo later	1 dose at 6 yr of age after primary series, or before travel to endemic area	Oral	>95%	None
3	Rubella	Live, attenuated virus grown in duck embryos, 1,000 $TCID_{50}$/dose	One yr to puberty	1 dose	None	Subcutaneous	>95%	Mild fever, arthralgia, arthritis, local induration
4	Yellow fever	Live, attenuated yellow fever virus from chick embryos	>6 mo	0.5 ml	0.5 ml every 10 yr if in endemic area	Subcutaneous	95%	Occasional low-grade fever, malaise, headache, hypersensitivity to eggs & egg products
5	Influenza	Formalin-ethylene oxide inactivated multitypic, from chick embryos	>3 mo	0.5 ml (700 CCA type A, 500 CCA type B)/mo for 2 doses	0.5 ml annually	Subcutaneous	60-75%	Fever, malaise, head & muscle aches, hypersensitivity to eggs
6	Mumps	Attenuated, live 5,000 $TCID_{50}$/dose	>1 yr	1 dose	None	Subcutaneous	95%	Occasional mild induration

continued

	Disease	Agent	Age Applicable	Dose Basic	Dose Booster	Route	Value	Adverse Reactions
7	Measles	Live, attenuated virus from chick embryos 2,000 $TCID_{50}$/ml	>12 mo	0.5 ml	None	Subcutaneous	95%	Mild fever & rash in <15%
8	Rabies	Rabies virus grown in duck embryos, inactivated with β-propiolactone	Preexposure / Postexposure	1 ml/mo for 3 doses / 1 ml/d for 14 d	1 ml, 6 mo after basic course; 1 ml, 10 & 20 d after basic course	Subcutaneous; different sites for each injection	∿80%	Local tenderness, induration, hypersensitivity

Rickettsial Diseases

	Disease	Agent	Age Applicable	Dose Basic	Dose Booster	Route	Value	Adverse Reactions
9	Typhus	Formalin-killed *Rickettsia prowazekii*, from chick embryos	>6 mo	0.2-1.0 ml every month for 2 doses	0.5-1.0 ml every 6-12 mo	Subcutaneous	High	Hypersensitivity to eggs, chickens
10	Rocky Mountain spotted fever	Formalin-killed *R. rickettsii*, from chick embryos	>6 mo	0.5-1.0 ml every week for 3 doses	0.5-1.0 ml annually	Subcutaneous	Decreased severity	Hypersensitivity to eggs, chickens

Bacterial Diseases

	Disease	Agent	Age Applicable	Dose Basic	Dose Booster	Route	Value	Adverse Reactions
11	Tularemia	Live, attenuated *Francisella tularensis*	Usually >6 yr	1 drop	3-5 yr	Multiple-pressure acupuncture	High	Local inflammation, with scarring
12	Typhoid	Acetone-killed *Salmonella typhi*, 10^9 cells/ml	>6 mo	0.25-0.5 ml every 4 wk for 2 doses	0.25-0.5 ml on exposure, or triennially	Subcutaneous	70-90%	Local induration, rare ulceration
13	Plague	Formalin-killed *Yersinia pestis*	>6 mo	0.1-0.5 ml every 4 wk for 3 doses	0.04-0.2 ml every 6-12 mo if in endemic area	Intramuscular	High	Local inflammation
14	Cholera	Phenol-killed *Vibrio cholerae* 8×10^9 cells/ml	>6 mo	0.1-1.0 ml every 2-4 wk for 2 doses	0.3-1.0 ml every 6 mo if in endemic area	Subcutaneous	50-60%	Local inflammation, malaise, slight fever, headache
15	Anthrax	Cell-free; alum-concentrated protein antigen	>6 mo with high risk of exposure	1.0 ml every 2-3 wk, for 3 injections	1.0 ml every 6 mo	Subcutaneous	95%	Local edema, induration
16	Diphtheria; pertussis; tetanus	Toxoid, 33 L_f/ml[1]; extracted *Bordetella pertussis*, Phase I, 8 units/ml[2]; toxoid, 10 L_f/ml[3]	2 mo-5 yr	0.5 ml each month for 3 doses	0.5 ml, 1 yr after basic, & at age 4	Intramuscular	>90%[1]; ∿85%[2]; ∿100%[3]	Mild local pain, induration
17	Tetanus; diphtheria	Toxoid, 10 L_f/ml[3]; toxoid, 4 L_f/ml[1]	>6 yr	0.5 ml each month for 2 doses	0.5 ml, 1 yr after basic, & every year thereafter	Intramuscular	∿100%[3]; >90%[1]	Mild local pain, induration; rare allergic reactions
18	Tuberculosis	BCG, an attenuated, live strain of *Mycobacterium bovis*	>3 mo	0.1-0.15 mg wet wt BCG	None	Subcutaneous or multiple percutaneous	80%	Local induration, rare ulceration

[1] Diphtheria. [2] Pertussis. [3] Tetanus.

Contributor: Hoeprich, Paul D.

Reference: Hoeprich, P. D., ed. 1977. Infectious Diseases. Ed. 2. Harper and Row, Hagerstown, MD.

II. IMMUNOLOGICAL FACTORS

50. MEDIATORS OF POTENTIAL IMPORTANCE IN HUMAN ANAPHYLAXIS

Mediator: derived from basophils and mast cells. **Structure:** n.d. = not determined. **Action:** H1 = Histamine-type 1 receptor.

	Mediator ⟨Synonym⟩	Preformed	Structure	Action	Reference
1	Histamine	Yes	2-(4-imidazolyl)-ethylamine	Contracts smooth muscle, increases vascular permeability (via H1 receptors)	3
2	Slow-reacting substance ⟨SRS⟩	No	Sulfated lipid, mol wt 500	Contracts smooth muscle, increases vascular permeability	5
3	Platelet-activating factor ⟨PAF⟩	Yes	Low mol wt phospholipid(s), mol wt <1100	Causes platelet release reactions	1
4	Eosinophil chemotactic factor of anaphylaxis ⟨ECF-A⟩	Yes[1]	2 tetrapeptides	Causes selective chemotaxis of eosinophils	2
5	Basophil kallikrein of anaphylaxis ⟨BK-A⟩	Yes	n.d.	Generates a kinin from serum kininogen	4

[1] A similar molecular weight ECF in basophils is not preformed.

Contributor: Lichtenstein, Lawrence M.

References

1. Henson, P. M. 1970. J. Exp. Med. 131:287-306.
2. Kay, A. B., et al. 1971. Ibid. 133:602-619.
3. Lichtenstein, L. M., and E. Gillespie. 1975. J. Pharmacol. Exp. Ther. 192:441-450.
4. Newball, H. H., et al. 1975. Nature (London) 254: 635-636.
5. Orange, R. P. 1974. Int. Congr. Immunol. Prog. Immunol. II, 4:29-39.

51. ASSAY OF SPECIFIC IMMUNOGLOBULIN-E ANTIBODY IN MAN

Part I. Methods of Detection

Methods in boldface type are considered current methods of choice in their respective categories.

	Site of Antibody	Method	Reference
	Tissue-fixed	Direct challenge of sensitized tissues or cells	
		In vivo	
1		**Skin: intradermal prick & scratch tests**	3,8
2		Bronchial challenge	1,2
3		Other: conjunctival, nasal, or oral challenge	1,2
		In vitro	
4		**Peripheral leukocytes—basophils: histamine release** (or other mediators)	6,7
5		Other: lung, nasal polyp, skin	1,2
	Serum	Passive sensitization	
		In vivo: Skin	
6		Pausnitz-Küstner transfer in man	1,2
7		Passive cutaneous anaphylaxis in monkey	1,2
		In vitro	
8		Peripheral leukocytes—basophils	1,2
9		Serological assay: **radioallergosorbent test** ⟨RAST⟩	4,5
10		Other: lung, skin	1,2

Contributor: Adkinson, N. Franklin, Jr.

continued

51. ASSAY OF SPECIFIC IMMUNOGLOBULIN-E ANTIBODY IN MAN

Part I. Methods of Detection

References
1. Adkinson, N. F., Jr., and L. M. Lichtenstein. 1977. Clinical Immunobiology. Academic Press, New York.
2. Augustin, R. 1973. In D. M. Weir, ed. Handbook of Experimental Immunology. B. H. Blackwell, London. pp. 42.1-42.42.
3. Becker, E. L., and B. Z. Rappaport. 1948. J. Allergy 19:317-328.
4. Gleich, G. J., and R. T. Jones. 1975. J. Allergy Clin. Immunol. 55:334-345, 346-357.
5. Johansson, S. G. O., et al. 1971. Int. Arch. Allergy Appl. Immunol. 41:443-451.
6. Lichtenstein, L. M., and D. A. Levy. 1970. In D. H. Campbell, et al., ed. Methods in Immunology. Ed. 2. W. A. Benjamin, New York. pp. 378-395.
7. May, C. D., et al. 1970. J. Allergy 46:12-20.
8. Norman, P. S., et al. 1973. J. Allergy Clin. Immunol. 52:210-214.

Part II. Comparison of Selected Methods

Titer Units: [Ag] = concentration of antigen. **Precision** indicates variability within an assay. **Reproducibility** indicates variability between assays.

	IgE Assay	Titer Units	Precision	Reproducibility	Sensitivity	Accuracy	Reference
1	Intradermal skin tests	[Ag] for 2+ response	± twofold	± threefold	Excellent	Good	1,6
2	Peripheral leukocytes: histamine release	[Ag] for 50% histamine release	± 10%	± twofold	Excellent	Good	4,5
3	Radioallergosorbent test (RAST)	Arbitrary reference units	± 15%	± 25%	Good to excellent	Good	2,3

Contributor: Adkinson, N. Franklin, Jr.

References
1. Becker, E. L., and B. Z. Rappaport. 1948. J. Allergy 19:317-328.
2. Gleich, G. J., and R. T. Jones. 1975. J. Allergy Clin. Immunol. 55:334-345, 346-357.
3. Johansson, S. G. O., et al. 1971. Int. Arch. Allergy Appl. Immunol. 41:443-451.
4. Lichtenstein, L. M., and D. A. Levy. 1970. In D. H. Campbell, et al., ed. Methods in Immunology. Ed. 2. W. A. Benjamin. New York. pp. 378-395.
5. May, C. D., et al. 1970. J. Allergy 46:12-20.
6. Norman, P. S., et al. 1973. J. Allergy Clin. Immunol. 52:210-214.

52. DIFFERENTIAL DIAGNOSIS OF ASTHMA

Condition: The order of presentation reflects, in general, the frequency of occurrence of the condition presenting as asthma. **Pulmonary Function:** FEV = forced expiratory volume; FEV_1 = forced expiratory volume during first second of FVC; FVC = forced vital capacity; RV = residual volume; $D_{L_{CO}}$ = diffusing capacity of lung for carbon monoxide (single-breath method); ↓ = decreased; ↑ = increased. **Immunology:** IgE = immunoglobulin E; RAST = radioallergosorbent test. **Clinical Manifestations:** ECG = electrocardiogram. Figures in heavy brackets are reference numbers.

	Condition	Pulmonary Function	Immunology	Eosinophilia	Clinical Manifestations
1	Asthma	Reversible obstruction. FEV, FVC, & FEV_1/ FVC ↓. RV ↑. $D_{L_{CO}}$ normal or ↑. [1,2]	Extrinsic (allergic): Type I (IgE-mediated); IgE ↑. Immediate skin tests positive. RAST positive.	Sputum, blood	Cough, wheezing, dyspnea. Onset usually in childhood. Personal & family history for atopy often positive. Attacks often self-limited.

continued

	Condition	Pulmonary Function	Immunology	Eosino-philia	Clinical Manifestations
2			Intrinsic: IgE normal. Immediate skin tests negative. RAST negative.	Sputum, blood	Cough, wheezing, dyspnea. Onset usually after age 35 yr. Atopic history usually negative. Attacks often fulminant.
3	Chronic bronchitis	FEV_1/FVC usually ↓. RV ↑. [3]	....	None	Chronic productive cough with or without wheezing, dyspnea. Occurs most often in male, middle-aged smoker. May progress to emphysema. May develop cor pulmonale (late).
4	Emphysema	Irreversible obstruction. FEV, FVC, & FEV_1/FVC ↓. RV ↑. $D_{L_{CO}}$ ↓. [4]	....	None	Cough, wheezing, dyspnea; hyperinflation of chest; distant breath sounds. Smoking history. Small number with deficient α_1-antitrypsin.
5	Congestive heart failure	FVC ↓. $D_{L_{CO}}$ may or may not be ↓. Lung compliance ↓.	....	None	History: often heart disease (atherosclerotic or valvular) or hypertension. Cardiac enlargement, gallop rhythm. Rales in dependent areas of lung. Roentgenogram: cardiomegaly, interstitial edema, with or without pleural effusions. Elevated pulmonary wedge pressure.
6	Pulmonary embolism [11]	FEV_1/FVC may or may not be ↓. $D_{L_{CO}}$ ↓. [7]	....	None	Cough, wheezing, dyspnea. Often history of long trip, pelvic disease, phlebitis, cardiac disease, or recent surgery. Pulmonary angiogram most often diagnostic. Chest roentgenogram & perfusion scan may be abnormal. Hypoxemia. Pulmonary artery pressure increased. ECG may show right heart strain.
7	Allergic bronchopulmonary aspergillosis [10]	FEV_1/FVC ↓ [10]	Types I + III. IgE ↑↑. Skin tests: Immediate & 6-8 h (Arthus) positive for *Aspergillus*. *Aspergillus* precipitins in serum.	Sputum, blood	Intermittent low-grade fever, cough; fluctuating pulmonary infiltrates. Expectoration of golden-brown mucus plugs containing *Aspergillus*; *Aspergillus* in sputum by stain & culture. Most often superimposed on long-standing asthma. Biopsy: chronic interstitial granulomatous pneumonitis. If chronic, proximal bronchiectasis.
8	Hypersensitivity pneumonitis [8]	FVC ↓. FEV_1 normal or ↓. Lung compliance ↓. [6]	Type III, ? type IV. Precipitins to offending antigen often positive.	Unusual	Recurrent fever, chills, cough, dyspnea, myalgias 4-6 h after inhalation of organic dust. Bibasilar moist rales. Chest roentgenogram: fine nodular densities & peripheral infiltrates. With chronic organic dust exposure, interstitial fibrosis may develop.
9	Cystic fibrosis	FEV_1 & FVC ↓. RV ↑. $D_{L_{CO}}$ normal. [5]	....	None	Bronchial obstruction & recurrent infection. Pancreatic insufficiency; viscous secretions. Abnormal sweat electrolytes—Na^+ & Cl^- increased.
10	Narrowing of upper airways	Variable, but FEV_1 usually ↓. Detected by analysis of flow-volume curves. [9]	....	None	Cough, wheezing, dyspnea. Roentgenogram may show foreign body, tumor, localized emphysema, or tracheal stenosis. History may reveal aspiration, malignancy, thyroid disease, old tracheostomy, etc.

Contributor: Rosenberg, Gary L.

continued

References

1. Aaronson, D. W. 1972. In R. Patterson, ed. Allergic Diseases: Diagnosis and Management. J. B. Lippincott, Philadelphia. p. 225.
2. Bates, D. V., et al. 1971. Respiratory Function in Disease. Ed. 2. W. B. Saunders, Philadelphia. pp. 129-130.
3. Bates, D. V., et al. 1971. Ibid. pp. 147-155.
4. Bates, D. V., et al. 1971. Ibid. pp. 177-200.
5. Bates, D. V., et al. 1971. Ibid. pp. 240-241.
6. Bates, D. V., et al. 1971. Ibid. pp. 338-339.
7. Bates, D. V., et al. 1971. Ibid. p. 346.
8. Fink, J. N. 1972. (Loc. cit. ref. 1). pp. 532-542.
9. Miller, R. D., and R. E. Hyatt. 1969. Mayo Clin. Proc. 44:145-161.
10. Slavin, R. G. 1972. (Loc. cit. ref. 1). pp. 543-546.
11. Windebank, W. J., et al. 1973. Br. Med. J. 1:90-94.

53. DRUGS USEFUL IN THE TREATMENT OF ALLERGIC DISEASE

Route: Parentheses indicate possible route. i.m. = intramuscular; i.v. = intravenous; s.c. = subcutaneous. *Abbreviations:* H1 = histamine type 1; H2 = histamine type 2; SRS-A = slow-reacting substance of anaphylaxis.

	Class & Agent ⟨Synonym⟩	Route	Clinical Use	Mechanism of Action	Remarks	Reference
			Drugs in Common Use			
1	Corticosteroids	Oral, i.m., or i.v.	Moderate & severe asthma; anaphylaxis; rhinitis; chronic urticaria	Uncertain. May involve: decreased circulating eosinophils; decreased circulating basophils; synergistic action with catecholamines (e.g., on cAMP levels); decreased synthesis of mediators (histamine, prostaglandins); "stabilization" of lysosomes; ? others.	Potent agent; delayed onset of action (not useful in acute anaphylaxis). Many side effects with long-term use.	8,9, 13, 18, 21, 24, 26
2		Intranasal	Rhinitis	Locally effective (with low systemic absorption)	Fewer systemic side effects than oral corticosteroids	28, 40
3		Inhaled	Asthma	Locally effective (with low systemic absorption)	Fewer systemic side effects than oral corticosteroids	43
4	Antihistamines Diphenhydramine; pyrilamine; chlorpheniramine; cyclizine; promethazine	Oral, (i.m.)	Allergic rhinitis; acute urticaria; chronic urticaria	Block histamine effects on end-organs (H1-receptors on smooth muscles & blood vessels)	Ineffective in anaphylaxis	14, 22, 41
5	Hydroxyzine; cyproheptadine	Oral, (i.m.)	Chronic urticaria; ? prophylaxis of serum sickness	Structurally distinct from other antihistamines; may have antiserotonin properties	....	14, 22, 41
6	β-Adrenergic agents Epinephrine (mixed β & α agent)	Inhaled, s.c., i.m., or i.v.	Acute anaphylaxis; acute urticaria; acute asthma	β-Adrenergic-induced smooth muscle relaxation (counteracting effect on end-organs of histamine & other mediators); complex vasoactive effects; β-adrenergic-induced elevation of basophil & mast cell cAMP levels inhibits release of histamine & other mediators. α-Adrenergic-induced vasoconstriction.	Treatment of choice of anaphylaxis	4,20, 31
7	Isoproterenol	Inhaled	Asthma	*See* entry 6, this column, first sentence	Excess use of inhaled isoproterenol is associated with deaths	12, 16, 20, 32

continued

53. DRUGS USEFUL IN THE TREATMENT OF ALLERGIC DISEASE

	Class & Agent ⟨Synonym⟩	Route	Clinical Use	Mechanism of Action	Remarks	Reference
8	Ephedrine (mixed β & α agent)	Oral	Asthma; rhinitis	Release of norepinephrine, an α-adrenergic agent, but actions are similar to that of epinephrine (see entry 6, this column, first sentence)	Frequently used in combination with theophylline	20
9	Selective β_2-adrenergic agents: metaproterenol; salbutamol [1]; terbutaline; isoetharine, etc.	Inhaled, oral, or s.c.	Asthma	Stimulate primarily β_2 (bronchodilator)-receptors	Apparently fewer β_1 effects (i.e., less tachycardia) than isoproterenol	20, 38
10	α-Adrenergic agents: ephedrine; pseudoephedrine; phenylephrine; phenylpropanolamine; mephentermine, etc.	Nasal spray, nose drops, or oral	Rhinitis	Stimulate α-receptors; vasoconstriction decreases nasal edema	Frequently used in conjunction with antihistamines	20
11	Cromolyn sodium	Spinhaler (inhaled) [2]	Chronic asthma; exercise-induced asthma	Uncertain. Presumed to inhibit mediator release	Valuable prophylactic but not useful in acute asthma	19, 23, 36, 39
12	Theophylline	Oral, i.v., or rectal suppository	Asthma	Relaxes smooth muscle; increases cAMP levels (inhibits cyclic-AMP phosphodiesterases), and thus inhibits release of histamine & other mediators; may be synergistic with β-adrenergic agents	Improved pulmonary function is directly related to blood level	29, 42
13	Expectorants: potassium iodide; guaiacol glyceryl ether ⟨glyceryl guaiacolate⟩; others	Oral	Asthma	Supposedly decrease sputum viscosity	Value not proven	12
	Recent or Experimental Treatment [3]					
14	Acetylsalicylic acid ⟨Aspirin⟩	Oral	?? Asthma; ? rhinitis	Inhibits prostaglandin synthesis; ? other effects	In rare patients is beneficial; but some patients have severe asthma from aspirin use	25, 35
15	Atropine	Oral or inhaled	Asthma (especially irritant-induced)	Blocks afferent vagus nerve	Uncertain value; perhaps useful in irritant-induced asthma	34
16	Colchicine	Oral	Anti-gout; ? other	Blocks microtubule aggregation, inhibits histamine release in vitro	Theoretical only; useful in vitro	15
17	Diethylcarbamazine	Oral	?	Inhibits histamine & SRS-A release in vitro	Useful in vitro, apparently not useful clinically	6
18	H2-receptor antagonist: cimetidine	Oral	Peptic ulcer disease; ? other	Blocks action of histamine on H2-receptors	Unknown effect on allergic disease	5, 11
19	Penicillin haptens	i.v.	Penicillin allergy	Compete with penicillin for IgE anti-penicillin antibodies	Only limited trials	10

[1] Not as yet in U.S.A. [2] Oral agents are in developmental stage. [3] Not in common use; some are being evaluated, some are only theoretical and not practical.

continued

	Class & Agent (Synonym)	Route	Clinical Use	Mechanism of Action	Remarks	Reference
20	Prostaglandins, E types	? (Oral or inhaled)	?? Asthma	Bronchodilators; increase cAMP levels and inhibit mediator release	Therapeutic trials in progress	17
21	Sedatives: phenobarbital; diazepam ⟨Valium⟩; others	Oral, i.m., or i.v.	? Asthma	Central nervous system sedation, etc.	Generally considered harmful except in very mild asthma; phenobarbital alters corticosteroid metabolism	7
22	SRS-A antagonists: FPL 55712	?	?	Block SRS-A action in vitro	Only in vitro data	3
23	Triacetyloleandomycin ⟨Troleandomycin⟩	Oral	? Asthma	Antibiotic; ? other mechanism (interacts with corticosteroids)	Uncertain value	37
	"Non-Drug" Treatment					
24	Immunotherapy	s.c.	Allergic disease in general	Immunologic changes	....	27, 30, 33

Contributor: Plaut, Marshall

General References

1. Goodman, L. S., and A. Gilman, ed. 1975. The Pharmacological Basis of Therapeutics. Macmillan, New York.
2. Patterson, R., ed. 1972. Allergic Diseases: Diagnosis and Management. J. B. Lippincott, Philadelphia.

Specific References

3. Augstein, J., et al. 1973. Nature (London) New Biol. 245:215-217.
4. Austen, K. F. 1974. N. Engl. J. Med. 291:661-664.
5. Beaven, M. A. 1976. Ibid. 294:30-36, 320-325.
6. Benner, M., and F. C. Lowell. 1970. J. Allergy 46:29-31.
7. Brooks, S. M., et al. 1972. N. Engl. J. Med. 286:1125-1128.
8. Claman, H. N. 1975. J. Allergy Clin. Immunol. 55:145-151.
9. Collins, J. V., et al. 1975. Q. J. Med. 174:259-273.
10. DeWeck, A. L., and C. H. Schneider. 1972. Int. Arch. Allergy Appl. Immunol. 42:782-797, 798-815.
11. Douglas, W. W. 1975. (Loc. cit. ref. 1). pp. 590-629.
12. Falleroni, A. E. 1972. (Loc. cit. ref. 2). pp. 237-291.
13. Falliers, C. J., et al. 1972. J. Allergy Clin. Immunol. 49:156-166.
14. Fink, J. N. 1972. (Loc. cit. ref. 2). pp. 341-354.
15. Gillespie, E., and L. M. Lichtenstein. 1972. J. Clin. Invest. 51:2941-2947.
16. Harris, L. H. 1970. Br. Med. J. 4:579-582.
17. Herxheimer, H., and I. Roetscher. 1971. Eur. J. Clin. Pharmacol. 3:123-125.
18. Horn, B. R., et al. 1975. N. Engl. J. Med. 292:1152-1155.
19. Hyde, J. S. 1973. Ann. Intern. Med. 78:966.
20. Innes, I. R., and M. Nickerson. 1975. (Loc. cit. ref. 1). pp. 477-513.
21. Kantrowitz, F., et al. 1975. Nature (London) 258:737-739.
22. Kniker, W. T. 1972. In I. H. Lepow and P. A. Ward, ed. Inflammation: Mechanisms and Control. Academic Press, New York. pp. 335-367.
23. Lavin, N., et al. 1976. J. Allergy Clin. Immunol. 57:80-88.
24. Lowell, F. C. 1975. N. Engl. J. Med. 292:1182-1183.
25. McDonald, J. R., et al. 1972. J. Allergy Clin. Immunol. 50:198-207.
26. McFadden, E. R., et al. 1976. Am. J. Med. 60:52-57.
27. Norman, P. S. 1974. Med. Clin. North Am. 58:111-126.
28. Norman, P. S., et al. 1967. J. Allergy 40:57-61.
29. Piafsky, K. M., and R. I. Ogilvie. 1975. N. Engl. J. Med. 292:1215-1222.
30. Platts-Mills, T. A. E., et al. 1976. J. Clin. Invest. 57:1041-1050.
31. Plaut, M., and L. M. Lichtenstein. 1974. Ration. Drug Ther. 8(7):1-6.
32. Reisman, R. E. 1970. J. Allergy 46:162-177.
33. Rose, B. 1974. Med. Clin. North Am. 58:127-134.
34. Rosenthal, R. R., et al. 1976. J. Appl. Physiol. 42: (in press).
35. Samter, M., and R. F. Beers, Jr. 1968. Ann. Intern. Med. 68:975-983.

continued

36. Sheffer, A. L., et al. 1975. N. Engl. J. Med. 293:1220-1224.
37. Spector, S. L., et al. 1974. J. Allergy Clin. Immunol. 54:367-379.
38. Tashkin, D. P., et al. 1975. Chest 68:155-161.
39. Taylor, A., et al. 1974. Int. Arch. Allergy Appl. Immunol. 47:175-193.
40. Turkeltaub, P. C., et al. 1975. J. Allergy Clin. Immunol. 55:120-121.
41. Valentine, M. D., et al. 1974. In F. G. McMahon, ed. Principles and Techniques of Human Research and Therapeutics. Futura, Mt. Kisco, NY. v. 9, pp. 227-237.
42. Weinberger, M. M., and E. A. Bronsky. 1974. J. Pediatr. 84:421-427.
43. Williams, M. H. 1974. Am. Rev. Resp. Dis. 110:122-127.

54. SURFACE MARKERS OF HUMAN LYMPHOCYTES

For additional information, consult references 11 and 13.

	Marker System ⟨Synonym⟩	Reactive Cells		Reference
		T Cells	B Cells	
1	Surface membrane immunoglobulin ⟨Sm Ig⟩	−	+ (M)[1]	9,16
2	Anti chronic lymphatic leukemia ⟨Anti CLL⟩	−	+	14,32
3	Human B lymphocyte ⟨HL-B⟩[2]	−	+	23,31
	Monkey erythrocyte			
4	Japanese ape	−	+	26
5	Rhesus	+	−	22
6	C3b[3], C3d[3]	−	+ (M)[1]	4,5,21,24,27
7	C4b[3]	−	+	6
8	Epstein-Barr virus ⟨EB virus⟩	−	+[4]	15,19
9	Heat-aggregated human immunoglobulin G (Fc portion)	+[5]	+ (M)[1]	3,8,12,35
	Anti T-cell			
10	Anti thymocyte	+	−	2,28-30
11	Anti peripheral blood T lymphocyte ⟨Anti PBL T-cell⟩	+	−	1
12	Anti brain	+	−	7
	Sheep erythrocyte rosette			
13	Total	+	−	10,20,25,33
14	Active	+	−	17,34
15	Morula	+	−	18

[1] Monocytes may react and give "+" reaction. [2] Detected by serum from women immunized during pregnancy. [3] Complement components. [4] May bind to C3 receptor of B cell. [5] Some cells.

Contributor: Hong, Richard

References

1. Aiuti, F., and H. Wigzell. 1973. Clin. Exp. Immunol. 13:171-181.
2. Balch, C. M., et al. 1975. Fed. Proc. Fed. Am. Soc. Exp. Biol. 34:994(Abstr. 4394).
3. Basten, A., et al. 1972. Nature (London) New Biol. 235:178-180.
4. Bianco, C., and V. Nussenzweig. 1971. Science 173:154-155.
5. Bianco, C., et al. 1970. J. Exp. Med. 132:702-720.
6. Bokisch, V. A., and A. T. Sobel. 1974. Ibid. 140:1336-1347.
7. Brown, G., and M. F. Greaves. 1974. Eur. J. Immunol. 4:302-310.
8. Dickler, H. B., and H. G. Kunkel. 1972. J. Exp. Med. 136:191-196.
9. Frøland, S., et al. 1971. Nature (London) New Biol. 234:251-252.
10. Frøland, S. S. 1972. Scand. J. Immunol. 1:269-280.
11. Frøland, S. S., and J. B. Natvig. 1973. Transplant. Rev. 16:114-162.
12. Frøland, S. S., et al. 1973. Scand. J. Immunol. 2:83.
13. Greaves, M. F. 1975. Prog. Hematol. 9:255-303.
14. Greaves, M. F., and G. Brown. 1973. Nature (London) New Biol. 246:116-119.
15. Greaves, M. F., et al. 1975. Clin. Immunol. Immunopathol. 3:514-524.

continued

16. Grey, H. M., et al. 1971. J. Clin. Invest. 50:2368-2375.
17. Horowitz, S., et al. 1975. Clin. Immunol. Immunopathol. 4:405-414.
18. Huang, S.-W., et al. 1976. Pediatr. Res. 10:120-126.
19. Jondal, M., and G. Klein. 1973. J. Exp. Med. 138:1365-1378.
20. Jondal, M., et al. 1972. Ibid. 136:207-215.
21. Lay, W. H., and V. Nussenzweig. 1968. Ibid. 128:991-1009.
22. Lohrmann, H.-P., and L. Novikovs. 1974. Clin. Immunol. Immunopathol. 3:99-111.
23. Mann, D. L., et al. 1975. J. Exp. Med. 142:84-89.
24. Michlmayr, G., and H. Huber. 1970. J. Immunol. 105:670-676.
25. Papamichail, M., et al. 1972. Lancet 2:64-66.
26. Pellegrino, M. A., et al. 1975. J. Immunol. 115:1065-1071.
27. Ross, G. D., et al. 1973. J. Clin. Invest. 52:377-385.
28. Smith, R. W., et al. 1973. J. Immunol. 110:884-887.
29. Touraine, J. L., et al. 1974. Clin. Exp. Immunol. 16:503-520.
30. Williams, R. C., Jr., et al. 1973. J. Clin. Invest. 52:283-295.
31. Winchester, R. J., et al. 1975. J. Exp. Med. 141:924-929.
32. Wortis, H. H., et al. 1973. Nature (London) New Biol. 243:109-111.
33. Wybran, J., et al. 1972. J. Clin. Invest. 51:2537-2543.
34. Wybran, J. M., et al. 1973. N. Engl. J. Med. 288:1036-1039.
35. Yoshida, T. O., and B. Andersson. 1972. Scand. J. Immunol. 1:401-408.

55. IMMUNOGLOBULIN CONCENTRATIONS IN EXTERNAL SECRETIONS

IgM: n.d. = not determined.

	Secretion	IgA mg/100 ml	IgG mg/100 ml	IgM mg/100 ml
1	Nasal washing	26.0	6.0	0.0
2	Expectorate sputum	27.0	11.0	0.0
3	Tracheobronchial secretions	17.0	0.0	0.0
4	Stimulated parotid secretion	3.95	0.036	0.043
5	Whole saliva	30.38	4.86	0.55
6	Jejunal secretions	27.6	34.0	n.d.
7	Colonic secretions	82.7	86.0	n.d.
8	Colostrum	1234.0	10.0	61.0

Contributor: Waldman, Robert H.

General References

1. Brandtzaeg, P., et al. 1970. Scand. J. Haematol., Suppl. 12.
2. Bull, D. M., et al. 1971. Gastroenterology 60:370-380.
3. Ganguly, R., and R. H. Waldman. 1977. In J. Clot, ed. Cinquièmes journées montpelliéraines de pneumologie. G. Masson, Paris.

56. SERUM IMMUNOGLOBULIN LEVELS IN NORMAL INDIVIDUALS

Geometric means are presented for each immunoglobulin at every age. The bounds, given in parentheses, are obtained by taking the mean logarithm ± twice the pooled standard deviations of the mean logarithms, and then taking the antilogs of the results. In the case of IgA, the first four age groups have a pooled standard deviation separate from the other ages. In the case of IgM, the bounds of the first four age groups are ± twice the individual group standard deviations.

Subjects		IgG		IgA		IgM	
Age	No.	mg/100 ml	% of Adult Level	mg/100 ml	% of Adult Level	mg/100 ml	% of Adult Level
1 Newborn	20	1004(598-1672)	95	<5(0-<5)	<2	9(6-15)	12
2 1-3 mo	10	365(218-610)	34	32(20-53)	12	24(11-51)	32

continued

56. SERUM IMMUNOGLOBULIN LEVELS IN NORMAL INDIVIDUALS

	Subjects		IgG		IgA		IgM	
	Age	No.	mg/100 ml	% of Adult Level	mg/100 ml	% of Adult Level	mg/100 ml	% of Adult Level
3	4-6 mo	12	381(228-636)	36	44(27-72)	17	38(25-60)	50
4	7-9 mo	10	488(292-816)	46	44(27-73)	17	47(18-124)	62
5	10-18 mo	13	640(383-1070)	60	67(27-169)	25	56(28-113)	74
6	2 yr	8	708(423-1184)	67	89(35-222)	33	65(32-131)	86
7	3 yr	6	798(477-1334)	75	100(40-251)	38	57(28-116)	75
8	4 yr	8	906(542-1515)	85	120(48-301)	45	41(20-82)	54
9	5 yr	5	901(539-1506)	85	134(53-336)	50	52(26-106)	68
10	6 yr	11	954(571-1597)	90	131(52-329)	49	57(28-115)	75
11	7 yr	11	1066 (638-1783)	100	223(89-559)	84	48(24-98)	63
12	8 yr	8	976(583-1631)	92	213(85-535)	80	55(27-112)	72
13	9 yr	7	1006(599-1673)	95	230(92-578)	86	56(28-113)	74
14	10 yr	7	991(593-1657)	93	188(75-472)	71	60(29-120)	79
15	11 yr	7	989(586-1637)	93	257(102-644)	97	56(28-113)	74
16	12 yr	7	855(511-1430)	81	232(92-581)	87	55(27-111)	72
17	13 yr	13	961(575-1607)	91	235(94-588)	88	52(26-105)	68
18	14 yr	8	940(562-1571)	89	217(86-544)	82	67(33-135)	88
19	Adult	30	1061(635-1775)	100	266(106-668)	100	76(37-154)	100

Contributor: Buckley, Rebecca H.

Reference: Buckley, R. H., et al. 1968. Pediatrics 41:600-611.

57. SERUM IMMUNOGLOBULIN CONCENTRATIONS IN PRIMARY IMMUNODEFICIENCY DISEASES

Part I. IgG, IgA, and IgM Concentrations

Means are geometric. Values in parentheses are ranges, estimate "c" (*see* Introduction).

	Condition	Subjects		IgG mg/100 ml	IgA mg/100 ml	IgM mg/100 ml
		No.	Age			
1	Transient hypogammaglobulinemia, of infancy	9	3-20 mo	146(50-305)	12(0-27)	25(12-95)
2	Severe combined immunodeficiency (SCID)	11	3-17 mo	20(0-250)	0.6(0-43)	1(0-120)
3	DiGeorge syndrome	2	3-5 mo	334(265-420)	51(46-57)	18(10-31)
4	X-linked agammaglobulinemia	13	3-16 yr	43(0-160)	0.2(0-7)	1(0-15)
5	Non-X-linked agammaglobulinemia	19	6-35 yr	32(0-230)	0.3(0-58)	5(0-48)
6	X-linked immunodeficiency with hyper-IgM	4	7 mo-21 yr	2(0-44)	0(0)	432(84-880)
7	Selective IgA deficiency	102	5 mo-50 yr	1019(320-3920)	0.3(0-10)	63(12-448)
8	Ataxia-telangiectasia syndrome	7	5-14 yr	738(390-1800)	0.97(0-500)	82(48-170)
9	Nezelof syndrome	5	5 mo-3 yr	906(312-1850)	245(55-1000)	151(72-360)
10	Wiskott-Aldrich syndrome	5	8 mo-12 yr	694(145-2400)	181(34-1168)	27(10-69)
11	Extreme hyperimmunoglobulinemia E syndrome	15	6 mo-31 yr	1539(580-4100)	185(30-570)	120(42-280)
12	Chronic granulomatous disease, of childhood	9	6 mo-17 yr	1625(375-2650)	553(22-1440)	143(46-320)

Contributor: Buckley, Rebecca H.

Reference: Buckley, R. H. Unpublished. Duke Univ. Medical Center, Durham, NC, 1976.

continued

57. SERUM IMMUNOGLOBULIN CONCENTRATIONS IN PRIMARY IMMUNODEFICIENCY DISEASES

Part II. IgD Concentrations

Ranges are geometric. *Abbreviations*: NS = not significantly different from normal. Values in parentheses are ranges, estimate "c" unless otherwise specified (*see* Introduction).

	Condition	Subjects		Range mg/100 ml	Mean mg/100 ml	p Value t Test	Median mg/100 ml	p Value Mann-Whitney
		No.	Age					
1	Normal infants	23	6 wk-19 mo	(<1-1.6)	0.1(0-0.6)[b]	....	0.1	....
2	Normal children	105	3-14 yr	(<1-36)	1.6(0-70)[b]	....	3.0	....
3	Normal adults	57	21-55 yr	(<1-11.2)	2.4(0-61)[b]	....	4.6	....
4	Transient hypogammaglobulinemia	8	3-20 mo	<0.1	<0.1	NS	0.1	NS
5	Severe combined immunodeficiency ⟨SCID⟩	9	3-17 mo	(<1-2)	0.1	NS	0.1	NS
6	X-linked agammaglobulinemia	10	3-16 yr	(<1-20.6)	0.4	0.02	0.1	NS
7	Non-X-linked agammaglobulinemia	15	6-35 yr	(<1-14.4)	0.2	<0.0001	0.1	0.0007
8	X-linked immunodeficiency with hyper-IgM	3	7 mo-21 yr	(<1-5.1)	0.4	NS	0.1	NS
9	Selective IgA deficiency	79	5 mo-50 yr	(<1-39.3)	0.7	<0.0001	0.1	0.0005
10	Ataxia-telangiectasia syndrome	7	5-14 yr	(<1-19.2)	2.6	NS	5.6	NS
11	Nezelof syndrome	3	8 mo-3 yr	(2-22)	7.0	NS	7.8	NS
12	Wiskott-Aldrich syndrome	4	8 mo-12 yr	(<1-7.8)	0.7	NS	1.4	NS
13	Extreme hyperimmunoglobulinemia E	11	3-31 yr	(2.7-159)	14.4	<0.0001	16.1	0.0004
14	Other variable immunodeficiency	6	1-14 yr	(<1-163.4)	3.6	NS	7.4	NS
15	Chronic granulomatous disease	10	6 mo-17 yr	(<1-53.1)	4.8	NS	4.6	NS

Contributor: Buckley, Rebecca H.

Reference: Buckley, R. H., and S. A. Fiscus. 1975. J. Clin. Invest. 55:157-165.

Part III. IgE Concentrations

Ranges are geometric. *Abbreviations*: NS = not significantly different from normal. Values in parentheses are ranges, estimate "c" unless otherwise specified (*see* Introduction).

	Condition	Subjects		Range IU/ml	Mean IU/ml	p Value t Test	Median IU/ml	p Value Mann-Whitney
		No.	Age					
1	Normal infants	12	2-19 mo	(3-81)	18(1-222)[b]	....	25	....
2	Normal children & adults	106	2-55 yr	(2-549)	55(5-621)[b]	....	55	....
3	Transient hypogammaglobulinemia	8	3-20 mo	(2-31)	6	0.05	5	0.0269
4	Severe combined immunodeficiency ⟨SCID⟩	9	3-17 mo	(<1-82)	2	<0.0001	2	0.0018
5	X-linked agammaglobulinemia	10	3-16 yr	(<1-5)	2	<0.0001	1	<0.0001
6	Non-X-linked agammaglobulinemia	15	6-35 yr	(1-10)	3	<0.0001	3	<0.0001
7	X-linked immunodeficiency with hyper-IgM	3	7 mo-21 yr	(<1-2)	1	<0.0001	1	0.0016
8	Selective IgA deficiency	74	5 mo-50 yr	(3-3800)	124	<0.0001	174	0.0001
9	Ataxia-telangiectasia syndrome	7	5-14 yr	(<1-54)	7	<0.0001	10	0.0005
10	Nezelof syndrome	3	8 mo-3 yr	(5-7000)	55	NS	5	NS
11	Wiskott-Aldrich syndrome	4	8 mo-12 yr	(135-720)	381	<0.0001	487	0.0020
12	Extreme hyperimmunoglobulinemia E	11	3-31 yr	(2150-40,000)	11,305	<0.0001	12,362	<0.0001
13	Other variable immunodeficiency	6	1-14 yr	(11-2880)	142	NS	70	NS
14	Chronic granulomatous disease	10	6 mo-17 yr	(<1-3160)	88	NS	100	NS

Contributor: Buckley, Rebecca H.

Reference: Buckley, R. H., and S. A. Fiscus. 1975. J. Clin. Invest. 55:157-165.

58. LYMPHOCYTE PROLIFERATION ASSAY

The values are not absolute, and results will vary from laboratory to laboratory with the age of the subject and the state of immunization. Proliferation was measured by incorporation of [^{3}H]thymidine having a specific activity of 6.7 mCi/mmole into cellular DNA, using 1 μCi per million cells (pulse period of 6-18 hours). Cells were cultured 3 days for mitogens and 6 days for antigens in the presence of 15% pooled normal AB serum. **Stimulation Index** is the ratio of the counts per minute in stimulated cultures to the counts per minute in control cultures, the latter usually having a range of 100-1000 CPM.

	Class	Stimulant	Range in Stimulated Cultures, counts/min	Stimulation Index
1	Mitogens	Phytohemagglutinin	⩾20,000	20
2		Concanavalin A	⩾20,000	20
3		Pokeweed	⩾10,000	10
4	Antigens	Tuberculin-purified protein derivative	1000-100,000	>3
5		*Candida albicans*	1000-100,000	>3
6		Streptokinase-streptodornase	1000-100,000	>3

Contributor: Rocklin, Ross E.

General References

1. Chalmers, D. G., et al. 1967. Int. Arch. Allergy Appl. Immunol. 32:117-130.
2. Chessin, L. N., et al. 1966. J. Exp. Med. 124:873-884.
3. Nowell, P. C. 1960. Cancer Res. 20(4):462-466.
4. Oppenheim, J. J. 1968. Fed. Proc. Fed. Am. Soc. Exp. Biol. 27:21-28.
5. Oppenheim, J. J., et al. 1967. Immunology 12:89-102.
6. Pearmain, G., et al. 1963. Lancet 1:637-638.
7. Rocklin, R. E., et al. 1970. Proc. 5th Leukocyte Cult. Conf., pp. 639-648.

59. LYMPHOCYTE MEDIATOR ASSAYS

The values are not absolute, and results will vary from laboratory to laboratory with the age of the subject and the state of immunization. *Abbreviation:* PMN = polymorphonuclear.

	Mediator	Variable & Units	Value	Reference
1	Migration inhibitory factor	Inhibition of macrophage migration, %	15-60	2
2	Leukocyte inhibitory factor	Inhibition of PMN leukocyte migration, %	15-60	3
3	Chemotactic factors	Chemotactic index: Total leukocytes (PMN or mononuclear) in 5 high-powered fields	50-300	5
4	Interferon	Titer: Reciprocal of dilution causing 50% reduction in viral plaques	20-400	1
5	Lymphotoxin	Titer: Reciprocal of dilution causing 50% cytotoxicity of target cells	10-100	4
6	Mitogenic factor	Counts/min due to "active" supernatant minus counts/min due to control supernatant	500-50,000	6

Contributor: Rocklin, Ross E.

References

1. Merigan, T. C. 1971. In B. R. Bloom and P. R. Glade, ed. In Vitro Methods in Cell-mediated Immunity. Academic Press, New York. pp. 489-499.
2. Rocklin, R., et al. 1970. J. Immunol. 104:95-102.
3. Søborg, M., and G. Bendixen. 1967. Acta Med. Scand. 181:247-256.
4. Spofford, B. T., et al. 1974. J. Immunol. 112:2111-2116.
5. Ward, P. A., et al. 1970. Cell. Immunol. 1:162-174.
6. Wolstencroft, R. A., and D. C. Dumonde. 1970. Immunology 18:599-610.

Absolute values for these tests vary among laboratories, depending on the specific conditions of the assay. All tests must be run parallel with control samples, or normal control values must be established prior to testing. **Principle of Test**: WBC = leukocytes. **Normal Values**: Rst = resting;

Phg = phagocytic; OD_{515} = optical density at 515 nm. *Abbreviation*: PMN = polymorphonuclear leukocyte(s). Values in parentheses are ranges, estimate "c" (*see* Introduction).

	Test Name	Principle of Test	Purpose of Test	Normal Values	Reference
		In Vitro			
1	Bacterial killing	Opsonified live bacteria are ingested and killed by phagocytic blood cells (PMN, monocytes)	Measures capacity of blood phagocytes to kill opsonified bacteria; may also be used to measure opsonic activity of sera	Less than 10% of most bacterial species remain viable after 60 min at 37°C incubation with an equal number of PMN	13
2	Oxygen consumption	Cyanide-insensitive O_2 consumption is associated with, but is not required for, phagocytosis by PMN & monocytes _____ hydroxyl radical $\langle OH^- \rangle$. Some or all of these reduction products are required for intraleukocyte bacterial killing.	Phagocytic blood cells reduce oxygen to hydrogen peroxide $\langle H_2O_2 \rangle$, superoxide anion $\langle O_2^- \rangle$, singlet oxygen $\langle O_2^* \rangle$, and	Rst: 7.4 ± 3.8 μl O_2 consumed per hour per 10^7 cells; Phg: 37.6 ± 22.5 μl O_2 consumed per hour per 10^7 cells	9
3	[1-^{14}C]Glucose oxidation	Oxidation of glucose through the hexose monophosphate shunt is stimulated in PMN & monocytes during phagocytosis	NADPH oxidation by O_2 and/or H_2O_2 occurs in PMN with an intact NADPH/NADH oxidase system activated during phagocytosis	Rst: 62.6 ± 10 nmoles glucose oxidized per 30 min per 5×10^6 cells; Phg: 169 ± 28 nmoles glucose oxidized per 30 min per 5×10^6 cells	15
4	[^{14}C]Formate oxidation	Oxidation of formic acid by PMN requires H_2O_2, and is catalyzed by catalase	This is an indirect quantitation of H_2O_2 produced during phagocytosis by PMN	Rst: $0.6(0.2-1.1)$ nmoles formate oxidized per hour per mg protein; Phg: $2.8(1.1-5.9)$ nmoles formate oxidized per hour per mg protein	5
5	Hydrogen peroxide release	Scopoletin fluorescence is extinguished when oxidized by H_2O_2 + horseradish peroxidase	Provides sensitive, direct quantitation of release of H_2O_2 from PMN during phagocytosis	Rst: 0.012 ± 0.003 nmole H_2O_2 released per min per 2.5×10^6 cells; Phg: 0.445 ± 0.064 nmole H_2O_2 released per min per 2.5×10^6 cells	16
6	Iodination of ingested particles	Bacteria and other particulate proteins are iodinated following their ingestion by PMN & monocytes. Biochemical requirements: halide ion, peroxidase, hydrogen peroxide. _____ assesses available pool of H_2O_2 in region of phagolysosomes to iodinate ingested particles	Measures capacity of specific granule peroxidase in blood phagocytes (PMN, monocytes) to be discharged into phagolysosomes, and	Rst: 0.04 ± 0.03 nmole iodide consumed per hour per 10^7 cells; Phg: 3.95 ± 0.82 nmoles iodide consumed per hour per 10^7 cells	12
7	Superoxide production	Univalent reduction product of oxygen is O_2^-; it & other substances reduce ferricytochrome c, and that amount of ferricytochrome c inhibited by purified superoxide dismutase $\langle SOD \rangle$ is due only to O_2^-	Measure release of O_2^- from PMN & monocytes at rest & during phagocytosis	Rst: 0.50 nmole O_2^- per 15 min per 10^7 cells; Phg: 1.0 nmole per 15 min per 10^7 cells	3

continued

	Test Name	Principle of Test	Purpose of Test	Normal Values	Reference
8	Chemiluminescence	The measurement of light produced by PMN & monocytes during phagocytosis of zymosan	Measures capacity of PMN & monocytes to reduce O_2 to H_2O_2, O_2^-, and O_2^*; all three are required for optimal chemiluminescence	$142.5 \pm 64 \times 10^3$ counts/min per 13 min per 10^7 PMN	1
9	Nitroblue tetrazolium ⟨NBT⟩ reduction	Solubilized redox dyes of tetrazolium salts when incubated with PMN are reduced to insoluble formazan. Reduction occurs to a larger extent during phagocytosis. Addition of superoxide dismutase ⟨SOD⟩ decreases amount of formazan formed, indicating that NBT reduction, in large part, reflects O_2^- generated by PMN.	Detects carriers of the X-linked form of chronic granulomatous disease ⟨CGD⟩; detects all affected patients with CGD	Rst: 0.088 ± 0.040 OD_{515} per 15 min per 10^7 cells; Phg: 0.319 ± 0.112 OD_{515} per 15 min per 10^7 cells	4
10	Phagocytic uptake of oil red O particles	Liquid petrolatum[1/], stained by oil red O dye and emulsified by sonication, is coated with *Escherichia coli* lipopolysaccharide, requiring opsonification by alternative pathway for efficient uptake by PMN	Sensitive measure of the rate of uptake of particles by PMN; also measures functional alternative pathway opsonic capacity	$0.138(0.121-0.157)$ mg liquid petrolatum[1/] taken up per min per 10^7 cells	17
11	Chemotaxis assay	PMN are sedimented on Millipore filter, placed in Boyden chamber, and incubated 3 h at 37°C, with a source of chemotactic factor placed on the opposite side of the filter. Chemotactic index is calculated by assessing the number of PMN migrating completely through the filter.	Assay to study directed PMN movement in response to a variety of chemotactic factors. Test can be adapted to study either cells, serum, or the effects of pharmacologic agents on chemotaxis.	Chemotactic index: 13 ± 5 (without chemotactic factor); 67 ± 16 (with chemotactic factor)	8
	Degranulation of lysosomal enzymes:				
12	Into phagolysosomes	Emulsified liquid petrolatum[1/] containing oil red O is phagocytized by PMN. Phagocytic vesicles are isolated from homogenized cells on a density gradient. Vesicles float to the top of the gradient, and the other cell components sediment.	Assesses lysosomal movement in PMN, dependent, in part, on normal microtubule assembly	$14.5 \pm 2.2\%$ of total β-glucuronidase released into phagocytic vesicles in 45 min	18
13	Into media	Cytochalasin B inhibits microfilament polymerization, and converts PMN to "secretory" cells releasing lysosomal enzymes during incubation with opsonified zymosan particles	Assesses lysosomal movement in PMN, dependent, in part, on normal microtubule assembly	20% of total β-glucuronidase released in 30 min	19
14	Fluorescein-conjugated concanavalin A ⟨Con A⟩ capping of PMN	PMN incubated with fluorescein Con A; the movement of fluorescence into polar aggregates represents microtubule depolymerization	Tests for factors that control microtubule polymerization in PMN. Drugs (e.g., colchicine) and diseases (e.g., Chediak-Higashi syndrome) that interfere with microtubule assembly increase number of capped PMN.	Fluorescence distribution: random, >90%; capped, <10%	11

[1/] Synonym: Paraffin oil.

continued

	Test Name	Principle of Test	Purpose of Test	Normal Values	Reference
15	Antineutrophil antibody	Human leukocytes or rabbit macrophages phagocytize neutrophils previously opsonified with antineutrophil antibodies present in test sera. Rate of ingestion is measured by quantitation of the rate of oxidation of $[1\text{-}^{14}C]$glucose to $^{14}CO_2$ by phagocytizing leukocytes or alveolar macrophages incubated with serum-treated neutrophils.	Serologic test for antineutrophil antibodies	1732 ± 653 counts/min per 30 min incubation per 10^7 cells	6
			In Vivo		
16	Rebuck skin window	Following skin abrasion, glass #2 cover slips are applied to area, and removed every 3 h for Wright staining. Exudation of PMN occurs during first few hours, mononuclear cells appear at 6 h, and predominate by 12 h.	Assessment of the in vivo inflammatory response	3 h: PMN; 6 h: PMN + monocytes; 12 h: monocytes	14
17	Endotoxin stimulation	Endotoxin[2] from *Salmonella enteritidis*[3], 0.8 ng/kg i.v., or typhoid vaccine, 0.5 ml s.c., with counting of WBC and differentials over next 6 h	Assessment of bone marrow reserve pool of PMN	Mean increase of PMN/μl: 6060 ± 880	10
18	Hydrocortisone stimulation	Single i.v. injection of 200 mg hydrocortisone 21-sodium succinate, with counting of WBC and differentials over next 6 h	Assessment of bone marrow reserve pool of PMN	Mean increase of PMN/μl: 4220 ± 320	7
19	Epinephrine stimulation	Single s.c. injection of 0.1 ml aqueous epinephrine 1:1000, with counting of WBC and differentials over next 30 min	Assessment of marginating pool of PMN in circulation	Twofold increase of PMN/μl compared to pre-injection value	2

[2] Lipexal, from Dorsey Lab. [3] Synonym: *S. abortus-equi.*

Contributor: Baehner, Robert L.

References

1. Allen, R. C., et al. 1972. Biochem. Biophys. Res. Commun. 47:679-684.
2. Athens, J. W., et al. 1961. J. Clin. Invest. 40:159-164.
3. Babior, B. M., et al. 1973. Ibid. 52:741-744.
4. Baehner, R. L., and D. G. Nathan. 1968. N. Engl. J. Med. 278:971-976.
5. Baehner, R. L., et al. 1970. J. Clin. Invest. 49:692-700.
6. Boxer, L. A., et al. 1975. N. Engl. J. Med. 293:748-753.
7. Dale, D. C., et al. 1975. J. Clin. Invest. 56:808-813.
8. Hill, H. R., et al. 1975. J. Lab. Clin. Med. 86:703-710.
9. Holmes, B., et al. 1967. J. Clin. Invest. 46:1422-1432.
10. Marsh, J. C., and S. Perry. 1964. Blood 23:581-599.
11. Oliver, J. M., et al. 1975. Nature (London) 253:471-473.
12. Pincus, S. H., and S. J. Klebanoff. 1971. N. Engl. J. Med. 284:744-750.
13. Quie, P. G., et al. 1967. J. Clin. Invest. 46:668-679.
14. Rebuck, J. W., and J. H. Crowley. 1955. Ann. N.Y. Acad. Sci. 59:757-805.
15. Root, R. K., et al. 1972. J. Clin. Invest. 51:649-665.
16. Root, R. K., et al. 1975. Ibid. 55:945-955.
17. Stossel, T. P. 1973. Blood 42:121-130.
18. Stossel, T. P., et al. 1972. J. Clin. Invest 51:604-614.
19. Zurier, R. B., et al. 1973. Proc. Natl. Acad. Sci. USA 70:844-848.

61. AGE-RELATED ASSESSMENT OF FACTORS CONTRIBUTING TO THE DIAGNOSIS OF SEVERE COMBINED IMMUNODEFICIENCY

Diagnostic Feature: SCID = severe combined immunodeficiency; HTLA = human T-lymphocyte antigen; DH = delayed hypersensitivity; dtaa = dilution titer of agglutinating antibody; DPT = diphtheria-pertusis-tetanus; RIA = radioimmunoassay. **Age A** = age after which feature is significantly abnormal. **Diagnostic Significance if Absent at Age A**: Plus sign (+) indicates that absence of diagnostic feature (or presence of normal quantity, structure, or function) excludes the diagnosis. Minus sign (−) indicates that absence of diagnostic feature does *not* exclude the diagnosis.

	Diagnostic Feature	Age A	Fraction of Normals with Diagnostic Feature		Diagnostic Significance if		Reference
			at Birth[1]	at Age A	Present at Age A	Absent at Age A	
	General						
1	Family history of SCID	Whenever elicited	....	....	++	−	16
2	Lymphopenia: <1000 cells/µl	Birth	<0.05	<0.05	+++	−	2
3	Low proportion of T lymphocytes (E-rosetting lymphocytes)[2]	Birth	0.00	0.00	+++	−	10
4	Absence of lymphoid precursors inducible with thymic extract to HTLA+ & E-rosettes	Birth-4 mo	0.0	0.0	+++	+	1
5	Absent thymus shadow	Birth	....	....	++[3]	+	7,9
6	Thymus morphology: embryonal; no Hassall's corpuscles	Birth	0.0	0.0	++++	+	5,7,19
7	Lymph node morphology: lymphopenia; absence of normal corticomedullary differentiation, follicular architecture, & germinal centers	Birth[4]	0.0	0.0	++++	+	10,16,17
8	Absence of tonsils or palpable lymph nodes	6 mo	....	....	....	..	3
	Absence of plasma cells						
9	In intestinal lamina propria	2-4 mo	....	....	....	..	8
10	In bone marrow	3-5 yr	>0.50	<0.05	+	−	26
11	Deficiency of adenosine deaminase (in fibroblasts, erythrocytes, & leukocytes)	Birth	<<0.001[5]	<<0.001	++++	−	19,20
	Cell-mediated Immunity						
	Skin tests						
	Failure to develop positive biopsy-documented DH skin reaction to						
12	Phytohemagglutinin	Birth	0.00	0.00	++	?	6
13	Diphtheria-tetanus toxoid	7-10 mo[6]	1.00	0.00	+	?	13
14	*Candida albicans*	7-12 mo[7]	∼1.00	0.50	±	+	13
15	Streptokinase-streptodornase	6-10 yr[7]	1.00	(0.11-0.49)	±	+	13
16	Failure to develop DH response after sensitization with fluorodinitrobenzene[8]	2-12 mo	(0.75-0.80)	0.00	+++	+	28
17	Failure to reject allogeneic skin graft	Birth	0.0	0.0	++++	+	12
	Lymphocyte transformation						
18	Absent response to phytohemagglutinin	Birth	0.0	0.0	++++	+	18
19	Absent response to allogeneic cells	Birth	(0.0-0.14)	(0.0-0.14)	++++	−	18

[1] Unless otherwise indicated. [2] Variations in normal proportion of lymphocytes forming spontaneous rosettes with sheep erythrocytes (E-rosettes) are seen in different laboratories, depending on techniques. Normal values are usually at least >50%, while patients with SCID usually have <30% E-rosettes, on repeated analysis. [3] Significant only in the absence of fetal or neonatal distress. [4] After antigen stimulation. [5] One case recorded. [6] If immunized. [7] If exposed. [8] Synonyms: Dinitrofluorobenzene, DNFB.

continued

65

61. AGE-RELATED ASSESSMENT OF FACTORS CONTRIBUTING TO THE DIAGNOSIS OF SEVERE COMBINED IMMUNODEFICIENCY

	Diagnostic Feature	Age A	Fraction of Normals with Diagnostic Feature		Diagnostic Significance if		Refer- ence
			at Birth[1]	at Age A	Present at Age A	Absent at Age A	
	Production of lymphokines: failure to respond to concanavalin A by producing						
20	Leukocyte migration inhibitory factor	Birth	0.01	0.01	+++	?+	21
21	Lymphotoxin	Birth	<0.11	<0.11	++	?+	11
	Humoral Immunity						
	Markedly reduced or undetectable serum levels of						
22	Immunoglobulin G	6 mo	<0.001	<<0.01	+	−	27
23	Immunoglobulin M	Birth	<<0.01	<<0.01	+++	−	27
24	Immunoglobulin A	6 mo	(0.5-0.8)	0.002	−	−	27
25	Incapacity of lymphocytes to synthe- size and secrete immunoglobulin	Birth-1 mo	0.0	0.0	++++	−	22
	Absent isohemagglutinins						
26	Anti-A (in patients of group O or group B), with dtaa of <1:2	>6 mo	(0.04-0.20)[9]	0.0	++[10]	−	14
27	Anti-B (in patients of group O or group A), with dtaa of <1:2	>6 mo	(0.12-0.25)[9]	0.0	++[10]	−	14
	Humoral unresponsiveness to protein antigens						
28	Diphtheria in DPT	3-4 mo	0.25[11]	0.01[12]	±	+	4
29	Pertussis, with dtaa of <1:20	....	0.94[13]; 0.88[11]	....	±	+	23
30	In DPT	3-4 mo	0.50[13]; 0.33[11]	0.10[12]	±	+	4
31	Tetanus in DPT	Birth	<0.10[11]	<0.10[12]	++++	+	4
32	Typhoid H antigen agglutinins	Birth-1 mo	0.22	0.22	++++	+	25
33	Polio (Salk) neutralizing antibodies[14]	5-6 mo	(0.25-0.50)[15]	0.10[12]	++	..	4
34	φX 174 coliphage	Birth	0.0	0.0	++++	+	15
	Humoral unresponsiveness to capsular polysaccharide antigens						
35	Meningococcus C (by RIA)	3-7 mo	....	(0.0-0.10)	±	+	24
36	Polyribophosphate from *Haemophilus influenzae* (by RIA)	2 yr	0.78[16]	0.13	±	+	29

[1] Unless otherwise indicated. [9] At age 3 months. [10] IgG isohemagglutinins may be passed transplacentally from sensitized mothers. The level of these isohemagglutinins should be markedly reduced in infants by age 6 months. Repeated determinations may be necessary to demonstrate decline. IgG antibodies also resist treatment with 2-mercaptoethanol (which IgM do not). [11] After 3 immunizations given at monthly intervals, beginning at birth. [12] After 3 monthly immunizations beginning at age A. [13] After 1 immunization, given at birth. [14] Response to polio antigens is strongly influenced by maternal antibody level. [15] After immunization given at birth and 1, 2, & 9 months. [16] At 0-12 months.

Contributor: O'Reilly, Richard J.

References

1. Aiuti, F. 1976. Int. Arch. Allergy Appl. Immunol. 51: (in press).
2. Altman, P. L., and D. S. Dittmer, ed. 1961. Blood and Other Body Fluids. Federation of American Societies for Experimental Biology, Washington, D.C. pp. 125-126.
3. Barness, L. A. 1972. Manual of Pediatric Physical Diagnosis. Ed. 4. Year Book, Chicago.
4. Barrett, C. D., et al. 1962. Pediatrics 30:720-736.
5. Berry, C. L. 1968. Proc. R. Soc. Med. 61:867-871.
6. Bonforte, R. J., et al. 1972. J. Pediatr. 81:775-780.
7. Boyd, E. 1932. Am. J. Dis. Child. 43:1162-1214.
8. Bridges, R. A., et al. 1959. J. Lab. Clin. Med. 53:331-357.
9. Caffey, J. 1972. Pediatric X-Ray Diagnosis. Year Book, Chicago. pp. 443-457.
10. Campbell, A. C., et al. 1974. Clin. Exp. Immunol. 18:469-482.
11. Eife, R. F., et al. 1974. Cell Immunol. 14:435-442.
12. Fowler, R., Jr., et al. 1960. Ann. N.Y. Acad. Sci. 87: 403-428.
13. Franz, M. L., et al. 1976. J. Pediatr. 88:975-977.

continued

14. Gartner, O. T., et al. 1967. J. Am. Med. Assoc. 201(3): 206-207.
15. Gold, R., et al. 1975. J. Clin. Invest. 56:1536-1547.
16. Hoyer, J. R., et al. 1968. Medicine (Baltimore) 47:201-206.
17. Kyriazis, A. A., and J. R. Esterly. 1971. Arch. Pathol. 91:444-451.
18. Leikin, S., et al. 1968. J. Pediatr. 72:510-517.
19. Meuwissen, H. J., et al. 1975. Ibid. 86:169-181.
20. Moore, E. C., and H. J. Meuwissen. 1974. Ibid. 85: 802-804.
21. O'Reilly, R. J., et al. 1976. Clin. Res. 24:316A.
22. Polmar, S. H., and P. A. Chase. 1975. J. Pediatr. 87: 545-549.

23. Provenzano, R. W., et al. 1965. N. Engl. J. Med. 273: 959-965.
24. Smith, D. H., et al. 1973. Pediatrics 52:637-644.
25. Smith, R. T., and D. V. Eitzman. 1964. Ibid. 33:163-183.
26. Steiner, M. L., and H. A. Pearson. 1966. J. Pediatr. 68:562-568.
27. Stiehm, E. R., and H. H. Fudenberg. 1966. Pediatrics 37:715-727.
28. Uhr, J. W., et al. 1960. Nature (London) 187:1130-1131.
29. Uhr, J. W., et al. 1962. J. Clin. Invest. 41:1509-1513.

62. MECHANISMS OF IMMUNODEFICIENCY

Table adapted from Horowitz, S., and R. Hong, 1977, *The Pathogenesis and Treatment of Immunodeficiency*, S. Karger, Basel.

	Type of Failure	Level or Site of Defect	Fault	Clinical Disease
1	Differentiation (Central organ problem)	Yolk sac, fetal liver, or bone marrow	Inability to generate hemato-poietic & lymphopoietic stem cells	Reticular dysgenesis
2		Fetal liver, bone marrow	Inability to generate lympho-poietic stem cells	Combined immunodeficiency
3		Thymus: Whole gland	T-cell deficiency, with variable B-cell effect	DiGeorge; cartilage hair; Nezelof
4		T-cell subpopulation	T suppressors overactive	Common variable
5			T helper	Selective IgA deficiencies; combined IgA & IgG deficiency; cartilage hair; DiGeorge; Nezelof
6		"Bursa"[1]; non-bursal differentiation site	Lack of B-cells; immature B-cells	Bruton's; sporadic immunodeficiency; some common variable
7		Thymosin	T-cell deficiency, with variable B-cell effect	Various T deficiencies; possibly cancer; systemic lupus erythematosus
8	Maturation (Ineffective but partially differentiated T or B cell)	Surface receptors[2]	Unable to receive or process triggering signals	Wiskott-Aldrich; mucocutaneous candidiasis; selective subgroup deficiency
9			Unable to interact in lympho-cyte-macrophage collaboration	Intrinsic macrophage defect
10		Structural or regulatory gene	Intracellular assembly or se-cretion	Selective Ig deficiencies; IgA defect; myeloma[3]; other lymphoid malignancy
11		Extracellular assembly	Failure to combine secretory component with IgA	Protein calorie malnutrition; sudden infant death
12			Failure to synthesize secre-tory component[4]	....

[1] The human counterpart of this avian organ may not exist, but the fetal liver has been postulated as a mammalian homologue. [2] Due to Ir gene defect. [3] Heavy-or light-chain disease. [4] A disease has been described implicating failure of secretory component synthesis, but has not been named [3].

continued

	Type of Failure	Level or Site of Defect	Fault	Clinical Disease
13		Inappropriate homeostasis	T suppressors overactive	Protein calorie malnutrition; sudden infant death
14			Excess feedback of antibody	No disease yet known
15			α-fetoprotein excess	Tumor establishment
16	Traffic	Pre-differentiation	Failure to develop T- & B-cells	Combined immunodeficiency
17		Post-differentiation	Failure to achieve T-B interaction in lymphoid collections	Some selective IgA deficiencies
18			Failure to "peripheralize"	Some selective IgA deficiencies
19	Amplification	T lymphocyte mediators	Macrophage migration inhibition factor deficiency	Chronic mucocutaneous candidiasis
20		B cell	Complement deficiency	C3 disorders
21	Environmental	All lymphoid tissues	Purine-pyrimidine metabolism	Adenosine deaminase deficiency; hypoxanthine phosphoribosyltransferase[5] deficiency
22			Malnutrition	Iron deficiency; protein calorie malnutrition
23			Autoimmunity	Associated with systemic lupus erythematosus & other autoimmune states; anti-mu
24			Lymphotoxin	Episodic lymphopenia
25			Viruses	Antibody-associated lymphotoxin deficiency secondary to cytomegalovirus, Epstein-Barr virus, hepatitis, rubella
26			Excessive loss	Intestinal lymphangiectasis; other protein-losing enteropathy; nephrosis
27			Various inhibitors	Uremia; malignancy

[5] Synonym: Nucleoside phosphorylase.

Contributor: Hong, Richard

References
1. Cooper, M. D., et al. 1973. Transplant. Rev. 16:51-84.
2. Good, R. A. 1972. Clin. Immunobiol. 1:1-28.
3. Strober, W., et al. 1976. N. Engl. J. Med. 294:351-356.

63. REPRESENTATIVE HISTOCOMPATIBILITY LEUKOCYTE ANTIGEN GENE FREQUENCIES IN CAUCASIANS

The locus HLA-C has been identified, and five alleles (HLA-Cw1 through 5) designated. **Gene Symbol: New** refers to nomenclature agreed upon in July 1975.

	Gene Symbol		Frequency				Gene Symbol		Frequency	
	New	Previous	Phenotype	Genotype			New	Previous	Phenotype	Genotype
	A Locus[1]					8	HLA-Aw19[2]	W19	0.348	0.176
						9	Blank[3]	....	.....	0.027
1	HLA-A1	HL-A1	0.224	0.130			B Locus[4]			
2	HLA-A2	HL-A2	0.451	0.259						
3	HLA-A3	HL-A3	0.240	0.128		10	HLA-B5[2]	HL-A5	0.143	0.074
4	HLA-A9[2]	HL-A9	0.247	0.132		11	HLA-B7	HL-A7	0.224	0.119
5	HLA-A10[2]	HL-A10	0.117	0.060		12	HLA-B8	HL-A8	0.156	0.081
6	HLA-A11	HL-A11	0.094	0.048		13	HLA-B12	HL-A12	0.295	0.161
7	HLA-A28	W28	0.078	0.040		14	HLA-B13	HL-A13	0.036	0.018

[1] Previously called LA (or first). [2] Complex specificities; many specificities are included. [3] Refers to caucasians who have no histocompatibility leukocyte antigens. [4] Previously called FOUR (or second).

continued

63. REPRESENTATIVE HISTOCOMPATIBILITY LEUKOCYTE ANTIGEN GENE FREQUENCIES IN CAUCASIANS

	Gene Symbol		Frequency				Gene Symbol		Frequency	
	New	Previous	Phenotype	Genotype			New	Previous	Phenotype	Genotype
15	HLA-B14	W14	0.086	0.043		20	HLA-Bw22	W22	0.055	0.028
16	HLA-B18	W18	0.179	0.091		21	HLA-Bw35[2]	W5	0.149	0.078
17	HLA-B27	W27	0.056	0.029		22	HLA-Bw40	W10	0.090	0.046
18	HLA-Bw15	W15	0.084	0.043		23	Blank[3]		....	.....	0.155
19	HLA-Bw17	W17	0.062	0.032						

[2] Complex specificities; many specificities are included. [3] Refers to caucasians who have no histocompatibility leukocyte antigens.

Contributor: Borzy, Michael

General References

1. Amos, D. B., et al. 1975. Bull. WHO 52:261-265.
2. Bodmer, J., et al. 1975. In F. Kissmeyer-Nielsen, ed. Histocompatibility Testing, 1975. E. Munksgaard, Copenhagen. pp. 21-99.

64. HISTOCOMPATIBILITY LEUKOCYTE ANTIGENS AND DISEASE ASSOCIATION

HLA = histocompatibility leukocyte antigens. **Relative Risk** = ad/bc, where a = number of patients with antigen, b = number of patients without antigen, c = number of controls with antigen, d = number of controls without antigen.

Values were calculated from data in references. For additional information, consult references 1, 6, 8, 9, 11, and 12.

	Disease	HLA	Relative Risk	Reference			Disease	HLA	Relative Risk	Reference
	Arthropathies					15		B8	10.1	5
1	Ankylosing spondylitis	B27	120.9	5		16		Dw3	200	3
2	Reiter's syndrome	B27	40.3	5		17	Chronic active hepatitis	A1	2.08	5
	Arthritis					18		B8	3.6	5
3	Juvenile rheumatoid[1]	B27	17.9	3			Endocrine disease			
4	Psoriatic	B27	4.7	5		19	Addison's disease	B8	7.0	10
5	Rheumatoid	B13	1.96	5		20		Dw3	10.5	10
6		Bw40	1.68	5		21	Diabetes mellitus[4]	B8	2.1	5
7		Dw4	3.0	7		22		Bw15	3.0	5
8	Reactive[2]	B27	.....	5		23		Dw3	4.5	10
9	Eye disease: acute anterior uveitis	B27	23.6	5		24	Graves' disease	B8	3.55	5
	Skin disease					25		Dw3	4.0	4
10	Psoriasis vulgaris	B13	5.0	5			Neuromuscular disease			
11		Bw17	4.8	5		26	Myasthenia gravis	B8	4.45	5
12	Pemphigus	A10	3.14	5		27	Multiple sclerosis	A3	1.63	5
13	Dermatitis herpetiformis	B8	4.3	5		28		B7	1.43	5
	Gastrointestinal disease					29		B18	1.78	5
14	Celiac sprue[3]	A1	4.16	5		30		Dw2	5.0	2

[1] Pauciarticular type in males only. [2] Associated with *Yersinia*, *Salmonella*, and *Shigella* infections. [3] Adult and child. [4] Insulin-dependent.

Contributor: Borzy, Michael

continued

References

1. Dausset, J., et al. 1974. Clin. Immunol. Immuno-pathol. 3:127-149.
2. Jersild, C., et al. 1975. Transplant. Rev. 22:148-163.
3. Keuning, J. J., et al. 1976. Lancet 1:506-507.
4. McDevitt, H. O., and W. F. Bodmer. 1974. Lancet 1:1269-1275.
5. McMichael, A. J., et al. 1975. In F. Kissmeyer-Nielsen, ed. Histocompatibility Testing, 1975. E. Munksgaard, Copenhagen. pp. 769-772.
6. Ryder, L. P., et al. 1974. Humangenetik 25:251-264.
7. Schaller, J. G., and G. S. Omenn. 1976. J. Pediatr. 88:913-925.
8. Schaller, J. G., et al. 1976. Ibid. 88:926-930.
9. Stastny, P. 1974. Tissue Antigens 4:571-579.
10. Svejgaard, A., et al. 1975. Transplant. Rev. 22:343.
11. Thomsen, M., et al. 1975. Ibid. 22:125-147.
12. Vladutiu, A. O., and N. R. Rose. 1974. Immunogenetics 1:305-328.

65. GRAFT-VERSUS-HOST REACTIONS

Data have been adapted from reference 1 in Part I.

Part I. Clinical Grades of Graft-Versus-Host Disease

Grade is a clinical estimate of severity, with increasing mortality and poorer response to therapy as grade IV is approached.

	Organ Systems	Grade I	Grade II	Grade III	Grade IV
		Clinical Signs			
1	Skin	Mild	Severe	Severe	Exfoliation
2	Gastrointestinal tract	None	Mild diarrhea, nausea, emesis, malabsorption	More severe than grade II	Very severe
3	Liver	None	Slight elevation of aspartate aminotransferase ⟨SGOT⟩, bilirubin, alkaline phosphatase	More severe than grade II	Very severe
4	Clinical performance	No impairment	No impairment	Moderate impairment	Marked impairment
		Histological Signs			
5	Skin	Mostly basal cells involved	Spongiosis, dyskeratosis	Dermo-epidermal separation	Epidermal loss
6	Gastrointestinal tract	Mucous gland dilation & degeneration	Mucous gland loss	Mucosal denudation	Diffuse mucosal dilation
7	Liver	Less than 25% bile duct involvement	25-49% bile duct involvement	50-74% bile duct involvement	Greater than 75% bile duct involvement

Contributor: Hong, Richard

References

1. Slavin, R. E., and G. W. Santos. 1973. Clin. Immunol. Immunopathol. 1:472-498.
2. Storb, R., et al. 1974. Blood 44:56-75.

continued

Part II. Aggressor Lymphocyte Destructive Lesions

Pathological stages should not be confused with clinical grades (Part I), and do not necessarily correlate in any way (e.g., a patient having florid skin disease as his only manifestation of graft-versus-host reaction ⟨GVHR⟩ quite likely would not be classified as other than clinical grade I.) Clinical grading takes into account the number of organ systems involved and the whole general clinical status, whereas pathological stages indicate the degree of progression of of the GVHR in a given organ system. Figures in heavy brackets are reference numbers.

Tissues	Pathological Stages		Quiescent
	Early	Florid	
Lesions Involving Squamous Epithelia of Skin, Tongue, & Esophagus[1]			
1 Gross appearance[2]	Focal erythematous maculo-papular rash, frequently beginning on abdomen or chest [1]	Diffuse erythematous maculo-papular rash with desquamation [1] & occasional bullae [1,4]. Alopecia.	Thin, parchment-like, bronze-hued skin. Alopecia.
Microscopic changes[3]			
2 Epidermis & pilosebaceous units	Prominent liquefaction or hydropic degeneration of basal layer, with focal microvesicle formation [1-4]. Focal discrete coagulation necrosis of basal & malpighian layer cells as well as melanocytes [1,2,4,5]. Satellite lymphocytes adjacent to degenerate & necrotic epithelial cells [2,5]. Intercellular edema (spongiosis) [5].	Prominent coagulation necrosis of cells of basal & malpighian layers & melanocytes [1,5]. Single or small groups of acantholytic necrotic epithelial cells within intraepithelial lacunae (mummified cells[4]) [5]. Focal liquefaction degeneration of basal epithelial cells. Satellite lymphocytes adjacent to degenerate & necrotic epithelial cells [2,5]. Intercellular edema. Occasional intraepithelial bullae [4]. Ragged & indistinct epidermal-dermal junction secondary to loss of basal cells [1].	Focal loss of basal cells [1]. Epidermal atrophy [1,2]. Isolated mummified cells[4] in epidermis [1]. Focal separation of epidermis from dermis. Hyperkeratosis. Intercellular edema. Loss of pilosebaceous units [1,2,4].
3 Dermis ⟨corium⟩ or submucosa	Perivascular lymphoid infiltrates in upper dermis or submucosa, with beginning migration to epidermis [1,3-5]. Occasional severe edema of dermal papillae or upper submucosa [1].	Focal or diffuse subepithelial infiltrates (lymphoid cells, macrophages, eosinophils) [3]. Mummified cells[4] in upper dermis & submucosa free or phagocytosed by macrophages [1]. Free or phagocytosed melanin pigment in upper dermis. Sweat glands spared.	Inflammatory infiltrate disappears [1]. Occasional mummified cells[4] in upper dermis or upper submucosa. Phagocytosed mummified cells & melanin. Dilated lymphatics. Occasional marked thickening of dermis.
Lesions Involving Liver			
4 Gross appearance	No discernible abnormalities	No discernible abnormalities or tiny flecks of yellow necrosis [1]	No discernible abnormality
Microscopic changes			
5 Portal triads	Focal minimal lymphoid infiltrates, consisting primarily of large lymphocytes ⟨lymphoblasts⟩ & medium-sized lymphocytes [5]	Patchy, mild to moderate cellular infiltrates, consisting primarily of lymphocytes admixed with macrophages & transient eosinophils [1-4]. "Moth-eaten" limiting plate. Regenerating tubules of cells [1]. Necrosis of bile duct epithelium[5] [1,5].	Minimal or no inflammatory infiltrates. Occasional "moth-eaten" limiting plates. Occasional tubules of regenerating cells [1].

[1] In quiescent stage, lesions may be complicated by superimposed infections, primarily viral. [2] As seen in the skin. [3] Some changes in the skin are caused by conditioning regimens involving high-dose chemotherapy or X-radiation.

[4] A necrotic, shrunken, rounded epithelial cell, with a laminated eosinophilic cytoplasm and a pyknotic or absent nucleus located in the epidermis, upper dermis, and submucosa. [5] Not seen in this series.

continued

Part II. Aggressor Lymphocyte Destructive Lesions

	Tissues	Pathological Stages		Quiescent
		Early	Florid	
6	Parenchyma	Randomly distributed minute zones of coagulation necrosis of hepatocytes & Kupffer cells associated with lymphoid cells [1,2,5]. Focal Kupffer cell hyperplasia. Disassociation of liver cell plates[6]. Mitosis of hepatocytes [1,5].	Small or large foci of coagulation necrosis of hepatocytes & Kupffer cells [1,4]. Periportal piecemeal necrosis of parenchymal cells. Distended canals of Hering. Acidophilic bodies[7] in sinusoids [1,4]. Kupffer cell hyperplasia & hypertrophy, focal Kupffer cells containing phagocytosed necrotic parenchymal cells, iron & bile pigments, & red cells. Mitosis of hepatocytes [1,2].	Rare acidophilic bodies[7] in sinusoids. Occasional dilated canals of Hering. Foci of Kupffer cell hyperplasia.

Lesions Involving Small & Large Intestines[8]

	Tissues	Early / Florid	Quiescent
7	Gross appearance	No discernible lesions admixed with occasional small superficial erosions [1]	No discernible lesions from GVHR itself, but frequent complicating lesions[9]
	Microscopic changes		
8	Intestinal glands	Granular necrosis of glandular epithelium, primarily within crypts; focal, involving scattered glands; local, involving a few epithelial cells at any given moment within an individual gland [1,2,4,5]. Lymphoid cells, some showing cytokaryorrhexis, adjacent to glandular basement membrane & among crypt epithelial cells [2,5]. Ghost glands[10] [5]. Lesions, randomly distributed but most common in ileum & colon [1,5].	Stretches of mucosa, depopulated of glands (with focal loss of villi in small intestines) [1,2,4,5]. Scattered cystically dilated glands lined by flattened non-specific epithelium containing cellular debris within their lumina [1,2,5].
9	Lamina propria	Leukocyte-depopulated lamina propria patchily infiltrated by lymphoid cells, initially large (lymphoblasts) & medium-sized lymphocytes followed by small lymphocytes, macrophages, & plasma cells [1,5]. Lymphoid infiltrates most common adjacent to lymphoid aggregates in ileum & colon. Leukocytorrhexis in blood vessels & within lamina propria proper.	Almost total depletion of all lymphoid cells & other leukocytes [1]. Only cells present are those of the intrinsic cellular reticulum admixed with an occasional macrophage.

[6] Presumed related to chemotherapy. [7] Mummified liver cells, round smoky-red-to-orange bodies, frequently showing miniscule vacuoles, found extruded in sinusoids. [8] No distinction made between early and florid stages. [9] Ulcerations, necrosis, membranous enterocolitis associated with superimposed viral infections. [10] Non-collapsed glandular basement membranes depopulated of all glandular cells.

Contributor: Slavin, Richard E.

References
1. Bekkum, D. W. van, and M. J. de Vries. 1967. Radiation Chimaeras. Academic Press, New York.
2. Chomette, G., et al. 1970. Virchows Arch. A349:98-114.
3. Kersey, J. H., et al. 1971. Hum. Pathol. 2:389-402.
4. Krüger, G. R. F., et al. 1971. Am. J. Pathol. 63:179-202.
5. Woodruff, J. M., et al. 1969. Lab. Invest. 20:499-511.

66. KIDNEY TRANSPLANTS

Part I. Donor Source

	Year	No. of Transplants	Donor Source, %					Year	No. of Transplants	Donor Source, %			
			Cadaver	Parent	Sibling	Other				Cadaver	Parent	Sibling	Other
1	1970	1943	69.1	14.3	14.7	1.9	3	1972	3313	67.5	13.2	16.4	2.9
2	1971	2812	68.2	12.9	15.9	3.0	4	1973	3072	70.4	12.7	14.4	2.5

Contributor: Borzy, Michael

Reference: Advisory Committee to the Renal Transplant Registry. 1975. J. Am. Med. Assoc. 233:787-796.

continued

66. KIDNEY TRANSPLANTS

Part II. Donor Source and Graft Transplant Survival

	Donor Source	Year of Transplant	No. of Patients	Survival, %			
				1 yr	2 yr	3 yr	4 yr
1	Sibling	1970	266	81.1 ± 2.4	78.2 ± 2.6	72.8 ± 2.9	69.6 ± 3.3
2		1971	406	73.7 ± 2.2	69.6 ± 2.3	67.7 ± 2.5	....
3		1972	447	79.9 ± 1.9	73.7 ± 2.5	....	....
4	Parent	1970	261	73.8 ± 2.7	68.3 ± 2.9	62.3 ± 3.1	57.3 ± 3.6
5		1971	326	73.7 ± 2.4	66.8 ± 2.7	62.3 ± 3.1	....
6		1972	359	71.7 ± 2.4	61.1 ± 3.1	....	....
7	Cadaver	1970	1147	55.3 ± 1.5	47.2 ± 1.5	42.0 ± 1.5	40.6 ± 1.6
8		1971	1559	53.1 ± 1.3	45.7 ± 1.3	41.8 ± 1.4	....
9		1972	1707	50.6 ± 1.2	42.6 ± 1.4	....	....

Contributor: Borzy, Michael

Reference: Advisory Committee to the Renal Transplant Registry. 1975. J. Am. Med. Assoc. 233:787-796.

Part III. Cadaver Transplant Survival

Graft Survival: **Grade 4**: Both sets of antigens at HLA-A and HLA-B match. **Grade 3a**: Two B and one A antigens match. **Grade 3b**: One B and two A antigens match. **Grade 2 or less**: At most two antigens match.

	Specification	Graft Survival, %		
		Grades 4 & 3a	Grade 3b	Grade 2 or less
1	All transplants in series[1]	46	37	26
	Influence of Previous Transplant[2]			
2	First transplant only	46	35	30
3	Previously transplanted[3]	64	...	28
	Influence of Tissue Type[4]			
4	HLA-D identical[5]	85[6]	...	...
5	HLA-D incompatible[7]	47[8]	...	...
	Influence of Previous Blood Transfusion[2]			
6	No previous blood transfusion	32	...	...
7	Previous blood transfusion	62	...	...

[1] 502 transplants. [2] 42 months after transplant. [3] Or cytotoxic antibodies present. [4] 18 months after transplant. [5] Less than 10% stimulation of donor cells in mixed leukocyte culture. [6] Value obtained from observation of 7 patients. [7] Greater than 25% stimulation of donor cells in mixed leukocyte culture. [8] Value obtained from observation of 21 patients.

Contributor: Borzy, Michael

Reference: Festenstein, H., et al. 1976. Lancet 1:157-161.

continued

66. KIDNEY TRANSPLANTS

Part IV. Mixed Leukocyte Reactivity and Graft Survival

Stimulation Index: <8 = negative reaction, and >8 = positive reaction, in two-way mixed leukocyte culture. **Adjusted Graft Survival:** Patients who died with normal renal function (serum creatinine <2 mg/dl) were not included in figuring percentage.

Subjects		Stimulation Index	Graft Survival %	Adjusted Graft Survival %
Condition	No.			
Related Donors				
1 All patients in series[1]	56	<8	83	91
2	3	>8	0	0
3 2-yr survivors	31	<8	80	92
Cadavers				
4 All patients in series[1]	85	<8	76	88
5	53	>8	32	33
6 2-yr survivors	28	<8	71	87
7	21	>8	23	23

[1] Time of observation: 6 months to 3 years.

Contributor: Borzy, Michael

Reference: Cochrum, K. C., et al. 1974. Ann. Surg. 180:617-622.

67. RESULTS OF BONE MARROW TRANSPLANTS

Part I. In Acute Leukemia

Data were adapted from reference 1. **Specification:** Fatal GVH = death from graft-versus-host disease; At risk = any survivor who has lived 100 or more days after transplantation.

Transplant Center	Conditioning	Specification	No.	Reference
1 Baltimore	Cyclophosphamide	Patients	20	5
2		Grafts	17	
3		Fatal GVH	1	
4		Recurrence At risk	13	
5		Cases	9 [70%]	
6		Symptom-free survivors	1 [4%]	
7		Survival time	7 mo	
8		Deaths from causes other than leukemia	3	
9 National	Cyclophosphamide	Patients	9	3
10 Cancer		Grafts	8	
11 Institute		Fatal GVH	1	
12		Recurrence At risk	5	
13		Cases	5 [100%]	
14		Symptom-free survivors	0 [0%]	

continued

Part I. In Acute Leukemia

	Transplant Center	Conditioning	Specification	No.	Reference
15		Total body irradiation	Patients	2	
16			Grafts	1	
17			Fatal GVH	1	
18			Recurrence	0	
19			Symptom-free survivors	0	
20		Cyclophosphamide & total body irradiation	Patients	5	
21			Grafts	3	
22			Fatal GVH	0	
			Recurrence		
23			At risk	3	
24			Cases	0 [0%]	
25			Symptom-free survivors	0 [0%]	
26			Deaths from causes other than leukemia	3	
27		BACT regimen (1,3-bis(2-chloroethyl)-1-nitrosourea ⟨BCNU⟩, arabinosyl-cytosine[1], cyclophosphamide, & 6-thioguanine)	Patients	5	
28			Grafts	5	
29			Fatal GVH	0	
			Recurrence		
30			At risk	4	
31			Cases	2 [50%]	
32			Symptom-free survivors	1 [14%]	
33			Survival time	36 mo	
34			Deaths from causes other than leukemia	1	
35	Seattle	Cyclophosphamide & total body irradiation	Patients[2]	16	2,4,6,
36			Grafts	16	7
37			Fatal GVH	0	
			Recurrence		
38			At risk	11	
39			Cases	4 [36%]	
40			Symptom-free survivors	6 [38%]	
41			Survival time	2-44 mo	
42			Deaths from causes other than leukemia	1	
43		Total body irradiation or cyclophosphamide & total body irradiation	Patients	68	
44			Grafts	63	
45			Fatal GVH	23	
			Recurrence		
46			At risk	41	
47			Cases	20 [50%]	
48			Symptom-free survivors	19 [28%]	
49			Survival time	3-49 mo	
50			Deaths from causes other than leukemia	2	
51	University of California at Los Angeles	Cyclophosphamide	Patients	1	1
52			Grafts	1	
53			Fatal GVH	0	
			Recurrence		
54			At risk	1	
55			Cases	1 [100%]	
56			Symptom-free survivors	0 [0%]	
57			Survival time	4 mo	
58		Cyclophosphamide & total body irradiation	Patients	5	
59			Grafts	5	
60			Fatal GVH	0	

[1] Synonym: Cytosine arabinoside. [2] Identical twins.

continued

67. RESULTS OF BONE MARROW TRANSPLANTS

Part I. In Acute Leukemia

	Transplant Center	Conditioning	Specification	No.	Reference
61			Recurrence		
62			At risk	3	
63			Cases	2 [66%]	
64			Symptom-free survivors	1 [20%]	
			Survival time	20 mo	
65		SCARI regimen (6-thioguanine,	Patients	8	
66		cyclophosphamide, arabinosyl-	Grafts	8	
67		cytosine [1]/, daunomycin [3]/, &	Fatal GVH	0	
		total body irradiation)	Recurrence		
68			At risk	8	
69			Cases	1 [12%]	
70			Symptom-free survivors	7 [90%]	
71			Survival time	2-7 mo	

[1]/ Synonym: Cytosine arabinoside. [3]/ Synonyms: Rubidomycin; Daunorubicin.

Contributor: Hong, Richard

References

1. Cline, M. J., et al. 1975. Ann. Intern. Med. 83:691-708.
2. Fefer, A., et al. 1974. N. Engl. J. Med. 290:1389-1393.
3. Graw, R. G., Jr., and G. P. Herzig. 1972. Schweiz. Med. Wochenschr. 102:1573-1581.
4. Powles, R. L., et al. 1971. Br. Med. J. 1:486-489.
5. Santos, G. W., et al. 1974. Transplant. Proc. 6:345-348.
6. Thomas, E. D., et al. 1957. N. Engl. J. Med. 257:491-496.
7. Thomas, E. D., et al. 1975. Ibid. 292:832-843, 895-902.

Part II. In Aplastic Anemia

Data were partially adapted from reference 3. **Fatal GVH**: Death from graft-versus-host disease.

	Center	Conditioning Program	Patients	Engraftment	Fatal GVH	Survivors	Reference
1	Baltimore	Cyclophosphamide	5	3	1	2	5
2	Boston	Cyclophosphamide	3	3	0	2	1
3		Antilymphocyte globulin	14	14	2	6	1
4	Cooperative	Cyclophosphamide; or cyclophosphamide, antilymphocyte globulin, & procarbazine	36	34	2	24	2
5	National Cancer	Antilymphocyte globulin	1	1	0	0	4
6	Institute	Plus total body irradiation	1	1	0	0	4
7		Cyclophosphamide	1	1	0	0	4
8	Seattle	Total body irradiation	8	7	2	1	6-8
9		Cyclophosphamide	27	26	8	15	6-8
10	UCLA	Cyclophosphamide	6	6	0	5	3

Contributor: Hong, Richard

continued

67. RESULTS OF BONE MARROW TRANSPLANTS

Part II. In Aplastic Anemia

References
1. Camitta, B. M., et al. 1975. Blood 45:355-363.
2. Camitta, B. M., et al. 1976. Ibid. 48:63-70.
3. Cline, M. J., et al. 1975. Ann. Intern. Med. 83:691-708.
4. Graw, R. G., Jr., and G. P. Herzig. 1972. Schweiz. Med. Wochenschr. 102:1573-1581.
5. Santos, G. W., et al. 1974. Transplant. Proc. 6:345-348.
6. Storb, R., et al. 1974. Blood 43:157-180.
7. Thomas, E. D., et al. 1971. Exp. Hematol. 21:16-18.
8. Thomas, E. D., et al. 1975. N. Engl. J. Med. 292:832-843, 895-902.

Part III. In Immunodeficiency

Matching at HLA-D = non-proliferative response in mixed leukocyte culture.

	Disease	Donor	Matching at HLA-A & HLA-B	HLA-D	Trans- planted	Survivors	Remarks	Refer- ence
1	Combined immuno- deficiency	Sibling	Yes	Yes	52	22	18 have surviving grafts	2,4
2		Mother	No	Yes	1	1	Poor take; child now aplastic	7
3		Uncle	Identical	Yes	1	1	Full B and T cell take	9
4			No	Yes	1	1	Partial B cell take; full T cell take	6
5		Unrelated	Match at HLA-B only	Yes	1	1	B and T cell take after 8 transplants	8
6					1	0	Died at 30 days of cytomegalovirus pneumonia	5
7	Bruton agammaglob- ulinemia	Sibling	Yes	Yes	3	3	No benefit	2
8	Wiscott-Aldrich	Sibling	Yes	Yes	2	1	"Cure" in survivor	1
9	Ataxia-telangiectasia	Sibling	Yes	Yes	1	1	No chimerism. IgA became normal. Neurological status unchanged.	3

Contributor: Hong, Richard

References
1. Bach, F. H., et al. 1968. Lancet 2:1364-1366.
2. Buckley, R. H. 1971. Prog. Immunol. 1:1061-1080.
3. Buckley, R. H. 1975. Birth Defects Orig. Artic. Ser. 11(1):421-424.
4. Cline, M. J., et al. 1975. Ann. Intern. Med. 83:691-708.
5. Horowitz, S. D., et al. 1975. Lancet 2:431-433.
6. Koch, C., et al. 1973. Ibid. 1:1146-1149.
7. Niethammer, D., et al. 1976. Proc. 3rd Workshop Int. Coop. Group Bone Marrow Transplant., Tarrytown, NY.
8. O'Reilly, R. J., et al. 1976. Clin. Res. 24:482A.
9. Vossen, J. M., et al. 1973. Clin. Exp. Immunol. 13: 9-20.

Part IV. Circumvention of Graft-Versus-Host Reaction

All marrow donors were HLA-incompatible.

	Method	Attempts	Failures	Reference
1	Enchancement	10	10	2,4,7,8
2	Removal of immunoreactive cells Gradient separation [1/]	6	6	1,3,4,7
3	"Suicide" techniques [2/]	3	3	9,10

[1/] Stem cells enriched fraction obtained by albumin gradient. [2/] Immunoreactive cells removed by techniques designed to cause self-destruction.

continued

67. RESULTS OF BONE MARROW TRANSPLANTS

Part IV. Circumvention of Graft-Versus-Host Reaction

	Method	Attempts	Failures	Reference
4	Incubation of graft [3/]	2	2	1
5	Limitation of cell number	5	5	1,5
6	Chemotherapy after transplantation	2	2	6

[3/] Cell infusion incubated at 37°C, with or without antilymphocyte serum to destroy immunoreactive cells.

Contributor: Hong, Richard

References

1. Buckley, R. H. 1971. Prog. Immunol. 1:1061-1080.
2. Buckley, R. H., et al. 1971. N. Engl. J. Med. 285:1035-1042.
3. Dicke, K. A., et al. 1975. Birth Defects Orig. Artic. Ser. 11(1):391-396.
4. Gelfand, E. W., et al. 1974. Exp. Hematol. 2:122-130.
5. Huang, S. W., et al. 1973. Transplantation 15:174-176.
6. Meuwissen, H. J., et al. 1971. Am. J. Med. 51:513-532.
7. Park, B. H., et al. 1975. Birth Defects Orig. Artic. Ser. 11(1):380-384.
8. Rubenstein, A., et al. 1975. Ibid. 11(1):397-408.
9. Salmon, S. E., et al. 1970. Lancet 2:149-150.
10. Sieber, O., et al. 1974. Clin. Res. 22:230A.

68. RESULTS OF OTHER LYMPHOID REPLACEMENT THERAPY

Part I. Thymus Transplantation in Immunodeficiency

GVHR = graft-versus-host reaction. **Laboratory Findings**: **Chim** = chimerism; **PHA** = phytohemagglutinin; **MLC** = mixed leukocyte culture; **Ag** = antigen; **E-RFC** = E-rosette forming cells. *Abbreviations & Symbols*: + = present; 0 = absent; N = normal; ↑ = increased; ↓ = decreased; HLA = histocompatibility leukocyte antigens; PT = post-transplantation.

	Investigator	GVHR	Laboratory Findings						Clinical Status	Reference
			Chim	PHA	MLC	Ag	E-RFC	Skin Tests		
			Severe Combined Immunodeficiency ⟨SCID⟩							
1	Rachelefsky, et al.	Mild	+[1/];new HLA; ♂ karyotype	+[2/]; N[2/]	+[2/];N[2/]	..	↑	+	T-cell reconstitution. Chronic encephalopathy.	15
2	Ammann, et al.	Severe	+[3/]; new HLA	+[3/]; N[4/] ↓[5/]	N[6/]; ↓[5/]	..	...	0	Did well for 3 yr PT. Transient diarrhea at 3½ yr PT.	2
3	Shearer & Hong	Very severe	0	+[7,8/]	....	..	↑	0	Doing well 1½ yr PT	16
			Cellular Immunodeficiency with Immunoglobulin							
4	Ammann, et al.	0	0	+	+	..	...	....	Transient improvement	3
5		0	0	+	+	..	+	....	Satisfactory at 2½ yr PT	
6		0	0	0	0	..	...	....	No effect; died	
			DiGeorge Deficiency							
7	Biggar, et al.	0	0	+	....	..	...	....	Satisfactory	5
8	Steele, et al.	0	0	+	....	..	...	....	Died 9 days PT	17
9	August, et al.	0	0	+	....	+	...	....	Immunologic reconstitution; doing well	4

[1/] 3 mo PT. [2/] 3 wk PT. [3/] 4 mo PT. [4/] 9 mo PT. [5/] 3½ yr PT. [6/] 11 mo PT. [7/] 12 days PT. [8/] Stimulation index = 3 until 4 mo PT; no response from 4 mo until present.

continued

68. RESULTS OF OTHER LYMPHOID REPLACEMENT THERAPY

Part I. Thymus Transplantation in Immunodeficiency

	Investigator	GVHR	Laboratory Findings						Clinical Status	Reference
			Chim	PHA	MLC	Ag	E-RFC	Skin Tests		
10	Cleveland, et al.	0	0	+	....	+	...	....	Immunologic reconstitution; mental retardation	6
11	Gatti, et al.	0	0	+	+9/	+	...	....	Satisfactory	8
	Other T-Cell Defects 10/									
12	Aiuti, et al. 11/	0	0	+	....	..	+	....	Improved	1
13	Levy, et al. 11/	0	0	+	....	+	...	....	Transient improvement	14
14	Kirkpatrick & Gallin 11/	0	0	+	+	0	+	+12/	No effect	12,13
15	Foroozanfar, et al.	0	0	+	+	..	+	....	Satisfactory	7
16	Jose, et al.	0	0	+	+	..	+	+	Transient improvement	11
17	Aiuti, et al.	0	0	+	+	..	+	+	Improved	1
18	Hong, et al.	0	+13/	+	+	0	...	.....	Transient improvement	10
19	Githens, et al.14/	0	0	0	....	..	...	....	No effect; died	9

9/ Before transplant. 10/ Does not include ataxia-telangiectasia or Wiskott-Aldrich syndrome. 11/ Cases of chronic mucocutaneous candidiasis. 12/ Became negative 9 mo after transplant; became positive again after transfer factor. 13/ Transient. 14/ Two cases.

Contributor: Horowitz, Sheldon

References

1. Aiuti, F., et al. 1975. Birth Defects Orig. Artic. Ser. 11(1):370-376.
2. Ammann, A. J., et al. 1973. N. Engl. J. Med. 289(1):5-9.
3. Ammann, A. J., et al. 1975. Transplantation 20:457-466.
4. August, C. S., et al. 1968. Lancet 2:1210-1211.
5. Biggar, W. D., et al. 1975. Birth Defects Orig. Artic. Ser. 11(1):361-366.
6. Cleveland, W. W., et al. 1968. Lancet 2:1211-1214.
7. Foroozanfar, N., et al. 1975. Br. Med. J. 1:314-315.
8. Gatti, R. A., et al. 1972. J. Pediatr. 81:920-926.
9. Githens, J. H., et al. 1973. Transplantation 15:427-434.
10. Hong, R., et al. 1972. Clin. Immunol. Immunopathol. 1:15-26.
11. Jose, D. G., et al. 1974. Aust. N.Z. J. Med. 4:267-273.
12. Kirkpatrick, C. H. Unpublished. N.I.A.I.D., National Institutes of Health, Bethesda, MD, 1976.
13. Kirkpatrick, C. H., and J. I. Gallin. 1975. Cell. Immunol. 15:470-474.
14. Levy, R. L., et al. 1971. Lancet 2:898-900.
15. Rachelefsky, G. S., et al. 1975. Pediatrics 55:114-118.
16. Shearer, W. T., and R. Hong. Unpublished. Univ. Wisconsin Medical Center, Madison, 1976.
17. Steele, R. W., et al. 1972. N. Engl. J. Med. 287:787-791.

Part II. Fetal Liver Transplantation

All cases were diagnosed as having severe combined immunodeficiency. **ADA** = adenosine deaminase. **GVHR** = graft-versus-host reaction. **Laboratory Findings: Chim** = chimerism; **T-Cell Reconstitution**—E-R = E-rosettes, PHA =

continued

Part II. Fetal Liver Transplantation

phytohemagglutinin, Con A = concanavalin A, PWM = pokeweed mitogen. *Abbreviations & Symbols*: + = present or
positive; ± = minimal and transient; − = negative; 0 = absent; ↑ = increased; PT = post-transplantation.

	Investi-gator	ADA	Transplant	GVHR	Chim	T-Cell Reconstitution	B-Cell Reconstitution	Clinical Status	Reference
1	Rieger, et al.	+	3.7 ×10⁶ cells, i.p., from 1.7-cm, 4- to 5-wk fetus, at 5 mo of age	+[1]	?	+: ↑ total E-R, normal in vitro responses to allogeneic cells & *Candida*, significantly ↑ response to PHA & PWM	0	Normal height & weight. Doing well 15 mo PT. Fluctuating skin rash, alopecia, & eosinophilia.	4
2	Buckley, et al.	+	3.8 × 10⁸ cells, i.p., from 9-wk fetus, at 11 mo of age	+[2]	0	↑ total E-R	0	No change. Died of chronic pulmonary disease 10 mo PT.	2
3		+	8 × 10⁷ cells, i.p., from 8-wk fetus, at 13 mo of age	+[2]	+	+: ↑ total E-R, normal in vitro responses to PHA, Con A, & PWM; positive *Candida* skin test	+: Normal IgM, no IgA or IgG, no functional antibody	Clearing of oral candidiasis. Doing well 23 mo PT.	
4	Keightley, et al.	−	2.5 × 10⁸ cells, i.p., from 4.2-cm, 8.5-wk fetus, at 3 mo of age	±[2]	+	+: ↑ lymphocyte count, ↑ total E-R, normal in vitro response to mitogens, allogeneic cells, & *Candida*	+: B lymphocytes & serum IgG, IgM, & IgA present; poor antibody response to φX 174 & *Salmonella typhi*	Did well for 12 mo. Died of nephrotic syndrome secondary to immune complex nephritis 15 mo PT.	3
5	Ackeret, et al.	−	1.23 × 10⁹ cells, (liver & thymus), i.v., from 12-wk fetus, at 7½ mo of age	?	?	+: Normal B- and T-cell function post-transplant; rapid decline of immune function 18 mo PT		Did well until 18 mo PT. Died suddenly after viral infection.	1

[1] 3 wk post-transplant to present. [2] 7-10 wk post-transplant.

Contributor: Horowitz, Sheldon

References
1. Ackeret, C., et al. 1976. Pediatr. Res. 10:67-70.
2. Buckley, R. H., et al. 1976. N. Engl. J. Med. 294:1076-1081.
3. Keightley, R. G., et al. 1975. Lancet 2:850-853.
4. Rieger, C. H. L., et al. 1970. Fed. Proc. 35:791(Abstr. 3225).

Part III. Effects of Thymosin Treatment

E-R Assay = in vitro total E-rosette assay with thymosin;
+ = positive, − = negative, ± = equivocal. **In Vivo Effect of Thymosin**: ↑ = increased; ↓ = decrease(d); E-R = E-rosettes;
PHA = phytohemagglutinin; MLC = mixed leukocyte culture; Con A = concanavalin A; PWM = pokeweed mitogen.

	Investigator	Age	Sex	Duration of Therapy	E-R Assay	In Vivo Effect of Thymosin	Reference
		Patients					
		Severe Combined Immunodeficiency ⟨SCID⟩					
1	Griscelli	4 mo	♂	4 wk	+[1]	No change	2
2	Seeger	7 mo	♂	3 wk	−	No change	2

[1] Response also with hemolyzed erythrocytes.

continued

68. RESULTS OF OTHER LYMPHOID REPLACEMENT THERAPY

Part III. Effects of Thymosin Treatment

	Investigator	Patients		Duration of Therapy	E-R Assay	In Vivo Effect of Thymosin	Reference
		Age	Sex				
3	Goldman	10 mo	♂	18 d	−	No change. Thymosin stopped because of skin reaction. Developed hepatitis post-therapy.	2
4		11 mo	♂	1 mo	−	No change.	
5	August	1 yr	♀	2½ mo	+	No ↑ in T-cell marker or function. Clearing of *Pneumocystis* pneumonia.	2
	Cellular Immunodeficiency with Immunoglobulin						
6	Hill	8 mo	♂	1 mo	+	↑ total E-R. Clearing of *Pneumocystis* pneumonia. Child died; evidence of hepatitis at autopsy.	2
7	Reid	2½ yr	♂[2/]	2 mo	+	Clinical improvement. ↑ total E-R. + *Candida*, tetanus, & diphtheria skin tests. Lymphopenia persists.	2
8	Goldman	6 yr	♂	5 wk	±	Possible ↓ in total E-R. Possible ↑ lymphocyte blastogenesis. Disappearance of IgG (κ) gammopathy.	2
9	Wara, et al.	6 yr	♀	>21 mo	+	Normal IgG (no antibodies following immunization); no change in IgM & IgA. ↑ total E-R & PHA response; no MLC reactivity. + mumps & *Candida* skin tests. ↓ infections & diarrhea; weight gain.	3
10	August	11 yr	♂	2 d	+	+ skin tests to mumps & streptokinase-streptodornase. Treatment terminated due to hives at injection site.	2
	T-Cell Deficiency						
11	Griscelli	3 mo	♂[3/]	>3 mo	+	Clinical improvement; ↓ infections. ↑ total E-R; in vitro response to PHA, Con A, PWM. + PHA skin test.	2
12	Ammann & Wara	5 yr	♀[4/]	8 mo	+	No change in Ig. ↑ total E-R, PHA, & MLC response. No + skin tests. Clinical improvement. Thymosin stopped due to sensitization.	1
	Ataxia-Telangiectasia						
13	Ammann & Wara	4 yr	♂	3 mo	+	Skin test conversion. ↑ total E-R. No change in PHA or MLC response. No change in clinical status.	1
14	Waldman	6 yr	♀	5 mo	+	↑ total E-R. ↑ MLC reactivity. ↑ response to PWM & Con A. + tetanus skin test.	2
15		7 yr	♀	5 mo	+	↑ total E-R	
16		9 yr	♀	10 mo	+	↑ total E-R. ↑ total lymphocytes.	
	Wiskott-Aldrich Syndrome						
17	Ammann &	11 yr	♂	11 mo	+	↑ total E-R. Normal PHA response; ↑ MLC reactivity. Eczema improved. ↓ Herpes stomatitis; ↓ bacterial infections.	1

[2/] Adenosine deaminase negative. [3/] Partial DiGeorge deficiency. [4/] Nucleoside phosphorylase deficiency.

Contributor: Horowitz, Sheldon

References

1. Ammann, A. J., and D. W. Wara. Modulation of Host Resistance in the Prevention and Treatment of Induced Neoplasias. In press, 1976.

2. Goldstein, A. L., et al. 1976. Med. Clin. North Am. 60(3):591-606.

3. Wara, D. W., et al. 1975. N. Engl. J. Med. 292:70-74.

69. IMMUNOPATHOLOGIC MECHANISMS

Classification of hypersensitivity disorders for types I-V is according to Gell and Coombs [ref. 16]. **Major Ig Immune Response**: LATS = long-acting thyroid stimulator. **Mediator or Mechanism of Inflammation**: SRS-A = slow reactive substance of anaphylaxis. **Major Inflammatory Cells**: PMN = polymorphonuclear leukocyte(s). *Symbol*: Asterisk (*) indicates relevant but not as frequent.

	Disease	Antigens	Major Ig Immune Response	Complement Consumption	Mediator or Mechanism of Inflammation	Major Inflammatory Cells	Major Organ Involved	Reference
	Type I: Anaphylactic Hypersensitivity							
1	Asthma	Pollens, dust, molds, drugs, animal dander	IgE	None	Histamine, SRS-A	Eosinophils, plasma cells	Lung	2
2	Allergic urticaria & allergic dermatitis[1]	Foods, drugs, chemicals	IgE	None	Histamine	*Eosinophils, *mast cells	Skin, larynx, oral pharynx, intestine	10
3	Anaphylactic shock	Drugs, serum	IgE; *IgG	None; *+	Histamine	None	Cardiovascular system, lung, larynx	6
	Type II: Cytotoxic-cytolytic Reactions							
4	Erythroblastosis fetalis	Rh blood group[2]	Maternal IgG	None	None	None	Fetal erythrocytes	13
5	Autoimmune cytolysis	Cell surface	IgG, IgM	Maybe	None	None	Blood cells	29
6	Hapten-induced cytolysis	Drugs, viruses, *haptens	IgG, IgM	Maybe	None	None	Blood cells	21
7	Innocent-bystander cytolysis	Drugs	IgG, IgM	Maybe	None	None	Blood cells	14
	Type III: Immune-Complex Reactions							
8	Acute proliferative glomerulonephritis	Bacteria[3], viruses	IgG, IgM; *IgA	++	C-chemotaxis	PMN	Kidney	18,28
9	Membranous glomerulonephritis	Chemical drugs, renal tubular brush border, malaria	IgG, IgM	+	?	None	Kidney	37
10	Lupus nephritis	Nuclear antigens, ? others	IgG, IgM, IgA; *IgE	+++	C-chemotaxis	PMN	Kidney	20
11	Hypersensitivity vasculitis	Drugs, chemicals	IgG, IgM	+	C-chemotaxis	PMN, eosinophils	Arterioles	33
12	Polyarteritis nodosa	Hepatitis virus, ? drugs	IgG, IgM	+	C-chemotaxis	PMN, eosinophils, lymphocytes	Medium-sized arteries; *veins	17
13	Serum sickness	Foreign serum (antigen excess)	IgG, IgM; *IgE	++	C-chemotaxis, C-anaphylatoxin, histamine	PMN, eosinophils	Cardiovascular system, kidney, joints	19
14	Arthus reaction	Foreign serum	IgG, IgM; (antibody excess)	++	C-chemotaxis, leukocyte factors	PMN	Skin; venules	1,7

[1] Synonym: Atopic eczema. [2] Also AB types. [3] Group A β-hemolytic *Streptococcus, Staphylococcus*, etc.

continued

	Disease	Antigens	Major Ig Immune Response	Complement Consumption	Mediator or Mechanism of Inflammation	Major Inflammatory Cells	Major Organ Involved	Reference
15	Nephrotoxic serum (Masugi) nephritis	Foreign serum immunoglobulins (anti-glomerular basement membrane)	IgG, IgM	++	C-chemotaxis	PMN	Kidney	41
	Autoaggressive antibody-mediated reactions							
16	Systemic lupus erythematosus	Nuclear antigens, cell surface antigens, cytoplasmic antigens, plasma proteins	IgG, IgM, IgA, IgE	++	C-chemotaxis	PMN, eosinophils, plasma cells	Cardiovascular system, lung, skin, synovial membranes, mesothelia, blood cells	30
17	Rheumatoid arthritis	Cell surface antigens, immunoglobulins (presumable microbial agent unknown)	IgM, IgG; *IgA; rheumatoid factor	+[4]	Leukocyte factors	Plasma cells, lymphocytes	Joints, cardiovascular system, blood cells	32
18	Goodpasture's syndrome	Alveolar & renal glomerular basement membrane	IgG; *IgM	±	?	Monocytes, macrophages	Kidney	22,26
19	Pemphigus	Epithelial intercellular bridge	IgG	+	?	*PMN	Epidermis	4,5
	Type IV: Cell-mediated Reactions							
20	Contact dermatitis	Drugs, chemicals, plant oils	T-lymphocytes	None	Lymphokines	Lymphocytes, macrophages	Skin	12
21	Microbial hypersensitivity	*Mycobacterium tuberculosis*, viruses, fungi	T-lymphocytes	None	Lymphokines	Lymphocytes, macrophages, giant cells	Any organ	36
22	Graft rejection	Histocompatibility leukocyte antigens	T-lymphocytes	None; ?±	Lymphokines	Lymphocytes, macrophages, plasma cells, PMN	Allografted organ	38
23	Graft-versus-host reaction	Histocompatibility leukocyte antigens	T-lymphocytes (mixed leukocyte reaction in vivo)	None	Lymphokines	Lymphocytes; *macrophages	Host lymphoid organs, skin	39
	Granulomatous diseases							
24	Wegener's granulomatosis	Unknown	Unknown	?	?	Lymphocytes, macrophages, giant cells, eosinophils	Arteries, veins, lung, kidney, skin	11
25	Regional ileitis[5]	Unknown	Unknown; *T-lymphocytes	None	?	Lymphocytes, macrophages	Small intestine	8,31

[4] Synovial fluid. [5] Synonyms: Crohn's disease; Granulomatous ileocolitis.

continued

	Disease	Antigens	Major Ig Immune Response	Complement Consumption	Mediator or Mechanism of Inflammation	Major Inflammatory Cells	Major Organ Involved	Reference
26	Farmer's lung disease	Thermophilic actinomycetes	Immunoglobulin, T-lymphocytes	?	Lymphokines	Lymphocytes, macrophages, giant cells, PMN	Lung	25,35
	Autoaggressive lymphocyte-mediated reactions							
27	Struma lymphomatosa [6]	Thyroglobulin, cytoplasmic antigens	IgG; *IgA; T-lymphocytes	None	Lymphokines	Lymphocytes, macrophages	Thyroid	9
28	Encephalomyelitis	Central nervous system myelin	T-lymphocytes	None	?	Lymphocytes	Brain, spinal cord	34
29	Guillain-Barré-Strohl syndrome	Peripheral nerve	T-lymphocytes	None	?	Lymphocytes	Peripheral nerves	42
	Type V: Immuno-Neutralization & Immuno-Stimulation							
30	Diabetes mellitus	Islet cells, ? insulin	Immunoglobulins	None	None	None	? Pancreatic beta cells	23
31	Pernicious anemia	Intrinsic factor, gastric parietal cells	Immunoglobulins	None	?	Lymphocytes, PMN	Stomach	3
32	Hemophilia	Antihemophilic globulin	Immunoglobulins	None	None	None	....	24
33	Myasthenia gravis	Skeletal muscle acetylcholine receptor, thymic epithelioid reticular cells	Immunoglobulins	None; *±	?	....	Muscle, thymus	15,40 43
34	Thyrotoxicosis	Thyrotropin [7] receptor	Immunoglobulins; *LATS	None	None	None	Thyroid	27

[6] Synonym: Hashimoto's thyroiditis. [7] Synonym: Thyroid-stimulating hormone.

Contributor: Burkholder, Peter

References

1. Arthus, M. 1903. C. R. Soc. Biol. 55:817-820.
2. Austen, K. R., and L. M. Lichtenstein. 1973. Physiology, Immunopharmacology and Treatment. Academic Press, New York.
3. Beck, W. S. 1973. Hematology. M. I. T. Press, Cambridge, Mass.
4. Beutner, E. H., and R. E. Jordon. 1964. Proc. Soc. Exp. Biol. Med. 117:505-510.
5. Beutner, E. H., et al. 1968. J. Invest. Dermatol. 51:63-80.
6. Bloch, K. J. 1967. Prog. Allergy 10:84-150.
7. Cochrane, C. G. 1967. Ibid. 11:1-35.
8. Crohn, B. B. 1959. Gastroenterology 36:398-408.
9. Doniach, D., and I. M. Roitt. 1969. In P. A. Miescher and H. J. Müller-Eberhard, ed. Textbook of Immunopathology. Grune and Stratton, New York. v. 2, pp. 516-533.
10. Ellis, E. F. 1969. Adv. Pediatr. 16:65-98.
11. Fauci, A. S., and S. M. Wolff. 1973. Medicine (Baltimore) 52:535-561.
12. Freedman, S. O. 1971. Clinical Immunology. Harper and Row, New York. pp. 121-129.
13. Freedman, S. O. 1971. (Loc. cit. ref. 12). pp. 277-281.
14. Freedman, S. O. 1971. (Loc. cit. ref. 12). pp. 561-563.
15. Geld, H. van der, and H. J. G. H. Oosterhuis. 1963. Vox Sang. 8:196-204.
16. Gell, P. G. H., and R. R. A. Coombs. 1968. Clinical Aspects of Immunology. Ed. 2. B. H. Blackwell, Oxford.
17. Gocke, D. J., et al. 1971. J. Exp. Med. 134:330s-336s.
18. Good, R. A., and D. W. Fisher. 1971. Immunobiology. Sinauer, Sunderland, MA. pp. 167-172.

continued

19. Humphrey, J., and R. White. 1970. Immunology for Students of Medicine. B. H. Blackwell, Oxford. pp. 453-455.
20. Koffler, D., et al. 1971. J. Exp. Med. 134:169s-179s.
21. Levine, B., and A. Redmond. 1967. Int. Arch. Allergy Appl. Immunol. 31:594-606.
22. Lundberg, G. D. 1963. J. Am. Med. Assoc. 184:915-919.
23. Mancini, A. M., et al. 1964. Lancet 1:726.
24. Margolius, A., et al. 1961. Medicine (Baltimore) 40:145-202.
25. McCombs, R. P. 1972. N. Engl. J. Med. 286:1186-1245.
26. McIntosh, R., and W. Griswold. 1971. Arch. Pathol. 92:329-333.
27. McKenzie, J. M. 1968. Physiol. Rev. 48:252-310.
28. Metcoff, J. 1967. Acute Glomerulonephritis. Little, Brown; Boston.
29. Miescher, P. A. 1969. (Loc. cit. ref. 9). v. 2, pp. 458-468.
30. Miescher, P. A., and F. Paronetto. 1969. (Loc. cit. ref. 9). v. 2., pp. 675-712.
31. Morson, B. 1970. Trans. Med. Soc. London 86:177-192.
32. Park, B., and R. A. Good. 1974. Principles of Modern Immunobiology. Lea and Febiger, Philadelphia. pp. 389-398.
33. Paronetto, F. 1969. (Loc. cit. ref. 9). v. 2, pp. 722-732.
34. Paterson, P. Y. 1966. Adv. Immunol. 5:131-208.
35. Pepys, J. 1969. Monogr. Allergy 4.
36. Roitt, I. 1974. Essential Immunology. B. H. Blackwell, Oxford. pp. 148-155.
37. Rosen, S. 1971. Hum. Pathol. 2:209-231.
38. Sell, S. 1975. Immunology, Immunopathology and Immunity. Harper and Row, New York. pp. 221-233.
39. Simonsen, M. 1962. Prog. Allergy 6:349-467.
40. Simpson, J. A. 1960. Scott. Med. J. 5:419-436.
41. Unanue, E. R., and F. S. Dixon. 1967. Adv. Immunol. 6:1-90.
42. Wiederholt, W. C., et al. 1964. Mayo Clin. Proc. 39:427-451.
43. Woolf, A. L. 1966. Ann. N. Y. Acad. Sci. 135(1):35-56.

70. IMMUNOFLUORESCENCE TESTS OF AUTOIMMUNE DISEASE

Part I. Anti-nuclear Antibodies

Percent Positive indicates percent of patients with significant positive titer. Level of significant titer must be determined for each laboratory. For incidence of fluorescent antibodies in "normals," consult reference 6.

	Pattern	Antigen	Disease	Percent Positive	Remarks	Reference
1	Peripheral ("shaggy")	Double-stranded DNA & deoxyribonucleoprotein	Systemic lupus erythematosus—active	99	....	3
2	Homogeneous (diffuse)	Deoxyribonucleoprotein	Systemic lupus erythematosus—in remission	90	....	3
3			Chronic discoid lupus erythematosus	20	....	
4			Rheumatoid arthritis	40	....	
5			Juvenile	24	Usually positive with associated uveitis	
6			Chronic active hepatitis	24	....	
7			Dermatitis herpetiformis [ref. 4]	34	....	
8	Speckled (Ribonuclease I[1/] sensitive)	Saline-extractable ribonucleoprotein	Mixed connective tissue disease; systemic lupus erythematosus	99	....	3

[1/] Synonym: RNase.

continued

Part I. Anti-nuclear Antibodies

	Pattern	Antigen	Disease	Percent Positive	Remarks	Reference
9	Ribonuclease I[1/] insensitive	"Sm"	Systemic lupus erythematosus	20	Speckled fluorescent pattern may be obscured by homogeneous antibody pattern	1,5
10	Nucleolar	....	Progressive systemic sclerosis	60	....	2

[1/] Synonym: RNase.

Contributor: Hong, Richard

References

1. Northway, J. D., and E. M. Tan. 1972. Clin. Immunol. Immunopathol. 1:140-154.
2. Ritchie, R. F. 1970. N. Engl. J. Med. 282:1174-1178.
3. Rothfield, N. F. 1976. In N. R. Rose and H. Friedman, ed. Manual of Clinical Immunology. American Society for Microbiology, Washington, D.C. pp. 647-651.
4. Seah, P. P., et al. 1971. Lancet 1:834-836.
5. Sharp, G. C., et al. 1972. Am. J. Med. 52:148-159.
6. Shu, S., et al. 1975. J. Lab. Clin. Med. 86:259-265.

Part II. Skin

	Pattern	Disease	Remarks	Reference
1	"Band" fluorescence at dermal-epidermal junction	Systemic lupus erythematosus & other diseases	Present in uninvolved & involved skin	2
2		Discoid lupus erythematosus	Usually present in involved skin only; occasionally weakly positive in uninvolved skin	
3	Immunoglobulin A deposits in dermal papillae	Dermatitis herpetiformis	....	4
4	Intercellular	Pemphigus	Also seen occasionally in high-titered anti-blood-group sera or burns	1,2
5	Linear basement membrane	Pemphigoid	....	1,3

Contributor: Hong, Richard

References

1. Beutner, E. H., et al. 1968. J. Invest. Dermatol. 51:63-80.
2. Burnham, T. K., and G. Fine. 1971. Arch. Dermatol. 103:24-32.
3. Jordon, R. E. 1976. In N. R. Rose and H. Friedman, ed. Manual of Clinical Immunology. American Society for Microbiology, Washington, D.C. pp. 701-709.
4. van der Meer, J. B. 1969. Br. J. Dermatol. 81:493-503.

continued

Part III. Tissue-specific Antigens

Disease or Condition: HB$_S$ Ag = hepatitis B surface antigen. **Percent Positive** indicates percent of patients with significant positive titer. Level of significant titer must be determined for each laboratory. For additional information, consult reference 16.

	Antigen	Disease or Condition	Percent Positive	Reference
1	Thyroid colloid	Thyroiditis	40-70	1
2	Thyroid microsomes (in epithelial cells)	Chronic thyroiditis	70-90	1
3		Primary hypothyroidism	64	
4		Thyrotoxicosis	50	
5		Thyroid tumors	17	
6		Simple goiter	10	
7	Adrenal cortex	Idiopathic Addison's disease	38-60	2
8	Mitochondria	Primary biliary cirrhosis	90-94	4,5,8
9		Cryptogenic cirrhosis	25-30	
10		Chronic active hepatitis	25-28	
11	Smooth muscle	Chronic active hepatitis	40-70	5,6
12		Primary biliary cirrhosis	50	
13		Cryptogenic cirrhosis	28	
14	Gastric parietal cells	Pernicious anemia	90	14
15		Atrophic gastritis	60	
16		Chronic thyroiditis	33	
17		Sicca syndrome	15	
	Antiglomerular basement membrane			
18	None-linear	Chronic active hepatitis	....	9
19	Linear	Goodpasture's syndrome	....	12
20	Antitubular basement membrane	Methicillin-induced interstitial nephritis	....	3,13
21		Renal homografts; rapidly progressive nephritis	....	
22	Reticulin	Adult celiac disease	36	15
23		Dermatitis herpetiformis	17	
24	? Hepatitis B virus	Granular pattern, patient serum positive for HB$_S$ Ag	....	7
25	Liver membrane	Linear pattern, patient serum negative for HB$_S$ Ag	....	7
26	Islets of Langerhans cells: insulinoma	Insulin-dependent diabetes and coexistent autoimmunity	....	10,11

Contributor: Hong, Richard

References

1. Balfour, B. M., et al. 1961. Br. J. Exp. Pathol. 42:307-316.
2. Bigazzi, P. E., and N. R. Rose. 1974. In A. J. Laskin and H. A. Lechevalier, ed. Handbook of Microbiology. CRC Press, Cleveland. v. 4, pp. 765-794.
3. Border, W. A., et al. 1974. N. Engl. J. Med. 291:381-384.
4. Doniach, D. 1972. Br. Med. Bull. 28:145-148.
5. Doniach, D., et al. 1966. Clin. Exp. Immunol. 1:237-262.
6. Feizi, T., et al. 1972. Ibid. 10:609-622.
7. Hopf, U., et al. 1976. N. Engl. J. Med. 294:578-582.
8. Klatskin, G., and F. S. Kantor. 1972. Ann. Intern. Med. 77:533-541.
9. Levy, R. L., and R. Hong. 1974. J. Pediatr. 85:155-158.
10. MacCuish, A. C., et al. 1974. Lancet 2:1529-1531.
11. MacLaren, N. K., et al. 1975. Ibid. 1:997-1000.
12. McCluskey, R. T. 1971. J. Exp. Med. 134(3-2):242s-255s.
13. McCluskey, R. T. 1975. N. Engl. J. Med. 292:914-915.
14. Roitt, I. M., and D. Doniach. 1969. In P. A. Miescher and H. J. Müller-Eberhard, ed. Textbook of Immunopathology. Grune and Stratton, New York. v. 2, pp. 534-546.
15. Seah, P. P., et al. 1971. Lancet 1:834-836.
16. Shu, S., et al. 1975. J. Lab. Clin. Med. 86:259-265.

71. NORMAL VALUES OF PROTEINS OF THE COMPLEMENT SYSTEM

	Protein	Concentration in Serum μg/ml	Reference		Protein	Concentration in Serum μg/ml	Reference
	Primary complement pathway				Alternative complement pathway		
1	C1q	180	4	12	Factor D	Trace	4
2	C1r	97	1,2	13	Factor B	200	4
3	C1s	32; 110	1,2,4	14	Properdin	25	4
4	C4	640	4	15	Nephritic factor	Trace	4
5	C2	25	4		Inhibitory proteins		
6	C3	1600	4	16	C1-inhibitor[1]	180	5
7	C5	80	4	17	C3b-inactivator	25	5
8	C6	75	4	18	C3b-inactivator accelerator	225	6
9	C7	55	4	19	Anaphylatoxin inactivator	35	3
10	C8	80	4	20	Related proteins: C1t	47	1,2
11	C9	230	4				

[1] Synonym: C1-esterase inhibitor.

Contributor: Gewurz, Henry

References

1. Assimeh, S. N., and R. H. Painter. 1975. J. Immunol. 115:482-487.
2. Assimeh, S. N., and R. H. Painter. Unpublished. Dep. Biochemistry, Univ. Toronto, ON, 1976.
3. Bokisch, V. A., and H. J. Müller-Eberhard. 1970. J. Clin. Invest. 49:2427-2436.
4. Müller-Eberhard, H. J. 1975. Annu. Rev. Biochem. 44:697-724.
5. Ruddy, S., et al. 1972. N. Engl. J. Med. 287:489-495.
6. Whaley, K., and S. Ruddy. 1976. Science 193:1011-1013.

72. DISEASES ASSOCIATED WITH SECONDARY DECREASES OF SERUM COMPLEMENT LEVELS

Frequency indicates occurrence of depressed serum complement levels with active diesase.

	Disease	Frequency		Disease	Frequency
1	Systemic lupus erythematosus	Regularly	7	Hypergammaglobulinemic & dysgammaglobulinemic states	Frequently
2	Acute post-streptococcal glomerulonephritis	Regularly	8	Rheumatoid arthritis	Occasionally (10%)[1]
3	Membranoproliferative chronic glomerulonephritis	Regularly	9	Infections & endotoxemia	Occasionally
4	Chronic active hepatitis	Regularly	10	Rapidly rejecting allografts	Occasionally
5	Subacute bacterial endocarditis	Usually	11	Hemolytic anemia	Occasionally
6	Serum sickness (e.g., simple proteins, viruses, protozoa)	Frequently	12	Chronic liver disease	Occasionally
			13	Chronic renal disease	Occasionally

[1] Regularly depressed in synovial fluids.

Contributor: Gewurz, Henry

General References

1. Frank, M. M., and J. P. Atkinson. 1975. Dis. Mon. (Jan.):1-54.
2. Gewurz, H., and L. A. Suyehira. 1976. In N. R. Rose and H. Friedman, ed. Manual of Clinical Immunology. American Society for Microbiology, Washington, D.C. pp. 36-47.
3. Ruddy, S., et al. 1972. N. Engl. J. Med. 287:642-646.

73. INBORN ERRORS OF THE COMPLEMENT SYSTEM

Data represent only a partial listing of patients with apparent inherited deficiencies of the complement system. All of these deficiencies are very rare. **Symptoms or Disease: Description**—SLE = systemic lupus erythematosus; **No. of**

Individuals indicates the number of persons, in whom the error was detected (column 2), who displayed the specified symptoms or disease.

Error		Symptoms or Disease	
Type	No. of Individuals with Error Detected	Description	No. of Individuals
1 C1r deficiency	3	Chronic renal disease	1
2		SLE-like	1
3 C1s deficiency	2	SLE-like	2
4 C4 deficiency	2	SLE-like	2
5 C2 deficiency	30	SLE-like	10
6		Chronic membranoproliferative glomerulonephritis	2
7		Anaphylactoid purpura	2
8		Dermatomyositis	1
9 C3 deficiency	4	Repeated infections	3
10		Rash, arthralgias, & fevers	1
11 C5 deficiency	2	SLE	1
12 dysfunction	3	Leiner's disease	....
13 C6 deficiency	2	Recurrent meningococcal meningitis	1
14 C7 deficiency	3	Chronic renal disease	1
15		Raynaud's phenomenon	1
16 C8 deficiency	3	SLE	1
17		Gonococcal infections	1
18 C1-inhibitor deficiency	Many	Hereditary angioneurotic edema	....
19 C3b-inactivator deficiency	1	Repeated infections	....

Contributor: Gewurz, Henry

General References

1. Alper, C. A., and F. S. Rosen. 1971. Adv. Immunol. 14:251-290.
2. Day, N. K., and R. A. Good. 1975. Birth Defects Orig. Artic. Ser. 11:306-311.
3. Donaldson, V., and R. M. Stroud. 1974. Prog. Immunol. II, 1:288.
4. Gewurz, H., and L. A. Suyehira. 1976. In N. R. Rose and H. Friedman, ed. Manual of Clinical Immunology. American Society for Microbiology, Washington, D.C. pp. 36-47.
5. Ruddy, S., et al. 1972. N. Engl. J. Med. 287:592-596.
6. Stroud, R. M. 1974. Transplant. Proc. 6:59-65.

III. METABOLIC DISORDERS

74. PRENATAL DIAGNOSIS OF INHERITED DISEASE

Part I. Inborn Errors of Metabolism

IP = inheritance pattern; AD = autosomal dominant; AR = autosomal recessive; X-LR = X-linked recessive. For source of **Enzyme Commission No.**, *see* Introduction. **Heterozygote Detection** is applicable to autosomal recessive and X-linked recessive disorders only; NA = not applicable because the disorder is autosomal dominant; ± = published data are conflicting. **CNS Damage:** Var = variable. *Symbol:* 0 = attempts at detection have not been reported. Data in brackets refer to the column heading in brackets.

	Disorder ⟨Synonym⟩	IP	Enzyme Deficiency ⟨Synonym⟩ [Enzyme Commission No.]	Expressed in Fibroblasts	Prenatal Diagnosis Reported	Hetero-zygote Detection	CNS Damage	Refer-ence
1	Acatalasia, several types	AR	Catalase [1.11.1.6]	Yes[1]	No	±	No	1,73
2	Adenosine deaminase deficiency	AR	Adenosine deaminase [3.5.4.4]	Yes	Yes	Yes	No	45
3	Aspartylglucosaminuria	AR	4-L-Aspartylglycosylamine amidohydrolase [3.5.1.37][2]	Yes	No	Yes	Yes	3,5
4	Cholesterol ester storage disease[3]	AR	Acid lipase	Yes	No	Yes	No	8
5	Collagen, heritable disorders of Ehlers-Danlos syndrome ⟨EDS⟩ type IV	AR	Unknown; absence of type III collagen	Yes	No	Yes	No	76
6	EDS type V	X-LR	Lysyl oxidase	Yes	No	?	No	23
7	Hydroxylysine-deficient collagen disease ⟨EDS type VI⟩	AR	Lysine, 2-oxoglutarate dioxygenase ⟨Peptidyllysine, 2-oxoglutarate:oxygen 5-oxidoreductase; lysyl hydroxylase⟩ [1.14.11.4]	Yes	No	Yes	No	55
8	EDS type VII	AR	Procollagen peptidase	Yes	No	0	No	59
9	Cystinosis, infantile (nephropathic) form	AR	Unknown; increased cellular cystine content & retention	Yes	Yes	Yes	No	85,93
10	Cystinuria, three types	AR	Unknown; defective transport of dibasic amino acids	No	Yes[4]	No[5]; Yes[6]	No	52
11	Fabry's disease	X-LR	α-Galactosidase [3.2.1.22]	Yes	Yes	Yes	Var	17
12	Farber's disease	AR	Ceramidase	Yes	No	0	Yes	96
13	Fucosidosis, types 1 & 2	AR	α-L-Fucosidase [3.2.1.51]	Yes	No	Yes	Yes	53,74, 107
14	Galactosemia	AR	Hexose-1-phosphate uridylyltransferase ⟨UDPglucose:α-D-galactose-1-phosphate uridylyltransferase⟩ [2.7.7.12]	Yes	Yes	Yes	Yes	66
15	Gaucher's disease, several forms	AR	Glucocerebroside β-glucosidase ⟨Glucocerebrosidase⟩	Yes	Yes	Yes	Yes[7]; No[8]	83
16	G$_{m_1}$ gangliosidosis (at least two types) Type 1 ⟨Generalized gangliosidosis⟩	AR	G$_{m_1}$-ganglioside β-galactosidase	Yes	Yes	Yes	Yes	49,60
17	Type 2 ⟨Juvenile G$_{m_1}$ gangliosidosis⟩	AR	G$_{m_1}$-ganglioside β-galactosidase	Yes	Yes	Yes	Yes	14
18	G$_{m_2}$ gangliosidosis (at least three forms) Tay-Sachs disease	AR	β-N-Acetylhexosaminidase A ⟨Hexosaminedase A⟩ [3.2.1.52]	Yes	Yes	Yes	Yes	72,82

[1] Japanese & Swiss types. [2] Possibly 3.5.1.26, aspartylglucosaminase. [3] *See also* entry 71. [4] In amniotic fluid. [5] For type I. [6] For types II & III. [7] In infantile & juvenile forms. [8] In adult form.

continued

Part I. Inborn Errors of Metabolism

	Disorder ⟨Synonym⟩	IP	Enzyme Deficiency ⟨Synonym⟩ [Enzyme Commission No.]	Expressed in Fibroblasts	Prenatal Diagnosis Reported	Hetero-zygote Detection	CNS Damage	Refer-ence
19	Sandhoff's disease	AR	β-N-Acetylhexosaminidase A ⟨Hexosaminidase A⟩ & β-N-Acetylhexosaminidase B ⟨Hexosaminidase B⟩ [3.2.1.52]; deficient with both natural & synthetic substrates	Yes	Yes	Yes	Yes	22
20	AB variant	AR	β-N-Acetylhexosaminidase A ⟨Hexosaminidase A⟩ & β-N-Acetylhexosaminidase B ⟨Hexosaminidase B⟩ [3.2.1.52]; deficient with natural but not synthetic substrate	Yes	No	0	Yes	80
21	Glucose-6-phosphate dehydrogenase deficiency	X-LR	Glucose-6-phosphate dehydrogenase ⟨D-Glucose-6-phosphate:NADP⁺ 1-oxidoreductase⟩ [1.1.1.49]	Yes	No	Yes	No	21,65
22	Glucosephosphate isomerase ⟨Phosphohexose isomerase⟩ deficiency	AR	Glucosephosphate isomerase ⟨D-Glucose-6-phosphate-ketol-isomerase⟩ [5.3.1.9]	Yes	No	No	No	56
23	β-Glucuronidase deficiency	AR	β-Glucuronidase [3.2.1.31]	Yes	No	Yes	Var	9,35
24	Glutaric aciduria	AR	Glutaryl-CoA dehydrogenase [1.3.99.7]	Yes	No	Yes	Yes	40
	Glycogenosis ⟨Glycogen storage disease⟩							
25	Type II ⟨Pompe's disease⟩	AR	α-Glucosidase [3.2.1.20]	Yes	Yes	Yes	No	69,70
26	Type III	AR	Amylo-1,6-glucosidase [3.2.1.33]	Yes	No	±	No	25,48
27	Type IV	AR	Amylo-(1,4 → 1,6)transglucosidase	Yes	No	Yes	No	46
28	Hunter syndrome	X-LR	L-Iduronate sulfatase	Yes	Yes	Yes	Var	7,33
29	Hurler/Scheie syndromes	AR	L-Iduronidase [3.2.1.76]	Yes	Yes	Yes	Yes⁹/; No ¹⁰/	6,33
30	Hypercholesterolemia, familial, several forms	AD	None known; receptor or catabolic defect	Yes	No	NA	No	37,38
31	Hyperphenylalaninemia due to dihydropteridine reductase deficiency	AR	Dihydropteridine reductase [1.6.99.7]	Yes	No	Yes	Yes	51
32	Hyperprolinemia, type 2	AR	1-Pyrroline dehydrogenase ⟨Δ¹-Pyrroline-5-carboxylic acid dehydrogenase⟩ [1.5.1.12]	Yes	No	0	Var	103
33	3-Ketoacid CoA-transferase ⟨Succinyl-CoA:3-oxoacid CoA-transferase⟩ deficiency	AR	3-Ketoacid CoA-transferase ⟨Succinyl-CoA:3-oxoacid CoA-transferase⟩ [2.8.3.5]	Yes	No	0	0	91,101
34	Krabbe's disease	AR	Galactosylceramide β-galactosidase	Yes	Yes	Yes	Yes	97,106
35	Lesch-Nyhan syndrome	X-LR	Hypoxanthine phosphoribosyltransferase ⟨Hypoxanthine-guanine phosphoribosyltransferase⟩ [2.4.2.8]	Yes	Yes	Yes	Yes	15
	Lysine metabolic errors							
36	Hyperlysinemia	?AR	Saccharopine dehydrogenase (NADP⁺, lysine-forming) ⟨Lysine-ketoglutarate reductase; lysine:α-ketoglutarate:triphosphopyridine nucleotide oxidoreductase⟩ [1.5.1.8]; saccharopine dehydrogenase (NAD⁺, L-glutamate-forming) [1.5.1.9]; & saccharopine oxidoreductase	Yes	No	0	Var	19,20

⁹/ In Hurler syndrome. ¹⁰/ In Scheie syndrome.

continued

Part I. Inborn Errors of Metabolism

	Disorder ⟨Synonym⟩	IP	Enzyme Deficiency ⟨Synonym⟩ [Enzyme Commission No.]	Expressed in Fibro-blasts	Prenatal Diagnosis Reported	Hetero-zygote Detection	CNS Damage	Refer-ence
37	Saccharopinuria	?AR	Saccharopine dehydrogenase (NAD$^+$, L-glutamate-forming) [1.5.1.9]; saccharopine dehydrogenase (NADP$^+$, lysine-forming) ⟨lysine-ketoglutarate reductase⟩ [1.5.1.8]; and possibly other defects	Yes	No	0	Var	28,89
38	Lysosomal acid phosphatase deficiency	AR	Acid phosphatase (lysosomal) [3.1.3.2]	Yes	Yes	Yes	Yes	67
39	Mannosidosis	AR	α-Mannosidase [3.2.1.24]	Yes	No	Yes	Yes	98
40	Maple syrup urine disease, at least four forms	AR	Branched-chain α-ketoacid decarboxylase	Yes	Yes	±	Var; Yes[11]; No[12]	18,105
41	Maroteaux-Lamy syndrome	AR	Arylsulfatase B [3.1.6.1]	Yes	No	Yes	No	10,31, 95
42	Menke's disease	X-LR	Unknown; increased copper content of cultured Menke's fibroblasts	Yes	No	No	Yes	36
43	Metachromatic leukodystrophy, three or more forms	AR	Arylsulfatase A [3.1.6.1]	Yes	Yes	Yes	Yes	58,68
44	5,10-Methylenetetrahydrofolate reductase deficiency	AR	5,10-Methylenetetrahydrofolate reductase ⟨5-Methyltetrahydrofolate:NAD$^+$ oxidoreductase⟩ [1.1.1.68]	Yes	No	Yes	Yes	26,64
45	Methylmalonic acidemia Primary methylmalonyl-CoA ⟨MM-CoA⟩ mutase deficiency ⟨Apo-enzyme defect⟩	AR	Methylmalonyl-CoA mutase ⟨Methylmalonyl-CoA CoA-carbonylmutase⟩ [5.4.99.2]	Yes	Yes	0	Yes	61,63
46	Secondary MM-CoA mutase deficiency Secondary to deficient formation of adenosyl-cobalamin ⟨5'-deoxy-5'-adenosylcobalamin; AdoCbl⟩	AR	Unknown	Yes	Yes	0	Var	2
47	Secondary to deficient formation of both AdoCbl & methylcobalamin	?AR	Unknown	Yes	No	0	Yes	24
48	Methylmalonyl-CoA racemase deficiency	?AR	Methylmalonyl-CoA racemase [5.1.99.1]	Yes	No	0	0	50
49	Morquio's syndrome	AR	N-Acetylgalactosamine-6-sulfate sulfatase	Yes	No	0	No	90
50	Mucolipidosis Type II ⟨I-cell disease⟩	AR	Cellular deficiency of multiple lysosomal enzymes	Yes	Yes	0	Yes	4,62, 100
51	Type III ⟨Pseudo-Hurler polydystrophy⟩	AR	Cellular deficiency of multiple lysosomal enzymes	Yes	No	?Yes	Yes	47
52	Niemann-Pick disease, several forms	AR	Sphingomyelinase	Yes	Yes	Yes	Yes	16,84

[11] In "classical" form. [12] In thiamine-responsive form.

continued

Part I. Inborn Errors of Metabolism

	Disorder ⟨Synonym⟩	IP	Enzyme Deficiency ⟨Synonym⟩ [Enzyme Commission No.]	Expressed in Fibroblasts	Prenatal Diagnosis Reported	Heterozygote Detection	CNS Damage	Reference
53	Ornithine—oxoacid aminotransferase ⟨Ornithine-ketoacid transaminase⟩ deficiency	?AR	Ornithine—oxoacid aminotransferase ⟨Ornithine-ketoacid transaminase⟩ [2.6.1.13]	Yes	No	0	Yes	34
54	Orotic aciduria Type I	AR	Orotate phosphoribosyltransferase [2.4.2.10] & orotidine-5'-phosphate decarboxylase [4.1.1.23]	Yes	No	Yes	Var	57
55	Type II	AR	Orotidine-5'-phosphate decarboxylase [4.1.1.23]	0	No	Yes	Yes[13]	32
56	Porphyrias Acute intermittent porphyria	AD	Uroporphyrinogen I synthase [4.3.1.8]	Yes	Yes	NA	Yes	81
57	Congenital erythropoietic porphyria	AR	Uroporphyrinogen III cosynthase	Yes	No	0	No	79
58	Protoporphyria	AR	Ferrochelatase ⟨Heme synthetase; protoheme ferro-lyase⟩ [4.99.1.1]	Yes	No	0	No	13
59	Propionic acidemia	AR	Propionyl-CoA carboxylase [4.1.1.41]	Yes	No	No	Yes	39
60	Pyroglutamic aciduria ⟨5-Oxoprolinuria⟩	AR	Glutathione synthetase [6.3.2.3]	Yes	No	0	Var[14]	92,104
61	"Pyruvate dehydrogenase complex" deficiency E1 defect	?AR	Pyruvate dehydrogenase (lipoate) [1.2.4.1]	Yes	No	0	Yes	11,94
62	E2 or E3 defect[13]	?AR	Lipoate acetyltransferase ⟨Dihydrolipoyl transacetylase⟩ [2.3.1.12] or lipoamide dehydrogenase ⟨dihydrolipoyl dehydrogenase⟩ [1.6.4.3]	Yes	No	0	Yes	12
63	Refsum's disease	AR	Phytanic acid oxidase	Yes	No	Yes	Yes	43,44
64	Sanfilippo syndrome (two or more forms) A form	AR	Heparan N-sulfatase	Yes	Yes	0	Yes	42
65	B form	AR	α-N-Acetylglucosaminidase ⟨2-Acetamido-2-deoxy-α-D-glucoside acetamidodeoxyglucohydrolase⟩ [3.2.1.50]	Yes	No	Yes	Yes	29,71
66	Sulfatase deficiency, multiple	AR	Deficiency of multiple lysosomal & microsomal sulfatases	Yes	No	0	Yes	27
67	Sulfur pathway disorders Cystathionine synthase deficiency homocystinuria	AR	Cystathionine β-synthase ⟨L-Serine hydro-lyase (adding homocysteine)⟩ [4.2.1.22]	Yes	No	Yes	Var	30,102
68	Sulfite oxidase deficiency	?AR	Sulfite oxidase [1.8.3.1]	Yes	No	0	Yes	88
69	Urea cycle disorders Argininosuccinic aciduria	AR	Argininosuccinate lyase [4.3.2.1]	Yes	Yes	±	Yes	41,86, 87
70	Citrullinemia	AR	Argininosuccinate synthetase ⟨L-Citrulline:L-aspartate ligase (AMP-forming)⟩ [6.3.4.5]	Yes	No	±	Var	78,99
71	Wolman's disease[15]	AR	Acid lipase	Yes	Yes	No	Yes	75

[13] One patient only. [14] One of three patients. [15] See also entry 4.

continued

Part I. Inborn Errors of Metabolism

Disorder ⟨Synonym⟩	IP	Enzyme Deficiency ⟨Synonym⟩ [Enzyme Commission No.]	Expressed in Fibro- blasts	Prenatal Diagnosis Reported	Hetero- zygote Detection	CNS Damage	Refer- ence
72 Xeroderma pigmentosum, several forms	AR	Unknown; defective repair of DNA following ultraviolet irradiation	Yes	Yes	No	Var	54,77

Contributor: Erbe, Richard W.

References

1. Aebi, H., and H. Suter. 1971. Adv. Hum. Genet. 2: 143-199.
2. Ampola, M. G., et al. 1975. N. Engl. J. Med. 293:313-317.
3. Aula, P., et al. 1973. Clin. Genet. 4:297-300.
4. Aula, P., et al. 1975. J. Pediatr. 87:221-226.
5. Aula, P., et al. 1976. Pediatr. Res. 10:625-629.
6. Bach, G., et al. 1972. Proc. Natl. Acad. Sci. USA 69: 2048-2051.
7. Bach, G., et al. 1973. Ibid. 70:2134-2138.
8. Beaudet, A. L., et al. 1974. J. Lab. Clin. Med. 84:54-61.
9. Beaudet, A. L., et al. 1975. J. Pediatr. 86:388-394.
10. Beratis, N. G., et al. 1975. Pediatr. Res. 9:475-480.
11. Blass, J. P., et al. 1970. J. Clin. Invest. 49:423-432.
12. Blass, J. P., et al. 1972. Ibid. 51:1845-1851.
13. Bonkowsky, H. L., et al. 1975. Ibid. 56:1139-1148.
14. Booth, C. W., et al. 1973. Pediatrics 52:521-524.
15. Boyle, J. A., et al. 1970. Science 169:688-689.
16. Brady, R. O., et al. 1971. Am. J. Med. 51:423-431.
17. Brady, R. O., et al. 1971. Science 172:174-175.
18. Dancis, J. 1972. In A. Dorfman, ed. Antenatal Diagnosis. Univ. Chicago Press, Chicago. pp. 123-125.
19. Dancis, J., et al. 1969. J. Clin. Invest. 48:1447-1452.
20. Dancis, J., et al. 1976. Pediatr. Res. 10:686-691.
21. Davidson, R. G., et al. 1963. Proc. Natl. Acad. Sci. USA 50:481-485.
22. Desnick, R. J., et al. 1973. Biochem. Biophys. Res. Commun. 51:20-26.
23. DiFerrante, N., et al. 1975. Connect. Tissue Res. 3: 49-53.
24. Dillon, M. J., et al. 1974. Clin. Sci. Mol. Med. 47:43-61.
25. DiMauro, S., et al. 1973. Pediatr. Res. 7:739-744.
26. Erbe, R. W. 1975. N. Engl. J. Med. 293:753-757, 807-812.
27. Eto, Y., et al. 1974. Arch. Neurol. (Chicago) 30:153-156.
28. Fellows, F. C. I., and N. A. J. Carson. 1974. Pediatr. Res. 8:42-49.
29. Figura, K. von, and H. Kresse. 1972. Biochem. Biophys. Res. Commun. 48:262-269.
30. Fleisher, L. D., et al. 1974. J. Pediatr. 85:677-680.
31. Fluharty, A. L., et al. 1974. Biochem. Biophys. Res. Commun. 59:455-461.
32. Fox, R. M., et al. 1973. Am. J. Med. 55:791-798.
33. Fratantoni, J. C., et al. 1969. N. Engl. J. Med. 280: 686-688.
34. Garnica, A. D., et al. 1976. Pediatr. Res. 10:365 (Abstr. 383).
35. Glaser, J. H., and W. S. Sly. 1973. J. Lab. Clin. Med. 82:969-977.
36. Goka, T. J., et al. 1976. Proc. Natl. Acad. Sci. USA 73:604-606.
37. Goldstein, J. L., et al. 1974. Am. J. Hum. Genet. 26: 199-206.
38. Goldstein, J. L., et al. 1975. Proc. Natl. Acad. Sci. USA 72:1092-1096.
39. Gompertz, D., et al. 1975. Clin. Genet. 8:244-250.
40. Goodman, S. I., and J. G. Kohlhoff. 1975. Biochem. Med. 13:138-140.
41. Goodman, S. I., et al. 1973. Clin. Genet. 4:236-240.
42. Harper, P. S., et al. 1974. J. Med. Genet. 11:123-132.
43. Herndon, J. H., Jr., et al. 1969. J. Clin. Invest. 48: 1017-1032.
44. Herndon, J. H., Jr., et al. 1969. N. Engl. J. Med. 281: 1034-1038.
45. Hirschhorn, R., et al. 1975. Lancet 1:73-75.
46. Howell, R. R., et al. 1971. J. Pediatr. 78:638-642.
47. Huijing, F., et al. 1973. Clin. Chim. Acta 44:453-455.
48. Justice, P., et al. 1970. Biochem. Biophys. Res. Commun. 39:301-306.
49. Kaback, M. M., et al. 1973. J. Pediatr. 82:1037-1041.
50. Kang, E. S., et al. 1972. Pediatr. Res. 6:875-879.
51. Kaufman, S., et al. 1975. N. Engl. J. Med. 293:785-790.
52. Komrower, G. M. 1974. Pediatrics 53:182-188.
53. Kousseff, B. G., et al. 1976. Ibid. 57:205-213.
54. Kraemer, K. H., et al. 1975. Proc. Natl. Acad. Sci. USA 72:59-63.
55. Krane, S. M., et al. 1972. Ibid. 69:2899-2903.
56. Krone, W., et al. 1970. Humangenetik 10:224-230.
57. Krooth, R. S. 1964. Cold Spring Harbor Symp. Quant. Biol. 29:189-212.
58. Leroy, J. G., et al. 1973. N. Engl. J. Med. 288:1365-1369.
59. Lichtenstein, J. R., et al. 1973. Science 182:298-300.
60. Lowden, J. A., et al. 1973. N. Engl. J. Med. 288:225-228.

continued

74. PRENATAL DIAGNOSIS OF INHERITED DISEASE

Part I. Inborn Errors of Metabolism

61. Mahoney, M. J., et al. 1975. Acta Paediatr. Scand. 64: 44-48.
62. Matsuda, I., et al. 1975. Humangenetik 30:69-73.
63. Morrow, G., III, et al. 1970. J. Pediatr. 77:120-123.
64. Mudd, S. H., et al. 1972. Biochem. Biophys. Res. Commun. 46:905-912.
65. Nadler, H. L. 1968. Biochem. Genet. 2:119-126.
66. Nadler, H. L. 1968. Pediatrics 42:912-918.
67. Nadler, H. L., and T. J. Egan. 1970. N. Engl. J. Med. 282:302-307.
68. Nadler, H. L., and A. B. Gerbie. 1970. Ibid. 282:596-599.
69. Nadler, H. L., and A. M. Messina. 1969. Lancet 2: 1277-1278.
70. Niermeijer, M. F., et al. 1975. Pediatr. Res. 9:498-503.
71. O'Brien, J. S. 1972. Proc. Natl. Acad. Sci. USA 69: 1720-1722.
72. O'Brien, J. S., et al. 1971. Science 172:61-64.
73. Pan, Y.-L., and R. S. Krooth. 1968. J. Cell. Physiol. 71:151-160.
74. Patel, V., et al. 1972. Science 176:426-427.
75. Patrick, A. D., et al. 1976. J. Med. Genet. 13:49-51.
76. Pope, F. M., et al. 1975. Proc. Natl. Acad. Sci. USA 72:1314-1316.
77. Ramsay, C. A., et al. 1974. Lancet 2:1109-1112.
78. Roerdink, F. H., et al. 1973. Pediatr. Res. 7:863-869.
79. Romeo, G., et al. 1970. Biochem. Genet. 4:659-664.
80. Sandhoff, K., and H. Jatzkewitz. 1972. Adv. Exp. Med. Biol. 19:305-319.
81. Sassa, S., et al. 1975. J. Exp. Med. 142:722-731.
82. Schneck, L., et al. 1970. Lancet 1:582-583.
83. Schneider, E. L., et al. 1972. J. Pediatr. 81:1134-1139.
84. Schneider, E. L., et al. 1972. Pediatr. Res. 6:720-729.
85. Schneider, J. A., et al. 1974. N. Engl. J. Med. 290: 878-882.
86. Shih, V. E., and J. W. Littlefield. 1970. Lancet 2:45.
87. Shih, V. E., et al. 1969. Biochem. Genet. 3:81-83.
88. Shih, V. E., et al. 1976. Pediatr. Res. 10:371(Abstr. 423).
89. Simell, O., et al. 1973. J. Pediatr. 82:54-57.
90. Singh, J., et al. 1976. J. Clin. Invest. 57:1036-1040.
91. Spence, M. W., et al. 1973. Pediatr. Res. 7:394.
92. Spielberg, S. P., et al. 1976. Ibid. 10:372(Abstr. 426).
93. States, B., et al. 1975. J. Pediatr. 87:558-562.
94. Strömme, J. H., et al. 1976. Pediatr. Res. 10:62-66.
95. Stumpf, D. A., et al. 1973. Am. J. Dis. Child. 126: 747-755.
96. Sugita, M., et al. 1972. Science 178:1100-1102.
97. Suzuki, K., et al. 1971. Biochem. Biophys. Res. Commun. 45:1363-1366.
98. Taylor, H. A., et al. 1975. Clin. Chim. Acta 59:93-99.
99. Tedesco, T. A., and W. J. Mellman. 1967. Proc. Natl. Acad. Sci. USA 57:829-834.
100. Thomas, G. H., et al. 1973. Pediatr. Res. 7:751-756.
101. Tildon, J. T., and M. Cornblath. 1972. J. Clin. Invest. 51:493-498.
102. Uhlendorf, B. W., and S. H. Mudd. 1968. Science 160:1007-1009.
103. Valle, D. L., et al. 1974. Ibid. 185:1053-1054.
104. Wellner, V. P., et al. 1974. Proc. Natl. Acad. Sci. USA 71:2505-2509.
105. Wendel, U., et al. 1973. Humangenetik 19:127-128.
106. Wenger, D. A., et al. 1974. Proc. Natl. Acad. Sci. USA 71:854-857.
107. Zielke, K., et al. 1972. J. Exp. Med. 136:197-199.

Part II. Other Disorders

Prenatal diagnosis has been reported in all of these disorders. **IP** = inheritance pattern; **AR** = autosomal recessive; **AD** = autosomal dominant; **MF** = multifactorial.

	Disorder	IP	Defect Expressed in:	Detected by:	CNS Damage	Reference
1	Chromosome disorders, many types	Fn[1]	Amniotic fluid cells	Karyotyping of amniotic fluid cells	Yes, in many; no, in some	9
2	Hemoglobinopathies β-Thalassemia, several forms	AR	Fetal erythrocytes	Diminished globin β-chain synthesis in fetal blood cells	No	6
3	Sickle cell anemia	AR	Fetal erythrocytes	Synthesis of globin β^S-chain instead of globin β^A-chain	Unusual complication	1,7
4	Myotonic dystrophy	AD	Amniotic fluid	Linkage to the locus for ABH blood secretion (secretor locus)	No	4,5,10

[1] Most sporadic.

continued

74. PRENATAL DIAGNOSIS OF INHERITED DISEASE

Part II. Other Disorders

	Disorder	IP	Defect Expressed in:	Detected by:	CNS Damage	Reference
5	Neural tube defects Anencephalia	MF	Amniotic fluid	Elevated levels of α-fetoprotein; detection of cranial malformation by ultrasound	Yes	2,3,8
6	Meningomyelocele, "open" type	MF	Amniotic fluid	Elevated levels of α-fetoprotein	Yes	2,3,8

Contributor: Erbe, Richard W.

References
1. Alter, B. P., et al. 1976. Clin. Res. 24:293A.
2. Brock, D. J. H., and R. G. Sutcliffe. 1972. Lancet 2: 197-199.
3. Campbell, S., et al. 1972. Ibid. 2:1226-1227.
4. Harper, P., et al. 1971. J. Med. Genet. 8:438-440.
5. Insley, J., et al. 1976. Lancet 1:806.
6. Kan, Y. W., et al. 1975. Ibid. 2:790-791.
7. Kan, Y. W., et al. 1976. N. Engl. J. Med. 294:1039-1040.
8. Milunsky, A., and E. Alpert. 1976. Pediatr. Res. 10: 419(Abstr. 708).
9. Milunsky, A., and L. Atkins. 1975. In A. Milunsky, ed. The Prevention of Genetic Disease and Mental Retardation. W. B. Saunders, Philadelphia. pp. 221-263.
10. Schrott, H. G., et al. 1973. Clin. Genet. 4:38-45.

75. HEREDITARY AND ACQUIRED AMINOACIDOPATHIES

The aminoacidurias presented in this table are divided into acquired and inherited types. Disturbances related to perinatal adaptive phenomena of multifactorial origin are included. The classification recognizes physiological factors affecting amino acid distribution between plasma and urine, and whether the disorder primarily affects catabolism or membrane transport of the amino acid(s). Thus, the disorders are grouped according to mechanism and preferred fluid for detection. The data refer to those conditions associated with perturbation of the normal content of ninhydrin-reactive metabolites in plasma or urine; some exceptions have been made to include ninhydrin-negative metabolites.

Part I. Group IA

The primary defect is in catabolism. There is a low renal clearance of amino acid but a hyperaminoaciduria by saturation of transepithelial transport. Detection in the plasma is preferable unless otherwise indicated, but the use of urine for screening (or diagnosis) is not precluded; assignment to this group implies primarily that diagnosis (or screening) of the condition is feasible by virtue of significant metabolite accumulation in blood (or plasma). **Amino Acid Affected:**

↓ = decreased; ↑ = increased. For source of **Enzyme Commission No.**, *see* Introduction. **IP:** Apparent inheritance pattern; AR = autosomal recessive; (AR) = probably autosomal recessive; XL = X-linked. **Remarks:** CNS = central nervous system; CoA = coenzyme A; CSF = cerebrospinal fluid. Data in brackets refer to the column heading in brackets.

	Condition or Disease	Amino Acid Affected	Enzyme Affected ⟨Synonym⟩ [Enzyme Commission No.]	IP	Remarks
			Common Perinatal (Adaptive) Traits [1]		
1	Neonatal hyperphenylalaninemia	Phenylalanine	Phenylalanine 4-monooxygenase ⟨Phenylalanine-hydroxylating system⟩ [1.14.16.1]	...	Benign; may respond to folic acid. Often occurs with tyrosinemia.

[1] These conditions have been detected by screening methods applied in the newborn period of life. They should not be misdiagnosed as permanent disorders of amino acid metabolism also identifiable by screening.

continued

Part I. Group IA

	Condition or Disease	Amino Acid Affected	Enzyme Affected ⟨Synonym⟩ [Enzyme Commission No.]	IP	Remarks
2	Neonatal tyrosinemia	Tyrosine	4-Hydroxyphenylpyruvate dioxygenase ⟨p-Hydroxyphenyl pyruvic acid hydroxylase⟩ [1.13.11.27]	...	Benign; responds to ascorbic acid & reduced protein intake
3	Hypermethioninemia	Methionine	? Methionine adenosyltransferase ⟨ATP:L-methionine S-adenosyltransferase⟩ [2.5.1.6]	...	Benign; usually found with high protein intake
4	Hyperhistidinemia	Histidine	? L-Histidine ammonia-lyase [4.3.1.3]	...	Benign; related to high protein intake
			Inherited Traits		
	Hyperphenylalaninemias				
5	Classical phenylketonuria	Phenylalanine	Phenylalanine 4-monooxygenase ⟨L-Phenylalanine, tetrahydropteridine:oxygen oxidoreductase (4-hydroxylating)⟩ [1.14.16.1]	AR	Plasma phenylalanine >16 mg/100 ml; causes mental retardation. When treated, L-phenylalanine tolerance in diet is 250-500 mg/d.
6	Atypical phenylketonuria	Phenylalanine	Same as for entry 5	(AR)	Plasma phenylalanine >16 mg/100 ml; similar to entry 5, but dietary tolerance for L-phenylalanine is >500 mg/d
7	Transient phenylketonuria	Phenylalanine	Same as for entry 5	(AR)	Plasma phenylalanine >16 mg/100 ml; change in status to that for entry 8, or normal, several months or years after birth
8	Benign hyperphenylalaninemia	Phenylalanine	Same as for entry 5	AR	Plasma phenylalanine <16 mg/100 ml on normal diet. Benign trait.
9	Phenylketonuria (dihydropteridine reductase deficiency)	Phenylalanine	Dihydropteridine reductase [1.6.99.7]	(AR)	Resembles classical phenylketonuria, but no CNS response to diet. Enzyme can be assayed in cultured skin fibroblasts.
	Hypertyrosinemias				
10	Tyrosinosis (Medes)	Tyrosine	? Tyrosine aminotransferase ⟨L-Tyrosine:α-ketoglutarate aminotransferase⟩ [2.6.1.5]	(AR)	One case known; myasthenia gravis probably incidental finding
11	Hypertyrosinemia	Tyrosine	Soluble (cytosol) tyrosine aminotransferase [2.6.1.5]	(AR)	Associated with developmental retardation. Richner-Hanhart syndrome in some patients.
12	Hereditary tyrosinemia	Tyrosine (& methionine in acute stage)	4-Hydroxyphenylpyruvate dioxygenase 2/ [1.13.11.27]	AR	Hepatic cirrhosis, & renal tubular failure; usually fatal in absence of tyrosine restriction
	Hyperhistidinemias 3/				
13	Classical form	Histidine (alanine in some cases)	L-Histidine ammonia-lyase 4/ [4.3.1.3]	AR	Occasionally associated with mental retardation & speech defect
14	Variant form	Histidine	L-Histidine ammonia-lyase 5/ [4.3.1.3]	(AR)	Same as for entry 13
	Branched-chain hyperaminoacidemias 6/				
15	Classical "maple syrup urine disease"	Leucine, isoleucine, valine, alloisoleucine	Branched-chain α-ketoacid oxidase(s) (probably decarboxylase component)	AR	Postnatal collapse; mental retardation in survivors. Diet therapy can be effective.

2/ Probably secondary defect; primary unknown. 3/ Urine screening is as efficient as, or even more reliable than, blood screening in these conditions. 4/ Liver and epidermis. 5/ Liver only. 6/ A number of disorders of branched-chain amino acid catabolism cause accumulation of substances which are ninhydrin-negative. These compounds can usually be detected by gas-liquid chromatographic methods.

continued

Part I. Group IA

	Condition or Disease	Amino Acid Affected	Enzyme Affected ⟨Synonym⟩ [Enzyme Commission No.]	IP	Remarks
16	Intermittent form	Leucine, isoleucine, valine, alloisoleucine	Branched-chain α-ketoacid oxidase(s) 7/	(AR)	Intermittent symptoms; development may be otherwise normal
17	Mild form	Same as for entry 16	Same as for entry 16	(AR)	Unremittent; milder than for entry 15
18	Thiamine-responsive form	Same as for entry 16	Same as for entry 16	(AR)	Mild form; responsive to thiamine ⟨Vitamin B_1⟩
19	Hypervalinemia	Valine	Branched-chain-amino-acid aminotransferase ⟨Valine aminotransferase⟩ [2.6.1.42]	AR	Retarded development & vomiting; responds to diet
20	Hyperleucinemia	Leucine or isoleucine	Branched-chain-amino-acid aminotransferase ⟨Leucine/isoleucine aminotransferase⟩ [2.6.1.42]	(AR)	Retarded development
	Sulfur aminoacidemias				
21	Homocyst(e)inuria 3/ (cystathionine synthase deficiency)	Methionine & homocyst(e)ine	Cystathionine β-synthase ⟨L-Serine hydro-lyase (adding homocysteine)⟩ [4.2.1.22]	AR	Usually associated with thromboembolic disease, mental retardation, & Marfan-like phenotype
22	Homocyst(e)inuria (methylene THF reductase deficiency)	Methionine (low) & homocyst(e)ine (high)	5,10-Methylenetetrahydrofolate reductase [1.1.1.68]	AR	Defective remethylation of homocysteine to methionine. Neurologic & behavioral symptoms associated.
23	Homocyst(e)inuria (with methylmalonic aciduria)	Homocyst(e)ine (high), methionine (low); plus methylmalonate	Defective cobalamin coenzyme biosynthesis	(AR)	Defective remethylation of homocysteine & methylmalonyl-CoA mutase ⟨MMA mutase⟩ activity. Severe neurologic signs & acidosis after birth.
24	Cystathioninuria 3/	Cystathionine	Cystathionine γ-lyase [4.4.1.1]	AR	Probably benign trait. Vitamin B_6 corrects biochemical trait in most patients.
	Hyperglycinemias				
25	Ketotic form	Glycine & other glucogenic amino acids	Propionyl-CoA carboxylase (ATP-hydrolyzing) ⟨Propionyl-CoA:carbon-dioxide ligase (ADP-forming)⟩ [6.4.1.3]	AR	Ketosis, neutropenia, mental retardation; often fatal. Detectable in skin fibroblasts.
26			Methylmalonyl-CoA racemase [5.1.99.1] or methylmalonyl-CoA mutase [5.4.99.2]	(AR)	Symptoms are those of methylmalonic aciduria with acidosis. (Some mutase-affected patients are responsive to vitamin B_{12}.)
27			Acetyl-CoA acyltransferase ⟨β-Ketothiolase⟩ [2.3.1.16] deficiency 8/	(AR)	Symptoms are those of α-methyl-β-hydroxybutyric aciduria (with or without tiglic aciduria) & acidosis
28	Non-ketotic form	Glycine	Glycine cleavage reaction (CO_2, NH_3, & hydroxymethyltetrahydrofolate formed)	AR	Severe CNS depression soon after birth. High CSF:plasma glycine ratio. Benzoate decreases plasma glycine; no effect on CNS prognosis.
29	Sarcosinemia 3/	Sarcosine	Sarcosine oxidase ⟨Sarcosine:oxygen oxidoreductase (demethylating)⟩ [1.5.3.1]	AR	Benign trait (probably)

3/ Urine screening is as efficient as, or even more reliable than, blood screening in these conditions. 7/ Partial activity: <2% of normal. 8/ Hyperglycinemia observed only in some patients with this enzyme deficiency.

continued

Part I. Group IA

	Condition or Disease	Amino Acid Affected	Enzyme Affected ⟨Synonym⟩ [Enzyme Commission No.]	IP	Remarks
	Hyperprolinemias				
30	Type I	Proline	Pyrroline-5-carboxylate reductase ⟨L-Proline:NAD(P)$^+$ 5-oxidoreductase; proline oxidase⟩ [1.5.1.2]	AR	Benign trait, sometimes associated with hereditary nephritis
31	Type II	Proline	1-Pyrroline dehydrogenase ⟨Δ^1-Pyrroline-5-carboxylate:NAD$^+$ oxidoreductase⟩ [1.5.1.12]	AR	Possibly benign trait, sometimes associated with CNS disease; Δ^1-pyrroline-5-carboxylate & 3-hydroxy-1-pyrroline-5-carboxylate excreted in urine; proline concentration $>$ type I
32	Hydroxyprolinemia	Hydroxyproline	4-Oxoproline reductase ⟨4-Hydroxy-L-proline:NAD$^+$ oxidoreductase⟩ [1.1.1.104]	AR	Sometimes associated with CNS disease; probably benign
	Hyperlysinemias				
33	Type I	Lysine (& glutamine)	Saccharopine dehydrogenase (NADP$^+$, lysine-forming) [1.5.1.8]	AR	Associated with mental retardation & hypotonia
34	Type II	Lysine, arginine (sometimes NH$_3$)	? Partial defect of enzyme in entry 33 or different enzyme	(AR)	Hyperammonemia symptoms, related to protein intake
35	Saccharopinuria[3/]	Lysine, saccharopine, citrulline	? Saccharopine dehydrogenase (NADP$^+$, L-glutamate-forming) ⟨Saccharopine dehydrogenase⟩ [1.5.1.10]	(AR)	Two cases; associated with mental retardation
36	Hydroxylysinemia	Free hydroxylysine	? Hydroxylysine kinase [2.7.1.81]	(AR)	Mental retardation
37	α-Aminoadipic aciduria	α-Aminoadipic acid (& α-ketoadipic acid)	? "α-Ketoadipate dehydrogenase"	(AR)	Mental retardation
38	Pipecolic acidemia[3/]	Pipecolic acid	? L-Pipecolate dehydrogenase ⟨Pipecolate oxidase⟩ [1.5.99.3]	(AR)	Hepatomegaly & mental retardation
	Hyperammonemias[9/]				
39	Carbamyl-phosphate synthetase ⟨CPS⟩ deficiency	Glycine, glutamine	Carbamate kinase ⟨ATP:carbamate phosphotransferase⟩ [2.7.2.2]	AR	Group of diseases with ammonia intoxication, protein intolerance, hepatomegaly, vomiting, etc. Argininosuccinic aciduria also has trichorrhexis nodosa.
40	Ornithine transcarbamylase ⟨OTC⟩ deficiency	Glutamine	Ornithine carbamoyltransferase ⟨Carbamoylphosphate:L-ornithine carbamoyltransferase⟩ [2.1.3.3]	XL	
41	Hyperornithinemia	Ornithine	Carbamate kinase ⟨ATP:carbamate phosphotransferase I⟩ [2.7.2.2] (possibly); or mitochondrial ornithine transport system, or ornithine decarboxylase [4.1.1.17]	(AR)	
42	Citrullinemia	Citrulline	Argininosuccinate synthetase ⟨L-Citrulline:L-aspartate ligase (AMP-forming)⟩ [6.3.4.5]	AR	
43	Argininosuccinic aciduria[3/]	Argininosuccinic acid	Argininosuccinate lyase ⟨L-Argininosuccinate arginine-lyase⟩ [4.3.2.1]	AR	

[3/] Urine screening is as efficient as, or even more reliable than, blood screening in these conditions. [9/] *See also* entry 34.

continued

75. HEREDITARY AND ACQUIRED AMINOACIDOPATHIES

Part I. Group IA

	Condition or Disease	Amino Acid Affected	Enzyme Affected ⟨Synonym⟩ [Enzyme Commission No.]	IP	Remarks
44	Hyperargininemia	Arginine	Arginase ⟨L-Arginine amidinohydrolase⟩ [3.5.3.1]	(AR)	Deterioration of CNS function & IQ in childhood. Hyperammonemia (inconstant) aggravated by protein.
45	Hyperalaninemias	Alanine	Pyruvate dehydrogenase (lipoate) ⟨Pyruvate dehydrogenase⟩ [1.2.4.1] deficiency	(AR)	Lactic acidosis, intermittent ataxia, mental retardation
46			Pyruvate carboxylase [6.4.1.1] deficiency	(AR)	Intermittent lactic acidosis, intermittent hypoglycemia
47	Aspartylglycosaminuria	Glycoasparagines	Aspartylglucosylaminase ⟨2-Acetamido-1-(β¹-L-aspartamido)-1,2-dideoxyglucose amidohydrolase⟩ [3.5.1.26]	AR	? Lysosomal disease; mental retardation
48	"Glutathionemia"	Glutathione or related peptide	γ-Glutamyltransferase ⟨γ-Glutamyl-transpeptidase⟩ [2.3.2.2] deficiency	(AR)	Mental retardation associated with finding
	Other Conditions Which May Affect Amino Acids in Plasma				
49	Protein-calorie malnutrition	Tryptophan/leucine/ isoleucine/valine ↓; tyrosine/glycine/ proline ↑	....	...	Severity of change related to severity of malnutrition
50	Prolonged fasting	Alanine ↓; threonine, glycine ↑	....	...	Early fasting does not show same pattern
51	Obesity	Leucine/isoleucine/ valine/phenylalanine/tyrosine ↑; glycine ↓	....	...	Reflects insulin insensitivity
52	Hepatitis	Methionine/tyrosine ↑	....	...	Reflects severity of liver disease

Contributor: Scriver, Charles R.

Reference: Scriver, C. R., and L. E. Rosenberg. 1973. Amino Acid Metabolism and Its Disorders. W. B. Saunders, Philadelphia.

Part II. Group IB

The primary defect is in catabolism. There is a high renal clearance of amino acid and a hyperaminoaciduria by saturation of transepithelial transport. Detection in the urine is preferable. *See also* entries 21, 24, and 43 in Part I. For source of **Enzyme Commission No.**, *see* Introduction. **IP:** Apparent inheritance pattern; AR = autosomal recessive; (AR) = probably autosomal recessive; AD = autosomal dominant. Data in brackets refer to the column heading in brackets.

	Condition or Disease	Substance Affected ⟨Synonym⟩	Enzyme Affected ⟨Synonym⟩ [Enzyme Commission No.]	IP	Remarks
1	Hypophosphatasia	Phosphoethanolamine	? Deficiency of ethanolaminephosphate phospho-lyase ⟨O-phosphorylethanolamine phospho-lyase⟩ [4.2.99.7]	AR	"Rickets"—unresponsive to vitamin D; craniosynostosis; hypercalcemia

continued

Part II. Group IB

	Condition or Disease	Substance Affected ⟨Synonym⟩	Enzyme Affected ⟨Synonym⟩ [Enzyme Commission No.]	IP	Remarks
2	Pseudohypophosphatasia	Phosphoethanolamine	"Alkaline phosphatase" activity present but altered (K_m mutant)	(AR)	Same as for entry 1
3	β-Aminoisobutyric aciduria	β-Aminoisobutyric acid	?	AD/AR	Benign polymorphic trait
4	Hyper-β-alaninemia	β-Alanine	? β-Alanine—pyruvate aminotransferase ⟨β-Alanine transaminase⟩ [2.6.1.18]	(AR)	Seizures; somnolence; mental retardation
5	Carnosinemia	Carnosine	Aminoacyl-histidine dipeptidase ⟨Carnosinase⟩ [3.4.13.3]	AR	Seizures & mental retardation; or benign possibly
6	Pyroglutamic acid-uria [1/]	L-Pyroglutamic acid ⟨5-Oxo-L-proline; pyrrolidone-2-carboxylic acid⟩	Glutathione synthetase [6.3.2.3]	(AR)	L-Pyroglutamic acid ⟨5-Oxo-L-proline⟩ results from overproduction via modified γ-glutamyl cycle

[1/] Urine screening is as efficient as, or even more reliable than, blood screening in these conditions.

Contributor: Scriver, Charles R.

Reference: Scriver, C. R., and L. E. Rosenberg. 1973. Amino Acid Metabolism and Its Disorders. W. B. Saunders, Philadelphia.

Part III. Group II

There is a primary defect in catabolism and a secondary defect in transport. Hyperaminoaciduria is of combined origin—saturation and competition. Detection is possible in both plasma and urine.

	Disease	Amino Acids		Remarks
		Affected in Plasma	Present in Urine	
1	Hyperprolinemia, types I & II	Proline	Proline, + hydroxyproline & glycine	*See* entries 30 & 31 in Part I. Competition occurs on iminoglycine transport system (*see* Part IV).
2	Hyper-β-alaninemia	β-Alanine	β-Alanine, + β-aminoisobutyric acid & taurine	*See* entry 4 in Part II. Competition occurs on β-amino transport system.
3	Hyperlysinemia	Lysine	Lysine, + ornithine & arginine	*See* entries 33-36 in Part I. Competition occurs on "dibasic" transport system (*see* Part IV).
4	Hyperargininemia	Arginine	Ornithine & lysine; & sometimes generalized hyperaminoaciduria	*See* entry 44 in Part I. Competition occurs on "dibasic" transport system (*see* Part IV). Pathogenesis of generalized aminoaciduria unknown.

Contributor: Scriver, Charles R.

General References

1. Scriver, C. R., and L. E. Rosenberg. 1973. Amino Acid Metabolism and Its Disorders. W. B. Saunders, Philadelphia.

2. Scriver, C. R., et al. 1976. Kidney Int. 9:149-171.

continued

Part IV.   Group III

The primary defect is in the membrane transport site. There is a high renal clearance of amino acid, and detection is possible only in the urine. **Activity Affected:** Presumed gene product activity affected by mutant gene. **IP:** Apparent inheritance pattern; AD = autosomal dominant; (AD) = probably autosomal dominant; AR = autosomal recessive; (AR) = probably autosomal recessive; XL = X-linked. **Remarks:** hetz = heterozygote; homoz = homozygote. *Abbreviation:* PTH = parathyroid hormone.

	Trait	Substance Affected	Activity Affected	Other Tissues Affected	IP	Remarks
			Common Perinatal (Adaptive) Trait			
1	Neonatal imino-glycinuria	Proline, hydroxy-proline, glycine	Specific proline & specific glycine transport (probably)	....	......	Benign adaptive trait; prolinuria subsides at ∿100 d, glycinuria at ∿200 d after full-term birth
2	Neonatal cystine-lysinuria	Cystine & dibasic amino acids (lysine, ornithine, & arginine)	Specific dibasic transport system	....	......	Transient; evident in newborn period in some but not all infants
			Inherited Hyperaminoacidurias			
3	Selective Hyperdibasic aminoaciduria	Lysine, ornithine, arginine ("dibasic" group)	Shared "dibasic" amino acid transport system	Intestine; ? liver; ? brain	AD/AR	Two alleles (? different loci). Type I associated with protein intolerance, failure to thrive, hyperammonemia (? mitochondrial defect); hetz silent. Type II associated with mental retardation in recently discovered homoz. Hetz have modest dibasic aminoaciduria.
4	Cystinuria	Lysine, ornithine, arginine, & cyst(e)ine	Shared membrane system (? for efflux)	Intestine; ? brain. (Skin fibroblasts are normal.)	AR	"Negative" readsorption of affected amino acid can occur. Three alleles (? same locus), each causing different phenotypes: In type I hetz, no amino acids in urine ("silent"); in type III homoz, intestinal transport intact (or partial defect).
5	Hypercystinuria	Cystine	Specific system for cyst(e)ine	?	(AR)	One pedigree only
6	Iminoglycinuria	Proline; hydroxy-proline; glycine	Shared system for imino acids, glycine (& sarcosine)	Intestine	AR	Four alleles (? same locus). I & II are silent hetz; III & IV are hyperglycinuric hetz. I associated with intestinal defect; IV with K_m mutant.
7	Hartnup	Neutral amino acids (excluding imino acids & glycine)	Shared system for large neutral amino acid group (luminal membrane)	Intestine. (Skin fibroblasts are normal.)	AR	Two alleles (? same locus). I, intestine affected; II, intestine normal. Hetz "silent" in both.
8	Histidinuria	Histidine	? Specific histidine system	Intestine	(AR)	Associated with mental retardation in siblings
9	Dicarboxylic aminoaciduria (glutamate-aspartate transport defect)	Glutamic acid, aspartic acid	? Shared dicarboxylic acid transport system	? Intestine	(AR)	Hypoglycemia

continued

Part IV. Group III

	Trait	Substance Affected	Activity Affected	Other Tissues Affected	IP	Remarks
10	Generalized Idiopathic Fanconi's syndrome	Generalized effect on all solutes & water	? Coupling of energy; ? tight junction integrity	Secondary to renal phenotype	AR (& ?AD)	Adult onset and infantile-childhood forms are differentiated. Basic defect unknown; probably several alleles.
11	Symptomatic forms of Fanconi syndromes Cystinosis: type I, type II, & type III	Same as for entry 10 (secondary response)	Cystine storage (lysosomal defect), with secondary damage to tubule & glomerulus (later)	Secondary to renal phenotype	AR [1]	Several alleles. Infantile (type I) & adolescent (type II) forms have differing rates for onset of nephropathy. "Adult" form (type III) has no nephropathy.
12	Hereditary fructose intolerance	Same as for entry 10, + fructose	Fructose-1-phosphate aldolase ⟨Fructose-bisphosphate aldolase⟩ (with secondary effects on cellular ATP)	Secondary to renal phenotype (hepatic cirrhosis)	AR	Nephropathy dependent on intact PTH-cAMP axis in kidney. Responds to fructose withdrawal.
13	Galactosemia	Same as for entry 10, + galactose	Galactose-1-phosphate uridylyltransferase (with secondary effects on cellular ATP)	Secondary to renal phenotype (cataracts, CNS effects)	AR	"Galactosemia" due to galactokinase deficiency does not have Fanconi's syndrome. Fanconi's syndrome responds to galactose withdrawal.
14	Hereditary tyrosinemia	Same as for entry 10, + tyrosine metabolites	Unknown (with secondary effects on cellular ATP)	Secondary to renal phenotype (hepatic cirrhosis)	(AR)	Fanconi's syndrome responds to tyrosine restriction
15	Wilson's disease	Same as for entry 10, with proximal & distal renal tubular acidosis	Unknown (? secondary effects on cytochrome oxidase system)	Hepatolenticular degeneration	(AR)	Fanconi's syndrome responds to depletion of copper storage
16	Lowe's oculocerebrorenal syndrome	Generalized dysfunction with defective urinary NH_3 production	Unknown	An oculocerebro-intestinal-renal syndrome (? involving tissues with high γ-glutamyl cycle activity)	XL [2]	Basic defect still unknown. Treatment for tubular reclamation defects does not improve mental retardation or the cataracts & hydrophthalmia.
17	Vitamin D dependency (Pseudodeficiency rickets)	Generalized defect (secondary response)	25-Hydroxyvitamin D-1-α-hydroxylase	Vitamin D hormone synthesis occurs in kidney mitochondria; deficiency affects intestinal absorption of calcium & initiates PTH response	AR	Nephropathy dependent on PTH excess & hypocalcemia (phenocopy occurs in vitamin D deficiency)
18	Miscellaneous Glucoglycinuria	Glucose & glycine	Unknown (the two solutes do not share a common carrier)	....	(AD)	Asymptomatic. Normal-Tm (type B) glucosuria. Possibility that this is a heterozygous manifestation of a Fanconi-like tubulopathy merits consideration.

[1] For each type. [2] Recessive.

continued

75. HEREDITARY AND ACQUIRED AMINOACIDOPATHIES

Part IV. Group III

	Trait	Substance Affected	Activity Affected	Other Tissues Affected	IP	Remarks
19	Luder-Sheldon syndrome	Generalized amino acids, glucose, & phosphate	Unknown	....	(AD)	Same as for entry 18. Symptoms of Fanconi's syndrome have occurred in probands.
20	Rowley-Rosenberg syndrome	Generalized aminoaciduria	Unknown	....	(AR)	Associated components of syndrome: growth retardation, muscular hypoplasia, pulmonary involvement, & right ventricular hypertrophy

Contributor: Scriver, Charles R.

General References

1. Scriver, C. R., and L. E. Rosenberg. 1973. Amino Acid Metabolism and Its Disorders. W. B. Saunders, Philadelphia.

2. Scriver, C. R., et al. 1976. Kidney Int. 9:149-171.

Part V. Normal Amino Acid Concentrations in Plasma or Serum

Data were adapted from table 3-1 in reference 5. All data were obtained by elution chromatography on ion exchange resin columns. **Neonates:** Values were recalculated from the reference; subjects were 25 infants, weighing >2500 grams, studied before first feeding. **Infants:** Values were recalculated from the reference; subjects were 12 infants, 16 days-4 months old, studied after 6- to 8-hour fast. **Children:** Subjects were 9 children, 3-10 years old, studied after overnight fast. **Adults:** Subjects were 10 men and 10 women, 33-56 years old. Values in parentheses are ranges, estimate "c" (*see* Introduction).

	Amino Acid	Value, μmole/liter			
		Neonates	Infants	Children	Adults
1	Alanine	329 ± 55	292 ± 53	234(137-305)	360 ± 71 (205-496)
2	β-Alanine	14.5	....	....	....
3	Arginine	54 ± 17	62 ± 9	53(23-86)	82 ± 17 (53-115)
4	Asparagine	759 ± 136[1]	(*See* entry 19)	295(57-467)[1]	56 ± 15 (34-82)
5	Aspartic acid	8 ± 4	19 ± 2	10(4-20)	(Trace-5)
6	½ Cystine	62 ± 13	42 ± 9	60(45-77)	49 ± 9 (34-67)
7	Glutamic acid	52 ± 25	....	110(23-250)	24 ± 12 (10-67)
8	Glutamine	(*See* entry 4)	....	(*See* entry 4)	640 ± 58 (520-742)
9	Glycine	343 ± 69	213 ± 35	166(117-223)	284 ± 44 (162-335)
10	Histidine	77 ± 16	78 ± 14	55(24-85)	88 ± 16 (65-119)
11	Hydroxyproline	32	....	25	....
12	Isoleucine	39 ± 8	39 ± 8	43(28-84)	60 ± 12 (38-83)
13	Leucine	72 ± 17	77 ± 21	85(56-178)	115 ± 23 (77-162)
14	Lysine	200 ± 46	135 ± 28	111(71-151)	186 ± 36 (99-249)
15	Methionine	29 ± 8	18 ± 3	14(11-16)	21 ± 4 (13-32)
16	Ornithine	91 ± 25	50 ± 11	33(27-86)	58 ± 14 (32-88)
17	Phenylalanine	78 ± 14	55 ± 10	42(26-61)	48 ± 7 (37-61)

[1] Combined value for asparagine + glutamine.

continued

Part V. Normal Amino Acid Concentrations in Plasma or Serum

Amino Acid	Value, μmole/liter			
	Neonates	Infants	Children	Adults
18 Proline	183 ± 32	193 ± 52	106(68-148)	185 ± 48 (90-270)
19 Serine	163 ± 34	131 ± 27[2/]	94(79-112)	99 ± 19 (67-129)
20 Taurine	141 ± 40	....	80(57-115)	59 ± 12 (41-78)
21 Threonine	217 ± 21	177 ± 36	76(42-95)	138 ± 31 (75-189)
22 Tryptophan	32 ± 17	....	....	31 ± 6 (19-45)
23 Tyrosine	69 ± 16	54 ± 21	43(31-71)	54 ± 11 (40-80)
24 Valine	136 ± 39	161 ± 38	162(128-283)	225 ± 40 (151-302)
Reference	2	1	4	3

[2/] Includes asparagine.

Contributor: Scriver, Charles R.

References

1. Brodehl, J., and K. Gellissen. 1968. Pediatrics 42:395-404.
2. Dickinson, J. C., et al. 1965. Ibid. 36:2-13.
3. Perry, T. L., and S. Hansen. 1969. Clin. Chim. Acta 25:53-58.
4. Scriver, C. R., and E. Davies. 1965. Pediatrics 32:592-598.
5. Scriver, C. R., and L. E. Rosenberg. 1973. Amino Acid Metabolism and Its Disorders. W. B. Saunders, Philadelphia. p. 42.

Part VI. Endogenous Renal Clearance of Amino Acids

Data were adapted from reference 5. All data were obtained by elution chromatography on ion exchange resins. **Infants: 7 Subjects**—four premature and three full-term infants, 30-60 days old, short-term clearance after 4-hour fast; **12 Subjects**—16 days-4 months old, short-term clearance after fasting. **Children: 12 Subjects**—2-13 years old, short-term clearance after overnight fast; **9 Subjects**—3-12 years old, short-term clearance after overnight fast. **Adults: 4 Subjects**—short-term clearance after overnight fast. Values in parentheses are ranges estimate "c" (see Introduction).

Amino Acid	Value, ml·min^{-1}·(1.73 m^2)$^{-1}$				
	Infants		Children		Adults
	7 Subjects	12 Subjects	12 Subjects	9 Subjects	4 Subjects
1 Alanine	(1.5-4.2)	1.6 ± 0.7	0.8 ± 0.4	0.8(0.2-1.3)	(0.3-0.9)
2 Arginine	(Trace-1.0)	0.4 ± 0.1	0.3 ± 0.1	0.5(0.15-1.2)	(0.2-0.8)
3 Asparagine + glutamine[1/]	(1.2-3.6)	(See entry 19)	(See entry 19)	1.3(0.1-2.3)	(0.7-1.8)
4 Aspartic acid	(Trace-16)	....	3.6 ± 0.9	2.8(trace-8.8)	(0-2.4)
5 ½ Cystine	(2.5-8.8)	1.1 ± 0.3	0.8 ± 0.2	(1.0-1.4)	(0.7-2.9)
6 Glutamic acid	(0.1-3.0)	....	....	0.8(0.1-2.4)	(0.3-0.7)
7 Glycine	(12-44)	7.4 ± 3.2	4.2 ± 1.4	4.4(1.2-8.6)	(2.7-5.8)
8 Histidine	(12-29)	8.5 ± 4.4	9.5 ± 2.6	9.2(1.9-21.8)	(4.7-9.1)
9 Hydroxyproline	(Trace-34)	....	....	(0-trace)	0
10 Isoleucine	(0.4-1.7)	0.3 ± 0.2	0.3 ± 0.1	0.5(0.2-1.0)	(0.2-1.0)
11 Leucine	(0.4-1.3)	0.8 ± 0.5	0.5 ± 0.1	0.5(0.2-0.9)	(0.2-0.9)
12 Lysine	(1.6-6.3)	1.3 ± 0.4	1.2 ± 0.4	1.1(0.3-2.4)	(0.2-1.9)
13 Methionine	(2.3-5.8)	0.8 ± 0.5	0.8 ± 0.3	1.9(1.0-3.4)	1.1
14 Ornithine	(0.6-1.1)	0.4 ± 0.1	0.4 ± 0.1	0.5(0.2-0.8)	Trace

[1/] Measured as the amides.

continued

75. HEREDITARY AND ACQUIRED AMINOACIDOPATHIES

Part VI. Endogenous Renal Clearance of Amino Acids

| Amino Acid | Value, ml·min^{-1}·(1.73 m^2)$^{-1}$ | | | | |
| | Infants | | Children | | Adults |
	7 Subjects	12 Subjects	12 Subjects	9 Subjects	4 Subjects
15 Phenylalanine	(1.0-2.2)	1.7 ± 0.9	1.5 ± 0.3	1.2(0.3-2.3)	(0.7-1.4)
16 Proline	(1.7-14.0)	1.0 ± 0.7	0.3 ± 0.2	(0-0.3)	0
17 Serine	(4.5-13.0)	4.1 ± 1.9	2.4 ± 0.5	2.4(1.2-3.4)	(1.9-3.0)
18 Taurine	(0.1-3.8)	....	....	13.7(9.9-26.2)	(1.7-14)
19 Threonine	(3.0-8.2)	2.0 ± 1.4[2/]	1.0 ± 0.2[2/]	1.4(0.5-2.5)	(0.8-1.5)
20 Tyrosine	(0.5-2.6)	1.8 ± 0.4	2.0 ± 0.8	2.0(0.8-3.3)	(1.0-1.7)
21 Valine	(0.2-0.6)	0.3 ± 0.1	0.2 ± 0.1	0.2(0.18-0.3)	(0.1-0.3)
Reference	3	1	1	4	2

[2/] Includes asparagine.

Contributor: Scriver, Charles R.

References

1. Brodehl, J., and K. Gellissen. 1968. Pediatrics 42:395-404.
2. Cusworth, D. C., and C. E. Dent. 1960. Biochem. J. 74:550-561.
3. O'Brien, D., and L. J. Butterfield. 1963. Arch. Dis. Child. 38:437-442.
4. Scriver, C. R., and E. Davies. 1965. Pediatrics 32:592-598.
5. Scriver, C. R., and L. E. Rosenberg. 1973. Amino Acid Metabolism and Its Disorders. W. B. Saunders, Philadelphia. p. 50.

76. SCREENING FOR GENETIC DISORDERS IN THE NEWBORN

Specific information concerning the disorders listed below may be found in other tables, especially table 75. **Metabolite or Enzyme Sought:** Present in increased concentration, unless otherwise indicated. **Specimen Most Suitable:** All specimens, except meconium, are dried into filter paper.

TEST ABBREVIATIONS

AFA = automated fluorometric assay (Hill, et al.)
BA = bacterial assay
BIA = bacterial inhibition assay (Guthrie)
DNPH = dinitrophenylhydrazine reaction as modified for eluates of urine
MRBA = metabolite-requiring bacterial assay

PC = paper chromatography: one-dimensional for blood; two-dimensional methods preferred for urine
RIA = radioimmunoassay
SEA = spot enzyme assay
TLC = thin-layer chromatography
TLE = thin-layer electrophoresis

Disorder ⟨Synonym⟩	Metabolite or Enzyme Sought ⟨Synonym⟩	Specimen Most Suitable	Test
Inborn Errors of Amino Acid Metabolism			
Hyperphenylalaninemias 1 Classical phenylketonuria ⟨PKU⟩	Phenylalanine	Blood	BIA, AFA
2 Phenylketonuria—dihydropteridine reductase deficiency	Phenylalanine	Blood	BIA, AFA

continued

	Disorder ⟨Synonym⟩	Metabolite or Enzyme Sought ⟨Synonym⟩	Specimen Most Suitable	Test
3	Atypical phenylketonuria	Phenylalanine	Blood	BIA, AFA
4	Persistent mild hyperphenylalaninemia	Phenylalanine	Blood	BIA, AFA
	Hypertyrosinemias			
5	Neonatal tyrosinemia	Tyrosine	Blood	BIA, AFA
6		Tyrosine metabolites: *p*-hydroxyphenyllactic acid ⟨p-HPLA⟩, *p*-hydroxyphenylacetic acid ⟨p-HPAA⟩	Urine	PC, TLC
7	Hereditary tyrosinemia ⟨Tyrosinosis⟩	Tyrosine	Blood	BIA, AFA
8		Tyrosine metabolites: *p*-hydroxyphenyllactic acid ⟨p-HPLA⟩, *p*-hydroxyphenylacetic acid ⟨p-HPAA⟩	Urine	PC, TLC
	Hyperhistidinemias			
9	Histidinemia	Histidine	Blood	BIA
10		Histidine metabolites: imidazolelactic acid ⟨ILA⟩, imidazoleacetic acid ⟨IAA⟩	Urine	PC, TLC
11	Atypical histidinemias	Histidine	Blood	BIA
12		Histidine metabolites: imidazolelactic acid ⟨ILA⟩, imidazoleacetic acid ⟨IAA⟩	Urine	PC, TLC
	Branched-chain hyperaminoacidemias			
13	Maple syrup urine disease ⟨MSUD⟩	Leucine [1]	Blood	BIA
14		Branched-chain α-keto acids	Urine	DNPH
15	Intermediate MSUD	Leucine [1]	Blood	BIA
16	Hyperleucinemia	Leucine	Blood	BIA
17	Hypervalinemia	Valine	Blood	PC, TLC
	Sulfur aminoacidemias			
18	Cystathionine β-synthase deficiency	Methionine	Blood	BIA, PC, TLC
19		Homocystine	Urine	PC, TLC
20	5,10-Methylenetetrahydrofolate reductase ⟨Methylene THF reductase⟩ deficiency	Homocystine	Urine	PC, TLC
21	Cystathioninemia	Cystathionine	Urine	PC, TLC
	Hyperglycinemias			
22	Non-ketotic hyperglycinemia	Glycine	Urine	PC, TLC
23	Ketotic hyperglycinemia	Glycine	Urine	PC, TLC
24	Sarcosinemia	Sarcosine	Urine	PC, TLC
	Hyperprolinemias			
25	Type I	Proline (also glycine & hydroxyproline)	Urine	PC, TLC
26	Type II	Proline (also glycine & hydroxyproline)	Urine	PC, TLC
27	Hydroxyprolinemia	Hydroxyproline	Urine	PC, TLC
	Hyperlysinemias			
28	Hyperlysinemia	Lysine (also cystine)	Urine	PC, TLC
29	Saccharopinuria	Saccharopine	Urine	PC, TLC
30	Hydroxylysinemia	Hydroxylysine	Urine	PC, TLC
31	Pipecolic acidemia	Pipecolic acid	Urine	PC, TLC
	Hyperammonemias			
32	Carbamoylphosphate synthase (ammonia) ⟨Carbamylphosphate synthetase; CPS⟩ deficiency	Glutamine	Urine	PC, TLC
33	Ornithine carbamoyltransferase ⟨Ornithine transcarbamylase; OTC⟩ deficiency	Glutamine	Urine	PC, TLC
34	Ornithinemia	Ornithine	Urine	PC, TLC
35	Citrullinemia	Citrulline	Blood [2]	PC, TLC
36			Urine	PC, TLC

[1] Also isoleucine and valine, which can be detected in blood by PC and TLC. [2] Special stain required.

continued

	Disorder ⟨Synonym⟩	Metabolite or Enzyme Sought ⟨Synonym⟩	Specimen Most Suitable	Test
37	Argininosuccinic acidemia ⟨ASA⟩	Argininosuccinic acid	Urine	PC, TLC
38		Argininosuccinate lyase ⟨Argininosuccinase⟩[3/]	Blood	MRBA
39	Hyperargininemia	Arginine (also lysine & cystine)	Urine	PC, TLC
40		Arginase[3/]	Blood	SEA
41	Lysinuric protein intolerance	Lysine	Urine	PC, TLC
42	Hyperalaninemia	Alanine	Urine	PC, TLC
43	Hypophosphatasia	Phosphoethanolamine	Urine	PC, TLC
44	Pseudohypophosphatasia	Phosphoethanolamine	Urine	PC, TLC
45	Hyper-β-alaninemia	β-Alanine	Urine	PC, TLC
46	Carnosinemia	Carnosine	Urine	PC, TLC
47	Urocanic aciduria	Urocanic acid	Urine	PC, TLC
48	Formiminoglutamic aciduria	Formiminoglutamic acid ⟨FIGLU⟩, glutamic acid	Urine	PC, TLC
49	Pyroglutamic aciduria	Pyroglutamic acid	Urine	PC
50	Alkaptonuria	Homogentisic acid	Urine	PC, TLC

Inborn Errors of Organic Acid Metabolism

51	Isovaleric acidemia	Isovalerylglycine	Urine	PC, TLC
52	Methylmalonic acidemia	Methylmalonic acid	Urine	PC, TLC
53	Glutaric acidemia	Glutaric acid	Urine	PC, TLC
54	Pyruvic acidemias	Pyruvic acid (also lactic acid)	Urine	PC, TLC

Inborn Errors of Carbohydrate Metabolism

	Galactose defects			
55	Galactosemia	Galactose	Blood	BA
56		Galactose-1-phosphate uridylyltransferase[3/]	Blood	SEA
57	Galactokinase deficiency	Galactose	Blood	BA
58	UDPglucose 4-epimerase ⟨UDPGal 4-epimerase⟩ deficiency	Galactose	Blood	BA

Inborn Errors of Transport

59	Cystinuria	Cystine, lysine, ornithine, arginine	Urine	PC, TLC
60	Isolated cystinuria	Cystine	Urine	PC, TLC
61	Hyperdibasic aminoaciduria	Lysine, ornithine, arginine	Urine	PC, TLC
62	Iminoglycinuria	Proline, hydroxyproline, glycine	Urine	PC, TLC
63	Hartnup disorder	Neutral amino acids (excluding glycine, proline, & hydroxyproline)	Urine	PC, TLC
64	Glutamate-aspartic aciduria	Glutamic acid, aspartic acid	Urine	PC, TLC
65	Fanconi's syndrome	Virtually all amino acids	Urine	PC, TLC

Hemoglobinopathies

66	Sickle cell disease	Hemoglobin S	Blood	TLE
67	Others	Abnormal hemoglobins: C, F, etc.	Blood	TLE

Immunologic Disorders

68	Adenosine deaminase deficiency	Adenosine deaminase[3/]	Blood	Spot test

Endocrine Disorders

69	Congenital hypothyroidism ⟨Cretinism⟩	Thyroxine ⟨T_4⟩[3/]	Blood	RIA
70		Thyrotropic hormone ⟨TSH⟩	Blood	RIA
71	Thyroxine-binding globulin ⟨TBG⟩ deficiency	Thyroxine ⟨T_4⟩[3/]	Blood	RIA

[3/] Present in decreased concentration.

continued

	Disorder ⟨Synonym⟩	Metabolite or Enzyme Sought ⟨Synonym⟩	Specimen Most Suitable	Test
		Miscellaneous Disorders		
72	Cystic fibrosis	Albumin	Meconium	Spot test
73	Muscular dystrophy ⟨Duchenne's⟩	Creatine kinase ⟨Creatine phosphokinase; CPK⟩	Blood	SEA
74	Hereditary angioneurotic edema	Acetylesterase ⟨C₁-esterase⟩ inhibitor [3]	Blood	SEA
75	α₁-Antitrypsin deficiency	α₁-Antitrypsin [3]	Blood	SEA, TLE
76	Orotic aciduria	Orotidine 5′-phosphate decarboxylase ⟨Orotidine 5′-monophosphate decarboxylase⟩ [3]	Blood	MRBA

[3] Present in decreased concentration.

Contributor: Levy, Harvey L.

Reference: Levy, H. L. 1973. Adv. Hum. Genet. 4:1-104.

77. INHERITED DISEASES DIAGNOSED FROM BLOOD CELLS

For source of **Enzyme Commission No.**, *see* Introduction. **Mode of Inheritance:** AR = autosomal recessive; SL = sex-linked; AD = autosomal dominant. Data in brackets refer to the column heading in brackets.

	Preferred Cells for Diagnosis	Disease	Enzyme ⟨Synonym⟩ [Enzyme Commission No.]	Mode of Inheritance	Reference
1	Erythro-	Anemia, non-spherocytic hered-	Adenosinetriphosphatase ⟨ATPase⟩ [3.6.1.3]	AR	21
2	cytes	itary hemolytic	Adenylate kinase [2.7.4.3]	AR	10,46
3	(RBC)		Bisphosphoglyceromutase ⟨Diphosphoglyceromutase⟩ [2.7.5.4]	AR	13,41
4			Fructose-bisphosphate aldolase ⟨Aldolase⟩ [4.1.2.13]	AR	8
5			Glucose-6-phosphate dehydrogenase [1.1.1.49] [1]	SL	4
6			Glucosephosphate isomerase [5.3.1.9]	AR	9,37
7			γ-Glutamyl-cysteine synthetase [6.3.2.2] [1]	AR	33
8			Glutathione reductase (NAD(P)H) [1.6.4.2] [1,2]	AR	3,31
9			Glutathione synthetase [6.3.2.3] [1]	AR	27
10			Hexokinase [2.7.1.1]	AR	25,51
11			6-Phosphofructokinase [2.7.1.11]	AR	54
12			Phosphogluconate dehydrogenase [1.1.1.43]	AR	38
13			Phosphoglycerate kinase [2.7.2.3] [3]	SL	11,52
14			Pyrimidine 5′-nucleotidase	AR	53
15			Pyruvate kinase [2.7.1.40]	AR	48
16			Triosephosphate isomerase [5.3.1.1] [3]	AR	40
17		Galactosemia	Galactokinase [2.7.1.6]	AR	7,20
18			Galactose-1-phosphate uridylyltransferase [2.7.7.10]	AR	6,23
		Glycogen storage disease [4]			
19		Type III	Amylo-1,6-glucosidase ⟨Debrancher enzyme⟩ [3.2.1.33]	AR	34
20		Type VII	6-Phosphofructokinase [2.7.1.11]	AR	50
21		Immunodeficiency	Adenosine deaminase [3.5.4.4]	AR	18
22			Purine-nucleoside phosphorylase ⟨Nucleoside phosphorylase⟩ [2.4.2.1]	AR	19

[1] Associated with sensitivity to the hemolytic effect of drugs. [2] The vast majority of cases are due to riboflavin deficiency. [3] Associated with neurologic disorder. [4] For other glycogen storage diseases, *see* entries 30-32.

continued

	Preferred Cells for Diagnosis	Disease	Enzyme ⟨Synonym⟩ [Enzyme Commission No.]	Mode of Inheritance	Reference
23		Lesch-Nyhan syndrome	Hypoxanthine phosphoribosyltransferase ⟨Hypoxanthine-guanine phosphoribosyltransferase⟩ [2.4.2.8]	SL	2,42
24		Methemoglobinemia[5]	Cytochrome b_5 reductase ⟨NADH diaphorase; DPNH methemoglobin reductase⟩ [1.6.2.2]	AR	24,30
25		Oral ulcerations	Catalase [1.11.1.6]	AR	1,47
26		Porphyria, acute intermittent	Uroporphyrinogen I synthase [4.3.1.8]	AD	32
27	Leuko-	Fabry's disease	α-Galactosidase [3.2.1.22]	SL	26
28	cytes	Gangliosidosis, generalized	β-Galactosidase [3.2.1.23]	AR	43
29	(WBC)	Gaucher's disease	β-Glucosidase [3.2.1.21]	AR	5,39
		Glycogen storage diseases[6]			
30		Type IIa ⟨Pompe's disease⟩	α-Glucosidase [3.2.1.20]	AR	28
31		Type IV	1,4-α-Glucan branching enzyme ⟨Branching enzyme⟩ [2.4.1.18]	AR	29
32		Type VI	Phosphorylase [2.4.1.1]	AR	55
33		Hypervalinemia	Valine transaminase	AR	15
34		Hypophosphatasia	Alkaline phosphatase [3.1.3.1]	AR	28
35		Isovaleric acidemia	Isovaleryl-CoA dehydrogenase	AR	12
36		Ketotic hyperglycinemia	Propionyl-CoA carboxylase [4.1.1.41]	AR	22
37		Maple syrup urine disease	Branched-chain ketoacid decarboxylase	AR	14
38		Metachromatic leukodystrophy	Arylsulfatase A [3.1.6.1]	AR	49
39		Methylmalonic aciduria	Methylmalonyl-CoA mutase ⟨Methylmalonic-CoA isomerase⟩ [5.4.99.2]	AR	35
40		Mucopolysaccharidosis	β-Glucuronidase [3.2.1.31]	AR	44
41		Niemann-Pick disease	Acylsphingosine deacylase ⟨Sphingomyelinase⟩ [3.5.1.23]	AR	17,45
42		Orotic aciduria	Orotidine 5'-phosphate decarboxylase ⟨Orotidylic decarboxylase⟩ [4.1.1.23]	AR	16
43		Sandhoff's disease	β-N-Acetylhexosaminidase ⟨β-Hexosaminidases A & B⟩ [3.2.1.52]	AR	36
44		Tay-Sachs disease	β-N-Acetylhexosaminidase ⟨β-Hexosaminidase A⟩ [3.2.1.52]	AR	36

[5] Some cases are associated with mental retardation. [6] For other glycogen storage diseases, *see* entries 19-20.

Contributor: Beutler, Ernest

References

1. Aebi, H., et al. 1968. In E. Beutler, ed. Hereditary Disorders of Erythrocyte Metabolism. Grune and Stratton, New York. pp. 41-65.
2. Bakay, B., et al. 1969. Biochem. Med. 3:230-243.
3. Beutler, E. 1969. J. Clin. Invest. 48:1957-1966.
4. Beutler, E. 1977. In J. B. Stanbury, et al., ed. The Metabolic Basis of Inherited Disease. Ed. 4. McGraw-Hill, New York.
5. Beutler, E., and W. Kuhl. 1970. J. Lab. Clin. Med. 76:747-755.
6. Beutler, E., and C. K. Mathai. 1968. (Loc. cit. ref. 1). pp. 66-86.
7. Beutler, E., et al. 1973. N. Engl. J. Med. 288:1203-1206.
8. Beutler, E., et al. 1974. Trans. Assoc. Am. Physicians 86:154-166.
9. Biervliet, J. P. G. van. 1975. Glucosephosphate Isomerase Deficiency. Drukkerij B. W. Elinkwijk, Utrecht, Netherlands.
10. Boivin, P., et al. 1971. Presse Med. 79:215-218.
11. Boivin, P., et al. 1974. Nouv. Rev. Fr. Hematol. 14:496-508.
12. Budd, M. A., et al. 1967. N. Engl. J. Med. 277:321-326.
13. Cartier, P., et al. 1972. Nouv. Rev. Fr. Hematol. 12:269-288.
14. Dancis, J., et al. 1967. N. Engl. J. Med. 276:84-89.
15. Dancis, J., et al. 1967. Pediatrics 39:813-817.
16. Fallon, H. J., et al. 1962. Blood 20:700-709.
17. Gal, A. E., et al. 1975. N. Engl. J. Med. 293:632-636.
18. Giblett, E. R., et al. 1972. Lancet 2:1067-1069.
19. Giblett, E. R., et al. 1975. Ibid. 1:1010-1013.

continued

20. Gitzelmann, R. 1967. Pediatr. Res. 1:14-23.
21. Hanel, H. K., et al. 1971. Hum. Hered. 21:313-319.
22. Hsia, Y. E., et al. 1969. Lancet 1:757-758.
23. Isselbacher, K. J., et al. 1956. Science 123:635-636.
24. Jaffe, E. R., and H. S. Hsieh. 1971. Semin. Hematol. 8:417-437.
25. Keitt, A. S. 1969. J. Clin. Invest. 48:1997-2007.
26. Kint, J. A. 1970. Science 167:1268-1269.
27. Konrad, P. N., et al. 1972. N. Engl. J. Med. 286:557-561.
28. Kretchmer, N., et al. 1958. Ann. N. Y. Acad. Sci. 75:279-285.
29. Legum, C. P., and H. M. Nitowsky. 1969. J. Pediatr. 74:84-89.
30. Leroux, A., et al. 1975. Nature (London) 258:619-620.
31. Loos, H., et al. 1976. Blood 48:53.
32. Magnussen, C. R., et al. 1974. Ibid. 44:857-868.
33. Mohler, D. N., et al. 1970. N. Engl. J. Med. 283:1253-1257.
34. Moses, S. W., et al. 1968. J. Clin. Invest. 47:1343-1348.
35. Oberholzer, V. G., et al. 1967. Arch. Dis. Child. 42:492-504.
36. Padeh, B., and R. Navon. 1971. Isr. J. Med. Sci. 7:259-263.
37. Paglia, D. E., and W. N. Valentine. 1974. Am. J. Clin. Pathol. 62:740-751.
38. Parr, C. W., and L. I. Fitch. 1967. Ann. Hum. Genet. 30:339-353.
39. Peters, S. P., et al. 1975. Clin. Chim. Acta 60:391-396.
40. Schneider, A. S., et al. 1968. (Loc. cit. ref. 1). pp. 265-272.
41. Schroeter, W. 1965. Klin. Wochenschr. 43:1147-1153.
42. Seegmiller, J. B., et al. 1967. Science 155:1682-1684.
43. Singer, H. S., and I. A. Schafer. 1970. N. Engl. J. Med. 282:571.
44. Sly, W. S., et al. 1973. J. Pediatr. 82:249-257.
45. Snyder, R. A., and R. D. Brady. 1969. Clin. Chim. Acta 25:331-338.
46. Szeinberg, A., et al. 1969. Acta Haematol. 42:111-126.
47. Takahara, S. 1971. Semin. Hematol. 8:397-416.
48. Tanaka, K. R., and D. E. Paglia. 1971. Ibid. 8:367-395.
49. Taniguchi, N., and I. Nanba. 1970. Clin. Chim. Acta 29:375-379.
50. Tarui, S., et al. 1965. Biochem. Biophys. Res. Commun. 19:517-523.
51. Valentine, W. N., et al. 1968. (Loc. cit. ref. 1). pp. 288-302.
52. Valentine, W. N., et al. 1969. N. Engl. J. Med. 280:528-534.
53. Valentine, W. N., et al. 1974. J. Clin. Invest. 54:866-879.
54. Waterbury, L., and E. P. Frenkel. 1972. Blood 39:415-425.
55. Williams, H. E., and J. B. Field. 1961. J. Clin. Invest. 40:1841-1845.

78. ENZYMES OF CLINICAL IMPORTANCE ASSAYED IN BLOOD

For source of **Enzyme Commission No.**, *see* Introduction. **Enzyme Activity Units:** P_i = inorganic orthophosphate; O. D. = optical density. Data in brackets refer to the column heading in brackets. Values in parentheses are ranges, estimate "b" unless otherwise indicated (*see* Introduction).

	Enzyme ⟨Synonym⟩ [Enzyme Commission No.]	Value	Enzyme Activity Units [Method]	Remarks	Reference
			Erythrocytes		
1	Acetylcholinesterase ⟨Acetylcholine hydrolase⟩ [3.1.1.7]	36.9(29.2-44.6)	μmoles acetylthiocholine hydrolyzed per min per g hemoglobin, at 37°C	Low activity in paroxysmal nocturnal hemoglobinuria; 0.5 mM acetylthiocholine iodide substrate; maximal activity with 1.0 mM substrate	6
2	Adenosine deaminase ⟨Adenosine aminohydrolase⟩ [3.5.4.4]	1.11(0.65-1.57)	μmoles adenosine hydrolyzed per min per g hemoglobin, at 37°C	0.08 mM adenosine substrate; low or absent in several families with immune deficiency disease	6

continued

	Enzyme ⟨Synonym⟩ [Enzyme Commission No.]	Value	Enzyme Activity Units [Method]	Remarks	Reference
3	Adenylate kinase ⟨ATP:AMP phosphotransferase⟩ [2.7.4.3]	258(199-317)	μmoles ADP formed per min per g hemoglobin from ATP & AMP, at 37°C	1 mM ATP & AMP substrate; 5 mM Mg^{2+}; deficiency in congenital hemolytic anemia	6
4	Arginase ⟨L-Arginine amidinohydrolase⟩ [3.5.3.1]	21.0 ± 12.6	mg urea nitrogen formed per h per 10^{11} erythrocytes, at 37°C	18.8 mM L-arginine hydrochloride substrate; elevated activity in untreated pernicious & other nutritional macrocytic anemias, & in thalassemia major	43
5		♂, 5100(2500-7700)	units per 100 ml [Kochakian]	....	31
6		♀, 4400(1800-7000)			
7	Aspartate aminotransferase ⟨Glutamic oxaloacetic transaminase⟩ [2.6.1.1]	5.0(3.2-6.8)	μmoles oxaloacetate formed per min per g hemoglobin, at 37°C	10 mM L-aspartate & 10 mM 2-oxoglutarate ⟨α-ketoglutarate⟩ substrate; stimulated ∿60% by 20 μM pyridoxal 5-phosphate	6
8	Bisphosphoglyceromutase ⟨Diphosphoglycerate mutase; 3-phospho-D-glyceroylphosphate:3-phospho-D-glycerate phosphotransferase⟩ [2.7.5.4]	4.78(3.48-6.08)	μmoles 1,3-diphosphoglycerate converted per min per g hemoglobin to 2,3-diphosphoglycerate, at 37°C	5 mM fructose 1,6-bisphosphate used as substrate and converted to 1,3-diphosphoglycerate by added fructose bisphosphate aldolase, triosephosphate isomerase, & glyceraldehyde-phosphate dehydrogenase	6
9	Carbonate dehydratase ⟨Carbonic anhydrase; carbonate hydrolyase⟩ [4.2.1.1]	73,000	Amount of erythrocytes that will halve the time of uncatalyzed reaction under specified conditions, at 30°C	Activity parallels erythrocyte zinc concentration. Isoenzymes (A-B & C) can be measured by immunochemical technique—concentration ∿14 mg enzyme protein/mg hemoglobin	3,32
10	Catalase ⟨Hydrogen-peroxide:hydrogen peroxide oxidoreductase⟩ [1.11.1.6]	153.1(105.3-200.9)	mmoles H$_2$O$_2$ hydrolyzed per min per g hemoglobin, at 37°C	9 mM H$_2$O$_2$ substrate; deficient in congenital acatalasia	6
11	Enolase ⟨2-Phospho-D-glycerate hydrolyase⟩ [4.2.1.11]	5.39(3.73-7.05)	μmoles 2-phosphoglyceric acid converted per min per g hemoglobin to phospho*enol*pyruvic acid, at 37°C	1 mM 2-phosphoglyceric acid substrate	6
12	Fructose-bisphosphate aldolase ⟨Aldolase; D-fructose-1,6-bisphosphate D-glyceraldehyde-3-phosphate-lyase⟩ [4.1.2.13]	3.19(2.47-3.91)	μmoles fructose 1,6-bisphosphate cleaved per min per g hemoglobin, at 37°C	1 mM fructose 1,6-bisphosphate substrate; increased activity in hemolytic disease	6
13	Galactokinase ⟨ATP:D-galactose 1-phosphotransferase⟩ [2.7.1.6]	0.29(0.28-0.31)	μmoles galactose phosphorylated per min per g hemoglobin to galactose 1-phosphate, at 37°C	0.33 mM galactose substrate containing [^{14}C] galactose	6

continued

	Enzyme ⟨Synonym⟩ [Enzyme Commission No.]	Value	Enzyme Activity Units [Method]	Remarks	Reference
14	Glucose-6-phosphate dehydrogenase ⟨D-Glucose-6-phosphate:NADP⁺ 1-oxidoreductase⟩ [1.1.1.49]	8.34(5.16-11.52)	μmoles glucose 6-phosphate oxidized per min per g hemoglobin to 6-phosphogluconic acid, at 37°C	0.6 mM glucose 6-phosphate substrate; most common erythrocyte deficiency results in drug- & naturally-induced congenital hemolytic anemia. World Health Organization method uses 25°C & a different calculation to give a range of 12.1(9.9-14.3)	6
15	Glucosephosphate isomerase ⟨D-Glucose-6-phosphate ketol-isomerase⟩ [5.3.1.9]	60.8(38.8-82.8)	μmoles fructose 6-phosphate converted per min per g hemoglobin to glucose 6-phosphate, at 37°C	2 mM fructose 6-phosphate substrate; deficiency resulting in nonspherocytic congenital hemolytic anemia	6
16	Glutathione peroxidase ⟨Glutathione:hydrogen peroxide oxidoreductase⟩ [1.11.1.9]	30.82(21.36-40.28)	μmoles reduced glutathione converted per min per g hemoglobin to oxidized glutathione in presence of H_2O_2, at 37°C	20 mM reduced glutathione & 10 mM tert-butyl hydroperoxide substrate	6
17	Glutathione reductase (NAD(P)H) ⟨NAD(P)H:oxidized-glutathione oxidoreductase⟩ [1.6.4.2]	10.4(7.4-13.4)	μmoles oxidized glutathione converted per min per g hemoglobin to reduced glutathione in presence of excess FAD, at 37°C	3.3 mM oxidized glutathione substrate; nutritional adequacy of FAD may be determined by assay in presence & absence of FAD	6
18	Glyceraldehyde-phosphate dehydrogenase ⟨D-Glyceraldehyde-3-phosphate:NAD⁺ oxidoreductase (phosphorylating)⟩ [1.2.1.12]	226(142-310)	μmoles 1,3-diphosphoglycerate reduced & converted per min per g hemoglobin to glyceraldehyde 3-phosphate, at 37°C	1,3-diphosphoglycerate generated from 10.0 mM 3-phosphoglycerate substrate	6
19	Hexokinase ⟨ATP:D-hexose 6-phosphotransferase⟩ [2.7.1.1]	1.16(0.82-1.50)	μmoles glucose converted per min per g hemoglobin to glucose 6-phosphate, at 37°C	2 mM glucose substrate; activity declines during cell aging	6
20 21	Hypoxanthine phosphoribosyltransferase ⟨Hypoxanthine-guanine phosphoribosyltransferase; IMP:pyrophosphate phosphoribosyltransferase⟩ [2.4.2.8]	♂, 52(22-82) ♀, 67(23-111)	mmoles guanine converted per h per ml to guanylate, at 37°C	5.3 μM guanine substrate; deficient in Lesch-Nyhan syndrome	11
22	Lactate dehydrogenase ⟨L-Lactate:NAD⁺ oxidoreductase⟩ [1.1.1.27]	200(147-253)	μmoles pyruvate reduced per min per g hemoglobin, at 37°C	1 mM sodium pyruvate substrate	6
23	Lactoyl-glutathione lyase ⟨Glyoxalase; S-Lactoyl-glutathione methylglyoxal-lyase (isomerizing)⟩ [4.4.1.5]	1398(1320-1500)ᶜ	ml CO_2 per 20 min per 100 ml erythrocytes, at 26°C & pH 7.2, in presence of glutathione	Methylglyoxal substrate	16
24	NAD⁺ nucleosidase ⟨Nicotinamide adenine dinucleotidase:NAD⁺ glycohydrolase⟩ [3.2.2.5]	28(20-35)	μmoles NAD⁺ hydrolyzed per h per 100 ml blood, at 37°C & pH 6.5	....	1

continued

	Enzyme ⟨Synonym⟩ [Enzyme Commission No.]	Value	Enzyme Activity Units [Method]	Remarks	Reference
25	6-Phosphofructokinase ⟨ATP:D-fructose-6-phosphate 1-phosphotransferase⟩ [2.7.1.11]	11.01(6.35-15.67)	μmoles fructose 6-phosphate phosphorylated per min per g hemoglobin to fructose 1,6-bisphosphate, at 37°C	2 mM fructose 6-phosphate substrate; unstable in hemolysates	6
26	Phosphoglucomutase ⟨α-D-Glucose-1,6-bisphosphate:α-D-glucose-1-phosphate phosphotransferase⟩ [2.7.5.1]	5.50(4.26-6.74)	μmoles glucose 1-phosphate converted per min per g hemoglobin to glucose 6-phosphate, at 37°C	2.5 μM glucose 1-phosphate substrate & 0.14 mM glucose 1,6-bisphosphate coenzyme	6
27	Phosphogluconate dehydrogenase (decarboxylating) ⟨6-Phosphogluconic dehydrogenase; 6-phospho-D-gluconate:NADP⁺ 2-oxidoreductase (decarboxylating)⟩ [1.1.1.44]	8.78(7.22-10.34)	μmoles 6-phosphogluconate oxidized per min per g hemoglobin to ribulose 5-phosphate, at 37°C	0.6 mM 6-phosphogluconate substrate	6
28	Phosphoglycerate kinase ⟨ATP:3-phospho-D-glycerate 1-phosphotransferase⟩ [2.7.2.3]	320(248-392)	μmoles 1,3-diphosphoglycerate formed per min per g hemoglobin from 3-phosphoglycerate, at 37°C	10.0 mM 3-phosphoglycerate substrate	6
29	Phosphoglycerate phosphomutase ⟨Monophosphoglyceromutase; D-phosphoglycerate 2,3-phosphomutase⟩ [5.4.2.1]	19.3(11.62-26.98)	μmoles 3-phosphoglycerate converted per min per g hemoglobin to 2-phosphoglycerate, at 37°C	2 mM 3-phosphoglycerate substrate	6
30	Pyruvate kinase ⟨ATP:pyruvate 2-O-phosphotransferase⟩ [2.7.1.40]	15.0(11.08-18.92)	μmoles pyruvate formed per min per g hemoglobin from phosphoenolpyruvate & ADP, at 37°C	5 mM phosphoenolpyruvate, 1.67 mM ADP substrates; deficiency most common cause of nonspherocytic congenital hemolytic anemia	6,7
31	Triosephosphate isomerase ⟨D-Glyceraldehyde-3-phosphate ketol-isomerase⟩ [5.3.1.1]	2111(1317-2905)	μmoles glyceraldehyde 3-phosphate converted per min per g hemoglobin to dihydroxyacetone phosphate, at 37°C	3 mM glyceraldehyde 3-phosphate substrate; deficiency results in nonspherocytic congenital hemolytic anemia	6
32	UDPglucose 4-epimerase ⟨Epimerase⟩ [5.1.3.2]	0.23(0.11-0.35)	μmoles UDPgalactose converted per min per g hemoglobin to UDPglucose, at 37°C	0.25 mM UDPgalactose substrate	6
			Serum or Plasma		
33	Acetylcholinesterase ⟨Acetylcholine hydrolase⟩ [3.1.1.7]	0.703	Decrease in pH per h per ml, at 25°C	15 mM acetylcholine substrate	37
34		319(150-500)ᶜ	μmoles acetylcholine hydrolyzed per min per 100 ml, at 37.5°C	1-2 mM acetylcholine substrate	48
35		89.3(51-128)ᶜ	μl CO₂ formed per min per ml, at 38°C	10 mM acetylcholine substrate	12
36 37		78(51-121)ᶜ[1,2] 105(71-166)ᶜ[3]	μl CO₂ formed per min per ml, at 37°C	10 mM acetylcholine substrate	35

[1] Children. [2] 7-15 yr old. [3] Adults.

continued

	Enzyme ⟨Synonym⟩ [Enzyme Commission No.]	Value	Enzyme Activity Units [Method]	Remarks	Reference
38	β-N-Acetylhexosaminidase ⟨Hexamidase A; 2-acetamido-2-deoxy-β-hexoside acetamidodeoxyhexohydrolase⟩ [3.2.1.52]	57.3(46.5-67.1)	μmoles hymecromone ⟨4-methylumbelliferone⟩ formed per h per ml, at 37°C (per cent heat stable out of total activity)	4-Methylumbelliferone-β-D-N-acetylglucosaminide substrate; deficiency in Tay-Sachs disease	61
39	Acid phosphatase ⟨Orthophosphoric-monoester phosphohydrolase (acid optimum)⟩ [3.1.3.2]	0.55(0.0-1.1)[d]	mg P_i hydrolyzed per h per 100 ml from β-glycerophosphate, at 37°C [Bodansky]	14.4 mM β-glycerophosphate substrate; pH 5.0. To convert units to μmoles, multiply by 6.1.	8
40		1.25(0-2.5)[d]	mg phenol liberated per h per 100 ml, at 37°C [Gutman or King-Armstrong]	5 mM phenyl phosphate substrate; pH 4.9. To convert units to μmoles, multiply by 15.	21
41		1.54(0.86-2.22)	mmoles p-nitrophenol hydrolyzed per h per 100 ml, at 37°C [Bessey-Lowry]	4 mM p-nitrophenyl phosphate substrate, pH 5.4; 0.45 mM Mg^{2+}. To convert units to μmoles, multiply by 145.	26
42		1.0(0.7-1.6)[c]	Color equivalent of 10 ml 2-naphthol ⟨β-naphthol⟩ per h per 100 ml, at 37°C	0.33 mM 2-naphthyl phosphate ⟨β-naphthyl phosphate⟩ substrate; pH 4.8. To convert units to μmoles, multiply by 69.	53
43 44		♂, 2.0(0.6-3.4) ♀, 1.5(0.5-2.5)	mg 1-naphthol ⟨α-naphthol⟩ liberated per h per 100 ml, at 37°C [Babson]	0.67 mg 1-naphthyl phosphate ⟨α-naphthyl phosphate⟩ substrate per tablet; pH 5.2. To convert units to μmoles, multiply by 14.	4
45		5.9(3.0-10.0)[c]	mg phenolphthalein liberated per h per 100 ml, at 37°C [Huggins & Tallaly]	1 mM phenolphthalein phosphate substrate; pH 5.4. To convert units to μmoles, multiply by 18.	27
46		0.28 ± 0.09 (0.11-0.60)[c]	μmoles thymolphthalein monophosphate hydrolyzed per min per liter, at 37°C	2.2 mM thymolphthalein monophosphate substrate	47
47	Adenosine deaminase ⟨Adenosine aminohydrolase⟩ [3.5.4.4]	17.1(10.6-23.6)	μmoles adenosine hydrolyzed per min per liter, at 37°C	20 mM adenosine substrate; pH 6.2-6.8 (optimal conditions)	20
48		10.5(6.4-14.7)	μg NH_3 nitrogen liberated per h per ml, at 37°C	4.2 mM adenosine substrate; pH 7.8	51
49 50	Alanine aminotransferase ⟨Glutamic pyruvic transaminase; GPT⟩ [2.6.1.2]	♂, 25(12-53)[c] ♀, 16(6-40)[c]	Absorbancy decrease of 0.001·min^{-1}·ml^{-1}, at 32°C	6.67 mM 2-oxoglutarate ⟨α-ketoglutarate⟩ & 167 mM alanine substrate	23
51 52		♂, 45(13-77) ♀, 31(11-51)	μmoles pyruvate transaminated per min per liter, at 37°C	18 mM 2-oxoglutarate ⟨α-ketoglutarate⟩ & 800 mM L-alanine substrate	56
53	Alkaline phosphatase ⟨Orthophosphoric-monoester phosphohydrolase (alkaline optimum)⟩ [3.1.3.1]	55(20-90)	μmoles p-nitrophenyl phosphate hydrolyzed per min per liter, at 30°C	15 mM p-nitrophenyl phosphate substrate; 0.1 mM Mg^{2+}; 2-amino-2-methyl-1-propanol buffer	10

continued

	Enzyme ⟨Synonym⟩ [Enzyme Commission No.]	Value	Enzyme Activity Units [Method]	Remarks	Reference
54		(280-525) [1,4]	μmoles p-nitrophenyl phosphate hydrolyzed per min per liter, at 30°C	14 mM p-nitrophenyl phosphate substrate; 0.1 mM Mg²⁺; diethanolamine buffer	60
55		(195-335) [1,5]			
56		(220-510) [1,6]			
57		♂, 154(80-220)			
58		♀, 140(70-210)			
59		25(17-33) [1]	mg phenol liberated per 15 min per 100 ml, at 37°C [King-Armstrong]	9.5 mM phenyl phosphate substrate	29
60		10(4-17) [3]			
61	Amine oxidase (pyridoxal-containing) ⟨Diamine oxidase; amine:oxygen oxidoreductase (deaminating) (pyridoxal-containing)⟩ [1.4.3.6]	27.5(18-37)	μmoles polyamine deaminated per min per liter, at 37°C	8 mM putrescine or 1 mM histamine substrate. Markedly elevated in pregnant women.	17
62 63	Aminopeptidase (cytosol) ⟨Leucine aminopeptidase; LAP; 1-leucyl-peptide hydrolase⟩ [3.4.11.1]	♂, 16.5(10.1-22.9) ♀, 15.2(9.8-20.5)	μmoles leucine-p-nitroanilide hydrolyzed per min per ml, at 25°C	1.5 mM L-leucine-p-nitroanilide substrate	57
64 65	α-Amylase ⟨1,4-α-D-glucan glucanohydrolase⟩ [3.2.1.1]	♂, 79(34-118) ♀, 94(46-141)	mg reducing substance expressed as glucose formed per 30 min per 100 ml, at 37°C	∿1.5% starch solution substrate	22
66		78(30-126)	μg dye per min per ml, at 37°C	200 mg Cibachron Blue-amylose substrate per assay	30
67	Arginase ⟨L-Arginine ureohydrolase⟩ [3.5.3.1]	(0.8-7.9)	μmoles urea formed per min per liter, at 37°C	60 mM arginine substrate	36
68	Argininosuccinate lyase ⟨L-Argininosuccinate arginine-lyase⟩ [4.3.2.1]	(0-4)	μmoles arginine formed per h per 100 ml, at 37°C	0.49 mM argininosuccinate substrate	13
69 70 71	Aspartate aminotransferase ⟨Glutamic oxaloacetic transaminase; GOT⟩ [2.6.1.1]	34(13-55) ♂, 23(15-36)ᶜ ♀, 20(12-30)ᶜ	Absorbancy decrease of 0.001 per min per ml, at 32°C	6.7 mM 2-oxoglutarate ⟨α-ketoglutarate⟩ & 125 mM aspartate substrate; pyridoxal-5-phosphate may increase activity. For conversion to international units, multiply by 0.484.	23
72 73		♂, 37(15-60) ♀, 27(14-40)	μmoles oxaloacetate transaminated per min per liter, at 37°C	12 mM 2-oxoglutarate ⟨α-ketoglutarate⟩ & 200 mM L-aspartate substrate	56
74 75		♂, (15-57)ᶜ ♀, (12-50)ᶜ	Absorbancy decrease of 0.001 per min per ml, at 37°C	6.7 mM α-ketoglutarate & 125 mM aspartate substrate	41
76 77	Creatine kinase ⟨CPK; ATP:creatine N-phosphotransferase⟩ [2.7.3.2]	♂, 42 ± 21 (12-99)ᶜ ♀, 23 ± 11 (10-61)ᶜ	μmoles phosphocreatine ⟨creatine phosphate⟩ converted per min per liter, at 37°C	9.7 mM phosphocreatine ⟨creatine phosphate⟩ & 0.97 mM ADP substrate; 4.85 mM cysteine activator	44
78	Cystyl-aminopeptidase ⟨Oxytocinase; α-aminoacylpeptide hydrolase⟩ [3.4.11.3]	♂, 3.9(1.5-6.3)	μmoles p-nitroanilide formed per min per liter, at 25°C	0.48 mM S-benzyl-L-cysteine-p-nitroanilide substrate	39

[1] Children. [3] Adults. [4] 0-1 yr old. [5] 1-12 yr old. [6] 12-16 yr old.

continued

	Enzyme ⟨Synonym⟩ [Enzyme Commission No.]	Value	Enzyme Activity Units [Method]	Remarks	Reference
79		♀, 2.8(0.2-5.4)	μmoles p-nitroanilide formed per min per liter, at 25°C	0.48 mM S-benzyl-L-cysteine-p-nitroanilide substrate. Increases in activity during pregnancy according to regression equation y = 0.2104 + 0.0497 x, where y = cystyl-aminopeptidase ⟨oxytocinase⟩ activity, & x = week of pregnancy.	39
80	Dopamine β-monooxygenase ⟨Dopamine β-hydroxylase; 3,4-dihydroxyphenylethyl-	(3.6-22.9)c	μmoles tyramine hydroxylated per min per liter, at 37°C	2.5 mM tyramine substrate	34
81	amine, ascorbate:oxygen oxidoreductase (β-hydroxylating)⟩ [1.14.17.1]	42.6 ± 27 (3-100)c	μmoles tyramine converted per min per liter to octopamine, at 37°C	20 mM tyramine substrate	38
82	Ferroxidase ⟨Ceruloplasmin; iron (II):oxygen oxidoreductase⟩ [1.16.3.1]	425(280-570)	Absorbancy increase of 0.001 per 30 min per 0.1 ml in 3.1 ml reaction mixture, at 37°C	0.08% p-diphenylenediamine substrate	25
83 84	Fructose-bisphosphate aldolase ⟨Aldolase; D-fructose-1,6-bisphosphate D-glyceralde-	♂, 8.0(0-12)c ♀, 4.7(1.5-11.9)c	μmoles fructose 1,6-bisphosphate converted per min per liter	1.5 mM fructose 1,6-bisphosphate substrate	40
85	hyde-3-phosphate-lyase⟩ [4.1.2.13]	490(350-800)c	μl fructose bisphosphate per h per 100 ml, at 38°C & pH 8.6	0.8 mM fructose 1,6-bisphosphate substrate	55
86	Glucosephosphate isomerase ⟨GPI; PHI; D-glucose-6-phosphate ketol-isomerase⟩	20 ± 8 (8-40)c	units per 100 ml, at 37°C [Bodansky]	7 mM glucose 6-phosphate substrate	9
87	[5.3.1.9]	55(20-90)	μmoles glucose 6-phosphate converted per min per liter to fructose 6-phosphate, at 37°C	7 mM glucose 6-phosphate substrate	52
88 89	β-Glucuronidase ⟨β-D-Glucuronide glucuronosohydrolase⟩ [3.2.1.31]	♂, (0-181) ♀, (37-230)	μg phenolphthalein per h per 100 ml, at 38°C & pH 4.5	Phenolphthalein glucuronide substrate	18
90	Glutamate dehydrogenase (NAD(P)+) ⟨L-Glutamate:NAD(P)+ oxidoreductase (deaminating)⟩ [1.4.1.3]	2.2(0.3-4.1)	μmoles α-ketoglutarate ⟨2-oxoglutarate⟩ converted per min per liter to glutamate, at 25°C	7 mM 2-oxoglutarate & 100 mM NH4+ substrate. For conversion to 37°C, multiply by 1.67.	49
91 92	γ-Glutamyltransferase ⟨γ-Glutamyl transpeptidase; γ-GTP; (γ-glutamyl)-peptide:amino-acid γ-glutamyl-	♂, 14.7(4.5-24.8) ♀, 8.4(3.2-13.5)	μmoles L-γ-glutamyl-p-nitroanilide hydrolyzed per min per liter, at 25°C	4 mM L-γ-glutamyl-p-nitroanilide substrate. For conversion to 37°C, multiply by 1.59.	58
93 94	transferase⟩ [2.3.2.2]	♂, 23.7 ± 14.8 ♀, 17.8 ± 14.8	μmoles L-γ-glutamyl-p-nitroanilide hydrolyzed per min per liter, at 37°C	5.6 mM L-γ-glutamyl-p-nitroanilide substrate; newborn	45
95	Glutathione reductase (NAD(P)H) ⟨NAD(P)H:oxidized-glutathione oxidoreductase⟩ [1.6.4.2]	40(10-70)	Absorbancy change per min per ml, at room temperature (26°C)	1.33 mg oxidized glutathione (substrate)/ml reaction mixture	33

continued

	Enzyme ⟨Synonym⟩ [Enzyme Commission No.]	Value	Enzyme Activity Units [Method]	Remarks	Reference
96	Guanine deaminase ⟨Guanase; guanine aminohydrolase⟩ [3.5.4.3]	2.1 ± 1.5	μmoles guanine converted per min per liter to xanthine, at 37°C	0.1 mM guanine substrate	14,19
97	4-Hydroxybutyrate dehydrogenase ⟨α-Hydroxybutyric dehydrogenase; 4-hydroxybutyrate:NAD$^+$ oxidoreductase⟩ [1.1.1.61]	118(67-169)	μmoles NADH oxidized per min per liter, at 32°C	1.9 mg sodium 2-oxoglutarate ⟨α-ketoglutarate⟩ (substrate)/ml reaction mixture	46
98 99	Isocitrate dehydrogenase (NADP$^+$) ⟨Isocitric dehydrogenase; ICD; *threo*-D$_s$-isocitrate:NADP$^+$ oxidoreductase (decarboxylating)⟩ [1.1.1.42]	♂, 110 ± 49 (55-324)^c ♀, 109 ± 56 (47-264)^c	μmoles NADPH formed per h per ml, at 25°C	3.2 mM isocitrate substrate	62
100	Lactate dehydrogenase ⟨LDH; L-lactate:NAD$^+$ oxidoreductase⟩ [1.1.1.27]	♂, 70(42-98)	Absorbancy change per min per ml, at 25°C	7.75 mM *dl*-lactate substrate; 7% increase in activity per degree temp	2
101 102		♂, 321(236-424)^c ♀, 297(212-420)^c	Absorbancy change per min per ml, at 32°C	0.6 mM pyruvate substrate	23
103	Lysozyme ⟨Muramidase; mucopeptide *N*-acetylmuramoyl hydrolase⟩ [3.2.1.7]	11.0(7.0-15.0)	Activity equivalent to μg of egg white lysozyme per min per ml, at 37°C	0.25 mg/ml suspension of *Micrococcus luteus* ⟨*M. lysodeikticus*⟩ substrate	63
104	Malate dehydrogenase ⟨Malic dehydrogenase; L-malate:NAD$^+$ oxidoreductase⟩ [1.1.1.37]	72(48-96)	μmoles oxaloacetate converted per min per liter, at 25°C	Oxaloacetate substrate formed from 1.2 mM α-ketoglutarate during aspartate aminotransferase reaction; added in excess	5
105	5'-Nucleotidase ⟨5'-Ribonucleotide phosphohydrolase⟩ [3.1.3.5]	7.4(3.2-11.6)	μmoles AMP hydrolyzed per min per liter, at 37°C	5 mM AMP substrate; assay in presence & absence of 10 mM Ni^{2+}	50
106	Ornithine carbamoyltransferase ⟨OCT; carbamoylphosphate:L-ornithine carbamoyltransferase⟩ [2.1.3.3]	<0.005	μmoles CO$_2$ formed per 0.5 ml per 2 h, at 37°C	50 μM citrulline substrate containing L-[*ureido*-^{14}C] citrulline	42
107	Ribonuclease I ⟨Alkaline ribonuclease; polyribonucleotide 2-oligonucleotidotransferase⟩ [3.1.4.22]	0.259(0.240-0.278)	Absorbancy change per min per ml, at 37°C. 0.1 O.D. unit equals 0.0027 μg crystalline bovine pancreatic ribonuclease I ⟨RNase⟩	0.4 mg ribonucleic acid/ml substrate	15
108	Sialyltransferase ⟨CMP-*N*-acetylneuraminate:D-galactosylglycoprotein *N*-acetylneuraminyltransferase⟩ [2.4.99.1]	281(197-365)	Counts per minute carbon-14 incorporated per mg protein per 30 min, at 37°C	1 nmole CMP-[^{14}C]sialic acid per reaction mixture containing 500 ng desialated fetuin as acceptor	28
109	Triacylglycerol lipase ⟨Lipase; glycerol ester hydrolase⟩ [3.1.1.3]	0.75(0-1.50)	ml 0.05 M NaOH required to neutralize liberated fatty acids per 16 h per ml, at 37°C	Olive oil emulsion substrate	24
110		0.34(0.02-0.66)	ml 0.05 M NaOH required to neutralize liberated fatty acids per 3 h per ml, at 37°C	Olive oil emulsion substrate; convert to international units by multiplying by 278	59
111		63.5(7-120)	Turbidity related to μmoles triglyceride bonds broken per min per liter, at 37°C	Olive oil emulsion substrate	54

continued

119

78. ENZYMES OF CLINICAL IMPORTANCE ASSAYED IN BLOOD

Contributor: Schwartz, Morton K.

References

1. Alivisatos, S. G. A., et al. 1956. Can. J. Biochem. Physiol. 34:46-60.
2. Amador, E., et al. 1963. Clin. Chem. 9:391-399.
3. Ashby, W. 1943. J. Biol. Chem. 151:521-527.
4. Babson, A. L., and P. A. Read. 1959. Am. J. Clin. Pathol. 32:88-91.
5. Bergmeyer, H. U., and E. Bernt. 1974. In H. U. Bergmeyer, ed. Methods of Enzymatic Analysis. Ed. 2. Academic Press, New York. v. 2, pp. 613-623.
6. Beutler, E. 1975. Red Cell Metabolism. Ed. 2. Grune and Stratton, New York.
7. Blume, K. G., et al. 1973. Clin. Chim. Acta 43:443-446.
8. Bodansky, A. 1933. J. Biol. Chem. 101:93-104.
9. Bodansky, O. 1954. Cancer (Philadelphia) 7:1191-1199.
10. Bowers, G. N., Jr., and R. B. McComb. 1975. Clin. Chem. 21:1988-1995.
11. Brewster, M. A., et al. 1974. In F. W. Sunderman, ed. Manual of Procedures for the Laboratory Diagnosis of Skeletal, Muscular and Nervous Disorders. Institute for Clinical Science and Association of Clinical Scientists, Philadelphia. pp. 81-87.
12. Callaway, S., et al. 1951. Br. Med. J. 2:812-816.
13. Campanini, R. Z., et al. 1970. Clin. Chem. 16:44-53.
14. Caraway, W. T. 1966. Ibid. 12:187-193.
15. Chretien, P. B., et al. 1973. Cancer (Philadelphia) 31:175-179.
16. Cohen, P. P., and E. K. Sober. 1945. Cancer Res. 5:631-632.
17. Dahlbäck, O., et al. 1968. Scand. J. Clin. Lab. Invest. 21:17-25.
18. Fishman, W. H., et al. 1948. J. Biol. Chem. 173:449-456.
19. Guisti, G. 1974. (Loc. cit. ref. 5). pp. 1086-1091.
20. Guisti, G. 1974. (Loc. cit. ref. 5). pp. 1092-1099.
21. Gutman, A. B., and E. B. Gutman. 1938. Proc. Soc. Exp. Biol. Med. 38:470-473.
22. Henry, R. J., and N. Chiamori. 1960. Clin. Chem. 6:434-452.
23. Henry, R. J., et al. 1957. Ibid. 3:77-89.
24. Henry, R. J., et al. 1960. Am. J. Clin. Pathol. 34:381-398.
25. Henry, R. J., et al. 1960. Proc. Soc. Exp. Biol. Med. 104:620-624.
26. Hudson, P. B., et al. 1947. J. Urol. 58:89-92.
27. Huggins, C., and P. Talalay. 1945. J. Biol. Chem. 159:399-410.
28. Kessel, D., and J. Allan. 1975. Cancer Res. 35:670-672.
29. Kind, P. R. N., and E. J. King. 1954. J. Clin. Pathol. 7:322-326.
30. Klein, B., et al. 1970. Clin. Chem. 16:32-38.
31. Kochakian, C. D., et al. 1948. Conf. Metab. Aspects Conval. 17:187-204.
32. Kondo, T., et al. 1975. Clin. Chim. Acta 60:347-353.
33. Manso, C., and F. Wroblewski. 1958. J. Clin. Invest 37:214-218.
34. Markianos, E. S., and I. E. Nyström. 1975. Z. Klin. Chem. Klin. Biochem. 13:273-276.
35. McArdle, B. 1940. Q. J. Med. 9:107-127.
36. Mellerup, B. 1967. Clin. Chem. 13:900-908.
37. Michel, H. O. 1949. J. Lab. Clin. Med. 34:1564-1568.
38. Nagatsu, T., and S. Udenfriend. 1972. Clin. Chem. 18:980-983.
39. Oudheusden, A. P. M. van. 1974. (Loc. cit. ref. 5). pp. 971-978.
40. Pinto, P. V. C., et al. 1969. Clin. Chem. 15:349-360.
41. Reed, A. H., et al. 1972. Ibid. 18:57-66.
42. Reichard, H. 1964. J. Lab. Clin. Med. 63:1061-1064.
43. Reynolds, J., et al. 1957. Ibid. 50:78-92.
44. Rosalki, S. B. 1967. Ibid. 69:696-705.
45. Rosalki, S. B. 1975. Adv. Clin. Chem. 17:53-107.
46. Rosalki, S. B., and J. H. Wilkinson. 1964. J. Am. Med. Assoc. 189:61-63.
47. Roy, A. V., et al. 1971. Clin. Chem. 17:1093-1102.
48. Sawitsky, A., et al. 1948. J. Lab. Clin. Med. 33:203-206.
49. Schmidt, E. 1974. (Loc. cit. ref. 5). pp. 650-656.
50. Schwartz, M. K. 1972. Stand. Methods Clin. Chem. 7:1-7.
51. Schwartz, M. K., and O. Bodansky. 1959. Proc. Soc. Exp. Biol. Med. 101:560-562.
52. Schwartz, M. K., et al. 1971. Clin. Chem. 17:656-657 (Abstr. 131).
53. Seligman, A. M., et al. 1951. J. Biol. Chem. 190:7-15.
54. Shihabi, Z. K., and C. Bishop. 1971. Clin. Chem. 17:1150-1153.
55. Sibley, J. A., and A. L. Lehninger. 1949. J. Biol. Chem. 177:859-872.
56. Siest, G., et al. 1975. Clin. Chem. 21:1077-1087.
57. Szasz, G. 1967. Am. J. Clin. Pathol. 47:607-613.
58. Szasz, G. 1969. Clin. Chem. 15:124-136.
59. Tietz, N. W., and E. A. Fiereck. 1972. Stand. Methods Clin. Chem. 7:19-31.
60. Tietz, N. W., et al. 1974. (Loc. cit. ref. 11). pp. 55-61.
61. Weisberg, H. F., et al. 1974. (Loc. cit. ref. 11). pp. 89-100.
62. Wolfson, S. K., and H. G. Williams-Ashman. 1957. Proc. Soc. Exp. Biol. Med. 96:231-234.
63. Zucker, S., and A. Webb. 1972. Stand. Methods Clin. Chem. 7:9-17.

All factors listed are present in plasma except III, and all are present in serum except for I, II, III, V, and VIII, although XIII is decreased to trace quantities. Factors I, VIII, and XIII are present in Cohn's fraction I; factors II, V, VII, IX, X, XI, and XII are present in Cohn's fraction III; and factors II, VII, IX, XI, and XII are present in Cohn's fraction IV. Recently the following not previously reported factors have been detected: Fletcher (pre-kininogenin ⟨pre-kallikrein⟩), Fitzgerald (high molecular weight kininogen, also designated as Williams trait, Flaujeac trait), Passovay (bleeding diathesis—prolonged partial thromboplastin time, normal known coagulation factors, autosomal dominant). Roman numerals have not yet been assigned. Factor VI is not listed because it is obsolete.

Physical & Chemical Properties: GP = glycoprotein; LP = lipoprotein; pI = isoelectric point; PPTA = degree of saturation of $(NH_4)_2SO_4$ solution necessary for precipitation of factor; AdK = adsorbed by Celite ⟨infusorial earth⟩, or kaolin, or carboxymethyl cellulose ⟨CMC⟩; AdB = adsorbed by $BaSO_4$, or $Al(OH)_3$, or $Ca_3(PO_4)_2$. **Volume of Distribution:** mpv = multiples of plasma volume, i.e., the number given, multiplied by the plasma volume, gives the total volume in which the factor is located. **Concentration for Hemostasis** gives the approximate concentration required to produce hemostasis, in per cent of normal concentration. **Deficiency State** is a condition in which the coagulation factor level in a given patient is below the acceptable normal level. IP = inheritance pattern; AD = autosomal dominant; AR = autosomal recessive; X-LR = sex-linked recessive.

	Factor ⟨Synonym⟩	Physical & Chemical Properties	Site of Synthesis	Biologic Half-Life h	Volume of Distribution mpv	Concentration for Hemostasis, %	Deficiency State	
							Prevalence cases/10^6 population	IP
1	I ⟨Fibrinogen⟩	GP; mol wt, 340,000; pI, 5.5; PPTA, 25%	Liver	95-120	2.5	20	Hypofibrinogenemia [1] or afibrinogenemia, <0.5	AR
2	II ⟨Prothrombin⟩	GP, α-globulin; mol wt, 73,000; pI, 4.2; PPTA, 50%; AdB, AdK	Liver [2]	72	1.5-2.5	20	Hypoprothrombinemia, <0.5	AR
3	III ⟨Thromboplastin⟩	LP	All body tissues	....	....	.....	Not reported	....
4	IV ⟨Calcium⟩	Divalent cation; mol wt, 40	....	....	....	.....	....	....
5	V ⟨Proaccelerin, plasma Ac-globulin⟩	GP; mol wt, 300,000; pI, 5.3; PPTA, 50%	Liver	12-36	2	10-20	Factor V deficiency, <0.5	AR
6	VII ⟨SPCA, proconvertin⟩	GP, α-β-globulin [3]; mol wt, 48,000-100,000; PPTA, 50%; AdB, AdK	Liver [2]	4-6	2-4	10	Factor VII deficiency, <0.5	AR
7	VIII ⟨Antihemophilic globulin, AHG, antihemophilic factor, AHF⟩	GP, α-β-globulin [3]; mol wt, 2,000,000 [4]; PPTA, 33%	? Endothelium, ? reticuloendothelial cells [5]	6-10 [6]; 15-18 [7]	1-1.5	30-40	Hemophilia A, 60-80	X-LR
8							von Willebrand's disease, 5-10	AD
9	IX ⟨Plasma thromboplastin component, PTC, Christmas factor⟩	GP, α-β-globulin [3]; mol wt, 55,000-70,000; pI, 4.50; PPTA, 50%; AdB, AdK	Liver [2]	6-10 [6]; 25-30 [7]	2-3	30-40	Hemophilia B ⟨Christmas disease⟩, 15-20	X-LR
10	X ⟨Stuart-Prower factor⟩	GP, α-globulin; mol wt, 100,000; pI, 5.5; PPTA, 50%; AdB, AdK	Liver [2]	40-50	1	10-20	Stuart-Prower deficiency, <0.5	AR
11	XI ⟨Plasma thromboplastin antecedent, PTA⟩	β- or γ-globulin; mol wt, 200,000; pI, 4-5.0; PPTA, 33%; AdK	Liver [5]	50-80	1	10-20	PTA trait, <1.0	AR [8]
12	XII ⟨Hageman factor⟩	Sialo-GP; β-γ-globulin [9]; mol wt, 100,000; PPTA, 50%; AdK	....	50-60	....	.....	Hageman trait, <1.0	AR

[1] Some pedigrees reported to have hypofibrinogenemia may be examples of dysfibrinogenemia; this condition is inherited as an autosomal dominant. [2] Synthesis is vitamin K dependent. [3] The factor migrates in an electrophoretic field between α- and β-globulins. [4] Molecular weight of procoagulant subunit is ∿200,000. [5] Data are suggestive, but conclusive evidence is not yet available. [6] Initial; the shorter initial half-lives for factors VIII & IX are probably due to distribution into extravascular compartments. [7] Secondary. [8] Reported to be inherited both as an autosomal recessive and as an autosomal dominant. [9] The factor migrates in an electrophoretic field between β- and γ-globulins.

continued

	Factor ⟨Synonym⟩	Physical & Chemical Properties	Site of Synthesis	Biologic Half-Life h	Volume of Distribution mpv	Concentration for Hemostasis, %	Deficiency State	
							Prevalence cases/10⁶ population	IP
13	XIII ⟨Fibrin-stabilizing factor⟩	α_2-globulin; mol wt, 350,000; PPTA, 33%	Liver[5]; ? megakaryocytes	95-120	1-2	1-2	Factor XIII deficiency, <0.5	AR

[5] Data are suggestive, but conclusive evidence is not yet available.

Contributor: Bell, William R., Jr.

General References

1. Austen, D. E. G., and C. R. Rizza. 1974. In A. C. Allison, ed. Structure and Function of Plasma Proteins. Plenum Press, New York. pp. 169-193.
2. Bang, N. U., et al. 1971. Thrombosis and Bleeding Disorders, Theory and Methods. Academic Press, New York.
3. Bidwell, E., et al. 1972. In R. Biggs, ed. Therapeutic Materials in Human Blood Coagulation. Blackwell Scientific Publications, Oxford. pp. 225-277.
4. Bocci, V. 1970. Arch. Fisiol. 67:363-374.
5. Cohn, E. J., et al. 1946. J. Am. Chem. Soc. 68:459-475.
6. Leavell, B. S., and D. A. Throup. 1976. Fundamentals of Clinical Hematology. Ed. 4. W. B. Saunders, Philadelphia. pp. 661-718.
7. Miale, J. B. 1972. Laboratory Medicine: Hematology. Ed. 4. C. V. Mosby, St. Louis. pp. 1062-1111.
8. Takeda, Y., et al. 1976. In R. Bianchi, et al., ed. Plasma Protein Turnover. Univ. Park Press, Baltimore. pp. 277-294.
9. Williams, W. J. 1972. In W. J. Williams, et al., ed. Hematology. McGraw-Hill, New York. pp. 1057-1098.
10. Wintrobe, M. M., et al. 1974. Clinical Hematology. Ed. 7. Lea and Febiger. Philadelphia. pp. 409-450.

80. FACTORS OF THE COMPLEMENT AND PROPERDIN SYSTEMS

Concentration in Serum gives the approximate concentration in human serum. **Function:** IgG = immunoglobulin G, IgM = immunoglobulin M; the bar above part of a factor symbol indicates the acquisition of enzyme activity.

	Factor Name	Molecular Weight daltons	Electrophoretic Mobility	No. of Chains	Concentration in Serum µg/ml	Function	Reference
	Classic activation						
1	C1q	400,000	γ	6[1]	140	Recognition subunit of C1; binds to IgG or IgM, and initiates classic activation	14,23,30
2	C1r	190,000	β_2	2	50	Protease: cleaves and activates C1s	14,31
3	C1s	86,000	α	1	50	Protease: cleaves C4 & C2, forming $C\overline{42}$, the classic C3-cleaving enzyme	14,25
4	C4	204,000	β_1	3	430	Substrate of $C\overline{1s}$: cleaved C4 provides binding site in formation of $C\overline{42}$	16,26
5	C2	117,000	β_2	...	25	Substrate of $C\overline{1s}$: cleaved C2 provides active site of $C\overline{42}$	3,22
6	Properdin activation Nephritic factor (Initiating factor)	150,000	γ	...	....	Initiating factor; stabilizes $C\overline{3B}$, the alternative pathway C3-cleaving enzyme	5,27,28

[1] Each chain consists of 3 polypeptides.

continued

	Factor Name	Molecular Weight daltons	Electro-phoretic Mobility	No. of Chains	Concentration in Serum μg/ml	Function	Reference
7	Factor D	25,000	α	1	....	Protease: cleaves factor B, forming $C\overline{3B}$	6,17
8	Properdin	220,000	γ	4	25	Binds to cleaved C3, stabilizing $C\overline{3B}$	8,20
9	Factor B	93,000	β_2	1	225	Substrate of factor $\overline{D}$: cleaved B provides active site of $C\overline{3B}$	1,7
10	Terminal sequence C3	191,000	β_1	2	1300	Substrate of $C\overline{42}$ & $C\overline{3B}$: cleavage products have biologic activity, modify $C\overline{42}$ & $C\overline{3B}$ for C5 cleavage	18,19
11	C5	200,000	β_1	2	75	Participates in formation of membrane-damaging complex, C5-C9. Substrate of $C\overline{423}$ & $C\overline{3B3}$; cleavage products have biologic activity, initiate assembly of cytolytic complex.	4,19
12	C6	128,000	β_2	1	10	Participates in formation of membrane-damaging complex, C5-C9	2,11
13	C7	121,000	β_2	1	60	Participates in formation of membrane-damaging complex, C5-C9	12,21
14	C8	163,000	γ	3	80	Participates in formation of membrane-damaging complex, C5-C9. Cytolysis proceeds slowly after union of C8 with C567.	15
15	C9	79,000	α	...	180	Participates in formation of membrane-damaging complex, C5-C9. Completes assembly of C5-C9; accelerates rate of cytolysis.	9
16	Control proteins $C\overline{1}$ inhibitor	105,000	α_2	1	180	Combines with and blocks activity of $C\overline{1s}$, $C\overline{1r}$, & several other plasma proteases	10,13
17	C3b inactivator	100,000	β_2	...	....	Protease: inactivates C3b fragment of C3 by further cleavage; also cleaves C4b	24,29

Contributor: Ruddy, Shaun

References

1. Alper, C. A., et al. 1973. J. Exp. Med. 137:424-437.
2. Arroyave, C. M., and H. J. Müller-Eberhard. 1971. Immunochemistry 8:995-1006.
3. Borsos, T., et al. 1961. J. Immunol. 87:310-325.
4. Cooper, N. R., and H. J. Müller-Eberhard. 1970. J. Exp. Med. 132:775-793.
5. Daha, M. R., et al. 1976. J. Immunol. 116:1-7.
6. Fearon, D. T., et al. 1974. J. Exp. Med. 139:355-366.
7. Götze, O., and H. J. Müller-Eberhard. 1971. Ibid. 134:90s-108s.
8. Götze, O., and H. J. Müller-Eberhard. 1974. Ibid. 139:44-57.
9. Hadding, U., and H. J. Müller-Eberhard. 1969. Immunology 16:719-735.
10. Harpel, P. C., and N. R. Cooper. 1975. J. Clin. Invest. 55:593-604.
11. Inoue, K., and R. A. Nelson, Jr. 1965. J. Immunol. 95:355-367.
12. Inoue, K., and R. A. Nelson, Jr. 1966. Ibid. 96:386-400.
13. Lepow, I. H., and M. A. Leon. 1962. Immunology 5:222-234.
14. Lepow, I. H., et al. 1963. J. Exp. Med. 117:983-1008.
15. Manni, J. A., and H. J. Müller-Eberhard. 1969. Ibid. 130:1145-1160.
16. Müller-Eberhard, H. J., and C. E. Biro. 1963. Ibid. 118:447-466.
17. Müller-Eberhard, H. J., and O. Götze. 1972. Ibid. 135:1003-1008.
18. Müller-Eberhard, H. J., et al. 1960. Ibid. 111:201-215.
19. Nilsson, U. R., et al. 1975. J. Immunol. 114:815-822.
20. Pillemer, L., et al. 1955. Science 122:545-549.
21. Podack, E. R., et al. 1976. J. Immunol. 116:263-269.

continued

22. Polley, M. J., and H. J. Müller-Eberhard. 1969. J. Exp. Med. 128:533-551.

23. Reid, K. B. M., and R. R. Porter. 1975. Contemp. Top. Mol. Immunol. 4:1-22.

24. Ruddy, S., and K. F. Austen. 1971. J. Immunol. 107: 742-750.

25. Sakai, K., and R. M. Stroud. 1973. Ibid. 110:1010-1020.

26. Schreiber, R. D., and H. J. Müller-Eberhard. 1974. J. Exp. Med. 140:1324-1335.

27. Schreiber, R. D., et al. 1975. Ibid. 142:760-772.

28. Spitzer, R. E., et al. 1969. Science 164:436-437.

29. Tamura, N., and R. A. Nelson, Jr. 1967. J. Immunol. 99:582-589.

30. Yonemasu, K., and R. M. Stroud. 1972. Immunochemistry 9:545-554.

31. Ziccardi, R. J., and N. R. Cooper. 1976. J. Immunol. 116:496-503.

81. DISACCHARIDASES OF THE SMALL INTESTINE IN SELECTED DISEASES

The enzymes lactase, sucrase, and maltase are confined to the brush border surface membrane of the small intestine. The peroral small intestinal biopsy is obtained from the upper jejunum. The tissue was preserved at $-20°C$ until analysis, then homogenized and assayed by specific measurement of glucose released from the disaccharide at $37°C$ [ref. 3]. A variety of non-gastrointestinal diseases have been reported to be associated with isolated lactase deficiency (ILD). These were not included because control populations are not available, and the prevalence of ILD in healthy adults ranges from 5-100% depending on the population group. **Patients below Normal** refers to percent of total patients with the specified disease who showed an enzyme level below the lower limits of the normal range. *Abbreviations*: IU = international units (μmoles substrate hydrolyzed/min). Values in parentheses are ranges, estimate "c" (*see* Introduction). Data in brackets refer to column headings in brackets.

	Condition	Lactase		Sucrase		Maltase		Sucrase / Lactase [Patients Abnormal %]	Reference
		Concentration IU/g protein [IU/g wt]	Patients below Normal %	Concentration IU/g protein [IU/g wt]	Patients below Normal %	Concentration IU/g protein [IU/g wt]	Patients below Normal %		
1	Normal	(15-95) [(1.0-6.5)]	...	(40-165) [(3.5-14)]	...	(130-460) [(8-36)]	...	(1.0-4.5)	4,10
2	Celiac sprue[1] Mild[2]	[(0.6-3.8)]	25	[(3.5-7.4)]	0	[(10-30)]	0	(1.7-6.9) [75]	10
3	Moderate[2]	[(0.1-0.8)]	100	[(0.1-2.4)]	80	[(0.4-12)]	20	(0.5-6.2) [70]	10
4	Severe[2]	(0-3.5) [(0-0.7)]	100	(6.7-24) [(0.1-1.9)]	100	(17-71) [(0.4-8.0)]	75	(1.3-10) [22]	7,10
5	Celiac sprue, treated[3] Excellent response[4]	(0.8-28) [(0.6-3.8)]	29	(12-74) [(3.5-7.4)]	0	(12-180) [(10-30)]	0	(1.7-6.2)	7,10
6	Good response[4]	[(0.2-0.6)]	100	[(0.6-1.7)]	100	[(2.3-7.8)]	43	(1.7-6.2)	7,10
7	Fair response[4]	[(0.1-0.7)]	100	[(0.1-2.3)]	86	[(0.4-7.6)]	43	(0.5-4.7) [29]	7,10
8	Kwashiorkor Acute[5]	(2.3-25)	80	(18-100)	50	(80-350)	30	(4.1-25) [70]	8
9	Past history of[6]	[(0.3-1.9)]	...	[(3.3-14)]	...	[(9-55)]	...	13	2
10	Tropical sprue[7]	[(0.1-0.5)]	100	[(0.2-4.0)]	65	[(0.4-12)]	68	7.2	5,9
11	Cholera Acute	(1.0-15)	86	(20-80)	57	(120-220)	20	11	6
12	Convalescent	(1.0-30)	86	(70-130)	0	(185-250)	0	14	6

[1] Synonyms: Gluten-sensitive enteropathy; non-tropical sprue. [2] Refers to degree of histological abnormality. [3] With gluten-free diet. [4] Refers to clinical condition of patient at time of biopsy rather than enzymatic response. [5] Bantu children, 3-6 wk into convalescent period; those with a history of Kwashiorkor in the remote past usually have normal enzyme levels. [6] Bahatu children with past history of disease; control group without history of disease had all assays within normal range. [7] Untreated patients; after treatment to remission, 63% remained lactase-deficient, but none had depressed activities for sucrase or maltase.

continued

81. DISACCHARIDASES OF THE SMALL INTESTINE IN SELECTED DISEASES

	Condition	Lactase		Sucrase		Maltase		Sucrase Lactase [Patients Abnormal %]	Ref-er-ence
		Concentration IU/g protein [IU/g wt]	Patients below Normal %	Concentration IU/g protein [IU/g wt]	Patients below Normal %	Concentration IU/g protein [IU/g wt]	Patients below Normal %		
	Gastroenteritis[8/]								
13	Acute	(0.5-2.0)	100	(15-80)	43	(40-210)	57	33	6
14	Convalescent	(0.5-7.0)	100	(55-110)	0	(210-300)	0	30	6
15	Infant diarrhea, acute	(0-33)	45	(0-92)	27	(0-324)	18	....	1
16	Pellagra	(1.3-4.7)	100	(30-77)	20	(84-256)	30	(8-35) [100]	8

[8/] Includes non-specific disease and that caused by bacteria.

Contributor: Gray, Gary M.

References

1. Burke, V., et al. 1965. Aust. Paediatr. J. 1:147-160.
2. Cook, G. C., and F. D. Lee. 1966. Lancet 2:1263-1267.
3. Dahlqvist, A. 1964. Anal. Biochem. 7:18-25.
4. Gray, G. M. 1971. Annu. Rev. Med. 22:391-404.
5. Gray, G. M., et al. 1968. Gastroenterology 54:552-558.
6. Hirschhorn, N., and A. Molla. 1969. Johns Hopkins Med. J. 125:291-300.
7. Plotkin, G. R., and K. J. Isselbacher. 1964. N. Engl. J. Med. 271:1033-1037.
8. Prinsloo, J. G., et al. 1971. Arch. Dis. Child. 46:474-478.
9. Sheehy, T. W., and P. R. Anderson. 1965. Lancet 2:1-5.
10. Welsh, J. D., et al. 1969. Arch. Intern. Med. 123:33-38.

82. PLASMA PROTEINS

Data have not been included for plasma coagulation factors (*see* tables 79 and 100), complement factors (*see* table 80), fetoproteins, or pregnancy proteins. **Non-Peptide Content**: CHO = carbohydrate; LIP = lipid. **Normal Conc in Serum or Plasma**: Concentrations have been quoted in part from reference 62; values in parentheses are ranges, estimate "c" (*see* Introduction). **Biological Function**: Hb = hemoglobin; HLA = histocompatibility leukocyte antigens. *Abbreviation & Symbols*: Conc = concentration; ↓ = decrease(d) or reduced; ↑ = increase(d) or raised. Data in brackets refer to the column heading in brackets.

	Protein ⟨Synonym⟩	Mol Wt [Non-Peptide Content]	Normal Conc in Serum or Plasma mg/100 ml	Biological Function	Biomedical Significance	Genetic Aspects	Refer-ence
1	Prealbumin ⟨Tryptophan-rich prealbu-min; thyrox-ine-binding prealbumin⟩	50,000 [1.3% CHO]	25(10-40)	Binding of thyroxine & vitamin A[1/]	↓ in severe liver dis-ease & in inflam-mations; ↑ during adrenal steroid ad-ministration	....	5,54
2	Albumin	69,000 [None]	4400(3500-5500)	Osmoregulation; transport of ions, pigments, etc.	↓ in cirrhosis, in ne-phrosis, & in chronic infections	Genetic defect: Analbuminemia. Genetic variants: Bisalbuminemia (A1-types). Genetic deter-mination of albumin dimers.	43,50, 69

[1/] Synonym: Retinol.

continued

	Protein ⟨Synonym⟩	Mol Wt [Non-Peptide Content]	Normal Conc in Serum or Plasma mg/100 ml	Biological Function	Biomedical Significance	Genetic Aspects	Reference
3	α_1-Acid glyco-protein ⟨Oro-somucoid; α_1-seromucoid⟩	44,000 [38% CHO]	90(55-140)	Unknown	Acute phase reac-tant (↑ in inflam-matory conditions, in rheumatoid arthritis, & in malignant neoplasias)	Genetic variants: Or-types	34,66
4	High-density li-poprotein ⟨HDL; α_1-lipo-protein⟩	180,000-350,000 [45-58% LIP]	360(290-770)	Lipid transport & transport of lipid-soluble substances (hormones, vita-mins)	↓ in liver diseases & in chronic renal disease	Genetic defect: Tangier disease[2]	1,41,44
5	α_1-Antitrypsin	54,000 [14% CHO]	290(200-400)	Proteinase (trypsin) inhibitor	Acute phase reac-tant (*see* entry 3 above)	Genetic polymor-phism: Pi-types. Genetic defect of Pi^z or Pi^o asso-ciated with pulmonary disease or infantile liver cirrhosis.	35,37,38
6	α_1B-glycopro-tein ⟨Easily precipitable α_1-glycoprotein⟩	50,000 [11% CHO]	22(15-30)	Unknown	....	....	61
7	Transcortin ⟨Corticoste-roid-binding globulin; CBG⟩	55,700 [14% CHO]	∼7	Binding & transport of hydrocorti-sone[3]	....	Inherited decrease in transcortin	15,69
8	Thyroxine-bind-ing globulin ⟨TBG⟩	36,500 [15% CHO]	1.5(1-2)	Binding of thyroxine	....	Electrophoretic variants of TBG; inherited TBG deficiency	55
9	α_1T-glycopro-tein ⟨Trypto-phan-poor α_1-glycoprotein⟩	∼60,000 [13% CHO]	8(5-12)	Unknown	....	....	23
10	α_1-Antichymo-trypsin ⟨α_1X-glycoprotein⟩	68,000 [27% CHO]	45(30-60)	Chymotrypsin inhib-itor	Acute phase reac-tant (*see* entry 3 above)	....	27
11	9.5S α_1-glyco-protein ⟨α_1M-glycoprotein⟩	308,000 [9% CHO]	5.5(3-8)	Binding of metal ions	....	....	25,63
12	Retinol-binding protein	21,000 [None]	4(3-6)	Binding & transport of vitamin A[1]	....	....	51,63
13	Transcobalamin I	56,000	....	Binding & transport of vitamin B_{12}[4]	....	Inherited transco-balamin I defi-ciency	7
14	Group-specific component ⟨Gc-globulin⟩	50,800 [3.3% CHO]	40(20-55)	Binding & transport of vitamin D	↓ in severe liver dis-ease; ↑ during pregnancy	Genetic polymor-phism: Gc-types; common alleles: Gc^1 & Gc^2	9,11
15	Inter-α-trypsin inhibitor	160,000 [9% CHO]	45(20-70)	Proteinase (trypsin) inhibitor	....	....	26,67
16	Antithrombin III	65,000 [15% CHO]	30(20-40)	Thrombin inhibitor	↓ in liver disease	Inherited deficien-cy associated with thrombophilia	16,42

[1] Synonym: Retinol. [2] Synonym: Analphalipoproteinemia. [3] Synonym: Cortisol. [4] Synonym: Cobalamin.

continued

Protein ⟨Synonym⟩	Mol Wt [Non-Peptide Content]	Normal Conc in Serum or Plasma mg/100 ml	Biological Function	Biomedical Significance	Genetic Aspects	Reference
17 Ceruloplasmin	132,000 [8% CHO]	35(15-60)	Copper binding; oxidase activity	↓ in hepatolenticular degeneration[5]; ↑ in pregnancy & in women taking contraceptive hormones; acute phase reactant (see entry 3 above)	Electrophoretic variants: Cp-types	3,33
18 Zn-α_2-glycoprotein	41,000 [15% CHO]	5(2-15)	Unknown	....	....	59
19 α_2-HS-glycoprotein ⟨Ba-α_2-glycoprotein⟩	49,000 [13% CHO]	60(40-85)	Unknown	↓ in cancer & in rheumatoid arthritis	....	10,58
20 C̄Ī inhibitor ⟨C1s inactivator; α_2-neuraminoglycoprotein; C_1-esterase inhibitor⟩	86,200	18(12-24)	Inhibitor of C1r, C1s, plasminogen, kallikrein, & coagulation factor XII	↓ in angioneurotic edema	Inherited form of angioneurotic edema with defect of C̄Ī inhibitor	56
21 Histidine-rich 3.8S α_2-glycoprotein	58,500 [16% CHO]	9(5-15)	Unknown	....	....	28
22 Erythropoietin	30,000	....	Erythropoiesis	....	....	21
Haptoglobin ⟨Hp⟩						
23 Type 1-1	100,000 [19% CHO]	170(100-200)	Hemoglobin binding; peroxidase activity of Hb-Hp complex	↓ in hemolytic anemias & in liver disease; acute phase reactant (see entry 3 above)	Genetic polymorphism: Hp-types; common alleles: Hp^1, Hp^2 (α-chain variation); rare genetic β-chain variants	12,52
24 Type 2-1	100,000 [19% CHO]	235(160-300)				
25 Type 2-2	100,000 [19% CHO]	190(120-260)				
26 α_2-Macroglobulin	820,000 [8% CHO]	240(150-350)[6]; 290(170-420)[7]	Proteinase (plasmin, thrombin, trypsin) inhibitor	↑ in nephrotic syndrome & in some patients with diabetes mellitus	....	6,22
27 Serum cholinesterase ⟨Pseudocholinesterase⟩	350,000 [24% CHO]	∼1(0.5-1.5)	Cholinesterase	Succinylcholine[8] sensitivity (apnea following administration)	Genetic variants as cause of sensitivity	40
28 8S α_3-glycoprotein	220,000 [32% CHO]	4(3-5)	Unknown	....	....	24
29 4S α_2-β_1-glycoprotein	60,000 [30% CHO]	....	Unknown	....	....	32
30 Low-density lipoprotein ⟨LDL; β-lipoprotein⟩	2,400,000 [75% LIP]	440(200-700)[6]; 400(200-600)[7]	Transport of lipids (e.g., cholesterol, hormones)	Age-dependent variations in concentration; ↑ in nephrosis (e.g., familial hypercholesterolemia[9]). Genetic polymorphism: Ag- & Lp-systems.	Genetic defect: Abetalipoproteinemia. Genetic conditions with increased LDL	1,39, 44,57
31 Steroid-binding β-globulin	65,000 [12% CHO]	0.4(0.1-1.2)[6]; 0.8(0.3-1.5)[7]	Binding of 17β-hydroxysteroids	Strongly ↑ in pregnancy	....	14,49

[5] Synonym: Wilson's disease. [6] Males. [7] Females. [8] Synonym: Suxamethonium. [9] Synonym: Hypercholesterinemia.

continued

	Protein ⟨Synonym⟩	Mol Wt [Non-Peptide Content]	Normal Conc in Serum or Plasma mg/100 ml	Biological Function	Biomedical Significance	Genetic Aspects	Reference
32	Hemopexin ⟨β_1B-globulin⟩	70,000 [23% CHO]	75(50-115)	Heme binding	↓ in hemolytic anemias	....	45
33	Transferrin ⟨Siderophilin⟩	80,000 [5% CHO]	295(200-400)	Binding & transport of iron	↓ in nephrosis & in diseases with inflammatory or necrotic processes	Genetic defect: Atransferrinemia. Electrophoretic variants: Tf-types.	4,13, 68
34	Transcobalamin II	....	....	Binding of vitamin B_{12}[4]	....	Genetic defect associated with megaloblastic anemia	65
35	C-reactive protein	135,000 [None]	<1.2	Phagocytosis-promoting activity	Highly ↑ in acute inflammatory reactions	....	20
36	β_2-Glycoprotein I	40,000 [19% CHO]	20(15-30)	Unknown	↓ in severe liver disease	Genetic defect; common genetic variation of β_2-glycoprotein I conc (Bg-types)	8,60
37	C3 proactivator ⟨β_2-Glycoprotein II⟩	80,000 [11% CHO]	18(10-40)[10]	Proenzyme of C3 activator	....	....	19
38	β_2-Glycoprotein III	35,000 [10% CHO]	10(5-15)	Unknown	....	....	64
39	β_2-Microglobulin	11,600 [None]	0.15(0.1-0.2)	Structural homologue to constant part of Ig-L- & H-chains; constituent of HLA	↑ urinary excretion in renal tubular defects & in impending kidney transplant rejection	....	53
	Immunoglobulins						
40	IgG ⟨γG; γ_2; $7S\gamma$⟩	150,000 [3% CHO]	1250(650-1600)	Major serum immunoglobulin; antibody molecule	↓ in IgA myeloma, in Waldenström's macroglobulinemia, in malabsorption syndromes, & during extensive protein loss. Monoclonal ↑ in IgG myeloma; polyclonal ↑ after hyperimmunization in autoimmune disease, & in chronic infections.	↓ in immunodeficiency, especially in B-cell defects & combined defects. Genetic polymorphism: heavy-chain marker—Gm groups; light-chain marker—Inv groups.	18,36, 46
41	IgA ⟨γA; γ_1A; β_2A⟩	160,000[11] [8% CHO]	210(50-400)	Serum immunoglobulin & immunoglobulin of body secretions (secretory IgA)	↓ in gastrointestinal diseases with protein loss, & in certain leukemias. Monoclonal ↑ in IgA myeloma; polyclonal ↑ in some stages of autoimmune diseases & in many cases of liver cirrhosis.	↓ in several genetic immunodeficiencies (e.g., ataxia-telangiectasia). Genetic polymorphism: Am groups.	2,29

[4] Synonym: Cobalamin. [10] Determined as C3 activator. [11] And polymers.

continued

	Protein ⟨Synonym⟩	Mol Wt [Non-Peptide Content]	Normal Conc in Serum or Plasma mg/100 ml	Biological Function	Biomedical Significance	Genetic Aspects	Reference
42	IgM ⟨γM; β_2M; 19Sγ⟩	900,000[11]/ [11% CHO]	125(60-250)[6]/; 160(70-280)[7]/	First antibody after primary antigenic stimulus. Major immunoglobulin synthesized by neonate.	↓ in some IgG & IgA myelomas. Monoclonal ↑ in Waldenström's macroglobulinemia; polyclonal ↑ in some parasitic infections & in infectious hepatitis.	↓ in several genetic immunodeficiencies	17,30
43	IgD ⟨γD⟩	170,000 [12% CHO]	3(1-8)	Trace component of serum immunoglobulins	↑ in IgD myelomas, in some chronic infections, & in cases with discoid lupus erythematosus[12]/	....	47
44	IgE ⟨γE⟩	190,000 [11% CHO]	0.01(0.005-0.03)	Antibodies: Reagins	↑ in IgE myelomas, in allergic patients, & in parasitic infections	↓ in certain immunodeficiencies	31
45	Lysozyme ⟨Muramidase⟩	15,000 [None]	0.15(0.07-0.2)	Lysis of bacteria	Strongly ↑ in monocytic leukemias	....	48

[6]/ Males. [7]/ Females. [11]/ And polymers. [12]/ Synonym: Lupus erythematodis.

Contributor: Cleve, Hartwig

References

1. Alaupovic, P., et al. 1972. Biochim. Biophys. Acta 260:689-707.
2. Ammann, H. J., and R. Hong. 1973. In E. R. Stiehm and V. Fulginiti, ed. Immunologic Disorders in Infants and Children. W. B. Saunders, Philadelphia. pp. 199-214.
3. Bearn, A. G. 1972. In J. B. Stanbury, et al., ed. The Metabolic Basis of Inherited Disease. Ed. 3. McGraw-Hill, New York. pp. 1033-1050.
4. Bearn, A. G., and H. Cleve. 1972. Ibid. pp. 1629-1642.
5. Blake, C. C. F., et al. 1974. J. Mol. Biol. 88:1-12.
6. Bourrillon, R., and E. Razafimakaleo. 1972. In A. Gottschalk, ed. Glycoproteins. Their Composition, Structure and Function. Ed. 2. Elsevier, Amsterdam. pp. 699-716.
7. Carmel, R., and V. Herbert. 1969. Blood 33:1-12.
8. Cleve, H. 1968. Humangenetik 5:294-304.
9. Cleve, H. 1973. Isr. J. Med. Sci. 9:1133-1146.
10. Cleve, H., and H. Dencker. 1966. Protides Biol. Fluids Proc. Colloq. 14:379-384.
11. Daiger, S. P., et al. 1975. Proc. Natl. Acad. Sci. USA 72:2076-2080.
12. Dayhoff, M. O. 1972. Atlas of Protein Sequence and Structure 1972. National Biomedical Research Foundation, Washington, D.C. v. 5, pp. D309-D314.
13. Dayhoff, M. O. 1972. Ibid. v. 5, pp. D310-D317.
14. De Moor, P., et al. 1968. Excerpta Med. Int. Congr. Ser. 157:159(Abstr. 396)
15. Doe, R. P., et al. 1965. Metabolism 14:940-943.
16. Egeberg, O. 1965. Scand. J. Clin. Invest. 17:92.
17. Fragione, B. 1975. In B. Benacerraf, ed. Immunogenetics and Immunodeficiency. Univ. Park Press, Baltimore. pp. 1-53.
18. Gally, J. A. 1973. In M. Sela, ed. The Antigens. Academic Press, New York. v. 1, pp. 161-298.
19. Götze, O., and H. J. Müller-Eberhard. 1971. J. Exp. Med. 134(3-2):90s-108s.
20. Gotschlich, E. C., and G. M. Edelman. 1965. Proc. Natl. Acad. Sci. USA 54:558-566.
21. Hammond, D., et al. 1968. Ann. N.Y. Acad. Sci. 149:516-527.
22. Harpel, P. C., and M. W. Mosesson. 1973. J. Clin. Invest. 52:2175-2184.
23. Haupt, H., and K. Heide. 1964. Clin. Chim. Acta 10:555-558.
24. Haupt, H., et al. 1971. Eur. J. Biochem. 23:242-247.
25. Haupt, H., et al. 1972. Hoppe Seylers Z. Physiol. Chem. 353:1841-1849.
26. Heide, K., et al. 1965. Clin. Chim. Acta 11:82-85.
27. Heimburger, N., et al. 1971. Proc. Int. Res. Conf. Proteinase Inhibitors, pp. 1-22.
28. Heimburger, N., et al. 1972. Hoppe Seylers Z. Physiol. Chem. 353:1133-1140.
29. Heremans, J. F. 1974. (Loc. cit. ref. 18). v. 2, pp. 365-522.

continued

30. Hobbs, J. R. 1975. Birth Defects Orig. Artic. Ser. 11: 112-116.
31. Ishizaka, K., and D. H. Dayton, Jr., ed. 1973. U.S. Dep. HEW Publ. (NIH) 73-502.
32. Iwasaki, T., and K. Schmid. 1970. J. Biol. Chem. 245:1814-1820.
33. Jamieson, G. A. 1972. (Loc. cit. ref. 6). pp. 676-685.
34. Johnson, A. M., et al. 1969. J. Clin. Invest. 48:2293-2299.
35. Kueppers, F. 1973. Am. J. Hum. Genet. 25:677-686.
36. Kunkel, H. G. 1975. (Loc. cit. ref. 17). pp. 56-80.
37. Laurell, C. B., and S. Eriksson. 1963. Scand. J. Clin. Lab. Invest. 15:132-140.
38. Laurell, C. B., and J. O. Jeppson. 1975. In F. W. Putnam, ed. The Plasma Proteins. Structure, Function and Genetic Control. Ed. 2. Academic Press, New York pp. 232-245.
39. Lees, R. S., et al. 1973. Prog. Med. Genet. 9:237-290.
40. Lehmann, H., and J. Liddell. 1972. (Loc. cit. ref. 3). pp. 1730-1736.
41. Lux, S. E., et al. 1972. J. Clin. Invest. 51:2502-2519.
42. Marciniak, E., et al. 1974. Blood 43:219-231.
43. Meloun, B., et al. 1975. FEBS Lett. 58:134-137.
44. Morrisett, J. D., et al. 1975. Annu. Rev. Biochem. 44:183-207.
45. Muller-Eberhard, U. 1970. N. Engl. J. Med. 283:1090-1094.
46. Nisonoff, A., et al. 1975. The Antibody Molecule. Academic Press, New York. pp. 86-99.
47. Nisonoff, A., et al. 1975. Ibid. pp. 119-124.
48. Osserman, E. F., and D. P. Lawler. 1966. J. Exp. Med. 124:921-952.
49. Pearlman, W. H., et al. 1969. J. Biol. Chem. 244:1373-1380.
50. Peters, T., Jr. 1975. (Loc. cit. ref. 38). pp. 133-181.
51. Peterson, P. A. 1971. J. Biol. Chem. 246:34-43.
52. Pintera, J. 1971. Ser. Haematol. 14:1-183.
53. Poulik, M. D. 1975. (Loc. cit. ref. 38). pp. 433-454.
54. Putnam, F. W. 1975. (Loc. cit. ref. 38). pp. 70-72.
55. Rivas, M. L., et al. 1971. Birth Defects Orig. Artic. Ser. 7(6):34-41.
56. Rosen, F. S., et al. 1971. J. Clin. Invest. 50:2143-2158.
57. Scanu, A. M., and C. Wisdom. 1972. Annu. Rev. Biochem. 41:703-730.
58. Schultze, H. E., and J. F. Heremans. 1966. Molecular Biology of Human Proteins. Elsevier, Amsterdam. p. 207.
59. Schultze, H. E., and J. F. Heremans. 1966. Ibid. p. 208.
60. Schultze, H. E., et al. 1961. Naturwissenschaften 48: 719.
61. Schultze, H. E., et al. 1963. Nature (London) 200: 1103.
62. Schwick, H. G., ed. 1975. Table of Human Blood Plasma Proteins. Hoechst A. G. Behring Institute, Frankfurt, Germany.
63. Schwick, H. G. 1976. Protides Biol. Fluids Proc. Colloq. 23:309-315.
64. Schwick, H. G., et al. 1968. Klin. Wochenschr. 46: 981-986.
65. Scott, C. R., et al. 1972. J. Pediatr. 81:1106-1111.
66. Spiro, R. G. 1973. Adv. Protein Chem. 27:350-367.
67. Steinbuch, M., et al. 1976. Protides Biol. Fluids Proc. Colloq. 23:115-118.
68. Sutton, H. E. 1972. (Loc. cit. ref. 6). pp. 653-666.
69. Weitkamp, L. R., et al. 1973. Ann. Hum. Genet. 36: 381-392.

83. VARIATIONS IN THE PLASMA PROTEINS IN SELECTED DISEASES

Method: Rid = radial immunodiffusion. **Fluid**: S = measured in serum; P = measured in plasma. Data in brackets refer to the column heading in brackets.

	Plasma or Serum Protein ⟨Synonym⟩	Disease ⟨Synonym⟩	Method [Fluid]	Value	Reference
1	Acetylesterase inhibitor	Hereditary angioneurotic edema	Biochemical [S]	0 units/ml	6,14
2	⟨C_1-esterase inhibitor⟩		Immunological [S]	3.15(0.9-5.6) mg/100 ml[1/]	16
3	Albumin	Analbuminemia	Chemical [S]	(<0.1-0.29) g/100 ml	19
4	α_1-Antitrypsin	α_1-Antitrypsin deficiency ⟨ZZ homozygote⟩	Rid [S]	14.5% of normal trypsin inhibitory activity	9,13
5			Trypsin inhibitory capacity [S]	0.27(0.07-0.47) mg trypsin inhibited by 1 ml serum	7,12

[1/] The majority of cases have decreased acetylesterase ⟨C_1-esterase⟩ inhibitor levels; however, some cases with elevated values of a functionally impaired inhibitor have been reported [ref. 16].

continued

83. VARIATIONS IN THE PLASMA PROTEINS IN SELECTED DISEASES

	Plasma or Serum Protein ⟨Synonym⟩	Disease ⟨Synonym⟩	Method [Fluid]	Value	Reference
6	Coagulation factors VIII ⟨Antihemophilic globulin⟩ & IX	Hemophilia A & B	Clot-promoting or procoagulant activity [P]	(0-2) % of control[2]; (2-5) % of control[3]; (5-25) % of control[4]	20
7	Complement component C1q	Deficiency associated with hypogammaglobulinemia	Rid [S]	<134 μg/ml[5]	10,11
8	C1r	Systemic lupus erythematosus & other connective tissue diseases	Immunological [S]	None detectable	5
9	C2	Systemic lupus erythematosus & other connective tissue diseases	Immunological [S]	<0.5 μg/ml	1
10	C3	Recurrent infections Homozygous C3 deficiency	Immunological [S]	<2.5 μg/ml[6]	2
11		Type I essential hypercatabolism of C3	Immunological [S]	30 mg/100 ml[7]	
12	Ferroxidase ⟨Ceruloplasmin⟩	Hepatolenticular degeneration ⟨Wilson's disease⟩	Chemical [S]	(1-20) mg/100 ml	4
13	Fibrinogen	Afibrinogenemia	Electrophoresis [P]	Absent	15
14			Immunodiffusion [P]	Trace	
15	Immunoglobulin IgG	Immunodeficiency	Rid [S]	<569 mg/100 ml	17,18
16	IgA	Immunodeficiency	Rid [S]	<61 mg/100 ml	17,18
17	IgM	Immunodeficiency	Rid [S]	<47 mg/100 ml	17,18
18	Lipoproteins α-	Tangier disease	Electrophoresis [P]	None detectable	8
19	β-	Abetalipoproteinemia	Electrophoresis [P]	None detectable	8
20	Transferrin	Transferrin deficiency	Immunoelectrophoresis [S]	None detectable	3

[2] Severe disease. [3] Moderate disease. [4] Mild disease. [5] In some cases. [6] Normal values are 1000-2000 μg/ml. [7] Normal values are 100-200 mg/100 ml.

Contributor: Litwin, Stephen D.

References

1. Agnello, V., et al. 1975. Birth Defects Orig. Artic. Ser. 11(1):312-316.
2. Alper, C. A., and F. S. Rosen. 1975. Ibid. 11(1):301-305.
3. Bearn, A. G., and S. D. Litwin. 1977. In J. B. Stanbury, et al., ed. The Metabolic Basis of Inherited Disease. Ed. 4. McGraw-Hill, New York. (In press).
4. Beeson, P. B., and W. McDermott, ed. 1975. Textbook of Medicine. Ed. 14. W. B. Saunders, Philadelphia. pp. 1878-1879.
5. Day, N. K., and R. A. Good. 1975. Birth Defects Orig. Artic. Ser. 11(1):306-311.
6. Donaldson, V. H. 1966. J. Lab. Clin. Med. 68:369-382.
7. Erlanger, B. F., et al. 1961. Arch. Biochem. Biophys. 95:271-278.
8. Frederickson, D. S., et al. 1972. In J. B. Stanbury, et al., ed. The Metabolic Basis of Inherited Disease. Ed. 3. McGraw-Hill, New York. pp. 493-530.
9. Ganrot, P. O., et al. 1967. Scand. J. Clin. Lab. Invest. 19:205-208.
10. Hanauer, L. B., and C. L. Christian. 1967. Am. J. Med. 42:882-890.
11. Kohler, P. F., and H. F. Muller-Eberhard. 1969. Science 163:474-475.
12. Kueppers, F., and L. F. Black. 1974. Am. Rev. Resp. Dis. 110:176-194.
13. Laurell, C. B., and S. Eriksson. 1963. Scand. J. Clin. Lab. Invest. 15:132-140.
14. Levy, L. R., and I. H. Lepow. 1959. Proc. Soc. Exp. Biol. Med. 101:608-611.
15. Ratnoff, O. D. 1972. Prog. Hemostasis Thromb. 1:41-47.
16. Rosen, F. S., et al. 1971. J. Clin. Invest. 50:2143-2149.
17. Soothill, J. F. 1967. J. R. Coll. Physicians London 2:67-74.

continued

18. Stiehm, E. R., and H. H. Fudenberg. 1966. Pediatrics 37:715-727.

19. Waldmann, T. A., et al. 1964. Am. J. Med. 37:960-963.

20. Wintrobe, M. M., et al. 1974. Clinical Hematology, Ed. 7. Lea and Febiger, Philadelphia. p. 1164.

84. LIPID CONSTITUENTS OF PLASMA

Constituent—Symbol, *n:y*: Figures in brackets indicate a chain of *n* carbons with *y* double bonds. **Concentration**: Single values are means, unless otherwise indicated. Values in parentheses are ranges, estimate "c" unless otherwise indicated (*see* Introduction).

	Constituent [Symbol, *n:y*] ⟨Synonym or Abbreviation⟩	Subjects	Concentration	Reference
1	Total lipids	....	(360-1442) mg/100 ml[1]	2
2			(380-1600) mg/100 ml[2]	2
3			(415-1395) mg/100 ml[3]	2
4		At birth: cord blood	313(174-440) mg/100 ml	5
5		<1 yr old	606(240-800) mg/100 ml	5
6		2-14 yr old	838(490-1090) mg/100 ml	5
	Fatty acids			
7	Total	....	(100-500)[b] mg/100 ml	5
8			(150-500) mg/100 ml	21
9			(294-341) mg/100 ml	16
10	Free (non-esterified) ⟨FFA⟩	....	(8-20) mg/100 ml	14
11			(10-35) mg/100 ml	5
12	Palmitic [16:0]	Fasting	(21.6-28.7) % of FFA	13
13			(22.3-25.38)[4] % of FFA	9
14			(23.1-24.2) % of FFA	19
15	Oleic [18:1]	Fasting	(23.6-29.7) % of FFA	13
16			(32.6-45.0) % of FFA	19
17			(42.0-54.3)[4] % of FFA	9
18	Linoleic [18:2]	Fasting	(6.72-11.96)[4] % of FFA	9
19			(8.1-14.5) % of FFA	19
20			(12.9-21.5) % of FFA	13
21	Triglycerides	At birth	2.6 ± 0.8 (1.5-3.0) mmoles/liter	3
22		1-14 yr old	3.6 ± 1.9 (1.8-8.1) mmoles/liter	3
23		18-20 yr old, ♀	4.0 ± 0.8 (2.5-5.6) mmoles/liter	3
24		18-30 yr old	1.23 ± 0.30 (0.63-1.86)[b] mmoles/liter	22
25		18-49 yr old	0.98 ± 0.31 (0.36-1.60)[b] mmoles/liter	22
26		19-85 yr old	0.91 ± 0.27 (0.37-1.18)[b] mmoles/liter	22
27		20-40 yr old	1.39 ± 0.55 (0.29-2.49)[b] mmoles/liter	22
28		20-65 yr old	1.32 ± 0.62 (0.08-2.56)[b] mmoles/liter	22
29		30-69 yr old, ♂	4.6 mmoles/liter	1
30		Adult	(1.6-9.9) mmoles/liter	3
31		♂	5.1 ± 1.9 mmoles/liter	3
32		♀	4.6 ± 2.3 mmoles/liter	3
	Triglyceride fatty acids ⟨TFA⟩			
33	[<16:0]	Fasting	1.3 wt % TFA	19
34			3.5 wt % TFA	9
35	Palmitic [16:0]	Fasting	(22.10-27.10)[4] wt % TFA	9
36			25.6 wt % TFA	19
37			29.8 wt % TFA	13

[1] Colorimetric method. [2] Turbidimetric method. [3] Gravimetric method. [4] Range of means.

continued

84. LIPID CONSTITUENTS OF PLASMA

	Constituent [Symbol, *n:y*] ⟨Synonym or Abbreviation⟩	Subjects	Concentration	Reference
38	Palmitoleic [16:1]	Fasting	3.1 wt % TFA	19
39			3.7 wt % TFA	9
40	[>16:1 & <18:0]	Fasting	0.5 wt % TFA	19
41			1.1 wt % TFA	9
42	Stearic [18:0]	Fasting	2.9 wt % TFA	19
43			4.6 wt % TFA	9
44	Oleic [18:1]	Fasting	39.1 wt % TFA	13
45			(42.46-49.20)[4/] wt % TFA	9
46			45.1 wt % TFA	19
47	Linoleic [18:2]	Fasting	(12.56-18.22)[4/] wt % TFA	9
48			15.7 wt % TFA	13
49			16.1 wt % TFA	19
50	[>18:2 & <20:4]	Fasting	1.2 wt % TFA	9
51			1.3 wt % TFA	19
52	Arachidonic [20:4]	Fasting	1.3 wt % TFA	9
53			4.5 wt % TFA	19
	Phospholipids			
54	Total	<1 yr old	(122-276) mg/100 ml	5
55		2-14 yr old	(188-292) mg/100 ml	5
56		15-24 yr old	257[5/] mg/100 ml	5
57		25-34 yr old	276[5/] mg/100 ml	5
58		35-44 yr old	300[5/] mg/100 ml	5
59		45-54 yr old	309[5/] mg/100 ml	5
60		55-64 yr old	306[5/] mg/100 ml	5
61	Phosphatidyl choline ⟨Lecithin⟩	....	(80-200) mg/100 ml	14
62			(100-200) mg/100 ml	21
63		7-9 yr old	66% total phospholipids	19
64		17-40 yr old	(106-200) mg/100 ml	17
65		Adult	67% total phospholipids	19
66	Phosphatidyl ethanolamine	7-9 yr old	4% total phospholipids	19
67		Adult	4% total phospholipids	19
68	Sphingomyelin	....	(10-50) mg/100 ml	21
69		7-9 yr old	20% total phospholipids	19
70		17-40 yr old	(43-80) mg/100 ml	17
71		Adult	21% total phospholipids	19
72	Lysophosphatidyl choline ⟨Lysolecithin⟩	7-9 yr old	9% total phospholipids	19
73		25-35 yr old	(0.60-1.07) mg/100 ml	8
74		Adult	7% total phospholipids	19
	Phospholipid fatty acids ⟨PhFA⟩			
75	[<16:0]	Fasting	0.8% PhFA	19
76			2.0% PhFA	9
77	Palmitic [16:0]	Fasting	(32.32-37.50)[4/] % PhFA	9
78			33.2% PhFA	13
79			34.0% PhFA	19
80	Palmitoleic [16:1]	Fasting	0.5% PhFA	19
81			1.1% PhFA	9
82	[>16:1 & <18:0]	Fasting	0.5% PhFA	19
83			0.9% PhFA	9
84	Stearic [18:0]	Fasting	14.3% PhFA	9,19
85	Oleic [18:1]	Fasting	(10.32-12.42)[4/] % PhFA	9
86			11.9% PhFA	13,19

[4/] Range of means. [5/] 95% of male population in specified age group will have this value as upper limit for their total phospholipids level.

continued

	Constituent [Symbol, *n:y*] ⟨Synonym or Abbreviation⟩	Subjects	Concentration	Reference
87	Linoleic [18:2]	Fasting	(16.68-23.96)[4/] % PhFA	9
88			20.4% PhFA	19
89			21.9% PhFA	13
90	[>18:2 & <20:4]	Fasting	3.3% PhFA	9
91			4.0% PhFA	19
92	Arachidonic [20:4]	Fasting	9.3% PhFA	9
93			14.0% PhFA	19
94	[>20:4]	Fasting	2.0% PhFA	9
	Cholesterol			
95	Total	0-19 yr old, ♂♀	(120-230)[a] mg/100 ml	6
96		1-30 yr old, ♂	220[6/] mg/100 ml	20
97		♀	212[6/] mg/100 ml	20
98		12-55 yr old, ♂	202 ± 8 mg/100 ml	7
99		♀	194 ± 13 mg/100 ml	7
100		18 yr old, ♂	188 mg/100 ml	12
101		♀	195 mg/100 ml	12
102		20-29 yr old, ♂♀	(120-240)[a] mg/100 ml	6
103		25-35 yr old, ♂	217 mg/100 ml	12
104		♀	205 mg/100 ml	12
105		30 yr old, ♂	195.1 mg/100 ml	10
106		30-39 yr old, ♂♀	(140-270)[a] mg/100 ml	6
107		30-60 yr old, ♂	245[6/] mg/100 ml	20
108		♀	240[6/] mg/100 ml	20
109		40 yr old, ♂	219.4 mg/100 ml	10
110		40-49 yr old, ♂♀	(150-310)[a] mg/100 ml	6
111		50 yr old, ♂	248.3 mg/100 ml	10
112		50-55 yr old, ♂	245 mg/100 ml	12
113		♀	252 mg/100 ml	12
114		50-59 yr old, ♂♀	(160-330)[a] mg/100 ml	6
115		60 yr old, ♂	240 mg/100 ml	12
116			253.3 mg/100 ml	10
117		♀	270 mg/100 ml	12
118		60-80 yr old, ♂	259[6/] mg/100 ml	20
119		♀	280[6/] mg/100 ml	20
120		70 yr old, ♂	244.6 mg/100 ml	10
121	Free	....	(30-100)[b] mg/100 ml	5
122			(40-64)[b] mg/100 ml	7
123	Esterified	....	(69-77)[b] % total cholesterol	5
124	Cholestanol ⟨Dihydrocholesterol⟩	....	0.57% total cholesterol	15
125			0.7% total cholesterol	5
	Cholesterol ester fatty acids ⟨ChFA⟩			
126	Palmitic [16:0]	Fasting	(10.80-12.30)[4/] wt % ChFA	9
127			11.5 wt % ChFA	19
128	Oleic [18:1]	Fasting	(20.48-25.26)[4/] wt % ChFA	9
129			23.0 wt % ChFA	19
130	Linoleic [18:2]	Fasting	(50.04-57.3)[4/] wt % ChFA	9
131			53.5 wt % ChFA	19
	Steroids			
132	Estradiol	....	0.23(0.02-0.66) μg/100 ml	11
133	Estrone	....	0.07(0.01-0.18) μg/100 ml	11
134	17-Ketosteroids	....	0.171 mg/100 ml	4

[4/] Range of means. [6/] Median.

continued

84. LIPID CONSTITUENTS OF PLASMA

	Constituent [Symbol, *n:y*] ⟨Synonym or Abbreviation⟩	Subjects	Concentration	Reference
	Bile Acids			
135	Total	....	0.081(0.029-0.226) mg/100 ml	18
136	Deoxycholic acid	....	0.025(0.006-0.045) mg/100 ml	18
137	Chenodeoxycholic acid	....	0.036(0.005-0.13) mg/100 ml	18
138	Cholic acid	....	0.020(0.002-0.065) mg/100 ml	18

Contributor: Gotto, Antonio M., Jr.

References

1. Albrink, M. J., et al. 1962. N. Engl. J. Med. 266:484-489.
2. Blaton, V. H., and H. Peeters. 1972. In G. J. Nelson, ed. Blood Lipids and Lipoproteins: Quantitation, Composition and Metabolism. Wiley-Interscience, New York. pp. 275-314.
3. Brown, D. F., et al. 1963. Am. J. Clin. Nutr. 13:1-7.
4. Clayton, G. W., et al. 1955. J. Clin. Endocrinol. Metab. 15:693-701.
5. Diem, K., and C. Lentner, ed. 1972. Geigy Scientific Tables. Ed. 7. Ciba-Geigy, Basel. pp. 600-601, 603.
6. Fredrickson, D. S., et al. 1967. N. Engl. J. Med. 276:148-156.
7. Furman, R. H., et al. 1961. Am. J. Clin. Nutr. 9:73-102.
8. Gjone, E., et al. 1959. J. Lipid Res. 1:66-71.
9. Goodman, D. S., and T. Shiratori. 1964. Ibid. 5:307-313.
10. Keys, A., et al. 1950. J. Clin. Invest. 29:1347-1353.
11. Kroman, H. S., et al. 1966. J. Atheroscler. Res. 6:247-255.
12. Lewis, L. A., et al. 1957. Circulation 16:227-245.
13. Lindgren, F. T., et al. 1961. Am. J. Clin. Nutr. 9:13-23.
14. Masoro, E. J. 1968. Physiological Chemistry of Lipids in Mammals. W. B. Saunders, Philadelphia. pp. 186-187.
15. Mosbach, E. H. 1967. Int. Congr. Nutr. 7th 1966 Proc. 5:469-471.
16. Page, E., and L. Michaud. 1951. Can. J. Med. Sci. 29:239-244.
17. Petersen, P. V. 1950. Scand. J. Clin. Lab. Invest. 2:44-47.
18. Sandberg, D. H., et al. 1965. J. Lipid Res. 6:182-192.
19. Skipski, V. P. 1972. (Loc. cit. ref. 2). pp. 471-583.
20. Werner, M., et al. 1970. Z. Klin. Chem. Klin. Biochem. 8:105-115.
21. White, A., et al., ed. 1973. Principles of Biochemistry. Ed. 5. McGraw-Hill, New York. p. 802.
22. Witter, R. F., and V. S. Whitner. 1972. (Loc. cit. ref. 2). pp. 75-111.

85. ABNORMAL LIPOPROTEINEMIAS

Part I. Definitions of Major Plasma Lipoproteins

Method of Definition: Flotation by Analytic Ultracentrifuge—measured in a sodium chloride solution with a density of 1.063 g/ml at 26°C; S_f units = Svedberg units = 10^{-13}s.

	Terminology ⟨Synonym⟩	Major Lipid Components	Density by Ultracentrifuge g/ml	Flotation by Analytic Ultracentrifuge S_f units	Electrophoresis
			Method of Definition		
1	Chylomicrons	Exogenous glycerides	<0.95	>400	Remain at origin
2	Very low density lipoproteins ⟨VLDL⟩	Endogenous glycerides	0.95-1.006	20-400	Pre-β mobility[1/]: pre-β lipoproteins

[1/] LP(a) lipoprotein has a pre-β mobility, but usually has a density >1.006, and is sometimes referred to as a "sinking" pre-β lipoprotein.

continued

Part I. Definitions of Major Plasma Lipoproteins

Terminology ⟨Synonym⟩	Major Lipid Components	Method of Definition		
		Density by Ultracentrifuge g/ml	Flotation by Analytic Ultra-centrifuge S_f units	Electrophoresis
3 Low density lipoproteins 4 ⟨LDL⟩ 5	Cholesterol, phospholipids, cholesterol esters	1.006-1.063 1.006-1.019[2/] 1.019-1.063	0-20 12-20 0-12	β-Mobility: β-lipoproteins
6 High density lipoproteins 7 ⟨HDL⟩	Phospholipids, cholesterol esters	HDL_2: 1.063-1.12 HDL_3: 1.12-1.21	Fn[3/]	α_1-Mobility: α-lipoproteins

[2/] Sometimes referred to as intermediate density lipoproteins. [3/] They do not float at 1.063.

Contributor: Gotto, Antonio M., Jr.

General References

1. Albers, J. J., et al. 1975. Metabolism 24:1047-1054.
2. Dahlen, G., et al. 1975. Acta Med. Scand. 198:263-267.
3. Fredrickson, D. S., et al. 1972. In J. B. Stanbury, et al., ed. The Metabolic Basis of Inherited Disease. Ed. 3. McGraw-Hill, New York. pp. 493-530.
4. Gotto, A. M., Jr. 1972. Cardiovasc. Res. Cent. Bull. (Houston) 11(1):3-20.
5. Phillips, G. B. 1974. Clin. Chim. Acta 53:127-134.
6. Rider, A. K., et al. 1970. Circulation 42, Suppl. III-10(Abstr. 34).
7. Rifkind, B. M. 1973. Clin. Endocrinol. Metab. 2(1):3-10.

Part II. Hyperlipoproteinemias

Plasma Lipoprotein Fractions: Chylomicrons were observed during fasting conditions. Associated Genetic Hyperlipidemia lists genetic disorders in which the given phenotype may be present. Associated Secondary Disease lists other diseases that may cause the given lipoprotein defect. Data in brackets refer to the column heading in brackets.

ABBREVIATIONS & SYMBOLS

Ch = cholesterol
TG = triglycerides
VLDL = very low density lipoprotein
LDL = low density lipoprotein
HDL = high density lipoprotein
LPL = diacylglycerol lipase ⟨Lipoprotein lipase⟩
PHLA = post-heparin lipolytic activity
AR = autosomal recessive

AD = autosomal dominant
P = polygenic
N = normal
↑ = increased
↑↑ = greatly increased
↓ = decreased
+ = present
0 = absent

continued

Part II. Hyperlipoproteinemias

	Phenotype		Plasma Lipids			Plasma Lipoprotein Fractions				Appearance of Plasma	Associated Genetic Hyperlipidemia [Mode of Inheritance]	Associated Secondary Disease
	Type	Definition	Ch	TG	Ch/TG Ratio by wt	Chylo-microns	VLDL	LDL	HDL			
1	I	Hyperchylomi-cronemia, with absolute deficiency of LPL or PHLA	N or ↑	↑↑	<0.2	+	Mildly ↑, N, or ↓	N or ↓	0	"Cream" layer over a clear in-franatant	Familial LPL de-ficiency [AR]	Diabetic acidosis; hypothy-roidism; dysglob-ulinemia
2	IIA	Increased LDL	↑	N	>1.5	0	N or ↓	↑	N	Clear	Familial hypercho-lesterolemia [AD]; familial combined hyper-lipidemia [AD]; polygenic hyper-cholesterolemia [P]	Hypothy-roidism; dysglob-ulinemia; nephro-sis; ob-structive liver dis-ease; di-etary ex-cess; au-toim-mune dis-ease; Cushing's disease; acute intermittent porphyria
3	IIB	Increased LDL & increased VLDL	↑	↑	Var-iable	0	↑	↑	N	Clear or faintly turbid		
4	III	Floating β-lipo-proteins[1/]	↑	↑	∿1[2/]	+, may be ↑	↑[1,3/]	LDL₁, ↑; LDL₂, ↓[4/]	N or ↓	Usually tur-bid; may also be faint "cream" layer	Familial broad beta disease [AD]	Secondary causes are rare as: diabetes mellitus; autoim-mune hy-perlipo-protein-emia; hypothyroidism; renal insufficiency

1/ Indicate presence of an abnormal plasma lipoprotein, with a density <1.006 g/ml and β-electrophoretic mobility, in addition to pre-β migrating lipoprotein [ref. 5]. 2/ When the plasma triglyceride concentration is between 150 and 1000 mg/100 ml, a ratio of VLDL cholesterol to plasma tri-glyceride concentration of ≥0.30 is suggested to be diag-nostic of type III hyperlipoproteinemia [ref. 6]. A ratio of VLDL cholesterol to VLDL triglycerides of >0.42 is sug-gested to be diagnostic of type III in hypertriglyceridemic subjects [ref. 7]. 3/ The VLDL "arginine-rich" protein ⟨ApoE-III⟩ is missing one of its three polymorphic appear-ances in type III hyperlipoproteinemia, when using isoelec-tric focusing of this protein (deficiency of ApoE-III) [ref. 9]. 4/ LDL₂ refers to lipoproteins of density 1.019-1.063, while LDL₁ refers to lipoproteins of density 1.006-1.019. Recently, the term "intermediate density lipoprotein(s)" ⟨IDL⟩ has been used for this latter density class. In the postabsorptive plasma of type III subjects, it is typically present in increased concentration, and appears, on zonal ultracentrifugation in a density gradient, as a distinct lipo-protein between VLDL and LDL₂ [ref. 8].

continued

Part II. Hyperlipoproteinemias

	Phenotype		Plasma Lipids			Plasma Lipoprotein Fractions				Appearance of Plasma	Associated Genetic Hyperlipidemia [Mode of Inheritance]	Associated Secondary Disease
	Type	Definition	Ch	TG	Ch/TG Ratio by wt	Chylo-microns	VLDL	LDL	HDL			
5	IV	Increased VLDL	N or ↑	↑	Var-iable	0	↑	↓ or N	N or ↓	Usually tur-bid	Familial hypertri-glyceridemia [AD]; familial combined hyper-lipidemia [AD]	Diabetes mellitus; hypothy-roidism; dysglobu-linemia; obstruc-tive liver disease; nephrot-ic syn-drome; uremia; glycogen-storage disease;
6	V	Hyperchylomi-cronemia & increased VLDL, with LPL or PHLA present but reduced	N or ↑	↑↑	0.15-0.60[5/]	↑	↑	↓ or N	Usu-ally ↓	"Cream lay-er"	Familial hypertri-glyceridemia [AD]; familial mixed or type V hyperlipide-mia [AD]; rare-ly familial com-bined hyperlip-idemia [AD]	alcoholism; pancreatitis; drugs: estrogens, steroids, other hormones

[5/] TG/Ch >0.5.

Contributor: Gotto, Antonio M., Jr.

General References

1. Beaumont, J. L., et al. 1970. Bull. WHO 43:891-915.
2. Goldstein, J. L., et al. 1973. J. Clin. Invest. 52:1544-1567.
3. Goldstein, J. L., et al. 1977. In J. B. Stanbury, et al., ed. The Metabolic Basis of Inherited Disease. Ed. 4. McGraw-Hill, New York. (In press).
4. Gotto, A. M., Jr. 1974. In H. F. Conn, ed. Current Therapy. W. B. Saunders, Philadelphia. pp. 418-427.

Specific References

5. Fredrickson, D. S., and R. I. Levy. 1972. In J. B. Stanbury, et al., ed. The Metabolic Basis of Inherited Disease. Ed. 3. McGraw-Hill, New York. pp. 545-614.
6. Fredrickson, D. S., et al. 1975. Ann. Intern. Med. 82: 150-157.
7. Hazzard, W. R., et al. 1972. Metabolism 21:1009-1019.
8. Patsch, J. R., et al. 1975. Eur. J. Clin. Invest. 5:45-55.
9. Uterman, G., et al. 1975. FEBS Lett. 56:352-355.

Part III. Hypolipoproteinemias

Data were adapted from reference 2. **Mode of Inheritance**: AR = autosomal recessive; AD = autosomal dominant. **Plasma Lipoprotein Fractions**: VLDL = very low density lipoproteins; LDL = low density lipoproteins; HDL = high density lipoproteins. Data in brackets refer to the column heading in brackets.

continued

Part III.   Hypolipoproteinemias

Disease ⟨Synonym⟩ [Mode of Inheritance]	Major Clinical Findings	Laboratory Findings								
		Plasma Lipids, mg/100 ml			Plasma Lipoprotein Fractions					Vitamins A & E
		Cholesterol	Triglycerides	Phospholipids	Chylomicrons	VLDL	LDL	HDL		
1 Abetalipoproteinemia[1] [AR]	Malabsorption of fat; acanthocytosis; retinitis pigmentosa; ataxic neuropathy	Low, (35-54)	Low, <20	Low, <100	Absent	Absent	Absent[2]	Present		Reduced
2 Hypobetalipoproteinemia[1] ⟨Familial low-density lipoprotein deficiency⟩ [AD]	Generally asymptomatic	Low, (55-164)	Low or normal, (20-140)[3]	Low or normal, (110-170)[3]	Normal	Moderately reduced	Low: one-eighth to one-tenth of normal[2]	Normal		Normal to low normal
3 Tangier disease ⟨Familial high-density lipoprotein deficiency⟩ [AR]	Cholesterol deposits in other tissues (reticuloendothelial system); abnormal tonsils; splenomegaly; peripheral neuropathy	Low, (30-125)	High (rarely normal), (150-330)	Low, (70-140)	Normal	Abnormal β-migrating VLDL	Normal or elevated	Very low & abnormal (HDL$_T$)		Normal

[1] There is a variant in which a homozygote for hypobetalipoproteinemia has an abetalipoproteinemia pattern [ref. 1]. [2] Lipoprotein containing HDL apoprotein is present in the LDL density range. [3] Tendency toward lower limits.

Contributor: Gotto, Antonio M., Jr.

References
1. Cottrill, C., et al. 1974. Metabolism 23: 779-791.

2. Fredrickson, D. S., et al. 1972. In J. B. Stanbury, et al., ed. The Metabolic Basis of Inherited Disease. Ed. 3. McGraw-Hill, New York. pp. 493-530.

86. KETO ACIDS IN SELECTED CONDITIONS

β-Hydroxybutyrate ⟨bohb⟩ and acetoacetate ⟨acac⟩ are the principal keto acids in intermediary metabolism. Their production by the liver is largely determined by free fatty acid, insulin, and glucagon concentrations. In diabetic ketoacidosis a combination of overproduction and underutilization of keto acids leads to pathogenic concentrations. The ratio of bohb to acac is determined by the redox potential which is altered in diabetic ketoacidosis and lactic acidosis. Keto acids are the primary protein-sparing agents in prolonged fasting through their replacement of protein-derived glucose as a fuel for the brain, and by their action to reduce branched-chain amino acid oxidation in muscle. Providing amino

continued

acids parenterally or whole protein orally, free of carbohydrate, (protein-sparing, modified fast) maintains synthetic rates while not significantly limiting the contribution of ketone bodies to nitrogen economy. **bohb + acac:** Ranges are given only if quantities are calculated from individual values; otherwise, "bohb + acac" is derived from accompanying means. **bohb/acac:** Values are derived from accompanying means. Values in parentheses are ranges, estimate "c" unless otherwise specified (*see* Introduction).

	Condition	No. of Subjects	Time of Observation days	bohb, mM	acac, mM	bohb + acac	bohb/ acac	Reference
1	Normal: fasting	6	1	0.016(0.014-0.018)[b]	0.013(0.007-0.019)[b]	0.029	1.23	3
2			2	0.39(0.28-0.50)[b]	0.16(0.10-0.22)[b]	0.55	2.44	
3			3	1.64(1.36-1.92)[b]	0.51(0.37-0.65)[b]	2.15	3.22	
4			6	3.13(2.65-3.61)[b]	0.85(0.69-0.10)[b]	3.98	3.68	
5			8	4.23(3.55-4.91)[b]	1.09(0.87-1.31)[b]	5.32	3.88	
6	Obese Prolonged starvation	11	−3[1]	0.06(0.04-0.08)[b]	0.03(0.01-0.05)[b]	0.09	2.00	8
7			0	0.07(0.05-0.09)[b]	0.03(0.01-0.05)[b]	0.10	2.33	
8			3	1.21(0.83-1.59)[b]	0.41(0.29-0.53)[b]	1.62	2.95	
9			10	4.30(3.5-5.1)[b]	1.00(0.78-1.22)[b]	5.30	4.30	
10			17	5.10(4.58-5.62)[b]	1.12(0.90-1.34)[b]	6.22	4.55	
11			24	5.78(5.24-6.32)[b]	1.27(1.05-1.49)[b]	7.05	4.55	
12			31	5.84(5.06-6.62)[b]	1.37(1.11-1.63)[b]	7.21	4.26	
13			35-38	5.85(5.09-6.61)[b]	1.34(1.06-1.62)[b]	7.19	4.36	
14	Protein-sparing, modified fasting (1g protein·kg body wt^{-1}· d^{-1}, or 1.5 g·kg ideal wt^{-1}·d^{-1})	19	0	0.16(0.0-0.73)	0.02(0.0-0.09)	0.21(0.0-0.75)	8.0	2
15			7	1.43(0.46-3.10)	0.27(0.01-0.73)	1.66(0.47-3.41)	5.29	
16			14	1.72(0.22-3.34)	0.34(0.04-0.80)	2.06(0.26-3.81)	5.05	
17			21	2.01(0.36-4.39)	0.38(0.04-0.96)	2.39(0.40-4.99)	5.28	
18			28	1.73(0.27-3.98)	0.25(0.06-0.51)	1.84(0.33-4.49)	6.92	
19	Fasting, with exogenous glucocorticoid ⟨EG⟩ administered after 35 d	6	35[2]	6.12(4.92-7.32)[b]	1.20(0.50-1.90)[b]	7.32	5.1	6
20			37[3]	6.54(5.44-7.64)[b]	1.30(0.80-1.80)[b]	7.84	5.03	
21			39[4]	5.91(4.85-6.97)[b]	1.48(0.76-2.20)[b]	7.39	3.99	
22			42[5]	4.95(4.85-5.05)[b]	1.52(0.76-2.28)[b]	6.47	3.26	
23	Diabetic Non-obese; insulin requiring; fasting	2	1	0.056(0.054-0.058)	0.035(0.029-0.040)	0.091(0.083-0.098)	1.60	3
24			2	0.300(0.21-0.39)	0.140(0.08-0.20)	0.441(0.29-0.59)	2.02	
25			3	1.35(0.81-1.89)	0.355(0.22-0.49)	1.71(1.03-2.38)	3.80	
26			6	3.48(2.78-4.18)	0.875(0.78-0.97)	4.36(3.56-5.15)	3.98	
27			8	3.95(3.18-4.72)	0.94(0.77-1.11)	4.89(3.95-5.83)	4.20	
28	Ketoacidosis	7	During episode	7.60(3.3-10.80)	2.94(1.45-4.28)	10.54(6.56-14.91)	2.59	7
29	Concurrent ketoacidosis & lactic acidosis	2	During episode	5.4(2.5-8.3)	0.69(0.33-1.06)	6.09(2.83-9.36)	7.83	4
30	Elective surgery Electrolytes, i.v.	4	3[6]	0.808(0.20-1.80)	0.365(0.18-0.60)	1.17	2.21	1
31	5% glucose[7] solution, i.v.	7	3[6]	0.126(0.01-0.30)	0.026(0.01-0.12)	0.152	4.85	1
32		6	4[6]	0.150(0.0-0.91)	0.140(0.02-0.60)	0.290	1.07	1
33	60-90 g amino acids/d, as 3% solution, i.v.	10	4[6]	1.10(0.25-2.28)	0.37(0.01-0.80)	1.47	2.97	1
34	No infection	7	0	0.39(0.0-0.98)	0.19(0.02-0.45)	0.58(0.03-1.43)	2.05	5
35			2[6]	1.03(0.41-1.10)	0.36(0.29-0.80)	1.37(1.35-2.80)	2.86	
36			4[6]	1.73(0.91-2.50)	0.61(0.30-0.82)	2.34(1.52-3.32)	2.83	
37	Infection	7	0	0.20(0.04-0.56)	0.08(0.02-0.19)	0.28(0.08-0.75)	2.50	5
38			2[6]	0.46(0.12-0.60)	0.20(0.05-0.22)	0.64(0.17-0.86)	2.30	
39			4[6]	1.22(0.25-1.75)	0.49(0.14-0.64)	1.71(0.39-2.29)	2.48	

[1] Fed. [2] Pre-EG. [3] 2 days post-EG. [4] 4 days post-EG. [5] 7 days post-EG. [6] Post-surgery. [7] Synonym: Dextrose.

continued

86. KETO ACIDS IN SELECTED CONDITIONS

Contributors: Bistrian, Bruce R., and Trerice, Mary S.

References
1. Benotti, P. N., et al. 1976. Surg. Forum 27:7-10.
2. Bistrian, B. R., and M. S. Trerice. Unpublished. Harvard Medical School, Boston, MA, 1976.
3. Cahill, G. F., Jr., et al. 1966. J. Clin. Invest. 45:1751-1769.
4. Marliss, E. B., et al. 1970. N. Engl. J. Med. 283:978-980.
5. Miller, J. D., et al. In press, 1976.
6. Owen, O. E., and G. F. Cahill, Jr. 1973. J. Clin. Invest. 52:2596-2605.
7. Owen, O. E., and G. A. Reichard, Jr. 1975. Isr. J. Med. Sci. 11:560-570.
8. Owen, O. E., et al. 1969. J. Clin. Invest. 48:574-583.

87. LACTATE AND PYRUVATE LEVELS IN BLOOD

The collection technique was rapid, and the method was enzymatic in all cases. $A - V$ = arteriovenous difference, i.e., arterial blood level minus venous blood level. Values in parentheses are ranges, estimate "c" (*see* Introduction).

Part I. Normal Values

Subjects were at rest (overnight fasted or postabsorptive).

	Structure or Body Region	No. of Subjects	Lactate Concentration mmoles/liter blood		Pyruvate Concentration mmoles/liter blood		Lactate:Pyruvate Ratio		Reference
			Arterial	A − V	Arterial	A − V	Arterial	Venous	
1	Brain	4	0.604 ± 0.032 (0.588-0.652)	−0.014 ± 0.004 (−0.012 to −0.020)	0.051 ± 0.006 (0.043-0.058)	−0.003 ± 0.006 (−0.011 to +0.003)	12.0 ± 1.5 (10.1-13.7)	11.9 ± 2.3 (8.7-14.0)	2
2	Splanchnic bed	5	0.587 ± 0.135 (0.438-0.804)	0.253 ± 0.082 (0.153-0.378)	0.068 ± 0.016 (0.065-0.093)	0.018 ± 0.004 (0.013-0.024)	8.7 ± 1.0 (7.3-9.8)	6.9 ± 1.4 (6.1-9.3)	3
3	Heart	6	0.595 ± 0.184 (0.35-0.92)	0.183 ± 0.209 (0.03-0.59)	0.073 ± 0.022 (0.05-0.11)	0.003 ± 0.018 (−0.01 to +0.03)	8.9 ± 3.6 (3.2-13.1)	6.4 ± 2.9 (3.4-11.5)	4
4	Kidney	71	....	0.059 ± 0.136	....	0.009 ± 0.154	....		5
5	Forearm	29	0.499 ± 0.088 (0.394-0.716)	−0.143 ± 0.086 (0.031-0.318)	0.044 ± 0.011 (0.030-0.065)	−0.001 ± 0.009 (−0.015 to +0.018)	11.8 ± 2.6 (6.5-17.0)	14.5 ± 3.6 (7.4-22.3)	1
6	Leg	10	0.630 ± 0.158	−0.150 ± 0.096	0.065 ± 0.012	0.002 ± 0.009	9.7	11.6	6

Contributors: Aoki, Thomas T., and Cahill, George F., Jr.

References
1. Aoki, T. T., M. F. Brennan, et al. Unpublished. Harvard Medical School, P. B. Brigham Hospital, Boston, MA, 1976.
2. Aoki, T. T., S. S. Saltz, et al. Unpublished. Harvard Medical School, P. B. Brigham Hospital, Boston, MA, 1976.
3. Garber, A. J., et al. 1974. J. Clin. Invest. 54:981-989.
4. Krasnow, N., et al. 1962. Ibid. 41:2075-2085.
5. Nieth, H., and P. Schollmeyer. 1966. Nature (London) 209:1244-1245.
6. Wahren, J., et al. 1071. J. Clin. Invest. 50:2715-2725.

Part II. Selected Conditions

	Condition	No. of Subjects	Structure or Body Region	Lactate Concentration mmoles/liter blood	Pyruvate Concentration mmoles/liter blood	Lactate:Pyruvate Ratio	Reference
				Arterial Level			
1	Fasting, 21 d or more	3	Brain	0.533 ± 0.139	0.054 ± 0.007 (0.047-0.061)	9.7 ± 1.9 (8.1-11.8)	6

continued

87. LACTATE AND PYRUVATE LEVELS IN BLOOD

Part II. Selected Conditions

	Condition	No. of Sub-jects	Structure or Body Region	Lactate Concentration mmoles/liter blood	Pyruvate Concentration mmoles/liter blood	Lactate:Pyruvate Ratio	Ref-er-ence
2		5	Splanchnic bed	0.470 ± 0.090	0.055 ± 0.013	8.5	6
3		5	Kidney	0.470 ± 0.090	0.055 ± 0.013	8.5	6
4		5	Forearm	0.533 ± 0.098 (0.400-0.672)	0.037 ± 0.012 (0.018-0.048)	15.20 ± 4.00 (11-14)	1
5	Exercise, heavy	6	Leg	3.5 ± 2.82	0.154 ± 0.056	22.8	7
6	Diabetic ketoacidosis	9	Forearm	1.82 ± 1.17 (0.74-4.50)	0.085 ± 0.050 (0.046-0.216)	21.9 ± 7.4 (14.8-37.6)	2
7	Lactic acidosis	6	Forearm	22.96 ± 6.49 (15.00-29.00)	0.450 ± 0.170 (0.300-0.770)	57.7 ± 17.3 (38.0-82.0)	3
				Arteriovenous Difference[1]			
8	Fasting, 21 d or more	3	Brain	−0.200 ± 0.090 (−0.09 to −0.26)	−0.030 ± 0.005 (−0.023 to −0.033)	8.7 ± 0.9 (7.8-9.5)[2]	5
9		5	Splanchnic bed	0.190 ± 0.110	0.019 ± 0.020	7.8[2]	6
10		5	Kidney	0.043 ± 0.016	0.004 ± 0.002	8.4[2]	6
11		5	Forearm	−0.079 ± 0.019	0.006 ± 0.004 (−0.002 to +0.015)	19.3 ± 5.0 (16.6-27.9)[2]	1
12	Exercise, heavy	6	Leg	−0.120 ± 0.470	−0.070 ± 0.050	....	7
13	High carbohydrate diet, ∿700 g/d	2	Forearm	1.55[2]	0.160[2]	9.7[2]	4

[1] Unless otherwise indicated. [2] Venous level.

Contributors: Aoki, Thomas T., and Cahill, George F., Jr.

References
1. Aoki, T. T., et al. 1975. Adv. Enzyme Regul. 13: 329-336.
2. Assal, J. P., et al. 1974. Diabetes 23:405-411.
3. Marliss, E. B., et al. 1972. Am. J. Med. 52:474-480.
4. O'Connell, R. C., et al. 1974. J. Clin. Endocrinol. Metab. 39:555-563.
5. Owen, O. E., et al. 1967. J. Clin. Invest. 46:1589-1595.
6. Owen, E. O., et al. 1969. Ibid. 48:574-583.
7. Wahren, J., et al. 1971. Ibid. 50:2715-2725.

88. DISEASES WITH DISTURBANCES IN PIGMENT METABOLISM

Disorders in which pigment alteration is secondary to inflammation have been excluded. **Mechanism or Responsible Agent**: MSH = melanocyte-stimulating hormone; ACTH = adrenocorticotropic hormone; DOPA = 3, 4-dihydroxyphenylalanine. Symbols: ↑ = increase(d); ↓ decrease(d). Figures in heavy brackets are reference numbers.

	Disease State or Condition	Nature of Change	Mechanism or Responsible Agent
		Increased Pigmentation	
1	Acromegaly	Diffuse brown melanosis [20]; occurs in ∿40% of patients; ↑ usually not marked [12]	....

continued

88. DISEASES WITH DISTURBANCES IN PIGMENT METABOLISM

	Disease State or Condition	Nature of Change	Mechanism or Responsible Agent
2	Addison's disease	Diffuse brown melanosis; buccal & palmar crease accentuation	↑ MSH & ↑ ACTH [17,18]; ↑ melanin synthesis
3	Cushing's syndrome	Diffuse brown melanosis; occurs extremely rarely	↑ MSH and/or ↑ ACTH [1,5]
4	Diffuse melanosis of disseminated malignant melanoma	Generalized slate-blue-gray color	Spread of melanosomes & melanogens derived from melanoma cells throughout skin [10,15,24]
5	Ectopic ACTH syndrome	Diffuse brown melanosis	Malignant tumors of non-endocrine origin, producing ACTH and/or MSH [19]
6	Fanconi's syndrome [8]	Generalized hyperpigmentation[1]	Autosomal recessive
7	Hyperthyroidism	Diffuse brown melanosis [23]	....
	Liver, metabolic disturbances of [20]		
8	Biliary cirrhosis	Diffuse melanosis	....
9	Hemochromatosis	Diffuse melanosis; may have grayish hue [9]	....
10	Porphyria cutanea tarda	Diffuse melanosis	....
11	Progressive lenticular degeneration[2]	Diffuse melanosis	....
12	Melanism [4]	Diffuse brown, present at birth; ↑ in intensity during early childhood	Autosomal dominant; ↑ epidermal melanization
13	Nelson's syndrome [22]	Diffuse brown melanosis	↑ MSH and/or ↑ ACTH from functioning pituitary adenoma arising after bilateral adrenalectomy
14	Pregnancy	Darkening of nipples, genitalia, linea alba, nevi	↑ estrogens [7]
15		Melasma	↑ progesterones [27]
16	Vitamin B_{12} deficiency [2]	Diffuse brown hypermelanosis[3]	....
		Decreased Pigmentation	
17	Albinism, oculocutaneous [29]	Generalized decreased-to-absent pigmentation; iris translucency; nystagmus	Recessive inheritance, at least 2 types: defective (monophenol monooxygenase[4] positive), or absence (monophenol monooxygenase negative) of functional monophenol monooxygenase (converts tyrosine to DOPA & DOPA to DOPAquinone)
18	Chediak-Higashi syndrome	Diffuse depigmentation with photophobia & nystagmus; late lymphoma-like phase; increased susceptibility to infection [3]	Giant melanosomes; defect in packaging granules
19	Fanconi's syndrome [8]	Decreased pigment in hair[5]	Autosomal recessive
20	Histidinemia [30]	Light-colored hair	Autosomal recessive histidine ammonialyase[6] deficiency
21	Homocystinuria	Blond—fine fair hair & fair skin; premature graying; malar flush, livedo reticularis of extremities [13]	Absence of cystathionine β-synthase
22	Hypopituitarism [9]	Diffuse ↓ in pigment	↓ ACTH; ↓ MSH
23	Kwashiorkor & other chronic protein deficiency states [25]	Decreased pigmentation of hair & skin, especially face [20]	Protein malnutrition

[1] Also causes decreased pigment in hair. [2] Synonym: Wilson's disease. [3] Also causes loss of hair color. [4] Synonym: Tyrosinase. [5] Also causes generalized hyperpigmentation. [6] Synonym: Histidine deaminase.

continued

	Disease State or Condition	Nature of Change	Mechanism or Responsible Agent
24	Methionine malabsorption syndrome [7] [26]	White hair, mental deficiency	Urinary α-hydroxybutyric acid
25	Phenylketonuria	Decreased pigment in hair & iris, fair skin [11] — nin production possibly by competitive inhibition of monophenol monooxygenase [4] by ↑ levels of phenylalanine [21]	Deficiency of phenylalanine 4-mono-oxygenase [8] [28]; relative ↓ in mela-
26	Piebaldism	Congenital, discrete areas of absent pigmentation; white forelock, usually asymmetric [6]	Autosomal dominant; melanocytes absent from non-pigmented areas [14]
27	Vitamin B$_{12}$ deficiency [2]	Loss of hair color [9]	....
28	Vitiligo [16]	Discrete areas of absent pigmentation; accentuation about body orifices & points of trauma	Destruction of melanocytes; familial tendency

[4] Synonym: Tyrosinase. [7] Synonym: Oasthouse disease. [8] Synonym: Phenylalanine hydroxylase. [9] Also causes diffuse brown hypermelanosis.

Contributors: Sober, Arthur J., and Fitzpatrick, Thomas B.

References

1. Bahn, R. C., et al. 1960. Proc. Staff Meet. Mayo Clin. 35:623-629.
2. Baker, S. J., et al. 1963. Br. Med. J. 1:1713-1715.
3. Blume, R., and S. Wolff. 1972. Medicine (Baltimore) 51:247-280.
4. Bogaert, L. 1948. Bull. Acad. R. Med. Belg. 13:397.
5. Bricaire, H., et al. 1967. Presse Med. 75:2697-2702.
6. Comings, D. E., and G. F. Odland. 1966. J. Am. Med. Assoc. 195:519-523.
7. Davis, M. E., et al. 1945. J. Clin. Endocrinol. 5:138-146.
8. Findlay, G. H. 1958. Br. J. Dermatol. 70:148-149.
9. Fitzpatrick, T. B., and M. C. Mihm. 1971. In T. B. Fitzpatrick, et al., ed. Dermatology in General Medicine. McGraw-Hill, New York. pp. 1591-1637.
10. Fitzpatrick, T. B., et al. 1954. J. Invest. Dermatol. 22:163-172.
11. Fleisher, T., and I. Zeligman. 1960. Arch. Dermatol. 81:898-903.
12. Freinkel, R. K., and N. Freinkel. 1971. (Loc. cit. ref. 9). pp. 1434-1459.
13. Gaudier, B., et al. 1968. Arch. Fr. Pediatr. 25:541-560.
14. Jimbow, K., et al. 1975. J. Invest. Dermatol. 64:50-62.
15. Konrad, K., and K. Wolff. 1974. Br. J. Dermatol. 91:635-655.
16. Lerner, A. B. 1972. Prog. Dermatol. 6:1-6.
17. Lerner, A. B., and J. S. McGuire. 1961. Nature (London) 189:176-179.
18. Lerner, A. B., and J. S. McGuire. 1964. N. Engl. J. Med. 270:539-546.
19. Liddle, G. W., et al. 1965. Cancer Res. 25:1057-1061.
20. Lorincz, A. L. 1975. In S. L. Moschella, et al., ed. Dermatology. W. B. Saunders, Philadelphia. pp. 1096-1128.
21. Miyamoto, M., and T. B. Fitzpatrick. 1957. Nature (London) 179:199-200.
22. Nelson, D. H., et al. 1960. Ann. Intern. Med. 52:560-569.
23. Readett, M. D. 1964. Br. J. Dermatol. 76:126-139.
24. Silberberg, I., et al. 1968. Arch. Dermatol. 97:671-677.
25. Sims, R. T. 1968. Br. J. Dermatol. 80:822-832.
26. Smith, A. J., and L. B. Strang. 1958. Arch. Dis. Child. 33:109-113.
27. Thiers, H., et al. 1966. J. Med. Lyon 47:1815-1816, 1819-1820.
28. Wallace, H. W., et al. 1957. Proc. Soc. Exp. Biol. Med. 94:632-633.
29. Witkop, C. J. 1970. Adv. Hum. Genet. 2:61-142.
30. Woody, N. C., et al. 1965. Am. J. Dis. Child. 110:606-613.

89. CHEMICAL AGENTS IN DRUGS CAUSING ABNORMAL PIGMENTATION

Symbols: ↑ = increase(d); ↓ = decrease(d). Figures in heavy brackets are reference numbers.

	Drug ⟨Synonym⟩	Structure	Nature of Pigment Disturbance	Mechanism
	Increased Pigmentation			
1	Anticonvulsants Diphenylhydantoin sodium	5,5-Diphenyl-2,4-imidazolidinedione sodium	Melasma [16]	....

continued

89. CHEMICAL AGENTS IN DRUGS CAUSING ABNORMAL PIGMENTATION

	Drug ⟨Synonym⟩	Structure	Nature of Pigment Disturbance	Mechanism
2	Mephenytoin ⟨Mesantoin⟩	5-Ethyl-3-methyl-5-phenylhydantoin	Melasma [16]	....
	Antimalarial drugs		Bluish-gray pigmentation on face, neck, oral mucosa, forearms, & shins [33]	Drugs have affinity for melanin; in addition, produce a pigmented metabolite
3	Amodiaquin [2]	4-(7-Chloro-4-quinolylamino)-α-diethylamino-o-cresol		
4	Chloroquine [1/] ⟨Aralen⟩	7-Chloro-4-(4-diethylamino-1-methylbutylamino)quinoline		
5	Hydroxychloroquine sulfate [1/] ⟨Plaquenil⟩	7-Chloro-4-(4-[ethyl(2-hydroxyethyl)amino]-1-methylbutylamino)quinoline		
6	Quinacrine hydrochloride ⟨Atabrine dihydrochloride⟩	6-Chloro-9-([4-(diethylamino)-1-methylbutyl]amino)-2-methoxyacridine dihydrochloride		
	Antineoplastic agents			
7	Bleomycin sulfate ⟨Blenaxane⟩	Exact structure unknown	Linear streaks of hyperpigmentation on trunk; hyperpigmentation over small joints of hands, knees, & elbows [6]	Local ↑ in melanogenesis
8	Busulfan ⟨Myleran⟩ [17]	1,4-Di(methanesulfonoxyl)butane	Diffuse melanosis [19]	....
9	Cyclophosphamide ⟨Cytoxan⟩	2-[Bis(2-chloroethyl)amino]tetrahydro-2H-1,3,2-oxazaphosphorine 2-oxide	Diffuse melanosis [19]; ↑ pigmentation in areas subjected to X-radiation [10]	....
10	Dactinomycin ⟨Actinomycin-D; Cosmegen⟩ [7]	2-Amino-4,6-dimethylacridone-3-quinone + 2 polypeptide chains, each containing a lactone ring	Diffuse melanosis [19]	....
11	Doxorubicin hydrochloride ⟨Adriamycin⟩	(8s-cis)-10-[(3-Amino-2,3,6-trideoxy-α-L-lyxo-hexopyranosyl)oxy]-7,8,9,10-tetrahydro-6,8,11-trihydroxy-8-(hydroxyacetyl)-1-methoxy-5,12-naphthacenedione	Hyperpigmentation of nail beds & dermal creases, primarily in children [21]	....
12	Procarbazine ⟨Matulane⟩	N-Isopropyl-α-(2-methylhydrazino)-p-toluamide	Diffuse melanosis [19]	....
	Heavy-metal-containing agents			
13	Bismuth, trivalent	....	Slate-blue line at gum margin; may have blue-gray skin pigmentation [8]	Deposition of metal
14	Gold preparations Aurothioglucose ⟨Gold thioglucose; Solganal⟩	....	May have purplish tinge; light-exposed areas more intensely pigmented; folds are spared. Takes months to years [19].	↑ melanization of epidermis; prominent dermal melanophages. Metal particles deposited in connective tissue about blood vessels [19].
15	Gold sodium thiomalate ⟨Myochrysine⟩	[(1,2-Dicarboxyethyl)thio] gold sodium salt; $C_4H_3AuNa_2O_4S$		
16	Gold sodium thiosulfate ⟨Sanocrysin⟩	$Na_3Au(S_2O_3)_2 \cdot 2H_2O$		
17	Potassium arsenite solution ⟨Fowler's solution⟩	$KAsO_2$	Prolonged ingestion: Diffuse pigmentation, most intense on trunk where macular areas of depigmentation may produce distinctive "raindrop" appearance [8]	....

1/ See also entries under Decreased Pigmentation.

continued

145

	Drug ⟨Synonym⟩	Structure	Nature of Pigment Disturbance	Mechanism
18	Silver preparations Mild silver protein ⟨Silver proteinate; Argyrol⟩	Metallic silver, AgO, silver proteinates [26]	Generalized faintly violaceous, dusky hyperpigmentation	↑ melanization of epidermis; prominent dermal melanophages. Metal particles deposited in connective tissue adjacent to sweat glands [19].
19	Silver nitrate	$AgNO_3$		
20	Hormones ACTH ⟨Acthar⟩ [5]	39 amino acids in single polypeptide chain [31]	Diffuse hyperpigmentation	↑ melanin synthesis; stimulation of ↑ monophenol monooxygenase[2/] activity, ↑ melanosome synthesis, & ↑ pigment transfer [18]
21	Oral contraceptives Estrogens	....	↑ pigmentation on nipples	↑ melanin synthesis
22	Progestationals [32]	....	Melasma (blotchy, irregularly patterned, irregularly bordered, brown hyperpigmentation on flush areas of cheeks, forehead, & upper lip) [27]; occurs in light-exposed areas [9]	↑ epidermal melanization without melanocyte proliferation; ↑ size of melanosomes [15]
23	Phenothiazides Chlorpromazine [29] ⟨Thorazine⟩	2-Chloro-10-(3-dimethylaminopropyl)phenothiazine	Bluish-gray pigmentation in exposed areas after long term, high-dose use [11]; may have conjunctional & nail bed pigmentation	Phenothiazines have affinity for melanin. Pigment ↑ in dermal melanophages. Metabolism of drug [34] thought to produce a pigmented intermediate.
24	Psoralens ⟨Furocoumarins⟩ Methoxsalen ⟨8-Methoxypsoralen; oxsoralen⟩	6-Hydroxy-7-methoxy-5-benzofuranacrylic acid δ-lactone	↑ pigmentation in areas of long-wave ultraviolet light exposure	↑ melanocyte number; ↑ melanin synthesis; ↑ pigment transfer [13]
25	Trioxsalen ⟨4,5,8-Trimethylpsoralen; trisoralen⟩	6-Hydroxy-β,2,7-trimethyl-5-benzofuranacrylic acid δ-lactone		
			Decreased Pigmentation	
26	Antimalarial drugs Chloroquine ⟨Aralen⟩[3/]	7-Chloro-4-(4-diethylamino-1-methylbutylamino)quinoline	↓ pigment in scalp hair, eyebrows, & lashes [18]	....
27	Hydroxychloroquine sulfate ⟨Plaquenil⟩[3/]	7-Chloro-4-(4-[ethyl(2-hydroxyethyl)amino]-1-methylbutylamino)quinoline		
28	Hormones Steroids, intralesional fluorinated	....	Local hypopigmentation [23]	....

[2/] Synonym: Tyrosinase. [3/] *See also* entries under Increased Pigmentation.

continued

	Drug ⟨Synonym⟩	Structure	Nature of Pigment Disturbance	Mechanism
	Hydroquinones, phenols, & related compounds			
29	*p-tert*-Butylphenol [14,24]	....	Depigmentation at site of application; may have 4-6 mo incubation period	Competitive inhibitor of monophenol monooxygenase[2]; toxic to melanocytes [20,25,28]
30	4-Isopropyl catechol [4]	....	Depigmentation at site of application; may have 4-6 mo incubation period	Competitive inhibitor of monophenol monooxygenase[2]; toxic to melanocytes [20,25,28]
31	Hydroquinone ⟨Artra⟩ [1]	*p*-Dihydroxybenzene	Local depigmentation at site of application after weeks to months; reversible	Necrosis of melanocytes [12]; inhibition of enzyme monophenol monooxygenase[2] [1]
32	Monobenzone ⟨Monobenzyl ether of hydroquinone⟩ [25]	....	Permanent depigmentation at site of local application; may have depigmentation at distant sites	Competitive inhibitor of monophenol monooxygenase[2]; toxic to melanocytes
33	Pentylphenol ⟨Amylphenol⟩ [14]	....	Depigmentation at site of application; may have 4-6 mo incubation period	Competitive inhibitor of monophenol monooxygenase[2]; toxic to melanocytes [20,25,28]
	Other			
34	Guanofuracin[3]	1-(5-Nitro-2-furfurylideneamino)-guanidine sulfate	↓ pigmentation of eyelids [35]	....
35	Mephenesin carbamate	3-*o*-Tolyloxyl-1,2-propandiol 1-carbamate	Depigmentation of hair during oral usage [30]	....
36	Triparanol ⟨MER-29⟩	1-[*p*-(2-Diethylaminoethoxy)phenyl]-1-(*p*-tolyl)-2-(*p*-chlorophenyl)ethanol	Scalp hair becomes sparse & white [22]	Blocks conversion of desmosterol to cholesterol

[2] Synonym: Tyrosinase. [3] Trade name.

Contributors: Sober, Arthur J., and Fitzpatrick, Thomas B.

References

1. Arndt, K. A., and T. B. Fitzpatrick. 1965. J. Am. Med. Assoc. 194:965-967.
2. Baer, R. L., and B. B. Levine. 1971. In T. B. Fitzpatrick, et al., ed. Dermatology in General Medicine. McGraw-Hill, New York. pp. 1281-1341.
3. Beerman, H., and B. A. Kirshbaum. 1975. In S. L. Moschella, et al., ed. Dermatology. W. B. Saunders, Philadelphia. v. 1, pp. 350-384.
4. Bleehen, S., et al. 1968. J. Invest. Dermatol. 50:103-117.
5. Cass, L. J., et al. 1964. Curr. Ther. Res. 6:601-607.
6. Cohen, I. S., et al. 1973. Arch. Dermatol. 107:553-565.
7. Dantzig, P. I. 1974. Ibid. 110:393-406.
8. Ebling, F. J., and A. Rook. 1972. In A. Rook, et al., ed. Textbook of Dermatology. Blackwell Scientific, Oxford. pp. 1241-1288.
9. Fitzpatrick, T. B., and M. C. Mihm. 1971. (Loc. cit. ref. 2). pp. 1591-1637.
10. Goodman, L. S., and A. Gilman, ed. 1975. The Pharmacological Basis of Therapeutics. Ed. 5. Macmillan, New York. pp. 1287-1288.
11. Greiner, A. C., and K. Berry. 1964. Can. Med. Assoc. J. 90:663-665.
12. Jimbow, K., et al. 1974. J. Invest. Dermatol. 62:436-449.
13. Jimbow, K., et al. 1974. Ibid. 62:548.
14. Kahn, G. 1970. Arch. Dermatol. 102:177-187.
15. Konrad, K., and K. Wolff. 1973. Ibid. 107:853-860.
16. Kuske, H., and A. Krebs. 1964. Dermatologica 129:121-139.
17. Kyle, R. A., et al. 1961. Blood 18:497-510.
18. Lerner, A. B. 1971. In T. Kawamura, et al., ed. Biology of Normal and Abnormal Melanocytes. Univ. Tokyo Press, Tokyo. pp. 3-16.

continued

19. Lorincz, A. L. 1975. (Loc. cit. ref. 3). pp. 1096-1128.
20. McGuire, J., and H. Hendee. 1971. J. Invest. Dermatol. 57:256-261.
21. Medical Economics, Inc. 1976. Physicians' Desk Reference. Ed. 30. Oradell, NJ.
22. Minton, L., and G. W. Bounds, Jr. 1963. Am. J. Ophthalmol. 55:787-791.
23. Morris, W. J. 1972. Calif. Med. 116(1):55.
24. Natten, K., et al. 1971. Trans. St. John's Hosp. Dermatol. Soc. 57:115-134.
25. Oliver, E., et al. 1939. J. Am. Med. Assoc. 113:927-928.
26. Oster, K. A., and N. J. Giarman. 1965. In J. R. DiPalma, ed. Drill's Pharmacology in Medicine. Ed. 3. McGraw-Hill, New York. pp. 1279-1299.

27. Resnick, S. 1967. J. Am. Med. Assoc. 199:601-605.
28. Riley, P. 1970. J. Pathol. 101:163-169.
29. Satanove, A. 1965. J. Am. Med. Assoc. 191:263-268.
30. Spillane, J. 1963. Br. Med. J. 1:997-1000.
31. Stecher, P. G., et al., ed. 1968. The Merck Index. Ed. 8. Merck, Rahway, NJ. p. 18.
32. Thiers, H., et al. 1966. J. Med. Lyon 47:1815-1816, 1819-1820.
33. Tuffanelli, D., et al. 1963. Arch. Dermatol. 88:419-426.
34. Van Woert, M. H. 1968. Nature (London) 219:1054-1056.
35. Yamada, M. 1955. Jpn. J. Dermatol. Venereol. 65:187-202.

90. CHANGES RESULTING FROM TRAUMA

For a comprehensive review of the subject, consult the following general references: Ballinger, W. F., ed., 1975, Manual of Surgical Nutrition, W. B. Saunders, Philadelphia; Clowes, G. H., Jr., ed. 1976. Surg. Clin. North Am. 56(4 & 5); Kirklin, J. W., and J. P. Archie, 1974, Surg. Gynecol. Obstet. 139:17-23.

Part I. Effects on Metabolic Constituents

Trauma is characterized by a CNS sympathetic-mediated "fight or flight" response, culminating in release of "mobilizing" hormones. These include epinephrine, glucagon, hydrocortisone ⟨cortisol⟩, and growth hormone with a relative inhibition of insulin, the key "storage" peripheral anabolic hormone. The ensuing state is "hypercaloremic," and is secondary to glycogenolysis, gluconeogenesis, lipolysis, ketogenesis, and muscle proteolysis. The severity of trauma can be determined by the metabolic constituents of the blood that result from the magnitude of the above process. In addition, the magnitude of the injury will effect the "turning point" between the "acute" phase and the "ketoadaptive" phase of the injury. The latter is best identified by the presence of ketonemia and ketonuria, most readily observed during glucose- ⟨dextrose-⟩ free intravenous fluid therapy. All studies excluded patients with nutritional depletion, hepatic failure, or renal failure. **Mild Trauma** = elective surgery; glucose-free i.v. fluids administered. **Moderate Trauma** = major surgery; glucose-free i.v. fluids administered. **Severe Trauma** = burns over more than 35% of body surface; patients had stable course, uncomplicated by sepsis; blood values from overnight fast; diets designed to achieve positive caloric balance. **Sepsis:** Minimum of 8 hours on glucose-free i.v. fluids. *Symbols:* − = not present; + = small amount present; ++ = moderate amount present. Figures in heavy brackets are reference numbers. Values in parentheses are ranges, estimate "c" unless otherwise specified (*see* Introduction).

	Property or Constituent	Fasting Normal	Mild Trauma			Moderate Trauma			Severe Trauma		Sepsis	
			No. of Subjects	Acute Phase	Adaptive Phase	No. of Subjects	Acute Phase	Adaptive Phase	No. of Subjects	Values	No. of Subjects	Values
	Urine											
1	Total nitrogen, g/d	7-10	9 [5]	7(5-9)[b]	9(2-16)[b]	5 [5]	11(2-22)	13(7-20)	9 [8]	21(17-25)[b]	7 [1]	16(10-22)
2	Urea, g/d	5-8	9 [5]	6(4-8)[b]	8(1-15)[b]	5 [5]	9(2-21)	11(5-18)	9 [8]	18(14-22)[b]	7 [1]	12(6-18)
3	Creatinine, g/d	0.8-2.0	9 [5]	1.3(0.7-1.9)[b]	1.2(0.8-1.3)[b]	5 [5]	1.2(0.9-1.4)	1.2(0.9-1.4)	9 [8]	1.4(1.1-1.7)[b]	.....	....
4	Ketones	−	9 [5]	−	+	5 [5]	+	++	......	....	7 [1]	−
	Venous Blood											
5	Glucose, mM	3.9-5.6	9 [5]	5.9(5.6-6.2)[b]	4.1(3.9-4.2)[b]	5 [5]	8.9(5.9-11.4)	7.3(4.9-10.9)	9 [8]	5.7(5.2-6.2)[b]	7 [1]	7.6(5.8-10.6)
6	Lactate, mM	0.6-1.8	9 [5]	0.82(0.26-1.4)[b]	0.76(0.24-1.28)[b]	5 [5]	1.5(1.2-3.6)	1.10(0.84-1.4)	......	....	7 [1]	1.7(1.1-2.4)
7	Ketone bodies, mM	0-0.22	9 [5]	0.19 ± 0.16	0.15(0.03-0.27)[b]	5 [5]	0.39(0.16-0.86)	0.97(0.26-1.79)	......	....	7 [1]	0.01(0-0.03)

continued

Part I. Effects on Metabolic Constituents

	Property or Constituent	Fasting Normal	Mild Trauma			Moderate Trauma			Severe Trauma		Sepsis	
			No. of Subjects	Acute Phase	Adaptive Phase	No. of Subjects	Acute Phase	Adaptive Phase	No. of Subjects	Values	No. of Subjects	Values
8	Free fatty acids, meq/liter	200-900	9 [5]	740(220-1260)[b]	780(340-1220)[b]	5 [5]	790(240-1500)	680(630-710)	9 [8]	1000(600-1400)[b]	7 [1]	700(250-1200)
9	Amino acids Alanine, mM	0.32-0.48	9 [5]	0.24(0.08-0.40)[b]	0.20(0.08-0.32)[b]	5 [5]	0.37(0.30-0.49)	0.37(0.20-0.45)	......	....	7 [1]	0.29(0.16-0.39)
10	Branched-chain (valine, isoleucine, leucine), mM	0.30-0.61	9 [5]	0.33(0.23-0.43)[b]	0.41(0.29-0.53)[b]	5 [5]	0.46(0.37-0.50)	0.67(0.51-0.85)	......	....	.....	....
11	Sum of thirteen[1/]	2.1-2.9	9 [5]	1.4(1.0-1.8)[b]	1.5(1.2-1.8)[b]	5 [5]	2.7(2.3-3.0)	2.7(1.7-3.5)	......	....	.....	....
12	Insulin, μU/ml	6-26	9 [5]	14(5-18)	14(5-25)	5 [5]	32(16-55)	19(15-22)	11 [7]	43(6-200)	7 [1]	42(35-54)
13	Glucagon, pg/ml	20-200	7 [4]; 8 [3]	154(112-196)[b] [4]	293(203-383)[b][3]	7 [4]	209(173-245)[b]	572(322-822)[b]	11 [7]	327(185-662)	6 [6]	409(151-667)[b]
14	Resting metabolic expenditure, kcal·m^{-2}·d^{-1}	900	15 [2]	857(587-1127)[b]	805(553-1057)[b]	5 [2]	....	1046(682-1410)[b]	9 [8]	1559(960-1894)	4 [2]	969(613-1325)[b]

[1/] Aspartic acid, threonine, serine, glutamic acid, glutamine, glycine, alanine, valine, methionine, isoleucine, leucine, tyrosine, and phenylalanine.

Contributors: Blackburn, George L., and Trerice, Mary S.

References
1. Clowes, G. H., Jr., et al. 1976. Surg. Clin. North Am. 56:1169-1184.
2. Duke, J. H., et al. 1970. Surgery 68:168-174.
3. Freeman, J. B., et al. 1975. Surg. Forum 26:35-37.
4. Meguid, M. M., et al. 1974. Arch. Surg. 109:776-783.
5. O'Donnell, T. F., Jr., et al. 1976. Surgery 80:192-200.
6. Rocha, D. M., et al. 1973. N. Engl. J. Med. 288:700-703.
7. Wilmore, D. W., et al. 1973. Surg. Forum 24:99-101.
8. Wilmore, D. W., et al. 1974. Surg. Gynecol. Obstet. 138:875-884.

Part II. Effects on Hemodynamic Function and Blood Content During Maximal Response

Patients were without shock, as characterized by decreased blood pressure, cool skin temperature, decreased cardiac output, or pale skin color. **Property**: Pa = arterial pressure.

Abbreviations: n = number of subjects. Values in parentheses are ranges, estimate "b" (*see* Introduction).

	Property	Survival			Death		Reference
		Uneventful Convalescence n = 30	Trauma & Hemorrhage n = 16	Sepsis n = 22	Trauma & Hemorrhage n = 12	Sepsis n = 16	
1	Cardiac index, liters·m^{-2}·min^{-1}	3.1(2.9-3.3)	3.9(2.5-5.3)	4.2(1.8-6.6)	4.4(1.4-7.4)	4.9(2.9-6.9)	1,2
2	Central venous pressure, mm Hg	4(0-8)	8(0-16)	9(1-17)	11 ± 7	12(2-22)	1,2

continued

Part II. Effects on Hemodynamic Function and Blood Content During Maximal Response

	Property	Survival			Death		Refer-ence
		Uneventful Convalescence n = 30	Trauma & Hemorrhage n = 16	Sepsis n = 22	Trauma & Hemorrhage n = 12	Sepsis n = 16	
	Pulmonary arterial pressure						
3	Systolic, mm Hg	22(12-32)	32(20-44)	36(22-50)	33(17-49)	38(18-58)	2
4	Wedge (left ventricular filling pressure), mm Hg	8(2-14)	12(6-18)	14(6-22)	15(7-24)	17(3-30)	5
	Systemic arterial pressure						
5	Systolic, mm Hg	137(125-149)	137(107-167)	125(95-155)	126(76-176)	120(88-152)	3,4
6	Diastolic, mm Hg	74(68-80)	69(44-94)	65(45-85)	67(49-85)	62(42-82)	3,4
7	Mean, mm Hg	90(62-118)	86(58-114)	91(67-115)	88(50-126)	85(53-117)	3,4
	Arterial blood gases[1]						
8	Pa_{O_2}, mm Hg	85(73-97)	71(61-81)	65(41-89)	48(24-72)	53(27-81)	1,2
9	Pa_{CO_2}, mm Hg	38(28-48)	29(15-43)	31(19-43)	27(15-39)	26(8-44)	1,2
10	CO_2 content, ml/100 ml blood	49.1	44(39-49)	36(31-41)	34(28-40)	33(27-39)	3
11	Buffer base, meq/liter	1(−3 to +5)	−3(−9 to +3)	−2(−8 to +4)	−8(−18 to +2)	−7(−15 to +1)	1,2
12	Excess lactate, mM	0.5(0.1-0.9)	0.9(0.1-1.7)	1.4(0-2.8)	2.4(−1.0 to +5.8)	2.5(−1.1 to +6.1)	1,2
	pH						
13	Arterial	7.42(7.38-7.46)	7.39(7.31-7.47)	7.48(7.38-7.58)	7.43(7.32-7.55)	7.44(7.34-7.54)	3
14	Mixed venous	7.39(7.36-7.42)	7.36(7.33-7.39)	7.42(7.37-7.47)	7.37(7.27-7.47)	7.38(7.28-7.48)	3

[1] Breathing air.

Contributors: Blackburn, George L., and Trerice, Mary S.

References

1. Clowes, G. H., Jr. 1974. Surg. Clin. North Am. 54(5): 993-1013.
2. Clowes, G. H., Jr., et al. 1975. Ann. Surg. 181(5): 681-692.
3. Dill, D. B., et al. 1936. Am. J. Physiol. 115:530-538.
4. National Research Council, Committee on Aviation Medicine. 1944. Handbook of Respiratory Data in Aviation. Washington, D.C. charts A-1, B-1, B-3.
5. Weisel, R. D., et al. 1975. N. Engl. J. Med. 292:682-684.

IV. ORGAN SYSTEM DISEASES

91. BLOOD VOLUMES IN NORMAL ADULTS

Circulating blood volumes were measured in normal adult men and women. Predicted blood volumes (PBV) were calculated on the basis of three prediction formulas: (i) body weight formula—PBV = 75 ml/kg body weight; (ii) surface area formula—PBV = 2.68 liter/m^2 × S.A., where S.A. is surface area in square meters; (iii) height cubed-body mass formula—PBV = $a_1H^3 + a_2W + a_0$, where a_1, a_2, and a_0 are constants, H is height in meters, and W is body weight in kilograms. Significant statistical improvement was attained when the data were plotted against predicted volumes based on computer-corrected surface area and height cubed-body mass formulas. Both computer-corrected formulas yield the same prediction data when sex, height, and weight are the only parameters used [ref. 7]. Values in parentheses are ranges, estimate "c" (see Introduction).

	Method	No. of Subjects	Blood Volume ml/kg	Erythrocyte Volume ml/kg	Plasma Volume ml/kg[1]	Reference
			Males			
1	Chromium-51	42	60.4 ± 8.59	28.3 ± 4.11	33.5 ± 5.18	4
2		201	62.4 ± 7.8	28.2 ± 4.0	34.2 ± 4.5	9
3		71	69.0	29.2	38.7	1
4		6[2]	76.5 ± 11.6	30.9 ± 3.1	....	5
5		10[3]	70.5 ± 18.2	27.5 ± 8.8	....	5
6	Iodine-131 human	31	74.2	....	40.3 ± 4.2	8
7	serum albumin	10	....	....	42.3 ± 5.8	6
8		13	....	....	2780(1900-3160)[4]	3
			Females			
9	Chromium-51	20	58.3 ± 6.8	23.8 ± 2.8	34.4 ± 4.7	4
10		101	61.9 ± 6.3	25.3 ± 3.0	36.6 ± 4.3	2
11		16	64.4 ± 7.6	27.0 ± 3.4	37.0 ± 4.8	1
12		6[2]	63.7 ± 16.0	23.0 ± 5.3	....	5
13		27[3]	63.1 ± 18.9	24.3 ± 7.5	....	5

[1] Unless otherwise indicated. [2] Young. [3] Elderly. [4] Total plasma volume in milliliters.

Contributors: Kansu, Emin, and Erslev, Allan J.

References
1. Berlin, N. I., et al. 1952. N. Engl. J. Med. 247:675-684.
2. Brown, E., et al. 1962. J. Clin. Invest. 41:2182-2190.
3. Franks, J. J., and F. Zizza. 1958. J. Appl. Physiol. 13:299-302.
4. Huff, R. L., and D. D. Feller. 1956. J. Clin. Invest. 35:1-10.
5. Hurdle, A. D. F., and A. J. Rosin. 1962. J. Clin. Pathol. 15:343-345.
6. Jaenike, J. R., et al. 1957. J. Lab. Clin. Med. 49:172-181.
7. Nadler, S. B., et al. 1962. Surgery 51:224-232.
8. Storaasli, J. P., et al. 1950. Surg. Gynecol. Obstet. 91:458-464.
9. Wennesland, R., et al. 1959. J. Clin. Invest. 38:1065-1077.

92. PERIPHERAL BLOOD ERYTHROCYTE COUNTS AND CELL INDICES

MCV = mean corpuscular volume. **MCH** = mean corpuscular hemoglobin. **MCHC** = mean corpuscular hemoglobin concentration; **RBC** = erythrocytes ⟨red blood cells⟩.

Part I. Infants to Elderly

All measurements were made on venous blood samples, unless otherwise indicated. **Erythrocyte Count** was measured by electronic Coulter counter, unless otherwise indicated. **Hematocrit** was measured by micromethod, unless otherwise

continued

Part I. Infants to Elderly

indicated. **Hemoglobin** was measured by cyan methemoglobin technique, unless otherwise indicated. All erythrocyte indices, **MCV, MCH,** and **MCHC,** are calculated values.

Plus/minus (±) values are standard deviations, unless otherwise indicated. Values in parentheses are ranges, estimate "b" (*see* Introduction).

	Subjects		Erythrocyte Count $10^6/\mu l$	Hematocrit %	Hemoglobin g/100 ml blood	MCV μm^3	MCH pg	MCHC g/100 ml RBC	Reference
	Age	No. & Sex							
1	1 d	19[1]	5.14 ± 0.7	61 ± 7.4	19.0 ± 2.2	119 ± 9.4	36.7	31.6 ± 1.9	7
2	2d	19[1]	5.15 ± 0.8	60 ± 6.4	19.0 ± 1.9	115 ± 7.0	36.9	31.6 ± 1.4	7
3	3d	19[1]	5.11 ± 0.7	62 ± 9.3	18.7 ± 3.4	116 ± 5.3	36.6	31.1 ± 2.8	7
4	4d	10[1]	5.00 ± 0.6	57 ± 8.1	18.6 ± 2.1	114 ± 7.5	37.2	32.6 ± 1.5	7
5	5d	12[1]	4.97 ± 0.4	57 ± 7.3	17.6 ± 1.1	114 ± 8.9	35.4	30.9 ± 2.2	7
6	6d	15[1]	5.00 ± 0.7	54 ± 7.2	17.4 ± 2.2	113 ± 10.0	34.8	32.2 ± 1.6	7
7	7d	12[1]	4.86 ± 0.6	56 ± 9.4	17.9 ± 2.5	118 ± 11.2	36.8	32.0 ± 1.6	7
8	1-2 wk	32[1]	4.80 ± 0.8	54 ± 8.3	17.3 ± 2.3	112 ± 19.0	36.0	32.1 ± 2.9	7
9	2-3 wk	11[1]	4.20 ± 0.6	46 ± 7.3	15.6 ± 2.6	111 ± 8.2	37.1	33.9 ± 1.9	7
10	3-4 wk	17[1]	4.00 ± 0.6	43 ± 5.7	14.2 ± 2.1	105 ± 7.5	35.5	33.5 ± 1.6	7
11	4-5 wk	15[1]	3.60 ± 0.4	36 ± 4.8	12.7 ± 1.6	101 ± 8.1	35.3	34.9 ± 1.6	7
12	5-6 wk	10[1]	3.55 ± 0.2	36 ± 6.2	11.9 ± 1.5	102 ± 10.2	33.5	34.1 ± 2.9	7
13	6-7 wk	10[1]	3.40 ± 0.4	36 ± 4.8	12.0 ± 1.5	105 ± 12.0	35.3	33.8 ± 2.3	7
14	7-8 wk	17[1]	3.40 ± 0.4	33 ± 3.7	11.1 ± 1.1	100 ± 13.0	32.6	33.7 ± 2.6	7
15	8-9 wk	13[1]	3.40 ± 0.5	31 ± 2.5	10.7 ± 0.9	93 ± 12.0	31.5	34.1 ± 2.2	7
16	9-10 wk	12[1]	3.60 ± 0.3	32 ± 2.7	11.2 ± 0.9	91 ± 9.3	31.1	34.3 ± 2.9	7
17	10-11 wk	11[1]	3.70 ± 0.4	34 ± 2.1	11.4 ± 0.9	91 ± 7.7	30.8	33.2 ± 2.4	7
18	11-12 wk	13[1]	3.70 ± 0.3	33 ± 3.3	11.3 ± 0.9	88 ± 7.9	30.5	34.8 ± 2.2	7
19	4 mo	71	4.332 ± 0.061[2]	35.3 ± 0.4[2]	11.9 ± 0.12[2]	82 ± 0.7[2]	27.7 ± 0.26[2]	33.7 ± 0.17[2]	5
20	6 mo	62	4.483 ± 0.052[2]	34.8 ± 0.3[2]	11.6 ± 0.12[2]	78 ± 0.7[2]	26.1 ± 0.28[2]	33.5 ± 0.20[2]	5
21	8 mo	64	4.713 ± 0.063[2]	35.6 ± 0.4[2]	11.7 ± 0.17[2]	76 ± 0.7[2]	24.9 ± 0.33[2]	32.8 ± 0.22[2]	5
22	10 mo	57	4.834 ± 0.058[2]	34.9 ± 0.4[2]	11.3 ± 0.18[2]	73 ± 1.0[2]	23.7 ± 0.47[2]	32.4 ± 0.28[2]	5
23	12 mo	51	4.758 ± 0.072[2]	34.5 ± 0.6[2]	11.1 ± 0.24[2]	73 ± 1.1[2]	23.5 ± 0.51[2]	32.3 ± 0.32[2]	5
24	14 mo	53	4.700 ± 0.074[2]	34.6 ± 0.5[2]	11.1 ± 0.25[2]	74 ± 1.0[2]	23.8 ± 0.51[2]	31.8 ± 0.37[2]	5
25	16 mo	50	4.904 ± 0.073[2]	34.7 ± 0.5[2]	11.0 ± 0.22[2]	71 ± 1.2[2]	22.8 ± 0.55[2]	31.7 ± 0.31[2]	5
26	18 mo	53	4.868 ± 0.062[2]	34.8 ± 0.4[2]	11.2 ± 0.27[2]	72 ± 1.2[2]	23.2 ± 0.60[2]	31.9 ± 0.39[2]	5
27	20 mo	47	4.807 ± 0.072[2]	35.9 ± 0.4[2]	11.7 ± 0.22[2]	75 ± 1.1[2]	24.6 ± 0.52[2]	32.6 ± 0.31[2]	5
28	2 yr	103	4.777 ± 0.042[2]	35.8 ± 0.3[2]	11.7 ± 0.14[2]	75 ± 0.7[2]	24.7 ± 0.35[2]	32.6 ± 0.21[2]	5
29	2.5 yr	74	4.703 ± 0.041[2]	36.2 ± 0.3[2]	12.1 ± 0.16[2]	77 ± 0.7[2]	25.9 ± 0.35[2]	33.5 ± 0.22[2]	5
30	3 yr	56	4.691 ± 0.052[2]	36.6 ± 0.4[2]	12.4 ± 0.15[2]	78 ± 0.7[2]	26.6 ± 0.28[2]	34.0 ± 0.20[2]	5
31	4 yr	43	4.618 ± 0.051[2]	36.9 ± 0.4[2]	12.4 ± 0.21[2]	80 ± 0.8[2]	26.9 ± 0.41[2]	33.7 ± 0.27[2]	5
32	5 yr	97	4.651 ± 0.047[2]	37.2 ± 0.3[2]	12.7 ± 0.10[2]	80 ± 0.4[2]	27.5 ± 0.15[2]	34.2 ± 0.12[2]	5
33	7 yr	103	4.790 ± 0.051[2]	38.1 ± 0.4[2]	12.9 ± 0.18[2]	79 ± 0.9[2]	27.4 ± 0.20[2]	34.3 ± 0.13[2]	5
34	10 yr	111	4.804 ± 0.045[2]	38.5 ± 0.3[2]	13.2 ± 0.12[2]	81 ± 0.6[2]	27.6 ± 0.26[2]	34.3 ± 0.14[2]	5
35	14 yr	45	4.922 ± 0.077[2]	39.7 ± 0.5[2]	13.6 ± 0.22[2]	81 ± 1.1[2]	27.9 ± 0.48[2]	34.3 ± 0.27[2]	5
36	17-19 yr	950♂	5.14 ± 0.42	45.8 ± 2.5	14.9 ± 0.90	88.4 ± 4.0	28.8 ± 1.4	32.6 ± 1.1	4
37	17-24 yr	4550♀	4.56 ± 0.38	40.9 ± 2.63	13.4 ± 1.16	90.3 ± 5.2	29.3 ± 2.4	32.5 ± 2.3	6,10
38	Adult	200♂	5.22 ± 0.40	46.6 ± 2.5	15.4 ± 0.83	88.4 ± 3.4	29.4 ± 1.3	33.3 ± 1.0	4
39		86♂	5.40 ± 0.80[3,4]	47.0 ± 5.0[3]	16.0 ± 2.0[3]	87.0 ± 5.0[3]	29.0 ± 2.0[3]	34.0 ± 2.0[3]	12
40		744♂	5.40 ± 0.70[3]	47.0 ± 5.0[3,5]	16.0 ± 2.0[3,5]	90.0 ± 9.0[3]	29.0 ± 2.0[3]	34.0 ± 2.0[3]	1
41		101♀	4.80 ± 0.60[3,4]	42.0 ± 5.0[3]	14.0 ± 2.0[3]	87.0 ± 5.0[3]	29.0 ± 2.0[3]	34.0 ± 2.0[3]	12
42		642♀	4.80 ± 0.60[3]	42.0 ± 5.0[3,5]	14.0 ± 2.0[3,5]	90.0 ± 9.0[3]	29.0 ± 2.0[3]	34.0 ± 2.0[3]	1
	Elderly								
43	60-90 yr	50♀	4.71 ± 0.46[4]	40.8 ± 2.89[6]	13.7 ± 1.07[7]	87.3	29.2	33.5	11
44	60-94 yr	50♂	4.75 ± 0.57[4]	42.1 ± 3.98[6]	14.1 ± 1.53[7]	89.2	29.8	33.5	11

[1] Measurements were made on heel-prick blood samples. [2] Plus/minus (±) value is standard error. [3] Plus/minus (±) value is 2 standard deviations. [4] Erythrocyte count by hemocytometer. [5] Done by Coulter counter. [6] Macromethod hematocrit determination. [7] Sahli method for hemoglobin.

continued

92. PERIPHERAL BLOOD ERYTHROCYTE COUNTS AND CELL INDICES

Part I. Infants to Elderly

	Subjects		Erythrocyte Count $10^6/\mu l$	Hematocrit %	Hemoglobin g/100 ml blood	MCV μm^3	MCH pg	MCHC g/100 ml RBC	Reference
	Age	No. & Sex							
45	62-90 yr	213♂	....	44.82 ± 4.18	14.76 ± 1.53	....	....	33.05 ± 1.74	8
46		259♀	....	41.05 ± 3.99	13.53 ± 1.46	....	....	33.04 ± 1.78	
47	65 yr	229♂	....	45.7 ± 0.27[2]	14.6 ± 0.09[2]	....	....	31.94	3
48		304♀	....	41.8 ± 0.20[2]	13.4 ± 0.07[2]	....	....	32.05	
49	65-91 yr	50♂	4.40[4]	41.2[6]	12.65[7]	97.7	28.5	29.6	9
50	66-104 yr	50♀	4.10[4]	36.70[6]	11.7[7]	90.0	28.8	32.3	9
51	70-94 yr	200♂	4.42(3.27-5.33)	42.65(30.48-55.42)	14.90(10.11-19.75)	96.5	33.71	34.93	2
52		200♀	4.35(3.33-5.38)	41.40(31.69-51.03)	14.31(10.38-18.30)	95.2	32.90	34.56	

[2] Plus/minus (±) value is standard error. [4] Erythrocyte count by hemocytometer. [6] Macromethod hematocrit determination. [7] Sahli method for hemoglobin.

Contributors: Kansu, Emin, and Erslev, Allan J.

References

1. Coulter Diagnostics, Inc. Unpublished. Hialeah, FL, 1969.
2. Earney, W. W., and A. J. Earney. 1972. J. Am. Geriatr. Soc. 20:174-177.
3. Elwood, P. C., et al. 1971. Br. J. Haematol. 21:557-563.
4. Greendyke, R. M., et al. 1962. Am. J. Clin. Pathol. 37:429-436.
5. Guest, G. M., and E. W. Brown. 1957. AMA J. Dis. Child. 93:486-509.
6. Lewis, G. K., et al. 1947. J. Lab. Clin. Med. 32:419-422.
7. Matoth, Y., et al. 1971. Acta Paediatr. Scand. 60:317-323.
8. Milne, J. S., and J. Williamson. 1972. Geriatrics 27:118-126.
9. Newman, B., and S. Gitlow. 1943. Am. J. Med. Sci. 205:677-687.
10. Ohlson, M. A., et al. 1944. Am. J. Physiol. 142:727-732.
11. Shapleigh, J. B., et al. 1952. J. Gerontol. 7:207-219.
12. Wintrobe, M. M., et al. 1974. Clinical Hematology. Ed. 7. Lea and Febiger, Philadelphia.

Part II. Normal Values for Pregnant Women

	Subjects		Erythrocyte Count $10^6/\mu l$	Hematocrit %	Hemoglobin g/100 ml blood	MCV μm^3	MCH pg	MCHC g/100 ml RBC
	Condition	No. of Observation						
1	Nonpregnant	42	4.44 ± 0.38	41.5 ± 2.0	13.4 ± 0.83	93.4	30.2	32.3
	Pregnant[1]							
2	3 mo	7	4.49	40.6	13.2	90.4	29.4	32.5
3	4 mo	9	3.83	37.0	12.0	96.6	31.3	32.4
4	5 mo	9	3.98	34.8	12.1	87.4	30.4	34.7
5	6 mo	20	3.85	36.0	12.2	93.5	31.7	33.9
6	7 mo	24	3.90	36.0	12.1	92.3	31.0	33.6
7	8 mo	34	3.89	36.4	11.9	93.6	30.6	32.7
8	9 mo	38	3.97	37.5	12.3	94.5	31.0	32.8
9	Postpartum	16	4.14	38.7	12.7	93.5	30.7	32.8

[1] Total number of subjects was 102.

continued

Contributors: Kansu, Emin, and Erslev, Allan J.

Reference: Holly, R. G. 1953. Obstet. Gynecol. 2:119-126.

93. HUMAN ERYTHROCYTE ENZYMES AND INTERMEDIATE METABOLITES RELATED TO CLINICAL DISORDERS

Part I. Enzymes

Values are for normal adults. For source of **Enzyme Commission No.**, *see* Introduction. Data in light brackets refer to the column heading in brackets. Figures in heavy brackets are reference numbers.

	Enzyme ⟨Synonym⟩ [Enzyme Commission No.]	Enzyme Activity IU/g hemoglobin	Temp & pH	Remarks	Clinical Disorder
1	Acetylcholinesterase [3.1.1.7]	36.9 ± 3.83 [1]	37°C, 8.0	Membrane-bound enzyme	Enzyme decreased in paroxysmal nocturnal hemoglobinuria
2	Adenosine deaminase [3.5.4.4]	1.11 ± 0.23 [1,2]	37°C, 8.0	Multiple molecular forms	Enzyme decreased in immune deficiency disease
3	Adenylate kinase [2.7.4.3]	258 ± 29.3 [1,2]	37°C, 8.0	Multiple molecular forms	Hereditary deficiency causes mild hemolytic anemia
4	Bisphosphoglyceromutase ⟨2,3-Diphosphoglyceromutase⟩ [2.7.5.4]	4.78 ± 0.65 [1,2]	37°C, 8.0	Multiple molecular forms	Hereditary hemolytic anemia (rare)
5	Catalase [1.11.1.6]	(15.3 ± 2.39) × 10⁴ [1]	37°C, 8.0	Reaction linear for 3-4 min	Oral ulcerations
6	Fructose-bisphosphate aldolase ⟨Aldolase⟩ [4.1.2.13]	3.19 ± 0.86 [1,2]	37°C, 8.0	Partially membrane-bound	Hemolytic anemia & glycogen storage disease (rare)
7 8	Galactokinase [2.7.1.6]	0.079 ± 0.006 [1] 0.029 ± 0.006 [1]	37°C, 7.4 37°C, 7.4	Newborn erythrocytes Adult erythrocytes	Deficiency causes galactosemia & cataracts in early childhood
9	Galactose-1-phosphate uridylyltransferase [2.7.7.10]	28.4 ± 6.94 [1]	37°C, 8.0	Fluorometric method	Galactosemia, cataracts, liver disease, neurologic disorders
10	Glucose-6-phosphate dehydrogenase [1.1.1.49]	8.34 ± 1.59 [1,2]	37°C, 8.0	Influenced by erythrocyte age	Hereditary (sex-linked) & drug-induced hemolytic anemia
11	Glucosephosphate isomerase ⟨Phosphoglucose isomerase⟩ [5.3.1.9]	60.8 ± 11.0 [1,2]	37°C, 8.0	Multiple molecular forms	Hereditary hemolytic anemia
12	γ-Glutamyl-cysteine synthetase [6.3.2.2]	0.43 ± 0.04 [5]	37°C, 8.25	Radioisotope assay	Hereditary hemolytic anemia & neurologic disease. Activity increased in myeloproliferative disorders.
13	Glutathione peroxidase [1.11.1.9]	31.4 ± 2.97 [2]	37°C, 8.0	Ethnic variation	Mild hereditary hemolytic anemia

continued

93. HUMAN ERYTHROCYTE ENZYMES AND INTERMEDIATE METABOLITES RELATED TO CLINICAL DISORDERS

Part I. Enzymes

	Enzyme ⟨Synonym⟩ [Enzyme Commission No.]	Enzyme Activity IU/g hemoglobin	Temp & pH	Remarks	Clinical Disorder
14	Glutathione reductase (NAD(P)H) [1.6.4.2]	7.18 ± 1.09 [1,2]	37°C, 8.0	Dependent on FAD	Hereditary defect with hemolysis (rare)
15	Glutathione synthetase [6.3.2.3]	0.19 ± 0.03 [5]	37°C, 8.25	Radioisotope assay	Hereditary hemolytic anemia
16	Hexokinase [2.7.1.1]	1.16 ± 0.17 [1,2]	37°C, 8.0	Influenced by erythrocyte age	Hereditary hemolytic anemia
17	Hypoxanthine phosphoribosyltransferase ⟨Hypoxanthine guanosine-phosphoribosyltransferase⟩ [2.4.2.8]	1.72 ± 0.3 [3]	38°C, 7.4	Reaction with hypoxanthine	Lesch-Nyhan syndrome
18	Methemoglobin reductase	2.60 ± 0.71 [2]	25°C, 7.0	Identical to cytochrome b_5 reductase [1.6.2.2]	Hereditary methemoglobinemia with or without neurologic disorders
19	6-Phosphofructokinase [2.7.1.11]	11.0 ± 2.33 [1,2]	37°C, 8.0	Partially membrane-bound	Hereditary hemolytic anemia with or without glycogen storage disease type VII
20	Phosphogluconate dehydrogenase (decarboxylating) [1.1.1.44]	8.78 ± 0.78 [1,2]	37°C, 8.0	Multiple molecular forms	Mild hereditary hemolytic anemia
21	Phosphoglycerate kinase [2.7.2.3]	320 ± 36.1 [1,2]	37°C, 8.0	Multiple molecular forms	Hereditary hemolytic anemia with neurologic disorder (sex-linked)
22	Pyrimidine 5′-nucleotidase	0.11 ± 0.03 [6]	37°C, 8.0	Reaction with uridine monophosphate	Hereditary deficiency causes hemolytic anemia with basophilic stippling. Decreased activity observed in lead poisoning.
23	Pyruvate kinase [2.7.1.40]	15.0 ± 1.96 [1,2]	37°C, 8.0	Allosteric action with fructose 1,6-bisphosphate [1/]	Hereditary deficiency causes hemolytic anemia. Decreased activity observed in various hematologic disorders.
24	Triosephosphate isomerase [5.3.1.1]	2111 ± 397 [1,2]	37°C, 8.0	Multiple molecular forms	Hereditary hemolytic anemia with severe neurologic disease & infections
25	Uroporphyrinogen I synthase [4.3.1.8]	2.52 [4]	37°C, 8.2	Fluorometric method	Enzyme decreased in acute intermittent porphyria

[1/] Synonym: Fructose 1,6-diphosphate.

Contributors: Beutler, Ernest, and Blume, K.-G.

References

1. Beutler, E. 1975. Red Cell Metabolism: A Manual of Biochemical Methods. Ed. 2. Grune and Stratton, New York.

2. Beutler, E., et al. 1976. Br. J. Haematol. 34:(in press).
3. Kelley, W. N., et al. 1967. Proc. Natl. Acad. Sci. USA 57:1735-1739.

continued

93. HUMAN ERYTHROCYTE ENZYMES AND INTERMEDIATE METABOLITES RELATED TO CLINICAL DISORDERS

Part I. Enzymes

4. Magnussen, C. R., et al. 1974. Blood 44:857-868.
5. Minnich, V., et al. 1971. J. Clin. Invest. 50:507-513.
6. Paglia, D. E., and W. N. Valentine. 1975. J. Biol. Chem. 250:7973-7979.

Part II. Intermediate Metabolites

Data in brackets refer to the column heading in brackets.

	Intermediate Metabolite ⟨Synonym⟩	Concentration μmoles/liter erythrocytes[1]	Reference
1	Adenosine 5'-diphosphate	635 ± 105	3
2	Adenosine 5'-monophosphate	62 ± 10	3
3	Adenosine 5'-triphosphate	1200 ± 102[2]	3
4		1438 ± 99[3]	
5	Dihydroxyacetone phosphate	9.4 ± 2.8	3,4
6	2,3-Diphosphoglycerate	4171 ± 636	3
7	Fructose 1,6-bisphosphate ⟨Fructose 1,6-diphosphate⟩	1.9 ± 0.6	3,4
8	Fructose 6-phosphate	9.3 ± 2.0	3,4
9	Glucose 1,6-bisphosphate ⟨Glucose 1,6-diphosphate⟩	180-300	1
10	Glucose 6-phosphate	27.8 ± 7.5	3,4
11	Glutathione, oxidized	4.2 ± 1.5	3
12	reduced	2234 ± 354	
13	Lactate	748.6 ± 63.7[4]	3,4
14	Mannose 1,6-bisphosphate ⟨Mannose 1,6-diphosphate⟩	150	2
15	Phospho*enol*pyruvate	12.2 ± 2.2	3,4
16	2-Phosphoglyceric acid	7.3 ± 2.5	3,4
17	3-Phosphoglyceric acid	44.9 ± 5.1	3,4
18	Pyruvate	67.7 ± 7.8[4]	3,4

[1] Unless otherwise indicated. [2] Negro. [3] Caucasian. [4] μmoles/liter blood.

Contributor: Beutler, Ernest, and Blume, K.-G.

References

1. Bartlett, G. R. 1959. J. Biol. Chem. 234:449-458.
2. Bartlett, G. R. 1968. Biochim. Biophys. Acta 156:231-239.
3. Beutler, E. 1975. Red Cell Metabolism: A Manual of Biochemical Methods. Ed. 2. Grune and Stratton, New York.
4. Niessner, H., and E. Beutler. 1973. Biochem. Med. 8: 123-134.

94. RELATIVELY COMMON HEMOGLOBINOPATHIES

Hemoglobin: Abnormal—tr = trace; $G_\gamma : A_\gamma$ = ratio of G_γ-globin chain to A_γ-globin chain. **Hb Conc** = hemoglobin concentration; if the figures were not given in the reference cited, the values were obtained by dividing the hematocrit by three. *Abbreviations:* Hb = hemoglobin; RBC = erythrocytes ⟨red blood cells⟩; Var = variable; HPFH = hereditary persistence of fetal hemoglobin. Data in brackets refer to the column heading in brackets.

continued

94. RELATIVELY COMMON HEMOGLOBINOPATHIES

#	Condition [Prevalence (%) & Nationality]	Hemoglobin Type			Hb Conc g/dl[1] [Reticulocyte Count, %[1]]	Erythrocytes	Remarks	Reference
		Abnormal %	F, %[1] [$G\gamma$:$A\gamma$[1]]	A_2 %[1]				
1	Normal Newborn [USA]	....	60-90 [3:1]	<1	15-25 [3-7]	Macrocytic, nucleated RBC	About 10% of Hb F is acetylated (Hb F1). Nucleated RBC & reticulocyte counts fall to normal by 1 wk of age.	1,35, 41,49
2	Adult [USA]	....	<1 [2:3]	1.6-3.5	14-18[2] [0.8-2.5]	Normal	Hb A_{1c}, 4-5%. Hb F is confined to a few "F" cells. Hb A_2 is low in iron deficiency anemia, high in megaloblastic anemia.	2,4,14, 30,31, 59,67, 73
3	β-Thalassemia trait [0.5-38, Italy; 6-14, Greece; 5, US Greek; 5, Thailand; 4, US Italian; 1, US Negro]	....	0.9-9.4 [Var]	3.6-7.1	8.2-16.6 [1-5]	Microcytic; some hypochromia, stippling, & poikilocytosis	Patients with "thalassemia intermedia" can only be clearly distinguished from those with β-thalassemia trait (heterozygotes) or homozygous β-thalassemia on the basis of clinical severity	6,21, 40,42, 51,68, 69
4	β-Thalassemia, homozygous [0.3, Greece; 0.06, US Greek; 0.06, Thailand[3]; 0.04, US Italian; 3×10^{-5}, US Negro]	....	20-80 [(1-2):1]	Var (<1-8)	2.5-6.5 [2-15]	Hypochromia, microcytosis, marked poikilocytosis, nucleated RBC, stippling, target cells	Also called Cooley's anemia. Bone deformity, iron overload, transfusion dependence, splenomegaly, lowered resistance to infection.	27,40, 52,68, 69,71, 73
5	α-Thalassemia trait [52, Shiite Arab; 15-28, Thailand; 5, Greece; 2.4, US Greek; 2-3, US Negro]	Hb H, tr	Normal	Normal	Normal to mild anemia [Normal]	Mild microcytosis	Includes severe (α_1) & mild (α_2) forms; they are best distinguished by % Hb Barts at birth: α_1, 5%; α_2, 1-2%	6,21, 22,43, 68,69, 71
6	Hb H disease [0.01-5, Chinese; <1, Shiite Arab; 0.5, Thailand; 0.1, Yemenite & Iraqi Jews; 0.1, Greek; rare, northern Europe; very rare, US Negro]	Hb H, 4-30; Hb Barts, tr	1-3	<2	7-10 [4-5]	Hypochromia; misshapen microcytes; inclusion bodies after staining with oxidant dyes	Hepatosplenomegaly common; some patients have mongoloid facies. Oxidant drugs may precipitate acute hemolysis. May be acquired, in patients with hematologic disorders.	18,22, 24,29, 43,62, 68,69, 71,75
7	Constant Spring trait [4-5, Thailand; 0.2-3, Malaysia; rare, Greece]	Hb Constant Spring, 1-2	1	2.0	14 [1]	Normal	Elongation mutant. Has essentially the same effects as α_2-thalassemia gene, and produces Hb H disease in conjunction with α_1-thalassemia. Hb Koya Dora is similar.	10,12, 37

[1] Unless otherwise specified. [2] Males. [3] At birth.

continued

	Condition [Prevalence (%) & Nationality]	Hemoglobin Type			Hb Conc g/dl[1] [Reticulocyte Count, %[1]]	Erythrocytes	Remarks	Reference
		Abnormal %	F, %[1] [Gγ:Aγ[1]]	A2 %[1]				
8	HPFH trait Swiss type [1-2, Switzerland]	....	1-3	Normal	Normal [Normal]	Normal	Heterogeneous distribution of Hb F	34
9	Greek type [0.2, Greece]	....	10-20 [Aγ only]	1.2-3.0	Normal [Normal]	Normal	Homogeneous distribution of Hb F	19,28, 73
10	Negro type [0.1, US]	....	18-30 [2:3[4]]	1.0-2.1	Normal [Normal]	Occasional target cell & microcyte	Homogeneous distribution of Hb F	11
11	British type [Very rare, England]	....	4-13 [Aγ, mainly]	Normal	Normal [Normal]	Normal	Heterogeneous distribution of Hb F; homozygote has 20% Hb F	72
12	HPFH homozygote, Negro type [Rare, US; rare, Ghana]	....	100 [(1-1.5):1]	0	Normal to slight increase [Normal]	Microcytosis; target cells	Increased oxygen affinity	69
13	Hb Lepore trait [0.02-3.5, Italy; low, worldwide]	Hb Lepore, 5-15	1-13 [1:2]	1.7-3.6	6-15.5 [Normal to slight increase]	Slight hypochromia; mild microcytosis	Occasional patient with splenomegaly. Hb Lepore is a "crossover" between δ- and β-chain genes	15,45, 46,51, 69
14	Hb Lepore homozygote [Very low]	Hb Lepore, 8-30	61-90 [1:1]	0	6-9	Hypochromia, microcytosis, poikilocytosis, nucleated RBC	Similar to homozygous β-thalassemia ⟨Cooley's anemia⟩	15,45
15	Sickle cell trait [0-46, Africa; 0-32, Greece; 8-15, US Negro]	Hb S, 20-48%	Normal	2.3-4.3	Normal [Normal]	Rare target cell	% Hb S decreased in iron deficiency & megaloblastic anemias. Some patients have hyposthenuria, and a very few have hematuria. Splenic infarction may occur at high altitudes.	3,6,9, 13,17, 23,33, 38,53, 73,74
16	Sickle cell anemia [1, Africa[3]; 0.16, US Negro]	Hb S, 80-95%	0.6-20 [Var]	2.0-4.8	4-12 [3-29]	Sickled forms, target cells, nucleated RBC; Howell-Jolly bodies	Hemolytic anemia & vasoocclusive crises; aplastic crises; leg ulcers; pulmonary infarction; autosplenectomy; gallstones	13,25, 26,38, 73,74
17	Hb C trait [11-28, Ghana; 2-3, US Negro]	Hb C, 32-53	Normal	2.9-3.7	Normal [Normal]	Occasional target cell	No disability	6,13, 26,38, 53
18	Hb C homozygote [0.5, Ghana; 0.02, US Negro]	Hb C, >90	0.4-1.5	2.8-5.4	7-14.5 [1-9]	Target cells & microspherocytes; intraerythrocytic crystals of hemoglobin	Mild hemolytic anemia, often with splenomegaly	5,13, 26,53, 55
19	Hb D Punjab trait [3, India; 0.8, Iran; 0.04, US Negro; 0.02, England; 0.01, Canada]	Hb D, 36-40	Normal	Normal	Normal [Normal]	Normal	Must be distinguished from other α- & β-chain variants with similar electrophoretic properties	32,48, 63,66, 73

[1] Unless otherwise specified. [3] At birth. [4] Usually.

continued

94. RELATIVELY COMMON HEMOGLOBINOPATHIES

Condition [Prevalence (%) & Nationality]	Hemoglobin Type			Hb Conc g/dl[1] [Reticulocyte Count, %[1]]	Erythrocytes	Remarks	Reference
	Abnormal %	F, %[1] [Gγ:Aγ]	A$_2$ %[1]				
20 Hb D$_{Punjab}$ homozygote [Very rare]	Hb D, >90	0.2-2.4	3.3	9-15 [1.2-4]	Target cells & spherocytes in some patients	Mild hemolytic anemia in some patients	44,57
21 Hb E trait [16-52, Thailand]	Hb E, 35-49	Normal	.....	10.1-15.8 [0.2-1.9]	Normal	No disability	8,39, 60,64, 65
22 Hb E homozygote [6, Thailand]	Hb E, >90	1.2-6.4	.....	7.9-13.2 [0.4-1.4]	Target cells, microcytes	Mild hemolytic anemia. Slight splenomegaly in some patients.	8,39, 64-66
23 Hb S—β-thalassemia [0.1-1.0, Greece; 0.02, US Negro]	Hb S, 50-93	2-21	3-6.4	6.4-13.2 [1-17]	Sickled cells, nucleated RBC, poikilocytosis	Hepatosplenomegaly, leg ulcers in some. Includes S/β⁺ & S/β° thalassemia. Generally milder than sickle cell anemia.	50
Sickle cell anemia—α-thalassemia 24 [Shiite Arab]	Hb S, 41; Hb Barts, 14	44	1.6	8.9 [3.0]	Poikilocytosis, target cells, anisocytosis. Hypochromia may be marked.	Mild disease	70
25 [Ghana]	Hb S, 82-84; Hb Barts, tr	12-15	3.1-3.2	8.2-8.8	Similar to sickle cell anemia	Milder than sickle cell anemia	16
26 Hb SC disease [0.06, US Negro]	Hb C > Hb S	0.9-5 [2:3]	.....	7-14 [0.4-8]	Target cells, rare sickled forms	Splenomegaly common. Milder than SS disease, but vitreous hemorrhage & aseptic necrosis of femoral head more common in SC disease.	26,54, 61
27 Hb SD$_{Punjab}$ disease [Quite rare]	Hb S = Hb D	5-20	.....	7-13 [4-10]	Target cells, sickled forms, poikilocytosis	*See* comment under D$_{Punjab}$ trait. Similar clinically to sickle cell anemia.	47,56, 58
28 Hb SO$_{Arab}$ disease [Rare, US Negro]	Hb S > Hb O	2-7	.....	6.8-8.7 [3-13]	Sickled forms, nucleated RBC, target cells, poikilocytosis	Similar to sickle cell anemia clinically. Must be distinguished from SC disease (& SE disease) on electrophoresis.	7,36
29 Hb E—β-thalassemia [0.6, Thailand]	Hb E, 52	48	.....	5-6	Microcytosis, hypochromic target cells	Similar to homozygous β-thalassemia ⟨Cooley's anemia⟩: hepatosplenomegaly, bone changes, retarded development, iron overload	20,39

[1] Unless otherwise specified.

Contributor: Charache, Samuel

References
1. Armstrong, D. H., et al. 1963. Blood 22:554-565.
2. Boyer, S. H. 1975. Science 188:361-362.
3. Boyle, E., Jr., et al. 1968. Arch. Environ. Health 17: 891-898.
4. Bunn, H. F., et al. 1975. Biochem. Biophys. Res. Commun. 67:103-109.
5. Charache, S. 1967. J. Clin. Invest. 46:1795-1811.
6. Charache, S., et al. 1974. Ann. N.Y. Acad. Sci. 232: 125-134.
7. Charache, S., et al. 1976. Am. J. Med., v. 62.
8. Chernoff, A. I., et al. 1956. J. Lab. Clin. Med. 47: 455-489.

continued

9. Choremis, C., et al. 1957. Lancet 273:1333-1334.
10. Clegg, J. B., and D. J. Weatherall. 1974. Ann. N.Y. Acad. Sci. 232:168-178.
11. Conley, C. L., et al. 1963. Blood 21:261-281.
12. DeJong, W. W., et al. 1975. Am. J. Hum. Genet. 27:81-90.
13. Edington, G. M., and H. Lehmann. 1954. Trans. R. Soc. Trop. Med. Hyg. 48:332-336.
14. Efremov, C. D., et al. 1974. J. Lab. Clin. Med. 83:657-664.
15. Efremov, G. D., et al. 1974. Br. J. Haematol. 27:319-329.
16. Enk, A. van, et al. 1972. Br. Med. J. 4:524-526.
17. Esan, G. J. F., and T. A. O. Adesina. 1974. Scand. J. Haematol. 13:370-376.
18. Fessas, P. 1959. In J. H. P. Jonxis and J. F. Delafresnaye, ed. Abnormal Haemoglobins. Blackwell Scientific, Oxford. pp. 134-157.
19. Fessas, P., and G. Stamatoyannopoulos. 1964. Blood 24:223-240.
20. Flatz, G., et al. 1965. Ann. Hum. Genet. 29:151-170.
21. Fraser, G. R., et al. 1964. Ann. N.Y. Acad. Sci. 119:415-435.
22. Friedman, S., et al. 1974. Pediatr. Res. 8:955-959.
23. Gelpi, A. P. 1973. Ann. Intern. Med. 79:258-264.
24. Hamilton, R. W., et al. 1971. N. Engl. J. Med. 285:1217-1221.
25. Huisman, T. H. J. 1972. Clin. Chim. Acta 38:5-16.
26. Huisman, T. H. J. 1972. Ibid. 40:159-163.
27. Huisman, T. H. J. 1974. Ann. N.Y. Acad. Sci. 232:107-124.
28. Huisman, T. H. J., et al. 1970. J. Clin. Invest. 49:1035-1040.
29. Ing, R. Y. K., and J. H. Crookston. 1968. Can. Med. Assoc. J. 99:49-56.
30. Josephson, A. M., et al. 1958. Blood 13:543-551.
31. Kunkel, H. G., et al. 1957. J. Clin. Invest. 36:1615-1625.
32. Lehmann, H., and R. G. Huntsman. 1974. Man's Hemoglobins. Ed. 2. J. B. Lippincott, Philadelphia.
33. Livingstone, F. B. 1967. Abnormal Hemoglobins in Human Populations. Aldine, Chicago.
34. Marti, H. R. 1963. Normale und anomale Menschliche Hämoglobine. Springer-Verlag, Berlin. pp. 85-89.
35. Matsuda, G., et al. 1960. Blood 16:984-996.
36. Milner, P. F. 1970. N. Engl. J. Med. 283:1417-1425.
37. Milner, P. F., et al. 1971. Lancet 1:729-732.
38. Motulsky, A. G. 1973. N. Engl. J. Med. 288:31-33.
39. Na-Nakorn, S., and V. Minnich. 1957. Blood 12:529-538.
40. Neel, J. V., and W. N. Valentine. 1945. Am. J. Med. Sci. 209:568-572.
41. Oski, F. A., and J. L. Naiman. 1966. Hematologic Problems in the Newborn. W. B. Saunders, Philadelphia.
42. Pearson, H. A., et al. 1974. Ann. N.Y. Acad. Sci. 232:135-144.
43. Pembrey, M. E., et al. 1975. Br. J. Haematol. 29:221-234.
44. Politis-Tsegos, C., et al. 1975. J. Med. Genet. 12:269-274.
45. Quattrin, N., and V. Ventruto. 1974. Ann. N.Y. Acad. Sci. 232:65-75.
46. Quattrin, N., et al. 1967. Acta Haematol. 37:266-275.
47. Ringelhann, B., et al. 1967. Ibid. 38:324-331.
48. Rucknagel, D. L. 1974. (Loc. cit. ref. 73). p. 846.
49. Schroeder, W. A., et al. 1971. Pediatr. Res. 5:493-499.
50. Serjeant, G. R., et al. 1973. Br. J. Haematol. 24:19-30.
51. Silvestroni, E., and I. Bianco. 1975. Am. J. Hum. Genet. 27:198-212.
52. Silvestroni, E., et al. 1968. Br. J. Haematol. 14:303-308.
53. Smith, E. W., and C. L. Conley. 1953. Bull. Johns Hopkins Hosp. 93:94-106.
54. Smith, E. W., and C. L. Conley. 1954. Ibid. 94:289-318.
55. Smith, E. W., and J. R. Krevans. 1959. Ibid. 104:17-43.
56. Smith, E. W., et al. 1959. Ann. Intern. Med. 50:94-105.
57. Stout, C., et al. 1964. Arch. Intern. Med. 114:296-300.
58. Sturgeon, P., et al. 1955. Blood 10:389-404.
59. Trivelli, L. A., et al. 1971. N. Engl. J. Med. 284:353-357.
60. Tuchinda, S., et al. 1964. Am. J. Hum. Genet. 16:311-335.
61. Tuttle, A. H., et al. 1960. J. Pediatr. 56:331-342.
62. Vella, F. 1960. Acta Haematol. 23:393-397.
63. Vella, F., and H. Lehmann. 1974. J. Med. Genet. 11:341-348.
64. Wasi, P., et al. 1967. Br. Med. J. 4:29-32.
65. Wasi, P., et al. 1967. Nature (London) 214:501-502.
66. Wasi, P., et al. 1968. Acta Haematol. 39:151-158.
67. Wasi, P., et al. 1968. J. Lab. Clin. Med. 71:85-91.
68. Wasi, P., et al. 1969. Ann. N.Y. Acad. Sci. 165:60-82.
69. Weatherall, D. J., and J. B. Clegg. 1972. The Thalassaemia Syndromes. Ed. 2. Blackwell Scientific, Oxford.
70. Weatherall, D. J., et al. 1969. Br. J. Haematol. 17:517-526.
71. Weatherall, D. J., et al. 1974. Ann. N.Y. Acad. Sci. 232:88-106.
72. Weatherall, D. J., et al. 1975. Br. J. Haematol. 29:191-198, 205-220.
73. Wintrobe, M. M., et al. 1974. Clinical Hematology. Ed. 7. Lea and Febiger, Philadelphia.
74. Wrightstone, R. N., and T. H. J. Huisman. 1974. Am. J. Clin. Pathol. 61:375-381.
75. Zaizov, R., and Y. Matoth. 1972. Isr. J. Med. Sci. 8:11-17.

95. PERIPHERAL BLOOD LEUKOCYTES

Entries 8-10 are from individual studies of overlapping age ranges, and have been included to demonstrate the variations in data obtained by different investigators and to be expected from different clinical laboratories. Values are given in thousands per microliter of blood and as percent of total leukocytes. Values in parentheses are ranges, estimate "c" (*see* Introduction).

	Age	Leuko-cytes, Total	Neutrophils			Eosinophils	Basophils	Lymphocytes	Monocytes	Reference
			Total	Band	Segmented					
1	0[1/]	18.1(9.0-30.0)[2/]	11.0(6.0-26.0)[3/] 61%	1.65 9.1%	9.4 52%	0.40(0.02-0.85) 2.2%	0.10(0-0.64) 0.6%	5.5(2.0-11.0) 31%	1.05(0.4-3.1) 5.8%	2
2	7 d	12.2(5.0-21.0)	5.5(1.5-10.0) 45%	0.83 6%	4.7 39%	0.5(0.07-1.1) 4.1%	0.05(0-0.25) 0.4%	5.0(2.0-17.0) 41%	1.1(0.3-2.7) 9.1%	2
3	14 d	11.4(5.0-20.0)	4.5(1.0-9.5) 40%	0.63 5.5%	3.9 34%	0.35(0.07-1.0) 3.1%	0.05(0-0.23) 0.4%	5.5(2.0-17.0) 48%	1.0(0.2-2.4) 8.8%	2
4	4 yr	9.1(5.5-15.5)	3.8(1.5-8.5) 42%	0.27 3.0%	3.5 39%	0.25(0.02-0.65) 2.8%	0.05(0-0.20) 0.6%	4.5(2.0-8.0) 50%	0.45(0-0.8) 5.0%	2
5	6 yr	8.5(5.0-14.5)	4.3(1.5-8.0) 51%	0.25 3.0%	4.0 48%	0.23(0-0.65) 2.7%	0.05(0-0.20) 0.6%	3.5(1.5-7.0) 42%	0.40(0-0.8) 4.7%	2
6	10 yr	8.1(4.5-13.5)	4.4(1.8-8.0) 54%	0.24 3.0%	4.2 51%	0.20(0-0.60) 2.4%	0.04(0-0.20) 0.5%	3.1(1.5-6.5) 38%	0.35(0-0.8) 4.3%	2
7	15-18 yr	8.4(4.0-13.0)	4.0(1.5-7.5) 48%	0.08 1%	4.0 48%	0.15(0-0.4) 2%	0.05(0-0.2) 0.5%	3.2(1.5-5.0) 42%	0.3(0-0.8) 4%	7
8	19-38 yr	7.4(4.0-11.0)	4.0(1.5-7.5) 54%	0.05 1%	4.0 54%	0.15(0-0.4) 2%	0.05(0-0.2) 0.5%	2.8(1.0-4.5) 38%	0.3(0-0.8) 4%	6
9	16-49 yr	7.0(4.3-10)	3.6(1.8-7.2) 52%	0.5[4/] 7%	3.0 43%	0.15(0-0.7) 2%	0.03(0-0.15) 0.4%	2.5(1.5-4.0) 36%	0.4(0.2-0.95) 6%	5
10	15-≥70 yr	6.7(4.1-10.9)	4.2(2.2-7.6) 64%	....	....	0.13(0-0.5) 2%	0.03(0-0.16) 0.3%	1.8(0.8-3.1)[5/] 27%	0.4(0.1-0.8) 5%	9

[1/] At birth. [2/] At birth, ∿500 nucleated erythrocytes per μl of blood may be present. These cells disappear from the blood during the first 4 d after birth [ref. 8]. [3/] Metamyelocytes, myelocytes, and promyelocytes may be present in the peripheral blood in the first few hours after birth [ref. 8]. The highly variable total and segmented neutrophil count at birth precludes interpretation of increases as indicative of neonatal infection. However, increases in the number of band neutrophils appear to be a reliable indication of infection in the newborn [ref. 1, 10]. [4/] The higher proportion of band forms in this study is probably due to the criteria chosen for band cells. Although significantly fewer bands were found in Negroes, no clinically significant difference was found between Negroes and Caucasians. Other workers have reported significant granulocytopenia and leukopenia in about 25% of Negroes [ref. 3]. [5/] A statistically significant decrease in the lymphocyte count has been reported in old people (mean age, 78 yr; total lymphocyte count, 1775 ± 802), in comparison with mature younger individuals (mean age, 31 yr; total lymphocyte count, 2430 ± 890) [ref. 4].

Contributor: Williams, William J.

References

1. Akenzua, G. I., et al. 1974. Pediatrics 54:38-42.
2. Altman, P. L., and D. S. Dittmer, ed. 1974. Biology Data Book. Ed. 2. Federation of American Societies for Experimental Biology, Bethesda, MD. v. 3, pp. 1856-1857.
3. Broun, G. O., Jr., et al. 1966. N. Engl. J. Med. 275: 1410-1413.
4. Díaz-Jouanen, E., et al. 1975. Am. J. Med. 58:620-628.
5. Orfanakis, N. G., et al. 1970. Am. J. Clin. Pathol. 53: 647-651.
6. Osgood, E. E., et al. 1939. Arch. Intern. Med. 64:105-120.
7. Osgood, E. E., et al. 1939. J. Lab. Clin. Med. 24:905-912.
8. Oski, F. A., and J. L. Naiman. 1972. Hematologic Problems in the Newborn. Ed. 2. W. B. Saunders, Philadelphia. pp. 16, 18.
9. Zacharski, L. R., et al. 1971. Am. J. Clin. Pathol. 56: 148-150.
10. Zipursky, A., et al. 1976. Pediatrics 57:839-853.

Constituent or Property	Value μmoles/g wet wt platelets[1]	Reference
Physical properties		
1	Platelet count	249,700 ± 93,800/μl blood	12
2	Platelet number per unit weight	0.78 × 10^{11}/g wet wt platelets	10
3	Individual volume, mean	5.0 μm³	13
4		5.2 μm³	4
5		7.1 μm³	10
6		7.5 μm³	3
7	mode	4.38 μm³	13
Inorganic constituents		
8	Water	77 mg/g wet wt platelets	7
9	Calcium	16.8	5
10		26.4	17
11		32.0	14
12	Magnesium	2.9	5
13	Orthophosphate	1.2	11
14	Phosphorus	53.3	1
15	Potassium	118 meq/liter intracellular water	7
16	Sodium	38.8 meq/liter intracellular water	7
17	Sulfate	2.9	1
18	Zinc	0.36	6
19	Ash	22.1 mg/g wet wt platelets	15
20	Lipid	29.8 mg/g wet wt platelets	10
21		49.8 mg/g wet wt platelets	1
22	Carbohydrate	11.0 mg/g wet wt platelets	18
23		19.4 mg/g wet wt platelets	1
24	Glycogen	3.82 mg/g wet wt platelets	11
25		5.38 mg/g wet wt platelets	18
26		5.60 mg/g wet wt platelets	8
27	Protein	119 mg/g wet wt platelets	10
28		148 mg/g wet wt platelets	11
Non-protein nitrogenous compounds		
29	Adenosine 5'-monophosphate	0.36	11
30		0.37	16
31	Adenosine 5'-diphosphate	1.39	11
32		2.61	9
33		2.76	16
34	Adenosine 5'-triphosphate	2.52	11
35		2.96	2
36		3.74	9
37		4.36	16
38	Serotonin	59.3 μg/g wet wt platelets	19

[1] Unless otherwise specified.

Contributor: Karpatkin, Simon

References

1. Barber, A. J., et al. 1969. Fed. Proc. Fed. Am. Soc. Exp. Biol. 28:575(Abstr. 1761).
2. Born, G. V. R. 1958. Biochem. J. 68:695-704.
3. Bull, B. S., and M. B. Zucker. 1965. Proc. Soc. Exp. Biol. Med. 120:296-301.
4. Corash, L., et al. 1977. Blood 49:(in press).
5. Cousin, C., and J. Caen. 1964. Rev. Fr. Etud. Clin. Biol. 9:520-523.
6. Foley, B., et al. 1968. Proc. Soc. Exp. Biol. Med. 128:265-269.
7. Gorstein, F., et al. 1967. J. Lab. Clin. Med. 70:938-950.
8. Gross, R., et al. 1967. In E. Kowalski and S. Niewiarowski, ed. Biochemistry of Blood Platelets. Academic Press, New York. pp. 161-172.
9. Holmsen, H., et al. 1975. Blood 46:131-142.

continued

10. Karpatkin, S. 1969. J. Clin. Invest. 47:1073-1082.
11. Karpatkin, S., and R. M. Langer. 1968. Ibid. 47: 2158-2168.
12. Karpatkin, S., et al. 1971. Am. J. Med. 51:1-4.
13. Khan, I., et al. 1975. Br. J. Haematol. 31:449-460.
14. Lages, B., et al. 1975. J. Lab. Clin. Med. 85:811-825.
15. Maupin, B., et al. 1962. Rev. Fr. Etud. Clin. Biol. 7: 169-173.
16. Mills, D. C. B., and D. P. Thomas. 1969. Nature (London) 222:991-992.
17. Wallach, D. F. H., et al. 1958. Blood 13:589-598.
18. Woodside, E. E., and W. Kocholaty. 1960. Ibid. 16: 1173-1183.
19. Zucker, M. B., et al. 1958. Proc. 6th Congr. Int. Soc. Hematol. Boston 1956, pp. 540-552.

97. RED CELL LIFE SPANS

Both diisopropyl fluorophosphate ([^{32}P]DFP) and chromium-51 (^{51}Cr) isotopic techniques for measuring red cell life span are random label methods. [^{32}P]DFP measures mean life span as $\dfrac{100}{\text{turnover rate/day}}$. Most laboratories report ^{51}Cr survival in terms of a red cell ^{51}Cr half-life. This is the time required for red cell ^{51}Cr content to decrease by one-half [ref. 1]. The chromium method suffers from continuous elution of the isotope from intact surviving red cells, at a rate varying from 0.5-2.9%/day. Values in parenthesis are ranges, estimate "c" (see Introduction).

	Method	Subjects	Value	Reference
			Mean Life Span, days	
1	[^{32}P]DFP	6♂	122(106-142)	7
2		8♂	124.6 ± 11.0[1] (118-127)	3
3		5♂[2]	132(118-154)	4
4		4♂; 4♀	127(114-136)	6

	Method	Subjects	Value	Reference
			Mean Half-Life, days	
5	^{51}Cr	11	26.2	5
6		6♂[3]	(24.7-31.0)	8
7		2♂[4]; 9♀[4]	(25.0-30.6)	8
8		25♂; 4♀	32.5(27-35)	9
9		163♂♀	29.0(25.0-40.0)	2

[1] Plus/minus (±) value is 2 standard deviations. [2] Negro. [3] Young. [4] Elderly.

Contributors: Kansu, Emin, and Erslev, Allan J.

References

1. Berlin, N. I. 1972. In W. J. Williams, et al., ed. Hematology. McGraw-Hill, New York. pp. 152-162.
2. Berlin, N. I., et al. 1959. Physiol. Rev. 39:577-616.
3. Bove, J. R., and F. G. Ebaugh, Jr. 1958. J. Lab. Clin. Med. 51:916-925.
4. Brewer, G. J., et al. 1961. Ibid. 58:217-224.
5. Donohue, D. M., et al. 1955. Br. J. Haematol. 1:249-263.
6. Eernisse, J. G., and J. J. van Rood. 1961. Ibid. 7:382-404.
7. Garby, L. 1962. Ibid. 8:15-27.
8. Hurdle, A. D. F., and A. J. Rosin. 1962. J. Clin. Pathol. 15:343-345.
9. Mollison, P. L. 1961. Clin. Sci. 21:21-36.

98. BONE MARROW DIFFERENTIAL CELL COUNTS

The values reported for bone marrow differential cell counts vary widely, and it is impossible to present a meaningful "normal" differential count. Among other variables such as age and site of biopsy, aspiration of larger volumes of marrow increases the number of segmented cells in the differential count [ref. 2, 6]. In the first few days of life there is a marked decrease in erythropoietic cells. Erythropoietic cells reappear in the next 2-3 months, and thereafter the myeloid:erythroid ratio is not influenced by age [ref. 3]. Lymphocytes increase in the marrow during the first few weeks of life, and may comprise up to 50% of all marrow cells in a 1- to 3-month-old child [ref. 3]. Subsequently

continued

98. BONE MARROW DIFFERENTIAL CELL COUNTS

the number of lymphocytes falls, reaching adult levels in the first few years of life [ref. 4, 5]. The data presented are selective as representative of a large literature. Values in parentheses are ranges, estimate "c" (*see* Introduction).

	Specification ⟨Synonym⟩	Gairdner, et al.	Gairdner, et al.	Glaser, et al.	Osgood & Seaman	Vaughan & Brockmyre	Custer	Wintrobe, et al.
1	Age of subjects	0-24 h	8-10 d	1-20 yr	Adult	Adult	Adult	Adult ♂
2	Volume of marrow	0.25 ml	0.25 ml	1 ml	0.5-10 ml	3 ml	....	....
3	Site of aspiration	Tibia	Tibia	Sternum	Sternum	Sternum	"Aspirations & sections"	....
4	Cells, % of total count[1] Pronormoblasts ⟨Proerythroblasts⟩	0.5(0-1.0)	0	0.5(0-1.5)	0.2(0-1)	....	(0.1-3.5)	(0.2-1.3)
5	Normoblasts	....	....	....	....	9.5(2-18)	....	....
6	Early ⟨Basophilic⟩	3.0(0-6)	(0-0.5)	1.7(0-5)	2(0-4)	....	(1.7-5.5)	(0.5-2.4)
7	Intermediate ⟨Polychromatophilic⟩	10(5-19)	1.5(0-5)	18(5-34)	6(4-8)	....	(5.0-20.0)	(17.9-29.2)
8	Late ⟨Orthochromatic⟩	26(18-41)	6(0-15)	2.7(0-8)	3(1-5)	....	(5.0-23.8)	(0.4-4.6)
9	Myeloblasts	1.0(0.5-2.0)	1.0(0-3)	1.2(0-3)	0.4(0-1)	1.3(0-3)	(0-3.5)	(0.2-1.5)
10	Promyelocytes	1.5(0.5-5.0)	2.0(0.5-7)	1.8(0-4)	1.4(0-3)	....	(0.5-8.0)	(2.1-4.1)
11	Myelocytes	....	....	16.5(8-25)	4.2(0-12)	8.9(3-15)	....	....
12	Neutrophilic	4(1-9)	4(1-11)	....	....	....	(7.0-35)	(8.2-15.7)
13	Eosinophilic	1.0(0-2.5)	1.0(0-2)	....	....	....	(0.3-3.0)	(0.2-1.3)
14	Basophilic	(0-0.5)	(0-0.5)	....	....	....	(0.0-0.5)	....
15	Metamyelocytes	14(4.5-28)	19(7-37)	23(14-34)	6.5(3-10)	8.8(4-15)	(20.3-49.0)	(10-26.8)
16	Bands	....	....	....	24(17-33)	23.9(12-34)		(9.7-17.7)
	Segmented							
17	Neutrophilic	22(10-40)	20(11-45)	12.9(4.5-29)	15(5-25)	18.5(9-32)	(7.0-25.0)	(6.0-12.0)
18	Eosinophilic	1.5(1.0-3.0)	1.0(0-2)	....	2(0-4)	1.9(0-6)	(0.1-3.0)	(0.0-1.3)
19	Basophilic	0(0-0.5)	0	....	0.2(0-5)	0.2(0-1)	(0.0-1.0)	(0.0-0.2)
20	Lymphocytes	12(4-22)	37(20-62)	16(5-36)	14(3-25)	16.2(8-26)	(2.5-25)	(11.1-23.2)
21	Monocytes	1.5(0-3.0)	1.7(0-3.0)	....	2(0-4)	2.4(0-6)	(0.1-3.2)	(0.0-0.8)
22	Megakaryocytes	....	....	....	....	(1-38)/50 low power fields	(0.05-1.2)	(0.0-0.4)
23	Plasma cells	....	....	....	....	0.3(0-1.5)	(0.1-1.2)	(0.4-3.9)
24	Reticulum cells	....	....	....	....	0.3(0-1)	(0.3-2.6)	(0.0-0.9)
25	Disintegrated cells[2]	15(1-43)	20(0-40)	....	19(10-30)	7.9(2-16)	....	....
26	Myeloid:erythroid ratio[3]	1.2:1	6.3:1	(1-5):1	3.6(2-8):1	(3.5-30):1	....	(1.5-3.3):1
	Reference	3	3	4	6	7	1	8

[1] Unless otherwise specified. [2] Cells which have been damaged in preparation, and therefore cannot be positively identified. [3] Calculated from the number of myeloid cells (i.e., granulocytes, not total leukocytes) and the number of erythroid cells.

Contributor: Williams, William J.

References
1. Custer, P. R. 1974. An Atlas of the Blood and Bone Marrow. Ed. 2. W. B. Saunders, Philadelphia. p. 42.
2. Dresch, C., et al. 1974. J. Clin. Pathol. 27:106-108.
3. Gairdner, D., et al. 1952. Arch. Dis. Child. 27:128-133.
4. Glaser, K., et al. 1950. Pediatrics 6:789-824.
5. Miale, J. B. 1972. Laboratory Medicine: Hematology. Ed. 4. C. V. Mosby, St. Louis. p. 328.
6. Osgood, E. E., and A. J. Seaman. 1944. Physiol. Rev. 24:46-69.
7. Vaughan, S. L., and F. Brockmyre. 1947. Blood (Spec. Issue) 1:54-59.
8. Wintrobe, M. M., et al. 1974. Clinical Hematology. Ed. 7. Lea and Febiger, Philadelphia. p. 1796.

The normal values in the table are representative of published results which differ slightly from one laboratory to another. Since the distributions of normal values are non-Gaussian (skewed toward lower limit) for serum iron, ferritin, and vitamin B_{12} concentrations, the parameters indicated are, for the most part, median and central 95 percentile. Although most published data for ferritin give geometric (logarithmic) mean and standard deviation, these parameters correspond closely with median and central 95 percentile. Therefore, for simplicity and practical usefulness, the median and central 95 percentile range have also been listed for ferritin. Total iron-binding capacity appears to average about 100 μg/dl higher when measured directly than when estimated by addition of serum iron and isotopically measured unsaturated iron-binding capacity. Serum haptoglobin ⟨Hp⟩ concentration depends on haptoglobin genotype: Hp 1-1 has a distinctly higher mean and normal range than Hp 2-2 by any current method. The range given is based on random samples of normal sera without haptoglobin typing, and is broad enough to include the separate ranges of the major genotypes. Normal values reported for vitamin B_{12} and folate assays have varied considerably, depending on the method used. In general, microbiological assays for vitamin B_{12} give slightly lower results than do radioimmunoassays, whereas the microbiological assay for folate gives values substantially higher than those obtained by radioimmunoassay. **Method:** Spect = spectrophotometric. Values in parentheses are ranges, estimate "a" unless otherwise indicated (*see* Introduction).

	Factor ⟨Synonym⟩	Subjects	Method	Concentration	Reference
1	Ferritin	Newborn	Immunoradiometric	101[1] (25-200) ng/ml	29
2		1 mo old	Immunoradiometric	365[1] (200-600) ng/ml	29
3		2-5 mo old	Immunoradiometric	100[1] (50-200) ng/ml	29
4		6 mo-15 yr old	Immunoradiometric	30[1] (7-142) ng/ml	29
5		Adult, ♂	Immunoradiometric	60[1] (20-300) ng/ml	1,6,13,16,22, 33
6		♀	Immunoradiometric	30[1] (10-120) ng/ml	1,6,13,16,22, 33
7	Folate	Healthy adults, ♂♀	Competitive binding assay	8.2[1] (4.5-13) ng/ml[2]	26,30,34
8				5.6 ± 2.3 ng/ml[2]	28
9			Plus microbiological (*Lactobacillus casei*)	10[1] (6.0-24) ng/ml[2]	26,30,34
10				9.9 ± 5.6 ng/ml[2]	28
11	Haptoglobin	Adult, ♂♀	Radial immunodiffusion	130[1] (40-270) mg/dl	2,11,18,27,32
12			Hemoglobin-binding capacity	100[1] (20-200) mg/dl	2,11,17,21,23, 27,32
13	Iron	Newborn	Spect: *o*-phenanthroline	160 ± 65 μg/dl	31
14		1-6 mo old	Spect: *o*-phenanthroline	89 ± 27 μg/dl	12,19
15		4 mo-5 yr old	Spect: bathophenanthroline	85 ± 25 μg/dl	19
16		3-6 yr old	Spect: bathophenanthroline	117 ± 40 μg/dl	19
17		9-17 yr old	Spect: bathophenanthroline	100[1] (50-200) μg/dl	14
18		12-17 yr old	Spect: bathophenanthroline	110[1] (60-200) μg/dl	14
19		Adult, ♂	Spect: ferrozine or bathophenanthroline	95[1] (70-180) μg/dl; 105 ± 30 μg/dl	3,4,8,14,24
20		♀	Spect: ferrozine or bathophenanthroline	90[1] (60-180) μg/dl; 100 ± 39 μg/dl	3,4,8,14,24
21	Iron-binding capacity ⟨TIBC⟩	3-6 yr old	Spect: bathophenanthroline	402 ± 63 μg/dl	7,14
22		12-17 yr old	Spect: bathophenanthroline	380[1] (330-490) μg/dl	7,14
23		Adult, ♂	Spect: ferrozine	385[1] (240-490) μg/dl	8,14
24		♀	Spect: ferrozine	430[1] (300-520) μg/dl	8,14
25		♂♀	Radioisotopic, unsaturated binding capacity, plus serum iron	(250-450)[c] μg/dl	3,8,24
26	Transferrin	Unspecified[3]	Radial immunodiffusion	(200-300)[d] mg/dl	9
27	Transferrin saturation	Adult, ♂	100 × iron/TIBC	26[1] (18-48) %	3,4,8,14,24
28		♀	100 × iron/TIBC	24[1] (12-58) %	3,4,8,14,24
29	Vitamin B_{12} ⟨Cobalamin⟩	Adult, ♂♀	Competitive binding (radioimmunoassay)	425[1] (180-800) pg/ml	15,20
30			Microbiological (*Lactobacillus leichmannii* or *Euglena gracilis*)	425[1] (180-1145)[c] pg/ml	10,25
31	Vitamin B_{12} ⟨Cobalamin⟩ unsaturated binding capacity	Unspecified[3]	Radioisotope with charcoal adsorber	1149(980-1756)[c] pg/ml	5

[1] Median. [2] Moderate interlaboratory variability. [3] No recognized age or sex difference.

continued

99. SERUM CONCENTRATIONS OF HEMATOPOIETIC FACTORS

Contributor: Fairbanks, Virgil F.

References

1. Addison, G. M., et al. 1972. J. Clin. Pathol. 25:326-329.
2. Braun, H. J., and F. W. Aly. 1969. Clin. Chim. Acta 26:588-590.
3. Cartwright, G. E., and M. M. Wintrobe. 1949. J. Clin. Invest. 28:86-98.
4. Cartwright, G. E., et al. 1948. Blood 3:501-525.
5. Chikkappa, G., et al. 1971. Ibid. 37:142-151.
6. Cook, J. D., et al. 1974. Am. J. Clin. Nutr. 27:681-687.
7. DeWijn, J. F., and N. A. Pikaar. 1971. Nutr. Metab. 13:43-44.
8. Fairbanks, V. F. Unpublished. Mayo Clinic, Rochester, MN, 1976.
9. Goya, N., et al. 1972. Blood 40:239-245.
10. Green, R., et al. 1974. Br. J. Haematol. 27:507-526.
11. Grunbaum, B. W., and N. Pace. 1964. Microchem. J. 8:317-323.
12. Haddy, T. B., et al. 1974. Am. J. Dis. Child. 128:787-793.
13. Jacobs, A., et al. 1972. Br. Med. J. 2:206-208.
14. Kasper, C. K., and R. O. Wallerstein. 1966. Am. J. Clin. Nutr. 18:286-293.
15. Lau, K. S., et al. 1965. Blood 26:202-214.
16. Lipschitz, D. A., et al. 1974. N. Engl. J. Med. 290:1213-1216.
17. Malin, S. F., and R. P. Baker, Jr. 1972. Biochem. Med. 6:205-209.
18. Mancini, G., et al. 1965. Immunochemistry 2:235-254.
19. Marner, T. 1969. Acta Paediatr. Scand. 58:363-368.
20. Matthews, D. M., et al. 1967. J. Clin. Pathol. 20:683-686.
21. Nyman, M. 1959. Scand. J. Clin. Lab. Invest., Suppl. 39:1-169.
22. Prieto, J., et al. 1975. Gastroenterology 68:525-533.
23. Ramirez-Zorrilla, M. de J., et al. 1971. Sangre 16:127-133.
24. Rath, C. E., and C. A. Finch. 1949. J. Clin. Invest. 28:79-85.
25. Raven, J. L., et al. 1972. Br. J. Haematol. 22:21-31.
26. Rothenberg, S. P., et al. 1972. N. Engl. J. Med. 286:1335-1339.
27. Roy, R. B., et al. 1969. J. Lab. Clin. Med. 74:698-704.
28. Rudzki, Z., et al. 1976. Ibid. 87:859-867.
29. Siimes, M. A., et al. 1974. Blood 43:581-590.
30. Tajuddin, M., and H. A. Gardyna. 1973. Clin. Chem. 19:125-126.
31. Vahlquist, B. 1941. Acta Paediatr. (Stockholm), Suppl. 5:1-374.
32. Valeri, C. R., et al. 1965. Clin. Chem. 11:581-588.
33. Walters, G. O., et al. 1973. J. Clin. Pathol. 26:770-772.
34. Waxman, S., and C. Schreiber. 1973. Blood 42:281-290.

100. COAGULATION FACTORS

Figures in heavy brackets are reference numbers

Factor ⟨Synonym⟩	Molecular Weight	Normal Concentration in Blood (mg/100 ml)[1]	Function	In Vivo Half-Life	Disease Importance
1 I ⟨Fibrinogen⟩	340,000 [2]	2-5 mg/ml[2] [21]	Polymerizes to fibrin after enzymatic degradation by thrombin	4-6 d [16]	Major component of thrombi, especially in veins. An acute-phase reactant protein. Increased levels associated with occlusive arterial disease.
2 II ⟨Prothrombin⟩	65,000 [9]	336 ± 20 NIH units/ml [20]	Precursor of thrombin	3-4 d [16]	Vitamin K required for biosynthesis
3 III ⟨Tissue factor⟩	220,000[3] [13]	....	Forms complex with VII to activate X (extrinsic pathway)	....	....
4 V ⟨Ac-Globulin; labile factor⟩	200,000 [5]	85-110 [15]	Accelerator of conversion of prothrombin by Xa	15-24 h [16]	Deficiency results in mild bleeding disorder
5 VII ⟨Proconvertin⟩	60,000 [14]	69-144 [10]	Required for activation of X by tissue extracts	4-6 h [16]	Vitamin K required for biosynthesis. Deficiency results in mild bleeding disorder.
6 VIII ⟨Antihemophilic factor⟩	1,100,000[4] [17]	58-181 [11]	Forms complex with IX, Ca, & phospholipids to activate X	12-18 h [16]	Hemophilia-A (severe bleeding disorder)
7 VIII/vW ⟨von Willebrand factor⟩	1,100,000[5] [12]	....	Necessary for normal hemostatic function of platelets. Factor found in endothelial cells.	? 12-18 h [16]	von Willebrand's disease (mild bleeding disorder)

[1] Unless otherwise specified. [2] Progressive rise with age.
[3] Protein component. [4] Subunits: 200,000. [5] Molecular identity to VIII not firmly established. Subunits: 25,000-240,000.

continued

	Factor ⟨Synonym⟩	Molecular Weight	Normal Concentration in Blood (mg/100 ml)	Function	In Vivo Half-Life	Disease Importance
8	IX ⟨Christmas factor⟩	60,000 [7]	60-130 [10]	Forms complex with VIII to activate X	18-30 h [16]	Vitamin K required for biosynthesis. Hemophilia-B (severe bleeding disorder).
9	X ⟨Stuart factor⟩	55,000 [6]	65-180 [8]	Xa in presence of V, Ca, phospholipids converts prothrombin to thrombin	40-60 h [16]	Vitamin K required for biosynthesis. Deficiency results in moderate bleeding disorder.
10	XI ⟨Plasma thromboplastin antecedent⟩	160,000 [22]	91-108 [4]	XIa in presence of Ca activates IX	60 h [16]	Deficiency results in mild bleeding disorder
11	XII ⟨Hageman factor⟩	90,000 [3]	65-175 [19]	Activated by foreign surface. XIIa activates XI.	50-70 h [16]	Deficiency state essentially asymptomatic
12	XIII ⟨Fibrin-stabilizing factor⟩	350,000 [18]	50-150 [1]	XIIIa stabilizes fibrin by forming cross links between γ- & α-chains by transamidation	? 3 d [16]	Deficiency results in mild bleeding disorder

Contributor: Gurewich, Victor

References
1. Bohn, H., and H. Haupt. 1968. Thromb. Diath. Haemorrh. 19:309-315.
2. Caspary, E. A., and R. A. Kekwick. 1957. Biochem. J. 67:41-48.
3. Cochrane, C. G., et al. 1972. In I. H. Lepow and P. A. Ward, ed. Inflammation: Mechanisms and Control. Academic Press, New York. pp. 119-138.
4. Egeberg, O. 1961. Scand. J. Clin. Lab. Invest. 13:140-152.
5. Esnouf, M. P., and F. Jobin. 1967. Biochem. J. 102:660-665.
6. Fujikawa, K., et al. 1972. Biochemistry 11:4882-4891.
7. Fujikawa, K., et al. 1973. Ibid. 12:4938-4945.
8. Hougie, C. 1962. Proc. Soc. Exp. Biol. Med. 109:754-756.
9. Lanchantin, G. F., et al. 1968. J. Biol. Chem. 243:5479-5485.
10. Lewis, J. H., et al. 1957. J. Lab. Clin. Med. 49:211-232.
11. Lian, E. C.-Y., and D. Deykin. 1976. Am. J. Med. 60:344-356.

12. Mammen, E. F. 1975. Semin. Hemostasis Thromb. 2(2):61-84.
13. Nemerson, Y., and F. A. Pitlick. 1970. Biochemistry 9:5100-5105.
14. Prydz, H. 1965. Scand. J. Clin. Lab. Invest., Suppl. 84:78-87.
15. Quick, A. J. 1960. J. Clin. Pathol. 13:457-462.
16. Rizza, C. R. 1972. In R. Biggs, ed. Human Blood Coagulation, Haemostasis and Thrombosis. Blackwell Scientific Publications, Oxford. pp. 333-360.
17. Schmer, G., et al. 1972. J. Biol. Chem. 247:2512-2521.
18. Schwartz, M. L., et al. 1971. Ibid. 246:5851-5854.
19. Veltkamp, J. J., et al. 1965. Thromb. Diath. Haemorrh., Suppl. 17:181-189.
20. Wagner, R. H., et al. 1964. In L. M. Tocantins and L. A. Kazal, ed. Blood Coagulation, Hemorrhage and Thrombosis. Ed. 2. Grune and Stratton, New York. pp. 159-165.
21. Weisert, O., and M. Jeremic. 1974. Vox Sang. 27:176-185.
22. Wuepper, K. D. 1972. (Loc. cit. ref. 3). pp. 93-117.

101. CARDIAC CYCLE AND RELATED CARDIOVASCULAR EVENTS

Phases occurring in the right ventricle correspond to those in the left ventricle, but are asynchronous [ref. 1-3, 5]: right atrial contraction generally precedes left atrial contraction; right ventricular contraction begins after left ventricular contraction; right ventricle has a shorter isovolumic contraction phase and begins to eject before the left ventricle; right ventricular ejection ends after left ventricular ejection; tricuspid valve opening usually occurs slightly before mitral valve opening. The schematic presentation of the left ventricular cardiac cycle does not show the exact duration of events. Left ventricular pressure exceeds aortic pressure only during the initial 45% of the ejection period [ref. 6]. The aortic valve actually closes 5-15 ms before the incisura and the aortic component of the second heart

continued

sound [ref. 4]. In the aortic valve echogram, the superior (anterior) aortic valve leaflet corresponds to the right coronary cusp, and the inferior (posterior) aortic valve leaflet corresponds to the non-coronary cusp. In general, upward movement represents anterior motion in echocardiograms.

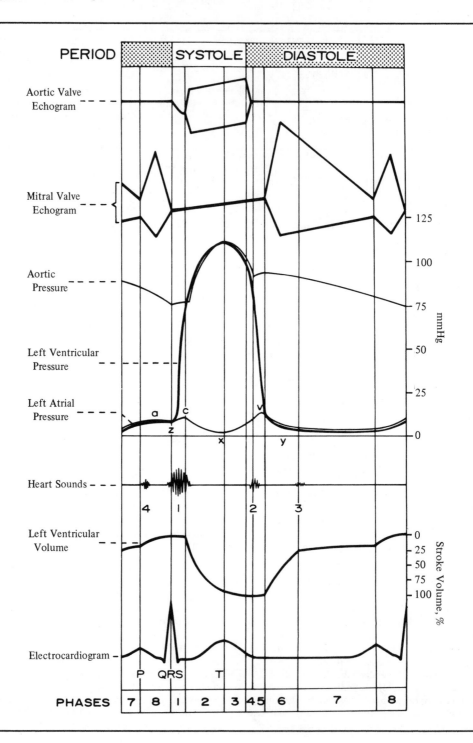

Contributor: Schlant, Robert C.

continued

References

1. Braunwald, E., et al. 1956. Circ. Res. 4:100-107.
2. Gribbe, P., et al. 1958. Cardiologia 33:293-304.
3. Leighton, R. F., et al. 1971. Am. J. Cardiol. 27:66-72.
4. MacCanon, D. M., et al. 1964. Circ. Res. 14:387-391.
5. Schlant, R. C. 1974. In J. W. Hurst, et al., ed. The Heart. Ed. 3. McGraw-Hill, New York. pp. 79-109.
6. Spencer, M. P., and F. C. Greiss. 1962. Circ. Res. 10:274-279.

102. CARDIAC OUTPUT

All subjects were resting. Values in parentheses are ranges, estimate "c" (*see* Introduction).

	Condition	Subjects Age yr	No.	Method	Cardiac Output liters·min^{-1}	Cardiac Index liters·min^{-1}·m^{-2}	Reference
1	Normal	6-9	9	Fick	3.8 ± 0.6	4.4 ± 0.6	23
2			2	Fick	3.8 ± 0.6	4.6 ± 0.8	7
3			17	Fick	6.1 ± 1.0	5.9 ± 1.1	14
4		10-19	12	Fick	4.8 ± 0.7	3.8 ± 0.3	23
5			8	Fick	5.9 ± 2.1	4.2 ± 1.1	7
6		20-29	9	Dye	6.5 ± 0.5	3.7 ± 0.3	4
7			6	Fick	....	3.8 ± 1.2	12
8			13	Dye	....	4.5 ± 1.1	6
9		30-39	10	Dye	6.6 ± 0.6	3.5 ± 0.3	4
10			9	Dye	6.5 ± 1.3	3.5 ± 0.7	13
11			5	Fick	5.6 ± 1.3	2.8 ± 1.0	15
12		40-49	11	Dye	5.3 ± 0.3	3.0 ± 0.2	4
13			18	Fick	7.0 ± 1.8	4.1 ± 1.0	3
14			11	Fick	....	3.8 ± 0.9	2
15			9	Fick	6.2 ± 1.5	....	20
16		50-59	11	Dye	4.6 ± 0.2	2.8 ± 0.1	4
17		60-69	10	Dye	4.3 ± 0.3	2.6 ± 0.2	4
18			8	Fick	6.0 ± 0.6	3.1 ± 0.3	11
19		70-79	9	Dye	4.0 ± 0.2	2.5 ± 0.2	4
20			7	Fick	5.7 ± 0.2	3.0 ± 0.1	11
21		>80	7	Dye	3.9 ± 0.4	2.4 ± 0.2	4
22			2	Fick	5.2 ± 0.2	3.0 ± 0.1	11
23	Anemia, severe	17-67	10	Fick	10.5 ± 2.7	6.4 ± 1.7	5
24	mild	19-45	8	Fick	5.6 ± 1.3	3.5 ± 0.8	5
25	Aortic valve insufficiency	32-58	9	Fick	....	2.5 ± 0.9	16
26	Arteriosclerosis	59	3	Dye	4.4 ± 1.6	2.4 ± 0.9	13
27	Cirrhosis, biliary	29-71	6	Dye	....	4.0 ± 0.8	17
28	portal	14-70	24	Dye	....	5.4 ± 2.0	17
29	Cor pulmonale	50-63	5	Dye	6.0 ± 1.9	3.3 ± 1.1	13
30		33-63	10	Fick	7.2 ± 1.8	....	8
31	Coronary artery disease	52 ± 8	26	Fick	5.1 ± 1.8	....	20
32	Heart failure	40-63	13	Fick	3.6 ± 0.9	2.2 ± 0.5	18
33		25-74	20	Fick	....	2.2 ± 0.6	2
34		58-66	5	Dye	4.4 ± 1.3	2.4 ± 0.7	13
35		57-65	3	Dye	4.0 ± 1.6	2.4 ± 0.9	13
36	Hepatitis, infectious	20-50	10	Dye	....	3.7(3.1-4.5)	1
37	Hypertension	58-66	5	Dye	4.4 ± 1.3	2.4 ± 0.7	13
38		29-58	18	Dye	....	4.4 ± 0.8	6
39		33-71	19	Fick	6.9 ± 3.1	4.0 ± 1.8	3

continued

Condition	Subjects Age yr	Subjects No.	Method	Cardiac Output liters·min^{-1}	Cardiac Index liters·min^{-1}·m^{-2}	Reference
40 Hyperthyroidism	25-78	5	Dye	8.2 ± 2.7	4.8 ± 1.8	13
41	....	15	Fick	....	5.6(3.3-8.5)	22
42	17-55	14	Fick	....	5.2 ± 0.8	19
43 Hypothyroidism ⟨Myx-	....	3	Fick	....	2.2(1.2-3.1)	22
44 edema⟩	25-74	7	Fick	....	1.9 ± 0.5	21
45	41-67	6	Fick	2.9 ± 0.3	....	9
46 Pulmonary fibrosis	22	1	Dye	6.4	4.2	13
47 Rheumatic heart disease	15-67	10	Fick	3.2 ± 0.6	....	9
48	15-48	8	Fick	3.3 ± 0.6	....	8
49	13-62	17	Fick	....	2.2 ± 0.6	16
50 Stenosis, aortic	31-61	5	Dye	4.9 ± 1.9	2.8 ± 1.1	13
51	44 ± 12	10	Fick	5.3 ± 1.3	2.9 ± 1.0	15
52 mitral	32-63	8	Dye	4.6 ± 1.8	2.6 ± 0.7	13
53	37	25	Fick	....	3.0 ± 0.6	10
54	32-58	8	Fick	....	3.5 ± 0.7	12
55	46 ± 2	6	Fick	3.3 ± 0.7	1.8 ± 0.5	15

Contributors: Tucker, Alan, and Reeves, John T.

Specific References
1. Abelmann, W. H., et al. 1954. Gastroenterology 27: 61-66.
2. Balin, J. M., et al. 1956. Am. J. Med. 20:820-833.
3. Bolomey, A. A., et al. 1949. J. Clin. Invest. 28:10-17.
4. Brandfonbrener, M., et al. 1955. Circulation 50:557-566.
5. Brannon, E. S., et al. 1945. J. Clin. Invest. 24:332-336.
6. Brod, J., et al. 1962. Clin. Sci. 23:339-349.
7. Brotmacher, L., and P. Fleming. 1957. Guy's Hosp. Rep. 106:268-272.
8. Davies, C. E., and J. A. Kilpatrick. 1951. Clin. Sci. 10:53-63.
9. Davies, C. E., et al. 1952. Br. Med. J. 2:595-597.
10. Dewar, H. A., and L. A. G. Davidson. 1958. Br. Heart J. 20:516-522.
11. Granath, A., et al. 1967. Acta Med. Scand. 176:447-466.
12. Kasalicky, J., et al. 1975. Cardiology 60:86-97.
13. Kattus, A. A., et al. 1955. Circulation 11:447-455.
14. Levin, A. R., et al. 1975. Pediatr. Res. 9:894-899.
15. Mark, A. L., et al. 1973. J. Clin. Invest. 52:1138-1146.
16. Merrill, A. J. 1946. Ibid. 25:389-400.
17. Murray, J. F., et al. 1958. Am. J. Med. 24:358-367.
18. Myers, J. D., and J. B. Hickam. 1948. J. Clin. Invest. 27:620-627.
19. Myers, J. D., et al. 1950. Ibid. 29:1069-1077.
20. Mymin, D., and G. P. Sharma. 1974. Ibid. 53:363-373.
21. Scheinberg, P., et al. 1950. Ibid. 29:1139-1146.
22. Sefidpar, M., et al. 1972. Experientia 28:915-916.
23. Sproul, A., and E. Simpson. 1964. Pediatrics 33:912-918.

General Reference
24. Wade, O. L., and J. M. Bishop. 1962. Cardiac Output and Regional Blood Flow. F. A. Davis, Philadelphia.

103. REGIONAL BLOOD FLOW

All subjects were resting. **Method:** A = helium breathing; B = nitrous oxide; C = p-aminohippurate; D = sulfobromophthalein sodium (bromsulphalein); E = plethysmography; F = thermocouple; G = dye dilution; H = xenon-133 washout; I = Rb uptake. Values in parentheses are ranges, estimate "c" (see Introduction).

Region	Condition	Subjects Age yr	Subjects No.	Method	Value ml·min^{-1}·100 g^{-1} or ml·min^{-1}·100 ml^{-1} [1/]	Reference
1 Skin	Normal	20-48	13	F	0.9 ± 0.4	5
2		19-36	12	E	3.0 ± 0.5	21

[1/] Unless otherwise indicated.

continued

	Region	Condition	Age yr	No.	Method	Value ml·min^{-1}·100 g^{-1} or ml·min^{-1}·100 ml^{-1} [1]	Reference
3		Hypertension	29-58	18	F	0.8 ± 0.4	5
4		Heart failure	28-44	8	E	1.5 ± 0.4	21
5	Cerebral	Normal	....	64	B	65 ± 16	18
6			32	8	B	50	15
7			21-24	6	B	56 ± 10	9
8		Cerebrovascular disease	28-69	23	B	41 ± 12	17
9		Emphysema	28-59	9	B	68 ± 21	15
10		Hypothyroidism	25-74	7	B	40 ± 10	18
11		Stenosis, mitral	17-52	25	B	39 ± 12	9
12	Splanchnic	Normal	....	9	D	1470 ± 340 [2]	12
13			....	50	D	1405 ± 360 [2]	13
14			19-63	91	D	1530 ± 300 [2]	4
15		Cirrhosis	17-67	39	D	1090 ± 380 [2]	4
16		Heart failure	40-63	13	D	926 ± 340 [2]	12
17		Hyperthyroidism	17-55	14	D	1521 ± 300 [2]	13
18	Coronary	Normal	17-48	20	A	70 ± 13	10
19			40 ± 6	9	I	386 ± 77 [2]	14
20			18-63	11	B	89 ± 16	2
21		Coronary artery disease	33-65	26	A	54 ± 11	10
22			52 ± 8	26	I	288 ± 124 [2]	14
23		Heart failure	25-74	20	B	74 ± 16	2
24		Rheumatic heart disease	54 ± 10	19	I	292 ± 111 [2]	14
25	Renal	Normal	17-48	14	C	1177 ± 161 [2]	7
26			20-48	13	C	1075 ± 68 [2]	5
27			21-62	18	C	1052 ± 259 [2]	3
28			....	14	C	1177(981-1483) [2]	8
29			....	11	G	1184 ± 193 [2]	16
30		Aortic valve insufficiency	32-58	9	C	325 ± 112 [2]	11
31		Cor pulmonale	33-63	10	C	528 ± 236 [2]	7
32	Muscle	Normal	20-48	13	E	1.2 ± 0.7	5
33			17-34	18	H	3.4 ± 0.9	1
34			35-49	14	H	3.2 ± 0.8	1
35			50-75	16	H	3.2 ± 0.6	1
36			19-36	12	E	3.3 ± 0.8	21
37		Hypertension	29-58	18	E	3.6 ± 2.1	5
38			17-34	24	H	4.2 ± 0.9	1
39			35-49	30	H	3.9 ± 0.8	1
40			50-75	28	H	3.8 ± 0.9	1
41		Heart failure	28-44	9	E	1.4 ± 0.1	21
42	Forearm	Normal	23-59	22	E	3.10 ± 1.27	22
43			21-43	7	E	3.31 ± 0.53	19
44			19-50	14	E	4.12 ± 1.98	20
45			18-22	5	E	2.83 ± 0.56	6
46		Heart failure	41-67	7	E	2.00 ± 0.82	22
47			23-56	17	E	2.09 ± 0.78	20

[1] Unless otherwise indicated.   [2] Values are ml/min.

Contributors: Tucker, Alan, and Reeves, John T.

Specific References

1. Amery, A., et al. 1969. Am. Heart J. 78:211-216.
2. Blain, J. M., et al. 1956. Am. J. Med. 20:820-833.
3. Bolomey, A. A., et al. 1949. J. Clin. Invest. 28:10-17.
4. Bradley, S. E., et al. 1952. Circulation 5:419-429.

continued

5. Brod, J., et al. 1962. Clin. Sci. 23:339-349.
6. Cruz, J. C., et al. 1976. J. Appl. Physiol. 40:96-100.
7. Davies, C. E., and J. A. Kilpatrick. 1951. Clin. Sci. 10:53-63.
8. Davies, C. E., et al. 1952. Br. Med. J. 2:595-597.
9. Dewar, H. A., and L. A. G. Davidson. 1958. Br. Heart J. 20:516-522.
10. Klocke, F. J., et al. 1974. Circulation 50:547-559.
11. Merrill, A. J. 1946. J. Clin. Invest. 25:389-400.
12. Myers, J. D., and J. B. Hickam. 1948. Ibid. 27:620-627.
13. Myers, J. D., et al. 1950. Ibid. 29:1069-1077.
14. Mymin, D., and G. P. Sharma. 1974. Ibid. 53:363-373.
15. Patterson, J. L., Jr., et al. 1952. Am. J. Med. 12:382-387.

16. Reubi, F. C., et al. 1966. Circulation 33:426-442.
17. Scheinberg, P. 1950. Am. J. Med. 8:139-147.
18. Scheinberg, P., et al. 1950. J. Clin. Invest. 29:1139-1146.
19. Weil, J. V., et al. 1971. Clin. Sci. 40:235-246.
20. Zelis, R., et al. 1968. J. Clin. Invest. 47:960-970.
21. Zelis, R., et al. 1969. Circ. Res. 24:799-806.
22. Zelis, R., et al. 1974. Circulation 50:137-143.

General References
23. Wade, O. L., and J. M. Bishop. 1962. Cardiac Output and Regional Blood Flow. F. A. Davis, Philadelphia.
24. Zelis, R. 1975. The Peripheral Circulations. Grune and Stratton, New York.

104. BLOOD PRESSURES

Data were collected in the resting, supine state, unless otherwise indicated. **Method:** Direct refers to measurement by catheter or indwelling needle; indirect refers to measurement of arterial pressure by sphygmomanometry. Values in parentheses are ranges, estimates "b" or "c" (*see* Introduction).

Part I. Systemic Arterial Pressures

	Location	Method	Subjects		Blood Pressure, mm Hg		Refer-ence
			Age & Sex	No.	Systolic Mean	Diastolic	
1	Aorta	Direct	Adult	12	126(106-146) 102(88-116)	81(69-93)	7
2		Tilt 70°	Adult	8	116(104-122) 98(89-105)	83(75-89)	7
3	Brachial artery	Direct	3-15 yr	37	105(71-139) 76(50-102)	57(33-81)	9
4			Adult	11	114(74-154)	63(47-79)	6
5				25	119(95-143)	69(53-85)	5,11
6				10	123(95-151) 93(79-107)	72(58-86)	2
7				33	145(85-205)	74(44-104)	10
8		Sitting	Adult	10	125(85-165) 98(82-114)	77(45-109)	2
9		Standing	Adult	11	128(86-170)	82(60-104)	6
10		Indirect	1 yr	31	90(67-113)	61(36-86)	1
11			5 yr	1470	94(80-108)	55(47-63)	3
12			10 yr	2320	109(93-125)	58(48-68)	3
13			15 yr	1657	121(103-139)	61(51-71)	3
14			Adult	25	118(86-150)	65(47-83)	5,11
15			20-24 yr, ♂	539	119	71	11
16				500+	123(95-151)	76(56-96)	8
17				60	123(97-149)	74(54-94)	4
18			♀	302	108	65	11
19				500+	116(92-140)	72(52-92)	8
20				68	119(93-145)	72(58-86)	4
21			40-44 yr, ♂	1064	120	76	11
22				99	127(91-163)	77(51-103)	4
23				500+	129(99-159)	81(61-101)	8

continued

104. BLOOD PRESSURES

Part I. Systemic Arterial Pressures

	Location	Method	Subjects		Blood Pressure, mm Hg		Reference
			Age & Sex	No.	Systolic	Diastolic	
					Mean		
24			♀	495	119	73	11
25				500+	127(93-161)	80(58-102)	8
26				122	134(94-174)	82(58-106)	4
27			60-64 yr, ♂	227	132	78	11
28				500+	142(100-184)	84(60-108)	8
29				52	154(88-220)	88(50-126)	4
30			♀	71	143	81	11
31				500+	144(100-188)	85(59-111)	8
32				87	159(105-213)	92(60-122)	4
33	Radial artery	Direct	Adult	12	140(116-164) 96(82-110)	75(65-85)	7
34	Femoral artery	Direct	3-15 yr	37	105(75-135) 77(49-105)	57(33-81)	9
35			Adult	33	148(88-208)	72(40-104)	10

Contributor: Nutter, Donald O.

References

1. Allen-Williams, G. M. 1945. Arch. Dis. Child. 20:125-128.
2. Bevegård, S., et al. 1960. Acta Physiol. Scand. 49:279-298.
3. Graham, A. W., et al. 1945. Am. J. Dis. Child. 69:203-207.
4. Hamilton, M., et al. 1954. Clin. Sci. 13:11-35.
5. Harrison, E. G., et al. 1960. Circulation 22:419-436.
6. Henschel, A., et al. 1954. J. Appl. Physiol. 6:506-508.
7. Kroeker, E. J., and E. H. Wood. 1955. Circ. Res. 3:623-632.
8. Master, A. M., et al. 1950. J. Am. Med. Assoc. 143:1464-1470.
9. Park, M. K., and W. G. Guntheroth. 1970. Circulation 41:231-237.
10. Pascarelli, E. F., and C. A. Bertrand. 1964. N. Engl. J. Med. 270:693-698.
11. Robinson, S. C., and M. Brucer. 1939. Arch. Intern. Med. 64:409-444.

Part II. Systemic Venous Pressures

All measurements were made by direct methods.

	Location	Subjects		Blood Pressure, mm Hg	Reference
		Age	No.		
1	Dorsal pedal vein	Adult	100	13(9-16)	1
2	Median basilic vein	Adult	100	7(4-10)	1
3	Portal vein (wedged hepatic venous pressure)	Adult	12	4.8	2
4			24	6.8(2.6-11.2)	3
5			6	12.0(9-16)	4
6	Unspecified	3-5 yr	....	3(2-5)	1
7		5-10 yr	....	4(2-6)	1

Contributor: Nutter, Donald O.

References

1. Burch, G. E. 1950. A Primer of Venous Pressure. Lea and Febiger, Philadelphia.
2. Myers, J. D., and W. J. Taylor. 1951. J. Clin. Invest. 30:662-663.
3. Paton, A., et al. 1953. Lancet 1:918-921.
4. Welch, G. E., et al. 1954. Am. J. Med. Sci. 228:643-645.

continued

Part III. Pressures in Cardiac Chambers and Pulmonary Circulation

All measurements were made by direct methods.

	Specification	Subjects		Blood Pressure, mm Hg		Reference
		Age & Sex	No.	Systolic Mean	End-Diastolic	
1	Right atrium	<4 d	8	−2(−8 to +2)[1]	0(−6 to +4)[2]	1
2		1-15 yr	50	4(1-8)		9
3		Adult	25	2.6(0-5.2)		8
4			11	4.6(2.0-7.5)[1] 2.9(1.0-4.5)	5.6(2.5-7.0)[2]	4
5		61-83 yr, ♂	8	6.0(2.6-9.4)		6
6	Right ventricle	<4 d	8	35(20-50)	0(−10 to +8)	1
7		1-15 yr	56	26(13-36)	5(1-10)	9
8		Adult	7	26(19-32)	3.6(2-6)	4
9			25	26(19-33)	3.4(0.9-5.9)	8
10		61-83 yr, ♂	17	26(19-32)	8(4-12)	6
11	Pulmonary artery	<10 h	51	56(40-76) 39(26-52)	27(16-40)	3
12		10-72 h		46(32-68) 29(20-52)	17(8-38)	
13		<4 d	8	30(16-50)	16(0-32)	1
14		1-9 mo	8	21(17-32)	11(6-18)	7
15		1-15 yr	61	24(11-36)	10(3-21)	9
16		Adult	25	22(15-29) 12(8-16)	6(1-11)	8
17			18	23(16-29) 14(10-18)	9(5-13)	4
18		61-83 yr, ♂	17	24(19-30) 16(11-21)	10(5-16)	6
19	Pulmonary capillary wedge	1-15 yr	44	9(4-13)		9
20		Adult	25	6.2(2.8-9.6)		8
21			16	8.4(4.5-13)		4
22		61-83 yr, ♂	17	9.9(5.3-14.5)		6
23	Left atrium	<4 d	8	0(−4 to +9)[1]	2(−2 to +10)[2]	1
24		Adult	18	12.8(6-21)[1] 7.9(2-12)	10.4(4-16)[2]	2
25			24	14(9-18)[1] 9(5-12)	11(7-16)[2]	11
26	Left ventricle	1-15 yr	19	106(85-125)	10(5-14)	9
27		Adult	18	....	8.7(5-12)	2
28			24	....	10(5-14)	11
29			20	109(71-147)	7(1.6-12.4)	5
30			7	113(98-140)	7.9(4-12)	10

[1] "v" wave. [2] "a" wave.

Contributor: Nutter, Donald O.

References

1. Adams, F. H., and J. Lind. 1957. Pediatrics 19:431-437.
2. Braunwald, E., et al. 1961. Circulation 24:267-269.
3. Emmanouilides, G. C., et al. 1964. J. Pediatr. 65:327-333.
4. Fowler, N. O., et al. 1953. Am. Heart J. 46:264-267.
5. Gorlin, R., et al. 1965. Circulation 32:361-371.
6. Grannath, A., et al. 1964. Acta Med. Scand. 176:425-446.

continued

104. BLOOD PRESSURES

Part III. Pressures in Cardiac Chambers and Pulmonary Circulation

7. James, L. S., and R. O. Rowe. 1957. J. Pediatr. 51:5-11.
8. Penaloza, D., et al. 1963. Am. J. Cardiol. 11:150-157.
9. Pongpanich, B., et al. 1969. Mayo Clin. Proc. 44:13-24.
10. Ross, J., Jr., et al. 1966. Circulation 34:597-608.
11. Samet, P., et al. 1965. Dis. Chest 47:632-635.

105. SYSTOLIC TIME INTERVALS MEASURED BY NON-INVASIVE METHODS

Data were derived from observations on 121 normal males and 90 normal females, from 15-65 years of age. Recordings were made between the hours of 0800 and 1000; subjects were supine and fasting. **Regression Equation:** HR = mean heart rate: ♂, 64 ± 10 beats/min; ♀, 70 ± 9 beats/min. **SDR** = standard deviation from regression. **SDRC** = standard deviation of the regression coefficient.

	Systolic Interval	Subjects	Duration, milliseconds			
			Value	Regression Equation	SDR	SDRC
1	QS$_2$ (total electromechanical systole)	♂	410 ± 25	−2.1 HR + 546	14	0.14
2		♀	411 ± 22	−2.0 HR + 549	14	0.16
3	PEP (pre-ejection period)	♂	104 ± 14	−0.4 HR + 131	13	0.13
4		♀	105 ± 12	−0.4 HR + 133	11	0.13
5	LVET (left ventricular ejection time)	♂	305 ± 19	−1.7 HR + 413	10	0.10
6		♀	306 ± 17	−1.6 HR + 418	10	0.12
7	S$_1$S$_2$ (interval between 1st & 2nd heart sounds)	♂	343 ± 22	−1.8 HR + 456	15	0.14
8		♀	345 ± 19	−1.6 HR + 461	12	0.14
9	Q-1 (interval between onset of ventricular de-	♂	67 ± 12	−0.4 HR + 90	11	0.10
10	polarization & 1st heart sound)	♀	66 ± 9	−0.3 HR + 89	9	0.10
11	ICT (calculated isovolumic contraction time)	♂	38 ± 11	....	....	.....
12		♀	39 ± 9			

Contributor: Weissler, Arnold M.

General References

1. Weissler, A. M., et al. 1968. Circulation 37:149-159.
2. Weissler, A. M., et al. 1969. Am. J. Cardiol. 23(4):577-583.

106. ECHOCARDIOGRAPHIC REPRESENTATION OF CARDIAC STRUCTURES

ABBREVIATIONS

AMV = anterior mitral valve cusp
AO = aorta
ARV = anterior right ventricular wall
AV = aortic valve
CW = chest wall
EN = inner surface of posterior left ventricular wall
EP = outer surface of posterior left ventricular wall
IVS = interventricular septum
LA = left atrium
LS = left surface of interventricular septum
LV = left ventricle

MV = mitral valve
PER = pericardium
PLA = posterior left atrial wall
PLV = posterior left ventricular wall
PMV = posterior mitral valve cusp
PPM = posterior papillary muscle
RA = right atrium
RS = right surface of interventricular septum
RV = right ventricle
S = sternum
T = transducer

continued

106. ECHOCARDIOGRAPHIC REPRESENTATION OF CARDIAC STRUCTURES

Echocardiography is a diagnostic examination which uses pulsed, reflected ultrasound to visualize cardiac structures in a non-invasive manner. So far as can be determined from all available information, the examination is harmless to the patient. The technique is enjoying increasing popularity, and is rapidly becoming a routine cardiologic examination.

Figure 1 illustrates how ultrasound can record cardiac structures and provide an "ice-pick" view of the heart. As the ultrasonic beam crosses an interface between two media of different acoustical impedance (which is roughly equivalent to density), part of the ultrasonic energy will be reflected and be recorded on the echocardiograph as a signal. Since all of the structures of the heart move, the distance between the transducer and the structures reflecting the ultrasound will vary, and wavy lines will be inscribed on the recording. Each of the cardiac structures has a characteristic pattern of motion. This pattern is a key to the identification of the individual echoes. As the ultrasonic beam travels through the chest and through the heart, echoes or returning signals will be recorded from the chest wall, the anterior right ventricular wall, the interventricular septum, parts of the mitral valve apparatus, the posterior left ventricular wall, and the lungs.

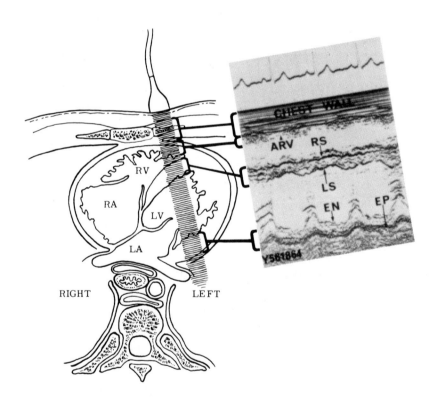

Figure 1

continued

One can enlarge on this "ice-pick" view by changing the direction of the ultrasonic beam. A fairly routine way of moving the transducer is to direct it toward the left ventricle in the vicinity of the posterior papillary muscle and then angle it toward the base of the heart (Figure 2A). As the ultrasonic beam is moved, it sweeps through the cavities of the right and left ventricles, across the mitral valve apparatus and into the base of the heart, including the root of the aorta, aortic valve, and left atrium (Figure 2B).

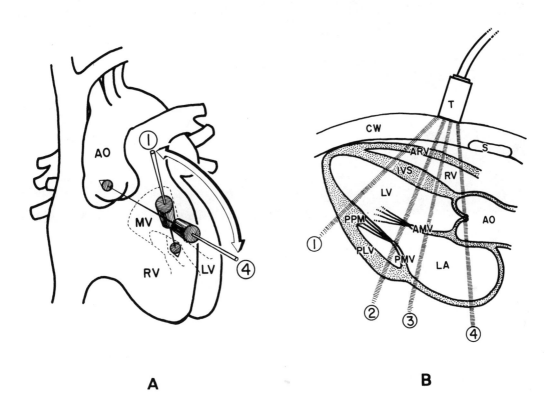

A

B

Figure 2

continued

An echocardiogram recorded by moving the transducer is known as a "scan." Figure 3 is a diagram of the echocardiogram which would be produced with such a scan of the ultrasonic beam. The various cardiac structures recorded by such a tracing are labeled on the illustration.

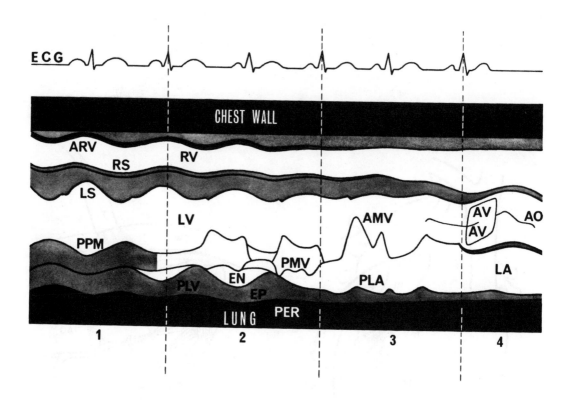

Figure 3

The ultrasonic beam can be directed in other directions, and the pulmonary and tricuspid valves can also be recorded. Thus echocardiography permits a recording of the cavities of the right ventricle, left ventricle, and left atrium, as well as parts of all four cardiac valves. Over the past 15-20 years, investigators have been looking at these echoes, and a large number of clinical applications have been developed.

The echocardiograms illustrated in Figures 1 and 3 are M-mode echocardiograms which represent the standard type of ultrasonic recording of the heart. There are a variety of techniques for creating cross-sectional or two-dimensional ultrasonic images of the heart. With these techniques the ultrasonic recording appears to be similar to that noted in the diagram in Figure 3. Such recordings can be obtained with a variety of instruments, and may be obtained either with a composite of multiple cardiac cycles, or by using real-time mechanical or electronic scanning probes.

Contributor: Feigenbaum, Harvey

General References

1. Edler, I., et al. 1961. Acta Med. Scand. 170(Suppl. 370).
2. Feigenbaum, H. 1972. Echocardiography. Lea and Febiger, Philadelphia.
3. Gramiak, R., and R. C. Waag, ed. 1975. Cardiac Ultrasound. C. V. Mosby, St. Louis.

Data were adapted from references 1 and 3. Lung volumes were measured in seated subjects. Method used was hydrogen in constant volume closed circuit [ref. 4]. Values for dead space are not included but can be calculated from the following formula: Anatomic dead space (in milliliters) = age (in years) + weight (in pounds) [ref. 2]

Subjects		Vital Capacity ⟨VC⟩ liters	Functional Residual Capacity ⟨FRC⟩ liters	Residual Volume ⟨RV⟩ liters	Total Lung Capacity ⟨TLC⟩ liters	RV/TLC %
Height, cm	Age, yr					
Males						
1	155	20	3.97	2.72	1.13	5.10	22
2		30	3.65	2.72	1.30	4.95	26
3		40	3.35	2.72	1.45	4.80	30
4		50	3.04	2.72	1.61	4.65	35
5		60	2.73	2.72	1.77	4.50	39
6		70	2.42	2.72	1.93	4.35	44
7	160	20	4.30	2.98	1.27	5.57	23
8		30	4.00	2.98	1.42	5.42	26
9		40	3.70	2.98	1.57	5.27	30
10		50	3.40	2.98	1.72	5.12	34
11		60	3.10	2.98	1.87	4.97	38
12		70	2.80	2.98	2.02	4.82	42
13	165	20	4.62	3.23	1.42	6.04	24
14		30	4.32	3.23	1.57	5.89	27
15		40	4.02	3.23	1.72	5.74	30
16		50	3.72	3.23	1.87	5.59	33
17		60	3.42	3.23	2.02	5.44	37
18		70	3.12	3.23	2.17	5.29	41
19	170	20	4.94	3.48	1.57	6.51	24
20		30	4.64	3.48	1.72	6.36	27
21		40	4.35	3.48	1.86	6.21	30
22		50	4.05	3.48	2.01	6.06	33
23		60	3.74	3.48	2.17	5.91	37
24		70	3.44	3.48	2.32	5.76	40
25	175	20	5.26	3.74	1.72	6.98	25
26		30	4.96	3.74	1.87	6.83	27
27		40	4.66	3.74	2.02	6.68	30
28		50	4.36	3.74	2.17	6.53	33
29		60	4.06	3.74	2.32	6.38	36
30		70	3.76	3.74	2.47	6.23	40
31	180	20	5.58	3.99	1.87	7.45	25
32		30	5.28	3.99	2.02	7.30	28
33		40	4.98	3.99	2.17	7.15	30
34		50	4.68	3.99	2.32	7.00	33
35		60	4.38	3.99	2.47	6.85	36
36		70	4.08	3.99	2.62	6.70	39
37	185	20	5.90	4.25	2.02	7.92	26
38		30	5.60	4.25	2.17	7.77	28
39		40	5.30	4.25	2.32	7.62	30
40		50	5.00	4.25	2.47	7.47	33
41		60	4.70	4.25	2.62	7.32	36
42		70	4.40	4.25	2.77	7.17	39
Females						
43	145	20	2.81	1.96	1.00	3.81	26
44		30	2.63	1.96	1.08	3.71	29

continued

Subjects		Vital Capacity ⟨VC⟩ liters	Functional Residual Capacity ⟨FRC⟩ liters	Residual Volume ⟨RV⟩ liters	Total Lung Capacity ⟨TLC⟩ liters	RV/TLC %
Height, cm	Age, yr					
45	40	2.45	1.96	1.16	3.61	32
46	50	2.27	1.96	1.24	3.51	35
47	60	2.09	1.96	1.32	3.41	39
48	70	1.91	1.96	1.40	3.31	42
49 150	20	3.08	2.20	1.05	4.13	25
50	30	2.89	2.20	1.14	4.03	28
51	40	2.71	2.20	1.22	3.93	31
52	50	2.53	2.20	1.30	3.83	34
53	60	2.35	2.20	1.38	3.73	37
54	70	2.17	2.20	1.46	3.63	40
55 155	20	3.34	2.43	1.19	4.53	26
56	30	3.15	2.43	1.28	4.43	29
57	40	2.97	2.43	1.36	4.33	31
58	50	2.79	2.43	1.44	4.23	34
59	60	2.61	2.43	1.52	4.13	37
60	70	2.43	2.43	1.60	4.03	40
61 160	20	3.60	2.67	1.32	4.92	27
62	30	3.41	2.67	1.41	4.82	29
63	40	3.22	2.67	1.50	4.72	32
64	50	3.05	2.67	1.57	4.62	34
65	60	2.87	2.67	1.65	4.52	37
66	70	2.69	2.67	1.73	4.42	39
67 165	20	3.88	2.90	1.44	5.32	27
68	30	3.68	2.90	1.54	5.22	30
69	40	3.50	2.90	1.62	5.12	32
70	50	3.32	2.90	1.70	5.02	34
71	60	3.14	2.90	1.78	4.92	36
72	70	2.96	2.90	1.86	4.82	39
73 170	20	4.13	3.14	1.58	5.71	28
74	30	3.94	3.14	1.67	5.61	30
75	40	3.76	3.14	1.75	5.51	32
76	50	3.58	3.14	1.83	5.41	34
77	60	3.40	3.14	1.91	5.31	36
78	70	3.22	3.14	1.99	5.21	38
79 175	20	4.38	3.37	1.80	6.18	29
80	30	4.20	3.37	1.90	6.10	31
81	40	4.02	3.37	2.00	6.02	33
82	50	3.84	3.37	2.10	5.94	35
83	60	3.66	3.37	2.20	5.86	38
84	70	3.48	3.37	2.30	5.78	40

Contributor: Briscoe, William A.

References

1. Bates, D. V., et al. 1971. Respiratory Function in Disease. Ed. 2. W. B. Saunders, Philadelphia. pp. 93-94.
2. Cotes, J. E. 1968. Lung Function. Ed. 2. F. A. Davis, Philadelphia. p. 255.
3. Goldman, H. I., and M. R. Becklake. 1959. Am. Rev. Tuberc. Pulm. Dis. 79:457-467.
4. McMichael, J. 1939. Clin. Sci. 4:167-173.

Data are for standing, healthy non-smokers, unless otherwise indicated. The spirometric data were derived from maximal forced expirations, and are corrected to BTPS. **Test:** FVC = forced vital capacity; FEV_1 = one-second forced expiratory volume; PEFR = peak forced expiratory flow rate; FEF200-1200 = mean forced expiratory flow between 200 and 1200 ml of FVC; FEF25-75% = mean forced expiratory flow during the middle half of FVC; FEF75-85% = mean forced expiratory flow between 75% and 85% of FVC; FEF25% = instantaneous forced expiratory flow after 25% of FVC has been exhaled (similarly for FEF50% and FEF75%); MVV = maximum voluntary ventilation at an unrestricted frequency; C_L = static lung compliance; G_{aw} = airway conductance; D_{sb} = single-breath carbon monoxide diffusing capacity of the lung; CV/VC% = ratio of closing volume to vital capacity, in percent. **Prediction Formula:** H = height in inches, unless otherwise indicated; A = age in years. Values in parentheses are ranges, estimate "c" (*see* Introduction).

	Test	Subjects Age, yr	Subjects No. & Sex	Prediction Formula	Standard Error of Estimate	Unit of Measurement	Reference
1	FVC	5-11[1]	274♂	$0.094H - 3.042$	0.18	liters	4
2			306♀	$0.077H - 2.371$	0.17	liters	4
3		12-18[2]	183♂	$0.164H + 0.174A - 9.425$	0.35	liters	4
4			198♀	$0.117H + 0.102A - 5.869$	0.30	liters	4
5		20-84	517♂	$0.148H - 0.025A - 4.241$	0.74	liters	8
6			471♀	$0.115H - 0.024A - 2.852$	0.52	liters	8
7		20-94	820♂[3,4]	$0.119H - 0.022A - 2.815$	0.46	liters	12
8			357♀[3,4]	$0.093H - 0.022A - 1.924$	0.36	liters	12
9	FEV_1	5-11[1]	274♂	$0.085H - 2.855$	0.16	liters	4
10			306♀	$0.074H - 2.482$	0.17	liters	4
11		12-18[2]	183♂	$0.143H + 0.121A - 7.864$	0.30	liters	4
12			198♀	$0.100H + 0.085A - 4.939$	0.29	liters	4
13		20-84	517♂	$0.092H - 0.032A - 1.260$	0.55	liters	8
14			471♀	$0.089H - 0.025A - 1.932$	0.47	liters	8
15		20-94	820♂[3,4]	$0.085H - 0.031A - 0.897$	0.39	liters	12
16			357♀[3,4]	$0.067H - 0.027A - 0.525$	0.29	liters	12
17	FEV_1/FVC%	20-79	509♂	$107.12 - 0.3118H - 0.242A$	7.79	%	9
18			454♀	$88.70 - 0.0679H - 0.1815A$	6.84	%	9
19	PEFR	4-18	139♂♀	$4.90H - 379.17$[5]	.....	liters/min	13
20		15-79	870♂	$0.144H - 0.024A + 0.2254$	.....	liters/s	3
21			452♀	$0.091H - 0.0178A + 1.132$	.....	liters/s	3
22	FEF200-1200	20-84	517♂	$0.109H - 0.047A + 2.010$	1.66	liters/s	8
23			471♀	$0.145H - 0.036A - 2.532$	1.19	liters/s	8
24		20-94	820♂[3,4]	$0.130H - 0.068A + 0.940$	1.65	liters/s	12
25			357♀[3,4]	$0.092H - 0.051A + 1.100$	1.02	liters/s	12
26	FEF25-75%	5-11[1]	274♂	$0.094H - 2.614$	0.39	liters/s	4
27			306♀	$0.087H - 2.389$	0.35	liters/s	4
28		12-18[2]	183♂	$0.135H + 0.126A - 6.498$	0.61	liters/s	4
29			198♀	$0.093H + 0.083A - 3.499$	0.62	liters/s	4
30		15-79	870♂	$0.059H - 0.037A + 2.612$	.....	liters/s	3
31			452♀	$0.049H - 0.031A + 2.256$	.....	liters/s	3
32		20-84	517♂	$0.047H - 0.045A + 2.513$	1.66	liters/s	8
33			471♀	$0.060H - 0.030A + 0.551$	0.80	liters/s	8
34		20-94	820♂[3,4]	$0.051H - 0.046A + 2.954$	0.84	liters/s	12
35			357♀[3,4]	$0.043H - 0.037A + 2.243$	0.58	liters/s	12
36	FEF75-85%	20-85	407♂	$0.013H - 0.023A + 1.21$	0.48	liters/s	10
37			396♀	$0.025H - 0.021A + 0.321$	0.45	liters/s	10
38	FEF25%	15-79	870♂	$0.090H - 0.0199A + 2.726$	.....	liters/s	3
39			452♀	$0.069H - 0.019A + 2.147$	.....	liters/s	3
40	FEF50%	15-79	870♂	$0.065H - 0.030A + 2.403$	.....	liters/s	3
41			452♀	$0.062H - 0.023A + 1.426$	.....	liters/s	3

[1] H = 42-59 inches. [2] H = 60-78 inches. [3] Subjects seated. [4] Smokers and non-smokers. [5] H = height in centimeters.

continued

	Test	Subjects		Prediction Formula	Standard Error of Estimate	Unit of Measurement	Reference
		Age, yr	No. & Sex				
42	FEF75%	15-79	870♂	$0.036H - 0.041A + 1.984$	.....	liters/s	3
43			452♀	$0.023H - 0.035A + 2.216$	.....	liters/s	3
44	MVV	4-18	139♂♀	$1.50H - 134.61$ [5]	27	liters/min	13
45		18-66	464♂	$3.39H - 1.26A - 21.4$	29	liters/min	6
46		18-71	549♀ [3]	$2.31H - 0.82A - 10.7$	15	liters/min	7
47	C_L	22-47	11♂♀ [3]	$0.150(0.08-0.18)$	.....	liters/cm H_2O	5
48	G_{aw}	....	53♂♀ [3,4]	$-1.846 + 0.0154H + 0.0032A$ [5]	0.296	liters·s^{-1}·cm H_2O^{-1}	11
49	D_{sb}	5-17	21♂♀ [3]	$0.126H + 0.897$ [5]	.....	ml CO·mm Hg^{-1}·min^{-1}	1
50		18-76	61♂♀ [3]	$0.53H - 61.9$ [5]	.....	ml CO·mm Hg^{-1}·min^{-1}	1
51	CV/VC%	16-85	284♂♀ [3]	$0.318A + 1.919$	4.61	%	2

[3] Subjects seated. [4] Smokers and non-smokers. [5] H = height in centimeters.

Contributor: Morris, James F.

References
1. Ayers, L. N., et al. 1975. West. J. Med. 123:255-264.
2. Buist, A. S., and B. B. Ross. 1973. Am. Rev. Resp. Dis. 107:744-752.
3. Cherniak, R. M., and M. B. Raber. 1972. Ibid. 106:38-46.
4. Dickman, M. L., et al. 1971. Ibid. 104:680-687.
5. Frank, N. R., et al. 1957. J. Clin. Invest. 36:1680-1687.
6. Kory, R. C., et al. 1961. Am. J. Med. 30:243-258.
7. Lindall, A., et al. 1967. Am. Rev. Resp. Dis. 95:1061-1064.
8. Morris, J. F., et al. 1971. Ibid. 103:57-67.
9. Morris, J. F., et al. 1973. Ibid. 108:1000-1003.
10. Morris, J. F., et al. 1975. Ibid. 111:755-762.
11. Pelzer, A., and M. L. Thomson. 1966. J. Appl. Physiol. 21:469-476.
12. Schmidt, C. D., et al. 1973. Am. Rev. Resp. Dis. 108:933-939.
13. Weng, T., and H. Levison. 1969. Ibid. 99:879-894.

109. CHARACTERISTIC CHANGES IN PULMONARY FUNCTION VALUES IN DISEASE

Data indicate typical directional changes in representative pulmonary function tests. The stage or degree of the disease, as well as associated or underlying diseases, will influence these changes. *Tests:* VC = vital capacity; FEV_1 = one-second forced expiratory volume; FEF25-75% = mean forced expiratory flow during the middle half of the forced vital capacity; FRC = functional residual capacity; RV = residual volume; TLC = total lung capacity; D_{sb} = single-breath carbon monoxide diffusing capacity of the lung. *Abbreviations & Symbols:* ↑ = increase; ↓ = decrease; NC = no change.

	Disease	Test						
		VC	FEV_1	FEF25-75%	FRC	RV	TLC	D_{sb}
1	Pulmonary emphysema	↓ or NC	↓	↓	↑	↑	↑	↓
2	Bacterial lobar pneumonia	↓	↓ or NC	↓ or NC	↓	NC	↓	↓
3	Bronchial asthma	↓	↓	↓	↑	↑	↑ or NC	NC
4	Diffuse interstitial fibrosis	↓	↓ or NC	↓ or NC	↓	↓ or NC	↓	↓
5	Acute respiratory distress syndrome	↓	↓	↓	↓	↓ or NC	↓	↓
6	Congestive heart failure	↓	NC	NC	↓	NC	↓	NC
7	Cystic fibrosis	↓	↓	↓	↑	↑	NC	NC
8	Respiratory muscle weakness	↓	↓	↓ or NC	↓	↑ or NC	↓	NC

Contributor: Morris, James F.

Reference: Bates, D. V., et al. 1971. Respiratory Function in Disease. W. B. Saunders, Philadelphia.

110. RESPIRATORY EXCHANGE VALUES

Part I. Alveolar and Arterial Oxygen and Carbon Dioxide Pressures

Specification: RT = room temperature. Plus/minus (±) values are standard deviations unless otherwise indicated.

	Subjects		Specification	Pressure mm Hg	Method	Reference
	Age	No. & Sex				
	Resting Alveolar Oxygen Pressure					
1	0-4 d	19♂♀	Sea level	107 ± 6.2	Alveolar air equation	5
2	7-19 yr	42♂♀	Sea level	104.9 ± 1.67	Paramagnetic O_2 analyzer	3
3	15-20 yr	12♂♀	Sea level	103.9 ± 4.0	Alveolar air equation	4
4	21-30 yr	16♂♀	Sea level	106.0 ± 6.4	Alveolar air equation	4
5	31-40 yr	12♂♀	Sea level	104.2 ± 3.5	Alveolar air equation	4
6	41-50 yr	16♂♀	Sea level	104.3 ± 3.8	Alveolar air equation	4
7	51-60 yr	12♂♀	Sea level	102.0 ± 6.1	Alveolar air equation	4
8	61-75 yr	12♂♀	Sea level	103.0 ± 6.7	Alveolar air equation	4
	Arterial Oxygen Pressure					
9	117-121 min	10♂♀	Ambient temp, 38°C	82 ± 5.0[1]	Clark electrode	10
10		6♂♀	Ambient temp, RT	74 ± 5.0[1]		
11	3-5 h	4♂♀	Premature	59.5 ± 7.7	Clark electrode	6
12	5 h	30♂♀	Full term	73.7 ± 12.0	Clark electrode	2
13	6-12 h	9♂♀	Premature	69.7 ± 11.8	Clark electrode	6
14	13-24 h	12♂♀	Premature	67.0 ± 15.2	Clark electrode	6
15	1 d	62♂♀	Full term	72.7 ± 9.5	Clark microelectrode	2
16	1-2 d	22♂♀	Premature	72.5 ± 20.9	Clark electrode	6
17	2 d	47♂♀	Full term	73.8 ± 7.7	Clark electrode	2
18	3-7 d	175♂♀	Full term	70-76	Clark electrode	2
19	7-19 yr	42♂♀	....	95.5 ± 3.68	Radiometer Po_2 electrode	3
20	21-30 yr	16♂♀	....	97.8 ± 6.6	Electrode	4
21	31-40 yr	12♂♀	....	93.1 ± 5.6	Electrode	4
22	41-50 yr	16♂♀	....	92.6 ± 9.1	Electrode	4
23	51-60 yr	12♂♀	....	87.9 ± 6.9	Electrode	4
24	61-75 yr	12♂♀	....	86.7 ± 8.3	Electrode	4
	Alveolar Carbon Dioxide Pressure					
25	1-4 d	18♂♀	....	29.88 ± 3.15	Scholander gas analyzer	8
26	Children	17♂♀	....	36-43	....	1
27	Adults	20♂♀	....	33-44	....	1
28		......	Supine	40.0	....	7
29			Sitting, reclined	39.2		
30			upright	37.3		
31			Standing	36.3		
32	68-89 yr	18♂	....	36.7 ± 3.7	Schol-Roughton (end tidal)	9
	Arterial Carbon Dioxide Pressure					
33	0.5-1.5 min	7♂♀	Ambient temp, 38°C	54 ± 3.2[1]	Micro Astrup equilibration	10
34		6♂♀	Ambient temp, RT	46 ± 2.3[1]		
35	3.5-6.5 min	8♂♀	Ambient temp, 38°C	52 ± 2.7[1]	Micro Astrup equilibration	10
36		5♂♀	Ambient temp, RT	46 ± 4.5[1]		
37	8.5-12 min	10♂♀	Ambient temp, 38°C	44 ± 1.7[1]	Micro Astrup equilibration	10
38		5♂♀	Ambient temp, RT	31 ± 2.1[1]		
39	29-32 min	10♂♀	Ambient temp, 38°C	35 ± 1.6[1]	Micro Astrup equilibration	10
40		6♂♀	Ambient temp, RT	28 ± 1.1[1]		

[1] Plus/minus (±) values are standard error.

continued

110. RESPIRATORY EXCHANGE VALUES

Part I. Alveolar and Arterial Oxygen and Carbon Dioxide Pressures

	Subjects		Specification	Pressure mm Hg	Method	Reference
	Age	No. & Sex				
41	2 h	10♂♀	Ambient temp, 38°C	34 ± 0.9[1]	Micro Astrup equilibration	10
42		6♂♀	Ambient temp, RT	29 ± 1.5[1]		
43	3-5 h	4♂♀	Premature	47.3 ± 8.5	Astrup	6
44	5 h	36♂♀	Full term	35.2 ± 3.6	Severinghaus electrode	2
45	6-12 h	9♂♀	Full term	28.2 ± 6.9	Astrup	6
46	13-24 h	12♂♀	Full term	27.2 ± 8.4	Astrup	6
47	25-48 h	22♂♀	Premature	31.3 ± 6.7	Astrup	6
48	5-7 d	117♂♀	Full term	35.2 ± 3.4	Severinghaus electrode	2
49	7-19 yr	42♂♀	....	37.09 ± 1.62	Radiometer P_{CO_2} electrode	3
50	21-30 yr	16♂♀	....	37.9 ± 3.6	Astrup interpolation	4
51	31-40 yr	12♂♀	....	38.4 ± 2.5	Astrup interpolation	4
52	41-50 yr	16♂♀	....	38.7 ± 1.7	Astrup interpolation	4
53	51-60 yr	12♂♀	....	39.0 ± 3.5	Astrup interpolation	4
54	61-65 yr	12♂♀	....	39.0 ± 2.3	Astrup interpolation	4
55	68-89 yr	18♂	....	38 ± 3.2	Calculated	9

[1] Plus/minus (±) values are standard error.

Contributors: Geiger, K., Laasberg, L. H., and Hedley-Whyte, J.

References

1. Graham, B. D., et al. 1959. Am. J. Dis. Child. 98:593-594.
2. Koch, G., and H. Wendel. 1968. Biol. Neonat. 12:136-161.
3. Levison, H., et al. 1970. Am. Rev. Respir. Dis. 101:972-974.
4. Mellemgaard, K. 1966. Acta Physiol. Scand. 67:10-20.
5. Nelson, N. M., et al. 1963. J. Appl. Physiol. 18:534-538.
6. Orzalesi, M. M., et al. 1967. Arch. Dis. Child. 42:174-180.
7. Rossier, P. H., et al. 1960. Respiration: Physiologic Principles and Their Clinical Applications. C. V. Mosby, St. Louis.
8. Stahlman, M. T. 1957. J. Clin. Invest. 36:1081-1091.
9. Tenney, S. M., and R. M. Miller. 1956. J. Appl. Physiol. 9:321-327.
10. Tunell, R. 1975. Acta Paediatr. Scand. 64:57-68.

Part II. Hematocrit and Hemoglobin Concentrations

Hemoglobin: Method—Cyanmeth = cyanmethemoglobin; Oxyhem = oxyhemoglobin.

	Subjects		Specification	Hematocrit		Hemoglobin		Reference
	Age	No. & Sex		Value, %	Method	Concentration g/100 ml	Method	
1	20 min	12♂♀[1]; 13♂♀[2]	Capillary blood; cord clamping immediately after delivery	55.2 ± 5.2	Micro	18.7 ± 1.6	Cyanmeth	2
2		30♂♀[1]; 27♂♀[2]	Capillary blood; cord clamping after cessation of pulsation	61.3 ± 5.6	Micro	20.0 ± 1.9	Cyanmeth	
3		12♂♀	Capillary blood; forced, late cord clamping	61.0 ± 3.1	Micro	20.4 ± 1.5	Cyanmeth	

[1] For hematocrit values. [2] For hemoglobin values.

continued

Part II. Hematocrit and Hemoglobin Concentrations

	Subjects			Hematocrit		Hemoglobin		Reference
	Age	No. & Sex	Specification	Value, %	Method	Concentration g/100 ml	Method	
4	1 d	19♂♀	Capillary blood	61 ± 7.4	Micro	19.3 ± 2.2	Oxyhem	3
5	3 d	19♂♀	Capillary blood	62 ± 9.3	Micro	18.8 ± 2.0	Oxyhem	3
6	5 d	12♂♀	Capillary blood	57 ± 7.3	Micro	17.6 ± 1.1	Oxyhem	3
7	7 d	12♂♀	Capillary blood	56 ± 9.4	Micro	17.9 ± 2.5	Oxyhem	3
8	2-3 wk	11♂♀[1]; 32♂♀[2]	Capillary blood Capillary blood	46 ± 7.3	Micro	15.6 ± 2.6	Oxyhem	3
9	4-5 wk	15♂♀	Capillary blood	36 ± 4.8	Micro	12.7 ± 1.6	Oxyhem	3
10	6-7 wk	10♂♀	Capillary blood	36 ± 4.8	Micro	12.0 ± 1.5	Oxyhem	3
11	8-9 wk	13♂♀	Capillary blood	31 ± 2.5	Micro	10.7 ± 0.9	Oxyhem	3
12	10-11 wk	11♂♀	Capillary blood	34 ± 2.1	Micro	11.4 ± 0.9	Oxyhem	3
13	3-3½ mo	168♂♀[1]; 165♂♀[2]	Capillary blood	36.7 ± 2.8	Micro	11.16 ± 0.83	Oxyhem & cyanmeth	4
14	8-10 mo	129♂♀[1]; 133♂♀[2]	Capillary blood	39.0 ± 2.2	Micro	11.76 ± 0.64	Oxyhem & cyanmeth	4
15	1½-3 yr	128♂♀[1]; 131♂♀[2]	Capillary blood	38.9 ± 2.2	Micro	11.8 ± 0.53	Oxyhem & cyanmeth	4
16	4-5 yr	143♂♀	Capillary blood	35.4 ± 2.2	Computed	11.8 ± 0.8	Coulter counter	7
17	7 yr	25♂	Capillary blood	38.9 ± 1.97	Micro	12.54 ± 0.83	Cyanmeth	6
18		29♀	Capillary blood	38.6 ± 2.83	Micro	12.47 ± 0.90	Cyanmeth	
19	10 yr	84♂	Capillary blood	39.3 ± 3.23	Micro	13.13 ± 0.82	Cyanmeth	6
20		80♀	Capillary blood	39.7 ± 2.74	Micro	13.24 ± 0.69	Cyanmeth	
21	13 yr	34♂	Capillary blood	41.2 ± 2.36	Micro	13.36 ± 0.94	Cyanmeth	6
22		37♀	Capillary blood	40.4 ± 2.77	Micro	13.31 ± 0.84	Cyanmeth	
23	16 yr	90♂	Capillary blood	43.7 ± 3.26	Micro	14.96 ± 1.07	Cyanmeth	6
24		83♀	Capillary blood	41.1 ± 3.17	Micro	13.87 ± 1.08	Cyanmeth	
25	19 yr	107♂	Capillary blood	45.4 ± 3.04	Micro	15.48 ± 0.90	Cyanmeth	6
26		77♀	Capillary blood	41.7 ± 2.95	Micro	14.04 ± 0.84	Cyanmeth	
27	20-29 yr	294♂	Venous blood	46.34 ± 3.0	Capillary tube	....	....	5
28		71♀	Venous blood	42.50 ± 2.84	Capillary tube	....	....	
29	21-30 yr	83♂	Capillary blood	....	....	15.1 ± 1.22	Cyanmeth	1
30		44♀	Capillary blood	....	....	12.7 ± 1.14	Cyanmeth	
31	30-39 yr	161♂	Venous blood	46.25 ± 2.96	Capillary tube	....	....	5
32		24♀	Venous blood	42.12 ± 3.57	Capillary tube	....	....	
33	31-40 yr	23♂	Capillary blood	....	....	14.6 ± 1.35	Cyanmeth	1
34		39♀	Capillary blood	....	....	13.2 ± 0.92	Cyanmeth	
35	40-49 yr	192♂	Venous blood	46.42 ± 3.34	Capillary tube	....	....	5
36		64♀	Venous blood	42.24 ± 3.16	Capillary tube	....	Cyanmeth	
37	41-50 yr	23♂	Capillary blood	....	....	14.7 ± 1.26	Cyanmeth	1
38		39♀	Capillary blood	....	....	13.2 ± 1.30	Cyanmeth	
39	50-59 yr	147♂	Venous blood	46.94 ± 3.66	Capillary tube	....	....	5
40		49♀	Venous blood	42.43 ± 2.83	Capillary tube	....	....	
41	51-60 yr	65♂	Capillary blood	....	....	14.4 ± 1.31	Cyanmeth	1
42		41♀	Capillary blood	....	....	13.1 ± 1.32	Cyanmeth	
43	61-70 yr	81♂	Capillary blood	....	....	13.9 ± 1.59	Cyanmeth	1
44		55♀	Capillary blood	....	....	12.9 ± 1.33	Cyanmeth	
45	65-69 yr	14♂	Capillary blood	44.90	Capillary tube	....	....	9
46		45♀	Capillary blood	40.87	Capillary tube	....	....	
47	65-74 yr	21♂♀	Arterial blood	....	....	13.4 ± 1.6	Calculated, Coulter counter	8

[1] For hematocrit values. [2] For hemoglobin values.

continued

Part II. Hematocrit and Hemoglobin Concentrations

Subjects		Specification	Hematocrit		Hemoglobin		Ref-er-ence
Age	No. & Sex		Value, %	Method	Concentration g/100 ml	Method	
48	70-74 yr	48♂	Capillary blood	44.76	Capillary tube	....	....	9
49		103♀	Capillary blood	41.59	Capillary tube	....	....	
50	71-80 yr	71♂	Capillary blood	....	....	13.4 ± 1.59	Cyanmeth	1
51		71♀	Capillary blood	....	....	13.0 ± 1.45	Cyanmeth	
52	75-79 yr	76♂	Capillary blood	44.32	Capillary tube	....	....	9
53		185♀	Capillary blood	40.85	Capillary tube	....	....	
54	75-84 yr	51♂♀	Arterial blood	....	....	12.9 ± 1.6	Calculated, Coulter counter	8
55	≥80 yr	199♂	Capillary blood	42.49	Capillary tube	....	....	9
56		589♀	Capillary blood	40.52	Capillary tube	....	....	
57	81-90 yr	28♂	Capillary blood	....	....	12.4 ± 1.73	Cyanmeth	1
58		23♀	Capillary blood	....	....	13.0 ± 1.24		
59	85-94 yr	20♂♀	Arterial blood	....	....	12.2 ± 1.4	Calculated, Coulter counter	8
60	91-100 yr	3♂	Capillary blood	....	....	11.2 ± 2.18	Cyanmeth	1
61		4♀	Capillary blood	....	....	11.4 ± 0.95		

Contributors: Geiger, K., Laasberg, L. H., and Hedley-Whyte, J.

References
1. Hawkins, W. W., et al. 1954. Blood 9:999-1007.
2. Künzel, W., and H. Wulf. 1970. Arch. Kinderheilkd. 180:150-165.
3. Matoth, Y., et al. 1971. Acta Paediatr. Scand. 60:317-323.
4. Moe, P. J. 1965. Ibid. 54:69-80.
5. Natvig, H., and O. D. Vellar. 1967. Acta Med. Scand. 182:193-205.
6. Natvig, H., et al. 1967. Ibid. 182:183-191.
7. Schmaier, A. H., et al. 1974. J. Pediatr. 84:559-561.
8. Smith, J. S., and D. M. Whitelaw. 1971. Can. Med. Assoc. J. 105:816-818.
9. Vellar, O. D. 1967. Acta Med. Scand. 182:681-689.

Part III. Arterial Base Excess and pH

Specification: RT = room temperature. Plus/minus (±) values are standard deviations unless otherwise indicated.

Subjects		No. & Sex	Specification	Value	Method	Ref-er-ence
Age						
	Arterial Base Excess, meq/liter					
1	Fetus, 38-42 wk gestation	65♂♀	Before labor; scalp	−1.2 ± 2.9	....	3
2	0.5-1.5 min	7♂♀	Ambient temp, 38°C	−2.6 ± 1.0 [L]	Micro Astrup equilibration	13
3		6♂♀	Ambient temp, RT	−3.6 ± 1.3 [L]		
4	3.5-6.5 min	8♂♀	Ambient temp, 38°C	−5.1 ± 1.0 [L]	Micro Astrup equilibration	13
5		5♂♀	Ambient temp, RT	−5.5 ± 1.5 [L]		
6	8.5-12 min	10♂♀	Ambient temp, 38°C	−5.8 ± 0.6 [L]	Micro Astrup equilibration	13
7		5♂♀	Ambient temp, RT	−5.2 ± 0.9 [L]		
8	14-20 min	10♂♀	Ambient temp, 38°C	−4.4 ± 0.5 [L]	Micro Astrup equilibration	13
9		6♂♀	Ambient temp, RT	−3.9 ± 1.0 [L]		

[L] Plus/minus (±) value is standard error.

continued

Part III. Arterial Base Excess and pH

	Subjects		Specification	Value	Method	Reference
	Age	No. & Sex				
10	29-32 min	10♂♀	Ambient temp, 38°C	−2.3 ± 0.7 [1]	Micro Astrup equilibration	13
11		6♂♀	Ambient temp, RT	−2.9 ± 0.7 [1]		
12	58-64 min	10♂♀	Ambient temp, 38°C	−0.9 ± 0.5 [1]	Micro Astrup equilibration	13
13		6♂♀	Ambient temp, RT	−1.2 ± 0.7 [1]		
14	2 h	10♂♀	Ambient temp, 38°C	−1.1 ± 0.6 [1]	Micro Astrup equilibration	13
15		6♂♀	Ambient temp, RT	−1.2 ± 0.7 [1]		
16	3-6 h	12♂♀	Premature, >1250 g	−4.82 ± 2.7	Micro Astrup—Siggaard-Andersen	2
17	7-12 h	22♂♀	Premature, >1250 g	−3.87 ± 2.7	Micro Astrup—Siggaard-Andersen	2
18		4♂♀	Premature, <1250 g	−2.20		
19	13-24 h	48♂♀	Premature, >1250 g	−2.44 ± 2.8	Micro Astrup—Siggaard-Andersen	2
20		7♂♀	Premature, <1250 g	−4.14 ± 2.5		
21	25-48 h	22♂♀	Premature, >1250 g	−2.3 ± 3.0	Astrup	10
22	48 h	54♂♀	Premature, >1250 g	−2.32 ± 2.0	Micro Astrup—Siggaard-Andersen	2
23		8♂♀	Premature, <1250 g	−4.76 ± 2.9		
24	3 d	41♂♀	Premature, >1250 g	−3.39 ± 2.1	Micro Astrup—Siggaard-Andersen	2
25		10♂♀	Premature, <1250 g	−5.18 ± 1.8		
26	4-5 d	40♂♀	Premature, >1250 g	−1.86 ± 2.2	Micro Astrup—Siggaard-Andersen	2
27		12♂♀	Premature, <1250 g	−6.15 ± 2.6		
28	5-10 d	12♂♀	Premature, >1250 g	−3.5 ± 2.3	Astrup	10
29	11-40 d	8♂♀	Premature, >1250 g	−2.1 ± 2.2	Astrup	10
30	Adult	5	In blood	−0.94 ± 2.79	Calculated	1
31		12	In plasma	−0.99 ± 0.059	Calculated	9

Arterial pH

32	Fetus, 15-4 min before birth	38	Scalp	7.35 ± 0.05	Micro glass electrode	14
33	0.5-1.5 min	8♂♀	Ambient temp, 38°C	7.30 ± 0.02 [1]	Micro Astrup equilibration	13
34		6♂♀	Ambient temp, RT	7.30 ± 0.02 [1]		
35	3.5-6.5 min	8♂♀	Ambient temp, 38°C	7.26 ± 0.01 [1]	Micro Astrup equilibration	13
36		5♂♀	Ambient temp, RT	7.29 ± 0.02 [1]		
37	8.5-12 min	10♂♀	Ambient temp, 38°C	7.29 ± 0.01 [1]	Micro Astrup equilibration	13
38		5♂♀	Ambient temp, RT	7.38 ± 0.02 [1]		
39	29-32 min	9♂♀	Ambient temp, 38°C	7.40 ± 0.01 [1]	Micro Astrup equilibration	13
40		6♂♀	Ambient temp, RT	7.44 ± 0.01 [1]		
41	2 h	10♂♀	Ambient temp, 38°C	7.42 ± 0.01 [1]	Micro Astrup equilibration	13
42		6♂♀	Ambient temp, RT	7.46 ± 0.01 [1]		
43	3-5 h	4♂♀	Premature	7.329 ± 0.038	Astrup	10
44	4 h	22♂♀	Full term	7.33 ± 0.009 [1]	Beckman, corrected to 38°C	11
45	5 h	36♂♀	Full term	7.339 ± 0.028	Micro glass electrode	6
46	6-12 h	9♂♀	Premature	7.425 ± 0.072	Astrup	10
47	13-24 h	12♂♀	Premature	7.464 ± 0.064	Astrup	10
48	24 h	34♂♀	Full term	7.38 ± 0.005 [1]	Beckman, corrected to 38°C	11
49	25-48 h	22♂♀	Premature	7.434 ± 0.054	Astrup	10
50	48 h	32♂♀	Full term	7.39 ± 0.006 [1]	Beckman, corrected to 38°C	11
51	3 d	29♂♀	Full term	7.38 ± 0.006 [1]	Beckman, corrected to 38°C	11
52	5-7 d	117♂♀	Full term	7.37 ± 0.03	Micro glass electrode	6
53	5-10 d	12♂♀	Premature	7.378 ± 0.043	Astrup	10
54	11-40 d	8♂♀	Premature	7.425 ± 0.033	Astrup	10
55	7-19 yr	42♂♀	....	7.39 ± 0.01	Astrup micro pH electrode	7
56	18-21 yr	7♂	....	7.389 ± 0.01	Electrode	8

[1] Plus/minus (±) value is standard error.

continued

Part III. Arterial Base Excess and pH

Subjects		Specification	Value	Method	Reference
Age	No. & Sex				
57	21-28 yr	7♂	....	7.396 ± 0.007[1/]	Electrode	4
58	27-40 yr	13♂	....	7.41 ± 0.02	Electrode	5
59	60-79 yr	61	....	7.36-7.44	....	12

[1/] Plus/minus (±) value is standard error.

Contributors: Geiger, K., Laasberg, L. H., and Hedley-Whyte, J.

References

1. Bellingham, A. J., et al. 1971. J. Clin. Invest. 50:700-706.
2. Bucci, G., et al. 1965. Biol. Neonat. 8:81-103.
3. Chang, A., and C. Wood. 1976. Am. J. Obstet. Gynecol. 125:61-64.
4. Forster, H. V., et al. 1975. J. Appl. Physiol. 38:1067-1072.
5. Goldring, R. M., et al. 1968. J. Clin. Invest. 47:188-202.
6. Koch, G., and H. Wendel. 1968. Biol. Neonat. 12:136-161.
7. Levison, H., et al. 1970. Am. Rev. Respir. Dis. 101:972-974.
8. Menn, S. J., et al. 1970. J. Appl. Physiol. 28:663-671.
9. Mitchell, R. A., et al. 1965. Ibid. 20:443-452.
10. Orzalesi, M. M., et al. 1967. Arch. Dis. Child. 42:174-180.
11. Reardon, H. S., et al. 1960. J. Pediatr. 57:151-170.
12. Rossier, P. H., et al. 1960. Respiration: Physiologic Principles and Their Clinical Applications. C. V. Mosby, St. Louis.
13. Tunell, R. 1975. Acta Paediatr. Scand. 64:57-68.
14. Wulf, H., et al. 1967. Z. Geburtshilfe Gynaekol. 167:113-155.

111. TOTAL BODY WATER, FLUID COMPARTMENTS, AND TISSUE WATER

Values in parentheses are ranges, estimate "c" (*see* Introduction).

Part I. Total Body Water

The hydrogen isotopes deuterium and tritium are used to estimate total body water by dilution techniques. Deuterium is favored for use in children because of its non-radioactivity; in adults, tritium is preferred because of simplicity of usage. A theoretical error exists due to exchange of the isotopes with hydrogen in organic molecules [ref. 1], but this error is insignificant in practice [ref. 2].

Subjects		Total Body Water liters/kg body wt	Reference	Subjects		Total Body Water liters/kg body wt	Reference
Age	No. & Sex			Age	No. & Sex		
		Deuterium		11	3 mo	19♂	0.625 ± 0.020	6,8
				12		18♀	0.618 ± 0.055	3,6-8
1	Newborn	41♂	0.784 ± 0.013	4-7,12	13	4 mo	11♂	0.646 ± 0.062	3,6,7
2		55♀	0.745 ± 0.023		14		11♀	0.614 ± 0.070	3,6,7,11
3	2-7 d	12♂	0.743 ± 0.010	3,6-8	15	5 mo	10♂	0.640 ± 0.047	3,6,11
4		10♀	0.788 ± 0.011		16		5♀	0.604 ± 0.024	
5	8-27 d	11♂	0.726 ± 0.052	3,5,6,8	17	6 mo	21♂	0.587 ± 0.028	6,8,11
6		11♀	0.707 ± 0.017		18		16♀	0.572 ± 0.027	
7	1 mo	23♂	0.720 ± 0.039	3,6,8	19	7 mo	6♂	0.605 ± 0.066	6,11
8		22♀	0.671 ± 0.053		20		7♀	0.570 ± 0.021	
9	2 mo	9♂	0.670 ± 0.049	6	21	8 mo	12♂	0.608 ± 0.060	3,6
10		7♀	0.627 ± 0.056		22		5♀	0.584 ± 0.056	

continued

111. TOTAL BODY WATER, FLUID COMPARTMENTS, AND TISSUE WATER

Part I. Total Body Water

	Subjects		Total Body Water liters/kg body wt	Reference		Subjects		Total Body Water liters/kg body wt	Reference
	Age	No. & Sex				Age	No. & Sex		
23	9 mo	4♂	0.572 ± 0.012	3,6,7	32	10-14 yr	11♂	0.572 ± 0.034	3,6,9
24		3♀	0.531 ± 0.020		33		11♀	0.562 ± 0.042	
25	12 mo	14♂	0.573 ± 0.060	6,8	34	14-18 yr	7♂	0.618 ± 0.018	3,6,9
26		8♀	0.571 ± 0.040		35		3♀	0.596 ± 0.002	
27	2 yr	9♂	0.616 ± 0.042	3,6,7		Tritium			
28		4♀	0.629 ± 0.053						
29	3 yr	10♂	0.590 ± 0.032	3,6,7	36	23-51 yr	10♀	0.486(0.407-0.559)	10
30	7 yr	6♂	0.583 ± 0.012	3,6,7	37	23-54 yr	10♂	0.543(0.460-0.595)	10
31		3♀	0.603 ± 0.009		38	60-74 yr	7♀	0.434(0.385-0.480)	10
					39	71-84 yr	7♂	0.508(0.468-0.580)	10

Contributors: Lewis, C., and Moore-Ede, M. C.

References

1. Culebras, J. M., and F. D. Moore. 1977. Am. J. Physiol. 232:(in press).
2. Culebras, J. M., et al. 1977. Ibid. 232:(in press).
3. Edelman, I. S., et al. 1952. Surg. Gynecol. Obstet. 95: 1-12.
4. Flexner, L. B., et al. 1947. J. Pediatr. 30:413-415.
5. Friis-Hansen, B. 1957. Acta Paediatr. (Stockholm) 46, Suppl. 110.
6. Friis-Hansen, B. 1965. In J. Brozek, ed. Human Body Composition. Pergamon Press, Oxford. pp. 191-209.
7. Friis-Hansen, B. J., et al. 1951. Pediatrics 7:321-327.
8. Hanna, F. M. 1963. Ann. N.Y. Acad. Sci. 110:840-848.
9. Hunt, E. E., Jr., and F. P. Heald. 1963. Ibid. 110:532-544.
10. Moore, F. D., et al. 1963. The Body Cell Mass and Its Supporting Environment. W. B. Saunders, Philadelphia. pp. 532-535.
11. Owen, G. M., et al. 1963. Ann. N.Y. Acad. Sci. 110:861-864.
12. Yssing, M., and B. Friis-Hansen. 1965. Acta Paediatr. Scand., Suppl. 159:117-118.

Part II. Extracellular Water

Method: ^{82}Br = bromine-82.

	Subjects		Extracellular Water liters/kg body wt	Method	Reference
	Age	No. & Sex			
1	Newborn, 1 d	1	0.439	Thiosulfate	1
2	23-51 yr	10♀	0.227(0.193-0.256)	^{82}Br dilution	2
3	23-54 yr	10♂	0.234(0.213-0.266)	^{82}Br dilution	2
4	60-74 yr	7♀	0.214(0.201-0.229)	^{82}Br dilution	2
5	71-84 yr	7♂	0.254(0.221-0.318)	^{82}Br dilution	2

Contributors: Lewis, C., and Moore-Ede, M. C.

References

1. Friis-Hansen, B. 1957. Acta Paediatr. (Stockholm) 46, Suppl. 110.
2. Moore, F. D., et al. 1963. The Body Cell Mass and Its Supporting Environment. W. B. Saunders, Philadelphia. pp. 532-535.

continued

111. TOTAL BODY WATER, FLUID COMPARTMENTS, AND TISSUE WATER

Part III. Plasma Volume

Method used was Evans Blue (T-1824) in all cases. To convert **Plasma Volume** to water volume, the value for water content of plasma from Part IV may be used.

	Subjects		Plasma Volume	Reference
	Age	No. & Sex	liters/kg body wt	
1	Newborn 15-30 min	50	0.0415 ± 0.004	2
2	24 h	61	0.0456 ± 0.004	2
3	3 mo	...	0.054	4
4	6 mo	1	0.055	4
5	12 mo	1	0.052	4
6	6 yr	1	0.051	4
7	10 yr	1	0.045	4

	Subjects		Plasma Volume	Reference
	Age	No. & Sex	liters/kg body wt	
8	15 yr	1	0.041	4
9	19-24 yr	12♂	0.044 ± 0.007	1
10		11♀	0.044 ± 0.005	1
11	23-51 yr	10♀	0.042(0.036-0.048)	3
12	23-54 yr	10♂	0.042(0.034-0.050)	3
13	60-74 yr	7♀	0.037(0.032-0.043)	3
14	71-84 yr	7♂	0.045(0.031-0.059)	3

Contributors: Lewis, C., and Moore-Ede, M. C.

References

1. Gibson, J. G., II, and W. A. Evans, Jr. 1937. J. Clin. Invest. 16:317-328.
2. Low, J. A., et al. 1963. Am. J. Obstet. Gynecol. 86: 886-892.
3. Moore, F. D., et al. 1963. The Body Mass and Its Supporting Environment. W. B. Saunders, Philadelphia. pp. 532-535.
4. Osgood, E. E. 1955. Pediatrics 15:733-751.

Part IV. Tissue Water

	Tissue	Subjects		Water Content	Method	Reference
		Age	No.	liters/kg tissue		
1	Bone: whole femur, excluding epiphyses	Fetus, 2-14 wk	3	0.0560	Dried to constant wt	3,5
2		Fetus, 20-24 wk	9	0.0546		
3		Newborn	8	0.0488		
4		2-4.5 mo	6	0.0492		
5		5-9 mo	5	0.0437		
6		12-14 mo	5	0.0397		
7		11-12 yr	2	0.0307		
8		18-35 yr	8	0.0227		
9	Skin: abdomen or thigh samples, fat removed	Fetus, 13-14 wk	2	0.917	Cut & dried to constant wt	7
10		Fetus, 20-22 wk	4	0.901		
11		Newborn	4	0.828		
12		3-6 mo	6	0.675		
13		Adult	5	0.694		
14	Striated (skeletal) muscle	Fetus, 14 wk	1	0.907	Cut & dried to constant wt	4
15		Fetus, 20-22 wk	2	0.887		
16		Newborn	2	0.804		
17		4-7 mo	3	0.785		
18		Adult	3	0.792		
19	Adipose tissue	Adult	90	0.147 ± 0.073	Cut & dried to constant wt	1
20	Erythrocytes	Adult	50	0.799 ± 0.042	Dried to constant wt	6
21	Plasma	Adult	15	0.925(0.910-0.930)	Karl Fischer method	2

continued

111. TOTAL BODY WATER, FLUID COMPARTMENTS, AND TISSUE WATER

Part IV. Tissue Water

Contributors: Lewis, C., and Moore-Ede, M. C.

References

1. Allen, T. H., et al. 1959. J. Appl. Physiol. 14:1005-1008.
2. Davis, F. E., et al. 1953. Science 118:276-277.
3. Dickerson, J. W. T. 1962. Biochem. J. 82:56-61.
4. Dickerson, J. W. T., and E. M. Widdowson. 1960. Ibid. 74:247-257.
5. Eastoe, J. E. 1961. In C. Long, ed. Biochemists' Handbook. Van Nostrand Reinhold, New York. p. 715.
6. Valberg, L. S., et al. 1965. J. Clin. Invest. 44:379-389.
7. Widdowson, E. M., and J. W. T. Dickerson. 1960. Biochem. J. 77:30-43.

112. IONIC COMPOSITION OF PLASMA, ERYTHROCYTES, INTERSTITIAL FLUID, LYMPH, AND MUSCLE TISSUE

Values in parentheses are ranges, estimate "c" unless otherwise specified (*see* Introduction).

	Body Compartment	Subjects Age	No.	Ion	Concentration meq/liter[1]	Method	Reference
1	Plasma	Adult	86	Calcium	4.30(3.04-5.27)	Spectrographic	9
2			151	Chloride	106(101-111)[b]	Volhard titrimetric (serum)	6
3			103	Magnesium	1.58(1.01-2.12)	Spectrographic	9
4			73	Potassium	4.06(3.61-4.85)	Flame photometry	9
5			70	Sodium	142(136-158)	Flame photometry	9
6	Erythrocytes	At birth, umbilical	3	Magnesium	4.4(4.3-4.6)	EDTA titration	11
7			3	Potassium	99.6(97-102)	Flame photometry	1
8		1 d	3	Potassium	105(100-108)	Flame photometry	1
9		2 d	3	Potassium	107(100-114)	Flame photometry	1
10		Before puberty	14	Magnesium	3.76(2.86-4.30)	Atomic absorption spectrophotometry	3
11		After puberty	13	Magnesium	4.26(3.68-5.26)	Atomic absorption spectrophotometry	3
12		Adult	50	Calcium	0.17 ± 0.05[2]	Flame spectroscopy	10
13			37	Chloride	67.9(58.9-76.9)	Argentometric	7
14			50	Magnesium	6.88 ± 0.98[2]	Emission spectroscopy	10
15			50	Potassium	136 ± 4.0[2]	Flame photometry	10
16			50	Sodium	12.9 ± 2.0[2]	Flame photometry	10
17	Interstitial fluid	....	....	Calcium	5	Gibbs-Donnan[3]	5,8
18				Chloride	102	Gibbs-Donnan[3]	8
19				Magnesium	2	Gibbs-Donnan[3]	5,8
20				Potassium	4	Gibbs-Donnan[3]	8
21				Sodium	141	Gibbs-Donnan[3]	8
22	Lymph	Adult	40	Calcium	4.2(2.9-5.0)	Autoanalyzer, N-21p	12
23			35	Chloride	103(85-112)	Autoanalyzer, N-21p	12
24			17	Magnesium	1.74(1.32-2.93)	Fluorometric	12
25			39	Potassium	3.8(2.5-4.7)	Autoanalyzer, N-21p	12
26			31	Sodium	138(119-151)	Autoanalyzer, N-21p	12

[1] Unless otherwise indicated. [2] meq/liter of intraerythrocytic fluid, corrected for 20% nonaqueous cell volume. [3] Calculated from plasma electrolyte concentrations, assuming a Gibbs-Donnan equilibrium which takes into account the effects of an excess of negatively charged impermeable molecules (mostly protein) within capillaries which must be counterbalanced by modifications in the ionic distribution of permeable ionic species between intravascular and interstitial fluids. For monovalent ions the correction is 0.95; there is none for bivalent ions.

continued

112. IONIC COMPOSITION OF PLASMA, RED BLOOD CELLS, INTERSTITIAL FLUID, LYMPH, AND MUSCLE TISSUE

	Body Compartment	Subjects		Ion	Concentration meq/liter[1]	Method	Reference
		Age	No.				
27	Striated ⟨skeletal⟩	Adult	3	Calcium	2.8(2.2-3.3)[4,5]	....	4
28	muscle		12	Chloride	0[4]	AgIO$_3$ titration	13
29			15	Magnesium	16.4 ± 2.1[4]	Clayton ⟨titan⟩ yellow	2
30			13	Potassium	165.7 ± 19.8[6]	Flame photometry	13
31			12	Sodium	13.1 ± 8.9[6]	Flame photometry	13

[1] Unless otherwise indicated.   [4] meq/kg muscle wet weight.   [5] Postmortem tissue into which bleeding had occurred.
[6] meq/liter intracellular water.

Contributors: Lewis, C., and Moore-Ede, M. C.

References

1. Acharya, P. T., and W. W. Payne. 1965. Arch. Dis. Child. 40:430-435.
2. Baldwin, D., et al. 1952. J. Clin. Invest. 31:851-858.
3. Boellner, S. W., et al. 1965. Am. J. Dis. Child. 110:172-175.
4. Dickerson, J. W. T., and E. M. Widdowson. 1960. Biochem. J. 74:247-257.
5. Diem, K., and C. Lentner, ed. 1970. Geigy Scientific Tables. Ed. 7. Ciba-Geigy, Ardsley, NY.
6. Flear, C. T. G., and P. Hughes. 1963. Br. Heart J. 25:166-172.
7. Marongiu, F., et al. 1966. Klin. Wochenschr. 44:1405-1412.
8. Muntwyler, E. 1968. Water and Electrolyte Metabolism and Acid-Base Balance. C. V. Mosby, St. Louis.
9. Smith, R. G., et al. 1950. Am. J. Clin. Pathol. 20:263-272.
10. Valberg, L. S., et al. 1965. J. Clin. Invest. 44:379-389.
11. Wallach, S., et al. 1962. J. Lab. Clin. Med. 59:195-210.
12. Werner, B. 1966. Acta Chir. Scand. 132:63-76.
13. Wilson, A. O. 1955. Br. J. Surg. 43:71-75.

113.   ACID-BASE BALANCE NOMOGRAM

This modified Siggaard-Andersen alignment nomogram [ref. 2] permits estimation of base excess (BE), both of blood and in vivo extracellular fluid (ECF). The arc (immediately left of the pH line) predicts the BE which an otherwise normal, chronically hypercapneic patient will eventually achieve in compensation.

In most circumstances, the first step is to measure the pH and P_{CO_2} of a blood sample at 37°C. A straight line on the graph through these two points intersects lines from which can be read total plasma CO_2, plasma HCO_3^-, whole blood BE (at the vertical line of appropriate hemoglobin), and in vivo ECF base excess (at the 3 g/100 ml hemoglobin line). A line drawn from a P_{CO_2} value tangent to the arc intersects the other lines at values expected if a patient with chronically elevated P_{CO_2} of that value were fully compensated metabolically at that P_{CO_2}. The body does not restore pH to 7.40 under these circumstances, the acidemia being a function of the P_{CO_2}, as shown in reference 1. In vivo ECF base excess, denoted BE$_3$, is read at an average hemoglobin of ECF of 3 g/100 ml. This is slightly below the healthy normal adult value, and slightly higher than the newborn or severely anemic subject, the differences being negligible.

$BE_c = BE_3$ at full compensation.

Example: A line drawn from P_{CO_2} = 80 mm Hg tangent to the arc predicts that a patient who maintained this P_{CO_2} over many weeks or months would be found to have pH = 7.323, BE$_3$ = BE$_c$ = 14.2 mmole/liter, BE of blood at 15 g/100 ml Hb of 10.5, plasma HCO_3^- = 40.8 mmole/liter and total CO_2 = 43.5 mmole/liter. If his measured values were: pH = 7.250 and P_{CO_2} = 80 mm Hg, then actual BE$_3$ = 7.1 mmole/liter, and he would have achieved 100 × (7.1/14.2) = 50% compensation.

BE$_3$ is the preferred clinical index of acid-base balance in patients for these reasons: (i) it is the index of metabolic acid-base balance least affected by acute alterations of P_{CO_2} in the patient; (ii) it does not require measurement of hemoglobin, being nearly independent of its value; (iii) it expresses the excess or deficit in the ECF compartment as a whole, and it is this compartment into which therapeutic buffers distribute. Thus, if BE$_3$ = −10.0 mmole/liter, in a 70 kg patient, the total deficit would be estimated to be 0.3 × 70 × −10 = −210 mmole, assuming ECF to occupy 30% of body weight.

continued

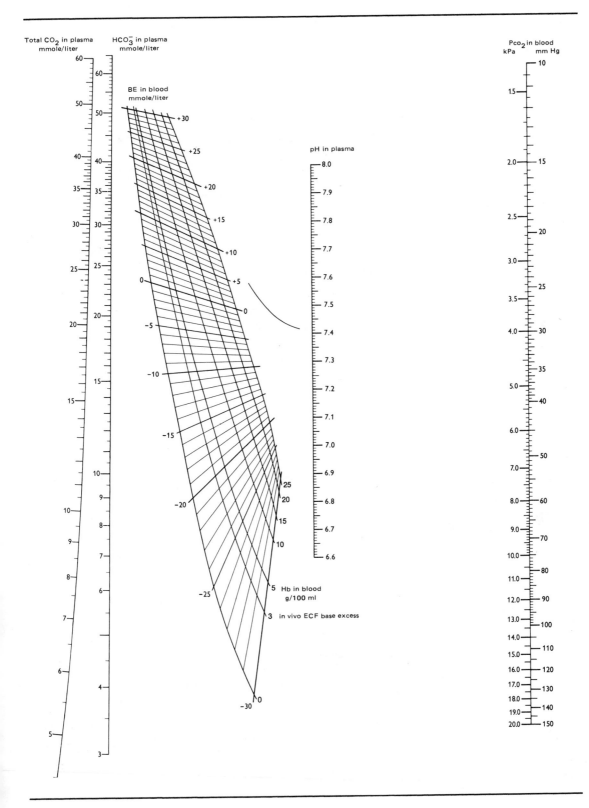

continued

113. ACID-BASE BALANCE NOMOGRAM

Contributor: Severinghaus, John W.

References

1. Brackett, N. C., et al. 1969. N. Engl. J. Med. 280:124-130.

2. Severinghaus, J. W. 1976. Anesthesiology 45:539-541.

114. NORMAL ACID-BASE VALUES FOR ARTERIAL OR ARTERIALIZED CAPILLARY BLOOD

All measurements were made at 37-38°C. Some investigators measure pH and CO_2 pressure, while others measure pH and total CO_2 content. Plasma bicarbonate, or plasma bicarbonate and CO_2 pressure, are then calculated, respectively, using the Henderson-Hasselbalch equation, $pK' = 6.10$, and the solubility coefficient for carbon dioxide, $\alpha = 0.030$ mmole CO_2/mm Hg. The results are comparable for each method. Data in brackets refer to the column heading in brackets.

	Subjects [No.]	CO_2 Pressure mm Hg	Plasma Bicarbonate Concentration mmole/liter	Hydrogen Ion Activity neq/liter	pH	Reference
1	Newborn, 1 d old [33]	33.4 ± 4.1	19.5 ± 2.3	42 ± 3	7.38 ± 0.03	3
2	Children, 5-12 yr old [33]	38 ± 2.6	23.1 ± 1.2	40 ± 2	7.40 ± 0.02	2
3	Adult, ♂ [8]	39 ± 2.4	24.4 ± 0.8	38 ± 1.6	7.42 ± 0.02	1
4	Adult, ♀ [20]	36 ± 2.8	23.1 ± 1.5	39 ± 1	7.41 ± 0.01	4
5	Pregnant, ♀ [305]	32 1/	21.3 1/	36 1/	7.44 1/	5

1/ Variance not provided in reference, but these are the only systematic data available for pregnant women.

Contributor: Lemann, Jacob, Jr.

References

1. Brackett, N. C., Jr., et al. 1965. N. Engl. J. Med. 272:6-12.
2. Cassels, D. E., and M. Morse. 1953. J. Clin. Invest. 32:824-836.
3. Reardon, H. S., et al. 1960. J. Pediatr. 57:151-170.

4. Siggaard-Andersen, O. 1974. The Acid-Base Status of the Blood. Ed. 4. Williams and Wilkins, Baltimore. pp. 103-104.
5. Sjöstedt, S. 1962. Am. J. Obstet. Gynecol. 84:775-779.

115. GLOMERULAR FILTRATION RATE, OTHER CLEARANCES, AND TUBULAR MAXIMA VALUES

Data in brackets are numbers of observations.

Part I. Clearances and Tubular Maxima

C_I = inulin clearance, measured by constant infusion method with urine collection. C_C = creatinine clearance. C_{PAH} = p-aminohippuric acid clearance, measured by constant infusion method. No correction was made for p-aminohippuric acid extraction (*see* Part II). Data include some values for diodone ⟨diodrast⟩ clearance, since available studies indicate values for p-aminohippuric acid clearance and diodone clearance are identical. F. F. = filtration fraction = $100 \times C_I/$ C_{PAH} (or $C_{diodone}$). Tm_{PAH} = p-aminohippuric acid tubular maxima. Tm_{GLU} = glucose tubular maxima. **Method A:** Values obtained using earlier methods (results depend on method used for measuring glucose) [ref. 20]. **Method B:** Glucose determined by methods utilizing glucose oxidase. Values in parentheses are ranges, estimate "b" unless otherwise specified (*see* Introduction).

continued

Part I. Clearances and Tubular Maxima

Subjects		C_I ml·min⁻¹·(1.73 m²)⁻¹	C_C ml·min⁻¹·(1.73 m²)⁻¹	C_{PAH} ml·min⁻¹·(1.73 m²)⁻¹	F.F. %	Tm_{PAH} mg·min⁻¹·(1.73 m²)⁻¹	Tm_{GLU} mg·min⁻¹·(1.73 m²)⁻¹	
Age	Sex						Method A	Method B
				Males & Females				
1	1-2 d	♂♀	18.3(8.0-28.6)[L] [12]	18.1(5.0-48.0)ᶜ [19]	52.9(23.5-128.0)ᶜ [13]	42.4(21.0-72.2)ᶜ [17]	....	28.0 [1]	....
2	3-7 d	♂♀	36.8(15.9-57.7)[L] [33]	39.7(15.0-89.0)ᶜ [28]	90.2(38.2-174.7)ᶜ [9]	36.5(25.8-52.9)ᶜ [9]	21.4(6.6-38.1)ᶜ [3]	50.5(49.0-52.0) [2]	....
3	8-14 d	♂♀	46.3(24.2-68.4)[L] [36]	58.8(30.3-87.3) [16]	132.9(54.3-210)ᶜ [13]	34.4(25.0-49.7)ᶜ [13]	17.6(3.7-57.0)ᶜ [10]	93.0 [1]	....
4	15-31 d	♂♀	52.9(31.0-125.3)ᶜ [15]	44.7(39.4-50.0)ᶜ [12]	150.2(59.3-373)ᶜ [17]	32.2(16.4-50.0)ᶜ [6]	21.7(6.7-46.0)ᶜ [7]	106.7(48.0-198)ᶜ [15]	62.0(37.0-129.0)ᶜ [8]
5	1-6 mo	♂♀	58.6(18.7-98.4) [47]	104.8(81.5-128.1) [9]	266(129-480)ᶜ [17]	29.0(19.6-42)ᶜ [17]	39.3(7.6-93.0)ᶜ [33]	113.2(60.0-175)ᶜ [19]	197.9(95.0-318.0)ᶜ [12]
6	7-12 mo	♂♀	99.0(95.0-103.0) [2]	137.6(93.5-181.7) [8]	461(268-781)ᶜ [11]	24.2(12.1-41.0)ᶜ [11]	61.2(21.3-108.0)ᶜ [10]	....	235 [1]
7	1-9 yr	♂♀	120.5(86.9-154.0) [36]	159.8(94.7-224.8) [12]	597(356-838) [42]	21.7(13.2-30.2) [42]	70.8(29.2-112.4) [30]	....	348(130-557)ᶜ [18]
8	10-19 yr	♂	123.3(94.5-152.1) [36]	138.9(83.9-193.9)[2] [10]	617(415-818) [17]	20.0(11.0-29.0) [16]	95.0 [1]	....	304(247-360) [8]
9		♀	116.2(83.0-149.4) [12]	....	608(336-881) [9]	19.6(13.1-26.1) [10]	88.5(82.0-95.0) [2]	364(313-432)ᶜ [3]	....
10	20-29 yr	♂	123.8(86.4-161.1) [106]	131.6(90.4-172.8) [37]	630(354-906) [67]	20.0(13.9-26.1) [65]	70.2(50.5-112.1)ᶜ [14]	352(276-428) [12]	340(234-446) [20]
11		♀	116.0(82.1-149.9) [43]	143.9(91.7-196.1) [19]	576(332-820) [28]	21.3(11.9-30.7) [28]	....	354(221-487) [23]	295(270-320)ᶜ [2]
12	30-39 yr	♂	124.0(86.6-161.3) [64]	130.6(87.4-173.8) [17]	652(380-924) [35]	19.5(11.4-27.6) [36]	....	348(194-502) [28]	292 [1]
13		♀	122.3(74.7-169.9) [17]	141.4(108.0-174.8) [7]	561(275-847) [13]	21.8(14.7-28.9) [13]	....	278(212-350)ᶜ [5]	....
14	40-49 yr	♂	119.6(76.4-162.9) [68]	122.5(65.6-179.4) [13]	619(339-899) [42]	19.9(13.4-26.4) [38]	79.8(46.4-113.2) [35]	335(170-499) [32]	300 [1]
15		♀	108.9(60.7-157.0) [19]	138.5(92.4-184.5) [8]	563(263-863) [13]	19.0(13.5-24.5) [15]	77.2(55.6-98.8) [16]	391(280-478)ᶜ [3]	....
16	50-59 yr	♂	106.6(62.6-150.6) [46]	117.3(87.2-147.8)ᶜ [4]	542(316-768) [25]	20.0(14.5-25.5) [24]	90.8(83.2-98.3)ᶜ [2]	311(172-451) [26]	....
17		♀	87.3(61.4-135.0)ᶜ [11]	92.3(87.0-103.0)ᶜ [3]	515(263-767) [5]	20.3(14.9-25.7) [6]	48.5 [1]	320(241-445)ᶜ [4]	....
18	60-69 yr	♂	95.9(50.6-141.1) [37]	99.7(75.5-123.0)ᶜ [5]	476(254-698) [16]	21.6(15.1-28.1) [18]	68.6(50.6-83.4)ᶜ [3]	....	....
19		♀	79.3(59.4-100.0)ᶜ [3]	64.3(35.0-93.6) [24]	....	26.0 [1]	....	270(143-398) [22]	
20	70-79 yr	♂	85.0(51.1-118.9) [25]	64.0(34.0-94.0) [18]	354(177-531) [9]	26.2(17.7-43.1)ᶜ [9]	....	238(144-331) [16]	....
21		♀	....	54.0(27.6-80.4) [27]	....	....	....	....	....
22	>80 yr	♂	72.0(29.8-114.2) [21]	47.0(15.7-78.3) [12]	289(105-473) [12]	22.9(14.9-30.9) [12]	....	219(113-326) [9]	....
23		♀	....	46.0(14.6-77.4) [32]	....	....	....	....	....

[L] Although studies have suggested that values for premature infants are lower than those for full-term, group data did not confirm this. All values pooled for analysis. [2] Includes values for males and females.

continued

Part I. Clearances and Tubular Maxima

Subjects		C_I ml·min^{-1}·(1.73 m^2)$^{-1}$	C_C ml·min^{-1}·(1.73 m^2)$^{-1}$	C_{PAH} ml·min^{-1}·(1.73 m^2)$^{-1}$	F. F. %	Tm_{PAH} mg·min^{-1}·(1.73 m^2)$^{-1}$	Tm_{GLU} mg·min^{-1}·(1.73 m^2)$^{-1}$	
Age	Sex						Method A	Method B
Pregnant Females								
24	16-45 yr 1st tri-mester	♀	166.4(117.3-215.6) [30]	187.1(107.0-267.3) [12]	794(506-1082) [15]	21.1(12.7-29.5) [14]	....	379(134-526)^c [6]	....
25	2nd tri-mester	♀	173.2(115.7-230.8) [23]	193.1(131.5-254.7) [24]	786(549-999)^c [4]	23.9(17.1-35.3)^c [4]	....	333(194-472) [16]	156(108-215)^c [3]
26	3rd tri-mester	♀	139.6(71.6-207.6) [75]	163.7(106.9-220.4) [26]	607(359-855) [39]	22.6(13.5-34.3)^c [27]	....	380(278-527)^c [9]	....
27	Postpar-tum	♀	125.3(76.9-173.7) [40]	123.6(83.4-163.8) [10]	572(359-785) [14]	22.4(17.0-32.5)^c [13]	....	....	....
Reference			2-5,7-9,11-13,17-19, 21-28,30, 31,33,34, 36-40,42, 44-46,48, 51-54	13,14,21,22, 31,32,34,37, 43-45,56	3,11-13,16, 19,23,24, 28,30,40, 41,44-46, 48,53	3,11-13,19, 23,24,30, 40,41,45, 46,48,49, 53	1-3,6,9,12, 13,15,35, 47,55	15,18,26, 28,33,35, 46,50-52, 54	10,20,25,27, 29,36,39

Contributor: Robson, Alan M.

References

1. Aurell, M., et al. 1966. Clin. Sci. 31:461-471.
2. Barnett, H. L., et al. 1948. J. Clin. Invest. 27:691-699.
3. Barnett, H. L., et al. 1948. Proc. Soc. Exp. Biol. Med. 69:55-57.
4. Barnett, H. L., et al. 1949. Pediatrics 3:418-422.
5. Berger, E. Y., et al. 1947. Proc. Soc. Exp. Biol. Med. 66:62-66.
6. Bolomey, A. A., et al. 1949. J. Clin. Invest. 28:10-15.
7. Broberger, U. 1973. Acta Paediatr. Scand. 62:625-629.
8. Brod, J., and J. H. Sirota. 1948. J. Clin. Invest. 27:645-654.
9. Brodehl, J., and K. Gellissen. 1968. Pediatrics 42:395-404.
10. Brodehl, J., et al. 1972. Acta Paediatr. Scand. 61:413-420.
11. Brun, C., et al. 1947. Acta Med. Scand. 127:464-470.
12. Brun, C., et al. 1947. Ibid. 127:471-479.
13. Bucht, H. 1951. Scand. J. Clin. Lab. Invest. 3(Suppl. 3).
14. Camara, A. A., et al. 1951. J. Lab. Clin. Med. 37:743-763.
15. Chasis, H., et al. 1945. J. Clin. Invest. 24:583-588.
16. Chesley, L. C., and E. R. Chesley. 1939. Am. J. Physiol. 127:731-737.
17. Chesley, L. C., and L. O. Williams. 1945. Am. J. Obstet. Gynecol. 50:367-375.
18. Christensen, P. J. 1958. Scand. J. Clin. Lab. Invest. 10:364-371.
19. Davies, D. F., and N. W. Shock. 1950. J. Clin. Invest. 29:496-507.
20. Davison, J. M., and G. A. Cheyne. 1972. Lancet 1:787-788.
21. Davison, J. M., and F. E. Hytten. 1974. J. Obstet. Gynaecol. Br. Commonw. 81:588-595.
22. Dean, R. F. A., and R. A. McCance. 1947. J. Physiol. (London) 106:431-439.
23. Denneberg, T. 1965. Acta Med. Scand., Suppl. 442.
24. Dill, L. V., et al. 1942. Am. J. Obstet. Gynecol. 43:32-42.
25. Elsas, L. J., and L. E. Rosenberg. 1969. J. Clin. Invest. 48:1845-1854.
26. Farber, S. J., et al. 1951. Ibid. 30:125-129.
27. Gekle, D., et al. 1967. Klin. Wochenschr. 45:416-419.
28. Goldring, W., et al. 1940. J. Clin. Invest. 19:739-750.
29. Grossmann, P., and K. Zoellner. 1968. Acta Biol. Med. Ger. 20:413-416.
30. Guignard, J. P., et al. 1975. J. Pediatr. 87:268-272.
31. Healy, J. K. 1968. Am. J. Med. 44:348-358.

continued

Part I. Clearances and Tubular Maxima

32. Kampmann, J., et al. 1974. Acta Med. Scand. 196: 517-520.

33. Letteri, J. M., and L. G. Wesson, Jr. 1965. J. Lab. Clin. Med. 65:387-405.

34. McCrory, W. W., et al. 1952. J. Clin. Invest. 31:357-366.

35. McDonald, R. K., and J. H. Miller. 1949. Proc. Soc. Exp. Biol. Med. 72:408-410.

36. McPhaul, J. J., Jr., and J. J. Simonaitis. 1968. J. Clin. Invest. 47:702-711.

37. Miller, B. F., and A. W. Winkler. 1938. Ibid. 17:31-40.

38. Miller, J. H., et al. 1952. J. Gerontol. 7:196-200.

39. Mogensen, C. E. 1971. Scand. J. Clin. Lab. Invest. 28: 101-109.

40. Robson, A. M., et al. 1974. J. Clin. Invest. 54:1190-1199.

41. Rubin, M. I., et al. 1949. Ibid. 28:1144-1162.

42. Schaffer, N. K., et al. 1943. Ibid. 22:201-206.

43. Sertel, H., and J. Scopes. 1973. Arch. Dis. Child. 48: 717-720.

44. Sirota, J. H., et al. 1950. J. Clin. Invest. 29:187-192.

45. Skov, P. E., and H. E. Hansen. 1974. Acta Med. Scand. 195:97-103.

46. Smith, H. W. 1943. Lectures on the Kidney. Univ. Kansas, Lawrence.

47. Smith, H. W. 1951. The Kidney. Oxford Univ. Press, New York.

48. Speck, B. 1967-69. Helv. Med. Acta 34:486-497.

49. Strauss, J., et al. 1965. Am. J. Obstet. Gynecol. 91: 286-290.

50. Tudvad, F. 1949. Scand. J. Clin. Lab. Med. 1:281-283.

51. Tudvad, F., and J. Vesterdal. 1953. Acta Paediatr. (Stockholm) 42:337-345.

52. Weintraub, D. H., et al. 1952. Proc. Soc. Exp. Biol. Med. 81:542-545.

53. Welsh, C. A., et al. 1942. J. Clin. Invest. 21:57-61.

54. Welsh, G. W., et al. 1960. Diabetes 9:363-369.

55. West, J. R., et al. 1948. J. Pediatr. 32:10-18.

56. Winberg, J. 1959. Acta Paediatr. (Stockholm) 48:443-452.

Part II. Other Functions

Data include values for both males and females. E_{PAH} = extraction ratio of p-aminohippuric acid. C_{osm} = osmolar clearance. Values for osmolar clearance are modified markedly by changes in diet [ref. 42]; those cited are for an average diet. C_{H_2O} (max) = maximal clearance of free water. $T^c_{H_2O}$ (max) = the maximal value for negative free water clearance—the value for water reabsorption in the collecting ducts of the kidneys which occurs under conditions of antidiuresis with endogenous vasopressin ⟨ADH⟩ release or after exogenous ADH administration. It is an important measure of the kidneys' ability to conserve water, and supplies more information than can be obtained by measuring urinary concentrating ability alone. U_{osm} (max) = maximal urinary osmolality (concentrating capacity). T. R. P. = tubular reabsorption of phosphate (glomerular filtration rate measured by clearance of inulin). These values vary according to dietary phosphate; those cited are for an "average" intake. **Titratable Acidity** was determined after 3-5 days of ammonium chloride administration. Values in parentheses are ranges, estimate "c" unless otherwise specified (*see* Introduction).

Age of Subjects	E_{PAH} %	C_{osm} ml·min^{-1} (1.73 m^2)$^{-1}$	C_{H_2O} (max) ml·min^{-1} (1.73 m^2)$^{-1}$	$T^c_{H_2O}$ (max) ml·min^{-1} (1.73 m^2)$^{-1}$	U_{osm} (max) mosmole/kg H$_2$O	T. R. P. % filtered load	Titratable Acidity µeq·min^{-1} (1.73 m^2)$^{-1}$
1	Newborn	....	....	3.0(0.9-6.2) [19]	....	426(350-460)[1] [7]	86.5(80.0-90.0) [6]	30.2(26.6-34.0)[2] [3]
2	<1 mo	60.0(34.1-74.5) [4]	1.08(0.24-2.25) [24]	....	3.8(1.6-5.2) [9]	728(401-1055)[b][3] [28]	76.1(65.0-90.4) [8]	....
3	1-12 mo	73.9(51.7-89.9) [5]	1.34(1.11-1.68) [3]	....	3.6 [1]	782(505-965)[4] [17]	79.3(60.0-93.0) [17]	54.7(20.6-95.2)[5] [16]
4	1-15 yr	91.6(81.4-98.6) [5]	....	15.4(10.3-23.0) [9]	6.7 [1]	1090(870-1309)[b] [255]	92.1(83.2-98.3) [11]	30.2(13.9-53.8) [14]

[1] First voided urine after delivery. [2] Premature infants.
[3] Results modified by altering dietary protein content.

[4] Ages 1-6 mo only; equivalent value for 7-12 mo: 906 ± 163 [18]. [5] Cow's milk diet.

continued

Part II. Other Functions

Age of Subjects	E_{PAH} %	C_{osm} ml·min^{-1}· (1.73 m^2)$^{-1}$	C_{H_2O} (max) ml·min^{-1}· (1.73 m^2)$^{-1}$	$T^c_{H_2O}$ (max) ml·min^{-1}· (1.73 m^2)$^{-1}$	U_{osm} (max) mosmole/kg H$_2$O	T. R. P. % filtered load	Titratable Acidity μeq·min^{-1}· (1.73 m^2)$^{-1}$
5 16-40 yr	91.0(81.0-100) [124]	2.54(0.80-4.28)[b] [125]	12.4(5.4-19.4)[b] [104]	5.9(3.4-8.3)[b] [106]	1040(736-1344)[b] [147]	82.0(76.0-87.0)[6/] [6]	34.5(18.0-51.0)[b] [7/] [20]
6 >40 yr	91.4(86.5-96.8) [23]	....	12.3(3.9-20.7)[b] [15]	5.2(3.7-6.6)[b] [12]	....	....	....
Reference	2,8,31,37	5,7,11,13,15, 17,18,22,27, 29,42	1,6,7,9,11,15, 26-29,36,38	3,5,6,10,13, 18,34,41	12-14,20,23-25,40	4,30,33,35, 39	16,19,21,32

6/ Using creatinine clearance as a measure of glomerular filtration rate [ref. 39] value is 88.4 ± 5.0 [45]. 7/ Adult patients, ages not specified.

Contributor: Robson, Alan M.

References

1. Aperia, A., et al. 1975. Acta Pediatr. Scand. 64:393-398.
2. Bergström, J., et al. 1959. Scand. J. Clin. Lab. Invest. 11:361-375.
3. Boyarsky, S., and H. W. Smith. 1957. J. Urol. 78:511-524.
4. Brodehl, J., and K. Gellissen. 1968. Pediatrics 42:395-404.
5. Brodsky, W. A., et al. 1952. J. Appl. Physiol. 5:62-72.
6. Buchborn, E., et al. 1959. Klin. Wochenschr. 37:347-355.
7. Burg, M. B., et al. 1961. J. Lab. Clin. Med. 57:533-545.
8. Calcagno, P. L., and M. I. Rubin. 1963. J. Clin. Invest. 42:1632-1639.
9. Cannon, P. J. 1968. Circulation 37:832-846.
10. Dorhout Mees, E. J. 1959. Br. Med. J. 1:1156-1158.
11. Dorhout Mees, E. J., and H. de Graaf. 1973. Clin. Sci. Mol. Med. 45:469-477.
12. Edelmann, C. M., Jr., and H. L. Barnett. 1960. J. Pediatr. 56:154-179.
13. Edelmann, C. M., Jr., et al. 1960. J. Clin. Invest. 39:1062-1069.
14. Edelmann, C. M., Jr., et al. 1967. Am. J. Dis. Child. 114:639-644.
15. Edwards, O. M., and R. I. S. Bayliss. 1973. Clin. Sci. Mol. Med. 45:495-504.
16. Elkinton, J. R., et al. 1960. Am. J. Med. 29:554-575.
17. Epstein, F. H., et al. 1957. J. Clin. Invest. 36:629-634.
18. Epstein, F. H., et al. 1957. Ibid. 36:635-641.
19. Fomon, S. J., et al. 1959. Pediatrics 23:113-120.
20. Frank, M. N., et al. 1957. Am. J. Med. Sci. 233:121-125.
21. Gordon, H. H., et al. 1948. Pediatrics 2:290-302.
22. Hanenson, I. B., et al. 1963. Circulation 28:867-876.
23. Heller, H. 1944. J. Physiol. (London) 102:429-440.
24. Isaacson, L. C. 1960. Lancet 1:467-468.
25. Jacobson, M. H., et al. 1962. Arch. Intern. Med. 110:83-89.
26. Kleeman, C. R., et al. 1956. J. Clin. Invest. 35:749-756.
27. Kleeman, C. R., et al. 1962. J. Lab. Clin. Med. 60:224-244.
28. Ladd, M. 1952. J. Appl. Physiol. 4:602-619.
29. Lindeman, R. D., et al. 1961. J. Clin. Invest. 40:152-158.
30. McCrory, W. W., et al. 1952. Ibid. 31:357-366.
31. Miller, J. H., et al. 1951. J. Gerontol. 6:213-216.
32. Peonides, A., et al. 1965. Arch. Dis. Child. 40:33-39.
33. Pronove, P., and F. C. Bartter. 1961. Metabolism 10:349-363.
34. Raisz, L. G., et al. 1959. J. Clin. Invest. 38:1725-1732.
35. Richmond, J. B., et al. 1951. Proc. Soc. Exp. Biol. Med. 77:83-87.
36. Robson, A. M., et al. 1971. J. Pediatr. 79:42-50.
37. Smith, H. W. 1951. The Kidney. Oxford Univ. Press, New York.
38. Steinmetz, P. R., et al. 1964. J. Lab. Clin. Med. 64:238-256.
39. Strott, C. A., and C. A. Nugent. 1968. Ann. Intern. Med. 68:188-202.

continued

40. Winberg, J. 1959. Acta Paediatr. (Stockholm) 48:318-328.

41. Zak, G. A., et al. 1954. J. Clin. Invest. 33:1064-1074.

42. Ziegler, E. E., and S. J. Fomon. 1971. J. Pediatr. 78: 561-568.

116.   URINE CONCENTRATION AND COMPOSITION

Part I.   Maximal Urine Concentration and Dilution

	Subjects	Condition	Urine Osmolarity mosmole/liter[1]	Reference
	Infants, premature	Renal solute load		
1		High	640-990	16
2		Low	300-500	16
3		Food & H_2O withheld	300-580	9
4			400-620	18
5			430-780	2
6			620	4
7		H_2O loading	50	2
8			50	4
9	premature & full-term	Varied food & H_2O	425-1200	8
10	full-term	Varied diets	70-450	9
11			70-490	3
12			230-1180	17
13			300-1200	7
14		Vasopressin administration	250-600	1
15	& children	H_2O restriction	200-1300	15
16			240-1300	6
17	Children	Vasopressin administration	500-1500	1
18		Plus H_2O restriction	800-1300	20
19	Adults	Varied conditions	750-1400	10
20		H_2O restriction	400-1200	12
21			860-1340	11
22			900-1400	14
23			1000-1300	5
24			1.015-1.038[2]	19
25		H_2O loading	150-1550	13
26			1.001-1.017[2]	19
27		Vasopressin administration	800-1100	5

[1] Unless otherwise indicated.   [2] Specific gravity.

Contributor: Van Pilsum, John

References
1. Aronson, A. S., and N. W. Svenningsen. 1974. Arch. Dis. Child. 49:654-659.

2. Barnett, H. L., and J. Vesterdal. 1953. J. Pediatr. 42: 99-119.

continued

Part I. Maximal Urine Concentration and Dilution

3. Calcagno, P. L., and M. I. Rubin. 1960. Ibid. 56:717-727.
4. Calcagno, P. L., et al. 1954. J. Clin. Invest. 33:91-96.
5. de Wardener, H. E. 1956. Lancet 270:1037-1038.
6. Donat, P. E., et al. 1970. J. Urol. 104:478-481.
7. Drescher, A. N., et al. 1962. Am. J. Dis. Child. 104:366-379.
8. Edelmann, C. M., Jr., et al. 1960. J. Clin. Invest. 39:1062-1069.
9. Fisher, D. A., et al. 1963. Am. J. Dis. Child. 106:137-146.
10. Goonaratna, C. de F. W., and O. M. Wrong. 1975. Clin. Sci. Mol. Med. 48:269-278.
11. Jacobson, M. H., and W. Newman. 1962. Arch. Intern. Med. 110:211-217.
12. Kaitz, A. L., and A. M. London. 1964. Am. J. Med. Sci. 248:7-15.
13. Mansberger, A. R., Jr., et al. 1968. Ann. Surg. 167:682-690.
14. Miller, M., et al. 1970. Ann. Intern. Med. 73:721-729.
15. Polacek, E., et al. 1965. Arch. Dis. Child. 40:291-295.
16. Pratt, E. L., and S. E. Snyderman. 1953. Pediatrics 11:65-69.
17. Pratt, E. L., et al. 1948. Ibid. 1:181-187.
18. Smith, C. A., et al. 1949. Ibid. 3:34-48.
19. Storey, W. E. 1951. Ann. Intern. Med. 34:737-746.
20. Winberg, J. 1959. Acta Paediatr. (Stockholm) 48:318-328.

Part II. Normal Major Urine Components

Data in brackets refer to the column heading in brackets.

	Constituent	Amount Excreted mg·kg body wt^{-1}·d^{-1} [μg·kg body wt^{-1}·d^{-1}]		Constituent	Amount Excreted mg·kg body wt^{-1}·d^{-1} [μg·kg body wt^{-1}·d^{-1}]
1	Solids	780-1000	18	Hexoses, bound, non-dialyzable	0.3-1.6
2	Water	7,000-42,000	19	Oligosaccharides, as fucose	0.6-2.4
3	Calcium	0.05-11.4	20	Amino sugars bound, non-dialyzable	[200-700]
4	Chloride	40-180	21	Sialic acids, bound, non-dialyzable	[370-800]
5	Magnesium	0.4-2.4	22	Oligosaccharides, as hexosamine	1-2.6
	Phosphorus		23	Acid mucopolysaccharides	[30-140]
6	Inorganic	10-15		Amino acids	
7	Organic	[90-190]	24	Total	20-40
8	Potassium	16-56	25	Free	13-20
9	Sodium	25-94	26	Creatinine	15-30
	Sulfur		27	Protein (non-enzymatic)	0.5-2.0
10	Total	5-21	28	Glycoprotein	[250-500]
11	Ethereal	0.6-1.4	29	Purine bases	[200-1000]
12	Inorganic	4-18		Nitrogen	
13	Neutral	1-3	30	Total	130-300
14	Bicarbonate	0.5-12	31	Ammonia	3-13
15	Lipids, non-dialyzable	[0-455]	32	Urea	200-500
16	Cholesterol	[0-70]	33	Ketone bodies	[600]
17	Glucose	[0-1.4]			

Contributor: Van Pilsum, John

Reference: Van Pilsum, J. 1974. In P. L. Altman and D. S. Dittmer, ed. Biology Data Book. Federation of American Societies for Experimental Biology, Bethesda, MD. v. 3, pp. 1496-1507.

Gastric secretion was measured as acid output, and reported as meq titratable acid/hour. Secretions were titrated with a glass electrode or phenol red to pH 7.0-7.2. **BAO** = basal acid output; one-hour basal collection. **Stimulants:** Pentagastrin—6 μg/kg body weight of pentagastrin ⟨Peptavlon⟩, administered subcutaneously; histamine—40 μg/kg body weight of histamine phosphate after an intramuscular injection of antihistamine during the basal collection; betazole dihydrochloride—1.5 mg/kg body weight of betazole di-hydrochloride ⟨Histalog⟩, administered subcutaneously. **PAO** = peak acid output—the highest half-hour acid output after stimulation, multiplied by 2. **MAO** = maximal acid output—the highest acid output collected during the hour after stimulation. Plus/minus (±) values are 2 standard deviations. Data in brackets refer to the column heading in brackets. Values in parentheses are ranges, estimate "c" (*see* Introduction). For additional information, consult reference 6.

	Subjects			BAO meq/h	Stimulants	PAO [MAO] meq/h	Reference
	Condition	Age yr	No. & Sex				
1	Normal	Adult	16	....	Pentagastrin	28(0.1-45)	5
2			♂	1(0-5)	Histamine, pentagastrin, betazole dihydrochloride	22(<1-45)	2
3			♀	1(0-5)	Histamine, pentagastrin, betazole dihydrochloride	12(<1-30)	2
4		13-80	42	....	Betazole dihydrochloride	[24.7(15-35)]	4
5		19-65	20♀	1.1 ± 1.75	Histamine	12.3 ± 8.95 [9.4 ± 7.2]	1
6		19-66	20♂	1.3 ± 1.59	Histamine	21.6 ± 13.8 [17.1 ± 11.94]	1
7		42.3	43♀	....	Histamine	[20.6]	3
8		49.7	89♂	....	Histamine	[25.6]	3
9	Gastric ulcer	Adult	6	....	Pentagastrin	8(0-12)	5
10			♂	1(0-5)	Pentagastrin, histamine, betazole dihydrochloride	23(3-40)	2
11			♀	1(0-2)	Pentagastrin, histamine, betazole dihydrochloride	10(1-30)	2
12		58.1	62♂	....	Histamine	[16.7]	3
13		61.5	97♀	....	Histamine	[12.9]	3
14	Duodenal ulcer	Adult	57	....	Pentagastrin	44(15-75)	5
15			♂	4(0-15)	Pentagastrin, histamine, betazole dihydrochloride	42(15-100)	2
16			♀	2(0-5)	Pentagastrin, histamine, betazole dihydrochloride	32(15-100)	2
17		13-80	48	....	Betazole dihydrochloride	[31.6(2-80)]	4
18		50.8	81♀	....	Histamine	[32.3]	3
19		54.2	268♂	....	Histamine	[43.9]	3

Contributor: Cerda, James J.

References
1. Baron, J. H. 1963. Gut 4:136-144.
2. Baron, J. H. 1973. Clin. Gastroenterol. 2(2):293-314.
3. Christiansen, P. M. 1968. In L. S. Semb and J. Myren, ed. The Physiology of Gastric Secretion. Williams and Wilkins, Baltimore. p. 570.
4. Goldenberg, J., et al. 1967. Am. J. Dig. Dis. 12:468-474.
5. Johnston, E., and K. Jepson. 1967. Lancet 2:585-588.
6. Kay, A. W. 1967. Gastroenterology 54:834-843.

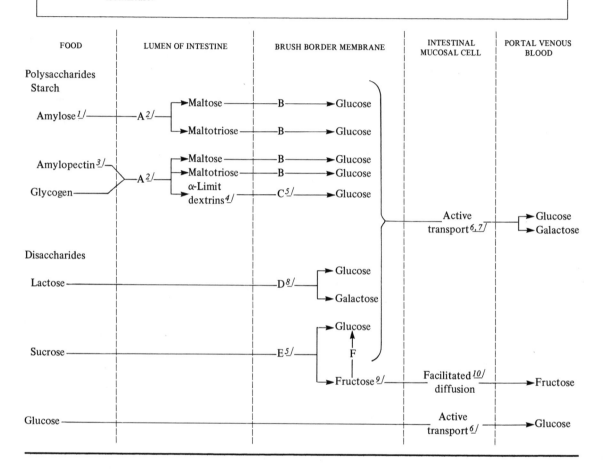

ENZYME ⟨SYNONYM⟩ KEY

A = α-amylase, salivary and pancreatic
B = α-glucosidase ⟨maltase⟩
C = oligo-1,6-glucosidase ⟨α-limit dextrinase, isomaltase⟩

D = β-galactosidase ⟨lactase⟩
E = β-fructofuranosidase ⟨sucrase⟩
F = glucosephosphate isomerase

1/ Amylose is a straight-chain polymer of glucose, with α-1,4-glucosidic linkages. 2/ α-Amylase hydrolyzes 1,4-glucosidic linkages in chains of glucose containing four or more residues; it does not split maltotriose or maltose. It does not split the 1,6-linkages in amylopectin, and acts only weakly on the 1,4-linkages adjacent to the 1,6-branching points, so that oligosaccharides with five-to-eight residues, the α-limit dextrins, are also formed as luminal end products. 3/ Amylopectin and glycogen are branched-chain polymers of glucose, with α-1,4-linkages in the straight-chain portions, and α-1,6-linkages at the points of branching. 4/ α-Limit dextrins consist of moderate-sized (molecular weight, 1500), branched saccharides having both 1,4- and 1,6-linkages. 5/ Sucrose and the α-limit dextrins are split by enzymes that are linked. There may be a rare congenital deficiency

of both enzymes, the so-called "sucrase-isomaltase deficiency." 6/ Active transport indicates "uphill" movement against a cell-to-lumen concentration gradient by a process that requires stereospecificity, energy, and Na⁺. 7/ However, there may rarely occur a congenital impairment of this active-transport system, i.e., the inability to transport glucose and galactose. 8/ Lactose hydrolysis may be diminished by congenital or acquired β-galactosidase ⟨lactase⟩ deficiency. 9/ Some fructose is transformed into glucose in the intestinal mucosal cell, and some passes through unchanged. 10/ Facilitated diffusion is a process requiring a specific entry mechanism, but in which the saccharide moves down its concentration gradient; energy and Na⁺ are not required.

continued

118. CARBOHYDRATE DIGESTION AND ABSORPTION

Contributor: Sleisenger, Marvin H.

Reference: Crane, R. K. 1974. Biomembranes 4A:541-553.

119. PROTEIN DIGESTION AND ABSORPTION

Pepsin, trypsin, and chymotrypsin are endopeptidases, i.e., they hydrolyze peptide bonds in the interior of the peptide chains as well as terminal bonds. The carboxypeptidases and aminopeptidase (cytosol) ⟨leucine aminopeptidase⟩ are exopeptidases, and can act only on terminal peptide bonds.

REACTIONS

I: Ingested protein is split by gastric pepsin into poly-peptides.

II: Polypeptides are hydrolyzed to oligopeptides by pancreatic proteases and peptidases.

III: Oligopeptides are split into di- and tri-peptides by brush border aminopeptidase.

IV: The bulk of di- and tri-peptides are actively transported into the cell.

V: A small amount is split on the brush border.

VI: Cytosol peptidases split di- and tri-peptides.

VII: Amino acids, released in reactions I, II, III, V, & VI, are actively transported into the mucosa unaltered except for transamination of glutamic acid. (The active transport of di- and tri-peptides (IV) is via a separate pathway.)

ENZYME KEY

A = pepsin A (hydrolyzes peptide bonds in which an aromatic amino acid is present)

B = trypsin (hydrolyzes peptide bonds to which L-arginine or L-lysine contributes the carbonyl group)

C = chymotrypsin (hydrolyzes peptide bonds in which an aromatic amino acid contributes the carbonyl group)

D = elastase (hydrolyzes peptide bonds in which an aliphatic amino acid contributes the carbonyl group)

E = carboxypeptidase A (acts on those linkages in which a non-basic amino acid, particularly a neutral aromatic amino acid, is C-terminal and has a free carboxyl group)

F = carboxypeptidase B (acts on those linkages in which a basic amino acid is C-terminal and has a free carboxyl group)

G = oligopeptidases (aminopeptidases) of brush border, most active against peptides containing bulky aliphatic or aromatic amino acids

H = di- and tri-peptidases; 15% in brush border, 85% in cytosol

---

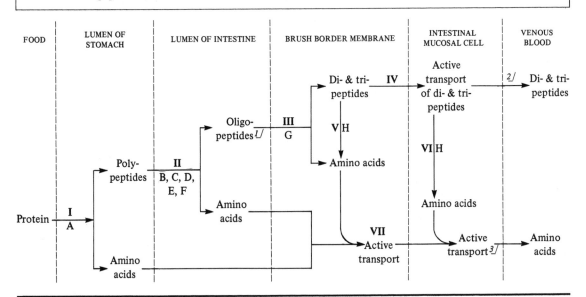

---

[1] Composed of 2-6 amino acids. [2] Whether di- and tri-peptides pass from cell to portal vein is a question at present. [3] In Hartnup disease, neutral amino acids are not transported, i.e., there is a congenital defect of transport. The same holds true for dibasic amino acids in congenital cystinuria.

Contributor: Sleisenger, Marvin H.

Reference: Matthews, D. M. 1975. Physiol. Rev. 55(4):537-608.

120. LIPID DIGESTION AND ABSORPTION

Abbreviations: ATP = adenosine 5'-triphosphate; CoA = coenzyme A; FAB = fatty-acid-binding protein.

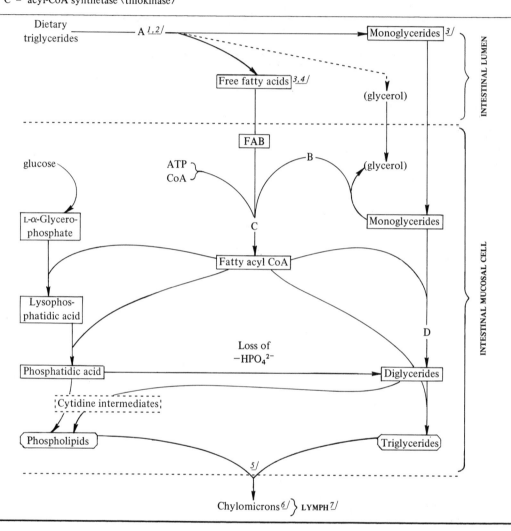

ENZYME ⟨SYNONYM⟩ KEY

A = triacylglycerol lipase ⟨pancreatic lipase⟩
B = monoacylglycerol lipase ⟨monoglyceride lipase⟩
C = acyl-CoA synthetase ⟨thiokinase⟩

D = acylglycerol palmitoyltransferase ⟨monoglyceride acylase⟩

[1]/ Triacylglycerol lipase ⟨pancreatic lipase⟩ acts preferentially on ester linkages at the terminal or 1 position of glycerol. Thus the major products of digestion are fatty acids and monoglycerides. In pancreatic disease, concentration of triacylglycerol lipase in the jejunum may be decreased. [2]/ Bile salts in their conjugated form participate in at least three reactions during fat digestion and absorption: (i) as a cofactor for triacylglycerol lipase ⟨pancreatic lipase⟩; (ii) to form micelles containing monoglyceride and fatty acid, as well as other lipids, including vitamins A, D, and K (these micelles are probably the form in which lipid is presented to the mucosal cell for absorption); (iii) as a cofactor for acyl-CoA synthetase in the intestinal mucosal cell. [3]/ Ab-

sorption of fatty acids and monoglycerides will be diminished if concentration of conjugated bile salts falls below a critical level. Cellular disease will also diminish absorption. [4]/ Fatty acids are transported into the cell by a protein, fatty-acid-binding protein. [5]/ Absorbed fatty acids go mainly into the triglycerides of chylomicrons, but small amounts are synthesized into cholesterol esters and phospholipids which also are constituents of chylomicrons. [6]/ Formation of chylomicrons may be impaired constitutionally (abetalipoproteinemia), and fat not pass into the lymphatics. [7]/ Fatty acids with chain lengths shorter than 10 carbon atoms are absorbed mainly into the portal blood, those with longer chain lengths mainly into the lymph.

continued

204

120. LIPID DIGESTION AND ABSORPTION

Contributor: Sleisenger, Marvin H.

Reference: Isselbacher, K. J. 1967. Fed. Proc. Fed. Am. Soc. Exp. Biol. 26:1420-1431.

121. VITAMIN AND MINERAL ABSORPTION

Part I. Folic Acid Absorption

Folic acid is a general name for pteroylglutamates. *Abbreviations & Symbols:* PPG = pteroylpolyglutamates; PMG = pteroylglutamate; 5-Me-THF = 5-methyltetrahydrofolate; A = hydrolyzing enzymes; B and C are reducing and methylating enzymes.

REACTIONS

I: PPG is broken down by A to PMG, probably at the cell surface, but possibly also in the lumen.

II: PMG enters the cell probably requiring a carrier for entry. Transport is probably active.

III: PMG attaches to receptors.

IV: PMG is acted on by B and C, and becomes 5-Me-THF.

V: 5-Me-THF passes into the portal blood.

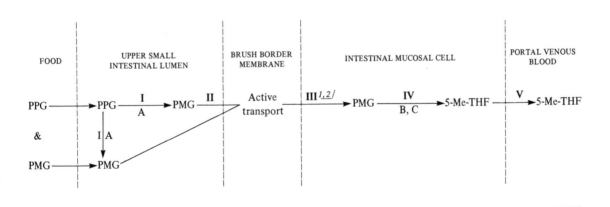

---

[1] Very rarely, receptors may be congenitally absent. [2] Transport may also be impaired by certain drugs, particularly diphenylhydantoin.

Contributor: Sleisenger, Marvin H.

Reference: Rosenberg, I. H. 1975. N. Engl. J. Med. 293:1303-1308.

continued

121. VITAMIN AND MINERAL ABSORPTION

Part II. Vitamin B_{12} Absorption

Abbreviations: B_{12} = vitamin B_{12}; I.F. = Castle's intrinsic factor; TC II = transcobalamin II.

MECHANISMS

I: B_{12} combines with I.F. secreted by the stomach.

II: Pancreatic trypsin is required for efficient I.F.-mediated B_{12} absorption. Mechanism is unclear. Recent works suggests that trypsin acts on the I.F.-B_{12} complex. It is not required for attachment to microvillus membrane. It probably influences transcellular transport of B_{12}.

III: Ca^{2+} and a pH of 5.5 are required for attachment of I.F.-B_{12} complex to ileal surface.

IV: Specific receptors for I.F.-B_{12} are located in the brush border membrane.

V: Little is known about transcellular transport or how or when B_{12} is released from I.F.-B_{12} complex. There is some evidence that some of the transported B_{12} is associated with mitochondria. Fate of I.F. is unknown.

VI: In plasma, B_{12} is bound to a protein, transcobalamin II.

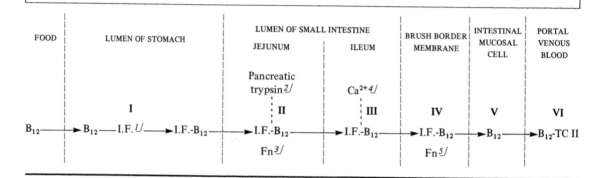

---

[1] Interference with absorption will occur if the stomach does not secrete I.F. (as in pernicious anemia, or total gastrectomy). [2] Pancreatic insufficiency may also be associated with failure of normal B_{12} absorption. [3] Aerobic and anaerobic gram-negative bacteria interfere with absorption in competing for dietary B_{12} by binding the I.F.-B_{12} complex, making it unavailable for ileal attachment. [4] Absorption will also be subnormal if concentration of Ca^{2+} is sub-optimal. [5] One child with TC II deficiency absorbed B_{12} poorly, thus raising the possibility of a role for TC II in B_{12} absorption. In selective malabsorption of B_{12}, the defect is unknown. The ileal receptors are normal.

Contributor: Sleisenger, Marvin H.

Reference: Donaldson, R. M. 1975. In B. M. Babion, ed. Cobalamin. J. Wiley, New York. pp. 335-368.

Part III. Calcium Absorption

For optimal transport of the calcium ion, 50 meq/liter of sodium ion is required in the intestinal lumen. In the brush border of the intestinal cell, Ca^{2+} combines with a binding protein, the synthesis of which is stimulated by $1\alpha,25$-dihydroxy-vitamin D_3. This in turn requires normal absorption of vitamin D_2 and its conversion to $1\alpha,25$-dihydroxy-vitamin D_3 by sequential action of the liver and kidney, respectively. (Thus absorption of Ca^{2+} is subnormal in disorders causing steatorrhea and in kidney disease.) Mode of extrusion of Ca^{2+} from cell into circulation is not known. *Symbols:* A = $1\alpha,25$-dihydroxy-vitamin D_3; B = binding protein.

continued

121. VITAMIN AND MINERAL ABSORPTION

Part III. Calcium Absorption

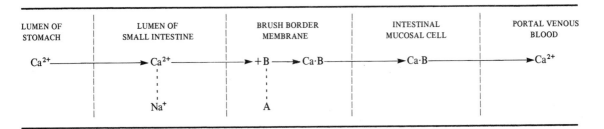

LUMEN OF STOMACH	LUMEN OF SMALL INTESTINE	BRUSH BORDER MEMBRANE	INTESTINAL MUCOSAL CELL	PORTAL VENOUS BLOOD

Contributor: Sleisenger, Marvin H.

Reference: DeLuca, H. F. 1976. J. Lab. Clin. Med. 87:7-26.

Part IV. Iron Absorption

Iron in the diet is absorbed both in inorganic form and as heme. The latter appears to be more important. Inorganic iron is released in the stomach from food. Hemoglobin is broken down by gastric pepsin A to heme, globin, and inorganic iron. Inorganic iron is absorbed from the upper small intestine by an active process as both Fe^{2+} and Fe^{3+}. Both are chelated before entering the cell. H^+ aids chelation and solution of Fe^{3+}, and Fe^{3+} may be reduced by ascorbic acid. This facilitates iron absorption, since Fe^{2+} is more readily transportable. Heme enters the duodenal and jejunal epithelial cells by an unknown process, possibly aided by Castle's intrinsic factor. Heme is broken down intracellularly by microsomal heme oxygenase (decyclizing), releasing Fe^{2+} which then passes into the portal circulation.

ABBREVIATIONS & SYMBOLS

Prec. che. = precipitating chelates, dietary
Hb = hemoglobin
A = pepsin A
Che = chelators: ascorbic acid, carbohydrates, amino
      acids, & pyrroles
Red. ag. = reducing agent, e.g., ascorbic acid

Glut. = glutathione, a reducing agent
I.F. = Castle's intrinsic factor
B = proteases
C = microsomal heme oxygenase (decyclizing)
Glob. = iron-binding globulins: transferrin ⟨siderophilin⟩

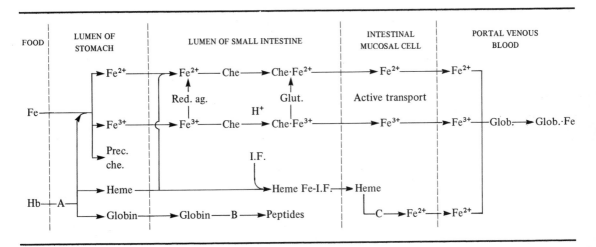

FOOD	LUMEN OF STOMACH	LUMEN OF SMALL INTESTINE	INTESTINAL MUCOSAL CELL	PORTAL VENOUS BLOOD

continued

Contributor: Sleisenger, Marvin H.

Reference: Callender, S. T. 1974. Biomembranes 4B:761-791.

122. STATISTICAL ANALYSIS OF RESPONSES TO SECRETIN TEST OF PANCREATIC FUNCTION

The range of response in normal patients following secretin administration (Secretin Test) depends on several factors: the type of secretin used, i.e., Boots (Warren-Teed), Vitrum, or synthetic; the method of administration, i.e., intravenous bolus or continuous intravenous infusion; the dosage, i.e., standard or augmented-maximum; and the length of collection of duodenal drainage. Data for the Standard Test, employing a bolus of 1.0-1.5 units per kilogram of Boots (Warren-Teed) secretin, is in general agreement with that using 1.0 (but not 2.0) units per kilogram of synthetic or Vitrum secretin, and is summarized below for 30-, 60-, and 80-minute collection periods. Since clinical usage in actual practice primarily involves diagnosis of deficiency states, the lower limits of normal, which have been accepted as minimizing minor variations in different states, have also been included. The Augmented Secretin Test [ref. 3, 4] attempts to define the maximum secretory capacity in regard to flow and bicarbonate secretion, i.e., the tubular secretory mass. This response can be obtained with a bolus dosage of 4.0 units per kilogram of Boots (Warren-Teed) secretin, or with 2.0 units per kilogram of synthetic or Vitrum secretin, or by intravenous infusion of secretin to a secretory plateau [ref. 5]. Data for normal patients using 4.0 units per kilogram Boots (Warren-Teed) secretin is given below. Figures in heavy brackets are reference numbers.

SYMBOLS	
D = duration of collection period	σ_x = standard deviation = $\sqrt{\dfrac{\Sigma x^2}{N} - \left(\dfrac{\Sigma x}{N}\right)^2}$
N = number of subjects	
x = observed value of variable	$\sigma_{\overline{x}}$ = standard deviation of sample mean = $\sigma_x/\sqrt{N}$
$\overline{x}$ = mean of sample = $(\Sigma x)/N$	V_c = coefficient of variation = $100 \cdot \sigma_x/\overline{x}$
	$\overline{x} \pm 2\sigma_x$ = calculated normal range

	Variable & Units	D min	N	Observed Range of x	$\overline{x} \pm \sigma_{\overline{x}}$	σ_x	V_c %	$\overline{x} \pm 2\sigma_x$
				Standard Test [2][1]				
1	Total volume of secretion, ml	30[2]	21	....	135 ± 6.24	28.6	21.2	78-192
2		30	123	54-220	104.7 ± 2.1	22.8	21.7	59-150
3		60	123	91-270	164.7 ± 2.7	29.2	18.3	106-223
4		80	123	117-392	200.3 ± 3.3	36.1	18.1	128-272
5	Total volume of secretion per unit body weight, ml/kg	30	123	1.0-2.8	1.73 ± 0.03	0.33	19.1	1.1-2.4
6		60	123	1.6-4.8	2.72 ± 0.05	0.53	19.2	1.7-3.8
7		80	123	2.0[3]-6.2	3.22 ± 0.05	0.55	17.0	2.1-4.3
8	Total bicarbonate secretion, meq	30[2]	21	....	11.35 ± 0.60	2.55	22.5	6.25-16.45
9		30	123	6.8-16.0	11.27 ± 0.10	1.13	10.0	9.0-13.6
10		60	123	13.2-23.7	17.81 ± 0.17	1.84	10.3	14.1-21.5
11		80	123	15.9[4]-32.6	20.83 ± 0.18	2.01	9.7	16.8-24.9
12	Maximum bicarbonate concentration, meq/liter	30;60; 80	123	88[5]-137	107.7 ± 0.7	8.3	7.7	91-125

[1] Unless otherwise indicated. [2] Data obtained using i.v. injection of 1.7 units secretin/kg body wt [1]. [3] Lower limit of normal. [4] Lower limit of normal is 15.0 meq. [5] Lower limit of normal is 90 meq/liter.

continued

	Variable & Units	D min	N	Observed Range of x	$\bar{x} \pm \sigma_{\bar{x}}$	σ_x	V_c %	$\bar{x} \pm 2\sigma_x$
13	Total amylase secretion, IU[1]	30[2]	21	....	624 ± 67.8[6]	303[6]	48.6	18-1230[6]
14		30	123	145-1254	480.7 ± 25.7	282.6	58.7	....
15		60	123	204-1621	722.4 ± 24.9	274.3	38.1	173-1270
16		80	123	439-1921	1055 ± 25.0	275.3	26.1	505-1605
17	Total amylase secretion per unit body weight, IU/kg	30	123	2.3-15.3	6.9 ± 0.4	3.6	52.6	....
18		60	123	3.7-22.8	10.3 ± 0.3	3.7	35.9	2.9-17.7
19		80	123	6.0[3]-27.2	14.9 ± 0.3	3.3	22.0	8.3-21.5
	Augmented Test [3-5]							
20	Total volume of secretion, ml	80	130	212-614	390	86	22.1	218-562
21	Total volume of secretion per unit body weight, ml/kg	80	130	4.0-8.9	6.3	0.9	14.3	4.5-8.1
22	Total bicarbonate secretion, meq	80	130	18.3-60.1	40.7	9.1	22.4	22.5-58.9
23	Maximum bicarbonate concentration, meq/liter	....	130	91-152	117	12	10.3	93-141
24	Total amylase secretion per unit body weight, IU/kg	80	130	12.0-71.3	36.7	14.2	38.8	8.3-65.1

[1] Unless otherwise indicated. [2] Data obtained using i.v. injection of 1.7 units secretin/kg body wt [1]. [3] Lower limit of normal. [6] Units are Nørby units.

Contributor: Dreiling, David A.

References

1. Burton, P., et al. 1960. Gut 1:111-124.
2. Dreiling, D. A. 1955. J. Mt. Sinai Hosp. N.Y. 21:363-372.
3. Dreiling, D. A., et al. 1974. Am. J. Gastroenterol. 61:433-442.
4. Hansky, J. 1971. Aust. N.Z. J. Med. 1(2):109-113.
5. Pascal, J. P., et al. 1968. Am. J. Dig. Dis. 13:213-221.

123. PRODUCTION, HEPATIC HANDLING, AND EXCRETION OF BILIRUBIN

Figures in parentheses refer to corresponding figures in diagram.

Plasma bilirubin turnover, which closely approximates total bilirubin production, is 3.9 ± 0.7 milligrams per kilogram per day in normal man. Of this amount, an average of 80% is derived from the death of circulating erythrocytes (1), and the remainder from ineffective erythropoiesis (2) and hepatic heme turnover (3). Transported to the liver from its sites of formation as an albumin complex (4), unconjugated bilirubin is taken into the liver cell across the sinusoidal membrane by a process which involves bi-directional flux and which is probably carrier-mediated (5). Net hepatic bilirubin clearance in normal man is 0.65 ± 0.18 milliliters plasma cleared per minute per kilogram. Binding to intracellular macromolecules (6) results in intrahepatic storage of an average of 30 milligrams bilirubin per mg/dl plasma concentration. Bilirubin is conjugated (7) by a specific microsomal UDPglucuronyltransferase, and then actively excreted across the canalicular membrane (8), principally as di- and mono-glucuronides. Because of intestinal bacterial action, hydrolysis and conversion (9) to urobilinogens and other unidentified products occur prior to fecal excretion. An enterohepatic circulation of urobilinogen results in excretion of 1-2% of this compound by the renal route.

Unconjugated hyperbilirubinemia due to increased bilirubin production occurs in hemolysis (1), and as a result of increased ineffective erythropoiesis (2)—such as occurs in vitamin B_{12} deficiency (and presumably also in folic acid deficiency)—erythropoietic porphyria, thalassemia major, sideroblastic anemia, or lead poisoning. Unconjugated hyperbilirubinemia due to reduced hepatic clearance occurs in Gilbert's syndrome, because of partial defects in either uptake (5) or conjugation (7); and in congenital non-hemolytic jaundice types I (Crigler-Najjar syndrome) and II (Arias syndrome), because of severely defective conjugation (7). Abnormal excretory transport (8) is the basis for the Dubin-Johnson syndrome, and possibly the Rotor syndrome, of conjugated hyperbilirubinemia. A conjugated hyperbilirubinemia may also occur in pure cholestatic states or in biliary tract obstruction. Most other acquired hepatobil-

continued

iary disorders result in a mixed hyperbilirubinemia due to multiple mechanisms.

Abbreviations: MHO = microsomal heme oxygenase; Alb = albumin; UCB = unconjugated bilirubin, GST = glutathione-*S*-transferase; UDPGT = bilirubin-UDPglucuronyltransferase; CB = conjugated bilirubin.

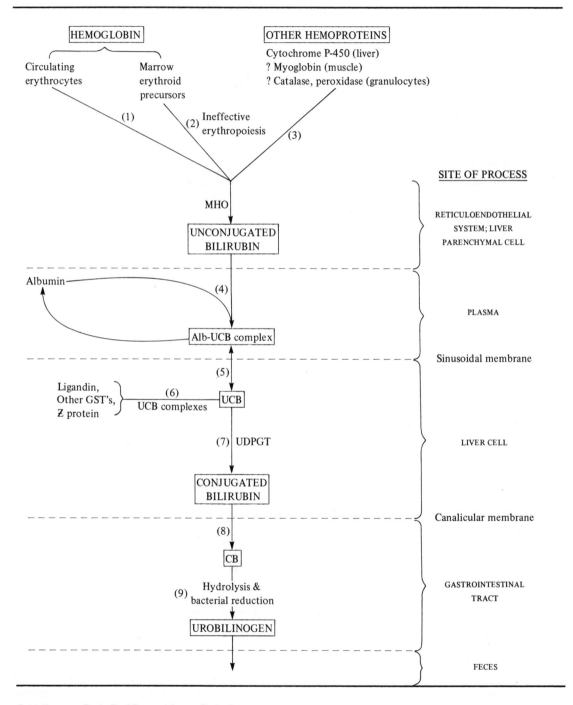

Contributors: Berk, Paul D., and Jones, E. Anthony

Reference: Berk, P. D., et al. 1974. In P. K. Bondy and L. Rosenberg, ed. Diseases of Metabolism. Ed. 7. W. B. Saunders, Philadelphia. pp. 825-880.

Class & Test: Serum autoantibodies (e.g., smooth muscle antibody, mitochondrial antibody, and nuclear antibody) and hepatitis-related immunologic tests (e.g., hepatitis B surface antigen) are not included. **Normal Value**: Many normal values, particularly those employed for enzyme activity determinations, are entirely dependent on the methods employed and on such conditions as reaction temperature. Normal values presented are principally those of the Clinical Chemistry Laboratories of the Clinical Center of the National Institutes of Health, using references cited. Laboratories employing other methods or conditions may have different normal ranges. **Remarks**: i.v. = intravenous.

	Class & Test ⟨Synonym⟩	Normal Value	Remarks	Reference
			Static Tests	
	Bile pigments Bilirubin Serum or plasma concentration			
1	Total	≤1.2 mg/100 ml	....	15
2	Direct reacting	≤0.2 mg/100 ml, if total bilirubin is normal. Otherwise, <15% of total.	Elevated direct reacting bilirubin with normal total is sensitive indicator of hepatic dysfunction or cholestasis	16
3	Indirect reacting[1]	≤1.0 mg/100 ml	May increase due either to overproduction of bilirubin (e.g., hemolysis) or hepatic dysfunction. Values >4.0 mg/100 ml indicate hepatic dysfunction even if hemolysis is present.	4
4	Urine	Negative	Bilirubinuria indicates increased conjugated bilirubin in serum. Positive early in viral hepatitis.	14
5	Urobilinogen Fecal ⟨Stercobilinogen⟩	40-280 mg/d indicates cholestasis.	Measured on pooled 3-d feces; unreliable in presence of current or recent antibiotic therapy. Virtual absence Elevated values suggest increased bilirubin production.	3
6 7	Urine	♂: <2.1 Ehrlich unit/2 h ♀: <1.1 Ehrlich unit/2 h	Measured on freshly voided urine collected from 14:00-16:00 h. Unreliable in presence of current or recent antibiotic administration. Absent in cholestasis, increased in either hemolysis or hepatocellular dysfunction.	43
8	Bile acids Serum concentration Fasting	<4 μmole/liter	Increased values sensitive indicator of hepatobiliary dysfunction	2,24, 26
9	2 h postprandial	<4 μmole/liter	Increased values very sensitive indicator of hepatobiliary dysfunction	2,24
10	Serum trihydroxy:dihydroxy ratio	....	Determined in jaundiced sera. Usually <1 in hepatocellular disease; >1 in cholestasis.	7,22
11	Serum enzyme activity Aspartate aminotransferase ⟨AST⟩	6-52 units/liter	Elevated values usually due to recent or continuing damage to hepatocytes, myocardium or striated ⟨skeletal⟩ muscle, or hemolysis. Markedly elevated values (>1000 units/liter) in some cases of acute viral- or drug-induced hepatitis. Mild or moderately increased values in cholestasis & most cases of hepatitis.	8,39, 45
12	Alanine aminotransferase ⟨ALT⟩	2-45 units/liter	Elevated values more hepato-specific than elevated AST (entry 11). Usually ALT exceeds AST in acute hepatitis, while AST exceeds ALT in alcoholic liver disease.	8,42, 45
13 14	Alkaline phosphatase	Adult: 25-78 units/liter Child: 75-115 units/liter	Physiological increase in late pregnancy, childhood, & particularly early puberty. Markedly elevated values in intrahepatic cholestasis, large duct biliary obstruction, infiltrative lesions of liver, & increased osteoblastic activity in bone. Mild or moderately increased values in hepatocellular disease.	23,31, 42

[1] Total concentration minus direct reacting concentration.

continued

	Class & Test ⟨Synonym⟩	Normal Value	Remarks	Reference
15	5'-Nucleotidase[2/]	2.2-15 units/liter	Physiological increase in late pregnancy. Markedly elevated values in intrahepatic cholestasis, large duct biliary obstruction, & infiltrative lesions of liver. Mild or moderately increased values in hepatocellular disease. Normal during growth & with bone disease.	10,18
16 17	Lactate dehydrogenase	♂: 115-340 units/liter ♀: 115-285 units/liter	Increased in hepatocellular disease & hemolysis. Markedly elevated values in hepatic neoplasia.	1,45
18	Plasma proteins Electrophoresis	Albumin: 3.0-4.8 g/100 ml	Reduced albumin & increased γ-globulin in chronic hepatocellular disease. Increased α_2- and β-globulin in cholestasis. Reduced α_1-globulin in α_1-antitrypsin deficiency. Reduced α_2-globulin in hemolysis.	20
19		α_1-Globulin: 0.1-0.3 g/100 ml		
20		α_2-Globulin: 0.4-0.9 g/100 ml		
21		β-Globulin: 0.7-1.2 g/100 ml		
22		γ-Globulin: 0.7-1.8 g/100 ml		
23	Albumin	3.0-4.8 g/100 ml	Increased plasma volume & decreased synthesis contribute to hypoalbuminemia of chronic hepatocellular disease. Long half-life precludes rapid fall in acute severe hepatocellular disease. Normal in cholestasis.	11,19
24	α_1-Antitrypsin	148-276 mg/100 ml	Markedly reduced in neonatal cholestasis, cirrhosis, liver cell carcinoma, & emphysema associated with α_1-antitrypsin deficiency	6,38
25	Ceruloplasmin[3/]	25-35 mg/100 ml	Physiological increase in pregnancy. Markedly reduced in most homozygotes & some heterozygotes for Wilson's disease & in severe hepatocellular disease. Increased values: large duct biliary obstruction & estrogen therapy.	17,40
26	Prothrombin time	1-2 s above control values	Depends on hepatic synthesis of fibrinogen ⟨coagulation factor I⟩, prothrombin ⟨coagulation factor II⟩, & coagulation factors V, VII, & X. Increased in severe hepatocellular disease & prolonged cholestasis. Parenteral vitamin K_1 corrects defect in cholestasis. Short half-life of coagulation factor VII permits rapid increase in prothrombin time in severe acute hepatocellular disease.	12,25, 35
27	α-Fetoprotein	<30 ng/liter	Physiological increased values in first yr of life & pregnancy. Markedly increased (e.g., >3000 ng/liter) in many patients with liver cell carcinoma & gonadal tumors. Less high values (e.g., 40-500 ng/liter) in chronic active hepatitis & during acute hepatitis. Increased values may reflect dedifferentiated hepatocytes or hepatic regeneration.	5,41
28 29 30	Immunoglobulins	IgG: 72-204 units/liter IgA: 30-261 units/liter IgM: 36-266 units/liter	Typically, IgG increased in chronic active hepatitis & cryptogenic cirrhosis, IgA in alcoholic cirrhosis, & IgM in primary biliary cirrhosis, & alcoholic cirrhosis. Wide ranges of values in each disease.	13
31	Lipoprotein-X	Not detectable	Detectable in intrahepatic cholestasis & large duct biliary obstruction	34,37
32	Other Cholesterol	Total: 150-270 mg/100 ml	Increased in intrahepatic cholestasis & large duct biliary obstruction. Also increased in association with diabetes mellitus, nephrotic syndrome, certain congenital hyperlipidemias, & hypothyroidism. Reduced in severe hepatocellular disease. Often reduced early & elevated later in the course of acute hepatitis.	29

[2/] Other enzymes behave like 5'-nucleotidase: leucine aminopeptidase and γ-glutamyl transpeptidase. [3/] A synonym for the enzyme ferroxidase, which may be measured as arbitrary units/ml.

continued

	Class & Test ⟨Synonym⟩	Normal Value	Remarks	Reference
33		Ester: 67-74% of total	Ester:free cholesterol ratio reduced in cholestasis (increase in free cholesterol), and in hepatocellular disease (decrease in ester)	
34	Plasma glucose	70-120 mg/100 ml	Hyperglycemia may occur in cirrhosis, alcoholic pancreatitis, pancreatic duct obstruction, hemochromatosis, & after portacaval shunt. Hypoglycemia may occur in massive hepatic necrosis, after portacaval shunts, after alcohol ingestion, in liver cell carcinoma & sarcoma, glycogenosis, & hereditary fructose intolerance.	28,30
35	Plasma ammonia	20-120 μg nitrogen/100 ml	Preferably determined in arterial blood. Elevated values, often associated with encephalopathy, found in severe acute & chronic hepatocellular disease, large portal-systemic shunts, & congenital hyperammonemia syndromes.	21,36
36	Serum vitamin B_{12}	200-900 pg/ml	Elevated in active hepatocellular disease & intrahepatic infections & space-occupying lesions. Normal in large duct biliary obstruction. Elevations may be due to increase in binding proteins.	32,33
			Dynamic Tests	
37	Sulfobromophthalein ⟨BSP⟩ retention	<5% at 45 min	Sensitive screening test for all types of hepatobiliary dysfunction. Unnecessary if existence of dysfunction already established.	9
38 39	Indocyanine green plasma disappearance rate	♂: 0.21 ± 0.02 %/min ♀: 0.24 ± 0.03 %/min	At standard dose (0.5 mg/kg, i.v.), less sensitive than BSP retention (entry 37)	27

Contributors: Jones, E. Anthony, and Berk, Paul D.

References
1. Amador, E., et al. 1963. Clin. Chem. 9:391-399.
2. Barnes, S., et al. 1975. J. Clin. Pathol. 28:506-509.
3. Bloomer, J. R., et al. 1970. Clin. Chim. Acta 29:463-471.
4. Bloomer, J. R., et al. 1971. J. Am. Med. Assoc. 218:216-220.
5. Bloomer, J. R., et al. 1975. Gastroenterology 68:342-350.
6. Brunt, P. W. 1974. Gut 15:573-580.
7. Carey, J. B., Jr. 1973. In P. P. Nair and D. Kritchevsky, ed. The Bile Acids. Plenum Press, New York. v. 2, pp. 55-82.
8. Clermont, R. J., and T. C. Chalmers. 1967. Medicine (Baltimore) 46:197-207.
9. Combes, B., and S. Schenker. 1975. In L. Schiff, ed. Diseases of the Liver. Ed. 4. J. B. Lippincott, Philadelphia. pp. 204-246.
10. Dixon, T. F., and M. Purdom. 1954. J. Clin. Pathol. 7:341-343.
11. Dykes, P. W. 1968. Clin. Sci. 34:161-183.
12. Dymock, I. W., et al. 1975. Br. J. Haematol. 29:385-395.
13. Feizi, T. 1968. Gut 9:193-198.
14. Free, A. H., and H. M. Free. 1972. CRC Crit. Rev. Clin. Lab. Sci. 3:481-531.
15. Gambino, S. R., and H. Schreiber. 1964. Autom. Anal. Chem. Technicon Symp. (White Plains, NY).
16. Gambino, S. R., et al. 1967. J. Am. Med. Assoc. 201:1047-1049.
17. Gault, M. H., et al. 1966. Gastroenterology 50:8-18.
18. Goldberg, D. M. 1973. Digestion 8:87-99.
19. Hasch, E., et al. 1967. Acta Med. Scand. 182:83-92.
20. Hobbs, J. R. 1967. Proc. R. Soc. Med. 64:1250-1254.
21. Hsia, Y. E. 1974. Gastroenterology 67:347-374.
22. Javitt, N. B. 1975. In L. Schiff, ed. Diseases of the Liver. Ed. 4. J. B. Lippincott, Philadelphia. pp. 111-145.
23. Kaplan, M. M. 1972. Gastroenterology 62:452-468.
24. Kaplowitz, N., et al. 1973. J. Am. Med. Assoc. 225:292-293.
25. Koller, F. 1973. Scand. J. Gastroenterol. 8(Suppl. 19):51-61.
26. Korman, M. G., et al. 1974. N. Engl. J. Med. 290:1399-1402.
27. Martin, J. F., et al. 1976. Proc. Soc. Exp. Biol. Med. 150:612-617.
28. McFadzean, A. J. S., and R. T. T. Yeung. 1969. Am. J. Med. 47:220-235.
29. McIntyre, N., et al. 1975. Gut 16:379-391.
30. Megyesi, C., et al. 1967. Lancet 2:1051-1055.
31. Morgenstern, S., et al. 1965. Clin. Chem. 11:876-888.
32. Neale, G., et al. 1966. Br. Med. J. 1:382-387.

continued

33. Rachmilewitz, M., and M. Eliakim. 1968. Isr. J. Med. Sci. 4:47-54.
34. Ritland, S. 1976. Scand. J. Gastroenterol. 10:785-789.
35. Roberts, H. R., and A. I. Cederbaum. 1972. Gastroenterology 63:297-320.
36. Schenker, S., et al. 1974. Ibid. 66:121-151.
37. Seidel, D., et al. 1973. Clin. Chem. 19:86-91;
38. Sharp, H. L. 1976. Gastroenterology 70:611-621.
39. Steinberg, D., et al. 1956. J. Lab. Clin. Med. 48:144-151.
40. Strickland, G. T., and M.-L. Len. 1975. Medicine (Baltimore) 54:113-137.
41. Waldmann, T. A., and K. R. McIntyre. 1974. Cancer 34:1510-1515.
42. Warnes, T. W. 1972. Gut 13:926-929.
43. Watson, C. J., et al. 1944. Am. J. Clin. Pathol. 14:605-615.
44. Wroblewski, F., and J. S. LaDue. 1956. Proc. Soc. Exp. Biol. Med. 91:569-571.
45. Zimmerman, H. J., and L. B. Seeff. 1970. In E. L. Coodley, ed. Diagnostic Enzymology. Lea and Febiger, Philadelphia. pp. 1-38.

125. LENGTH, WEIGHT, AND HEAD CIRCUMFERENCE FROM BIRTH TO THREE YEARS

All subjects were measured nude. For standardized techniques of measurement and method of development of growth charts, consult the appended reference.

	Age mo	Males, Percentile							Females, Percentile						
		5	10	25	50	75	90	95	5	10	25	50	75	90	95
		Length, cm													
1	Newborn	46.4	47.5	49.0	50.5	51.8	53.5	54.4	45.4	46.5	48.2	49.9	51.0	52.0	52.9
2	1	50.4	51.3	53.0	54.6	56.2	57.7	58.6	49.2	50.2	51.9	53.5	54.9	56.1	56.9
3	3	56.7	57.7	59.4	61.1	63.0	64.5	65.4	55.4	56.2	57.8	59.5	61.2	62.7	63.4
4	6	63.4	64.4	66.1	67.8	69.7	71.3	72.3	61.8	62.6	64.2	65.9	67.8	69.4	70.2
5	9	68.0	69.1	70.6	72.3	74.0	75.9	77.1	66.1	67.0	68.7	70.4	72.4	74.0	75.0
6	12	71.7	72.8	74.3	76.1	77.7	79.8	81.2	69.8	70.8	72.4	74.3	76.3	78.0	79.1
7	18	77.5	78.7	80.5	82.4	84.3	86.6	88.1	76.0	77.2	78.8	80.9	83.0	85.0	86.1
8	24	82.3	83.5	85.6	87.6	89.9	92.2	93.8	81.3	82.5	84.2	86.5	88.7	90.8	92.0
9	30	87.0	88.2	90.1	92.3	94.6	97.0	98.7	86.0	87.0	88.9	91.3	93.7	95.6	96.9
10	36	91.2	92.4	94.2	96.5	98.9	101.4	103.1	90.0	91.0	93.1	95.6	98.1	100.0	101.5
		Weight, kg													
11	Newborn	2.54	2.78	3.00	3.27	3.64	3.82	4.15	2.36	2.58	2.93	3.23	3.52	3.64	3.81
12	1	3.16	3.43	3.82	4.29	4.75	5.14	5.38	2.97	3.22	3.59	3.98	4.36	4.65	4.92
13	3	4.43	4.78	5.32	5.98	6.56	7.14	7.37	4.18	4.47	4.88	5.40	5.90	6.39	6.74
14	6	6.20	6.61	7.20	7.85	8.49	9.10	9.46	5.79	6.12	6.60	7.21	7.83	8.38	8.73
15	9	7.52	7.95	8.56	9.18	9.88	10.49	10.93	7.00	7.34	7.89	8.56	9.24	9.83	10.17
16	12	8.43	8.84	9.49	10.15	10.91	11.54	11.99	7.84	8.19	8.81	9.53	10.23	10.87	11.24
17	18	9.59	9.92	10.67	11.47	12.31	13.05	13.44	8.92	9.30	10.04	10.82	11.55	12.30	12.76
18	24	10.54	10.85	11.65	12.59	13.44	14.29	14.70	9.87	10.26	11.10	11.90	12.74	13.57	14.08
19	30	11.44	11.80	12.63	13.67	14.51	15.47	15.97	10.78	11.21	12.11	12.93	13.93	14.81	15.35
20	36	12.26	12.69	13.58	14.69	15.59	16.66	17.28	11.60	12.07	12.99	13.93	15.03	15.97	16.54
		Head Circumference, cm													
21	Newborn	32.6	33.0	33.9	34.8	35.6	36.6	37.2	32.1	32.9	33.5	34.3	34.8	35.5	35.9
22	1	34.9	35.4	36.2	37.2	38.1	39.0	39.6	34.2	34.8	35.6	36.4	37.1	37.8	38.3
23	3	38.4	38.9	39.7	40.6	41.7	42.5	43.1	37.3	37.8	38.7	39.5	40.4	41.2	41.7
24	6	41.5	42.0	42.8	43.8	44.7	45.6	46.2	40.3	40.9	41.6	42.4	43.3	44.1	44.6
25	9	43.5	44.0	44.8	45.8	46.6	47.5	48.1	42.3	42.8	43.5	44.3	45.1	46.0	46.4
26	12	44.8	45.3	46.1	47.0	47.9	48.8	49.3	43.5	44.1	44.8	45.6	46.4	47.2	47.6
27	18	46.3	46.7	47.4	48.4	49.3	50.1	50.6	45.0	45.6	46.3	47.1	47.9	48.6	49.1
28	24	47.3	47.7	48.3	49.2	50.2	51.0	51.4	46.1	46.5	47.3	48.1	48.8	49.6	50.1
29	30	48.0	48.4	49.1	49.9	51.0	51.7	52.2	47.0	47.3	48.0	48.8	49.4	50.3	50.8
30	36	48.6	49.0	49.7	50.5	51.5	52.3	52.8	47.6	47.9	48.5	49.3	50.0	50.8	51.4

continued

125. LENGTH, WEIGHT, AND HEAD CIRCUMFERENCE FROM BIRTH TO THREE YEARS

Contributor: Vaughan, Victor C., III

Reference: Hamill, P. V. V., et al. 1976. Mon. Vital Stat. Rep. 22(3):1-22.

126. HEIGHT AND WEIGHT FROM TWO TO EIGHTEEN YEARS

All subjects were measured wearing light clothing (~ 0.05 kg at 1-2 yr, ~ 0.1 kg at 3-5 yr, and ranging from 0.11 kg at 6 yr to 0.3 kg at 18 yr). For standardized techniques of measurement and method of development of growth charts, consult the appended reference.

	Age yr	Males, Percentile							Females, Percentile						
		5	10	25	50	75	90	95	5	10	25	50	75	90	95
		Height, cm													
1	2.0	82.5	83.5	85.3	86.8	89.2	92.0	94.4	81.6	82.1	84.0	86.8	89.3	92.0	93.6
2	2.5	85.4	86.5	88.5	90.4	92.9	95.6	97.8	84.6	85.3	87.3	90.0	92.5	95.0	96.6
3	3.0	89.0	90.3	92.6	94.9	97.5	100.1	102.0	88.3	89.3	91.4	94.1	96.6	99.0	100.6
4	3.5	92.5	93.9	96.4	99.1	101.7	104.3	106.1	91.7	93.0	95.2	97.9	100.5	102.8	104.5
5	4.0	95.8	97.3	100.0	102.9	105.7	108.2	109.9	95.0	96.4	98.8	101.6	104.3	106.6	108.3
6	4.5	98.9	100.6	103.4	106.6	109.4	111.9	113.5	98.1	99.7	102.2	105.0	107.9	110.2	112.0
7	5.0	102.0	103.7	106.5	109.9	112.8	115.4	117.0	101.1	102.7	105.4	108.4	111.4	113.8	115.6
8	5.5	104.9	106.7	109.6	113.1	116.1	118.7	120.3	103.9	105.6	108.4	111.6	114.8	117.4	119.2
9	6.0	107.7	109.6	112.5	116.1	119.2	121.9	123.5	106.6	108.4	111.3	114.6	118.1	120.8	122.7
10	6.5	110.4	112.3	115.3	119.0	122.2	124.9	126.6	109.2	111.0	114.1	117.6	121.3	124.2	126.1
11	7.0	113.0	115.0	118.0	121.7	125.0	127.9	129.7	111.8	113.6	116.8	120.6	124.4	127.6	129.5
12	7.5	115.6	117.6	120.6	124.4	127.8	130.8	132.7	114.4	116.2	119.5	123.5	127.5	130.9	132.9
13	8.0	118.1	120.2	123.2	127.0	130.5	133.6	135.7	116.9	118.7	122.2	126.4	130.6	134.2	136.2
14	8.5	120.5	122.7	125.7	129.6	133.2	136.5	138.8	119.5	121.3	124.9	129.3	133.6	137.4	139.6
15	9.0	122.9	125.2	128.2	132.2	136.0	139.4	141.8	122.1	123.9	127.7	132.2	136.7	140.7	142.9
16	9.5	125.3	127.6	130.8	134.8	138.8	142.4	144.9	124.8	126.6	130.6	135.2	139.8	143.9	146.2
17	10.0	127.7	130.1	133.4	137.5	141.6	145.5	148.1	127.5	129.5	133.6	138.3	142.9	147.2	149.5
18	10.5	130.1	132.6	136.0	140.3	144.6	148.7	151.5	130.4	132.5	136.7	141.5	146.1	150.4	152.8
19	11.0	132.6	135.1	138.7	143.3	147.8	152.1	154.9	133.5	135.6	140.0	144.8	149.3	153.7	156.2
20	11.5	135.0	137.7	141.5	146.4	151.1	155.6	158.5	136.6	139.0	143.5	148.2	152.6	156.9	159.5
21	12.0	137.6	140.3	144.4	149.7	154.6	159.4	162.3	139.8	142.3	147.0	151.5	155.8	160.0	162.7
22	12.5	140.2	143.0	147.4	153.0	158.2	163.2	166.1	142.7	145.4	150.1	154.6	158.8	162.9	165.6
23	13.0	142.9	145.8	150.5	156.5	161.8	167.0	169.8	145.2	148.0	152.8	157.1	161.3	165.3	168.1
24	13.5	145.7	148.7	153.6	159.9	165.3	170.5	173.4	147.2	150.0	154.7	159.0	163.2	167.3	170.0
25	14.0	148.8	151.8	156.9	163.1	168.5	173.8	176.7	148.7	151.5	155.9	160.4	164.6	168.7	171.3
26	14.5	152.0	155.0	160.1	166.2	171.5	176.6	179.5	149.7	152.5	156.8	161.2	165.6	169.8	172.2
27	15.0	155.2	158.2	163.3	169.0	174.1	178.9	181.9	150.5	153.2	157.2	161.8	166.3	170.5	172.8
28	15.5	158.3	161.2	166.2	171.5	176.3	180.8	183.9	151.1	153.6	157.5	162.1	166.7	170.9	173.1
29	16.0	161.1	163.9	168.7	173.5	178.1	182.4	185.4	151.6	154.1	157.8	162.4	166.9	171.1	173.3
30	16.5	163.4	166.1	170.6	175.2	179.5	183.6	186.6	152.2	154.6	158.2	162.7	167.1	171.2	173.4
31	17.0	164.9	167.7	171.9	176.2	180.5	184.4	187.3	152.7	155.1	158.7	163.1	167.3	171.2	173.5
32	17.5	165.6	168.5	172.4	176.7	181.0	185.0	187.6	153.2	155.6	159.1	163.4	167.5	171.1	173.5
33	18.0	165.7	168.7	172.3	176.8	181.2	185.3	187.6	153.6	156.0	159.6	163.7	167.6	171.0	173.6
		Weight, kg													
34	2.0	10.49	10.96	11.55	12.34	13.36	14.38	15.50	9.95	10.32	10.96	11.80	12.73	13.58	14.15
35	2.5	11.27	11.77	12.55	13.52	14.61	15.71	16.61	10.80	11.35	12.11	13.03	14.23	15.16	15.76
36	3.0	12.05	12.58	13.52	14.62	15.78	16.95	17.77	11.61	12.26	13.11	14.10	15.50	16.54	17.22
37	3.5	12.84	13.41	14.46	15.68	16.90	18.15	18.98	12.37	13.08	14.00	15.07	16.59	17.77	18.59

continued

	Age	Males, Percentile							Females, Percentile						
	yr	5	10	25	50	75	90	95	5	10	25	50	75	90	95
38	4.0	13.64	14.24	15.39	16.69	17.99	19.32	20.27	13.11	13.84	14.80	15.96	17.56	18.93	19.91
39	4.5	14.45	15.10	16.30	17.69	19.06	20.50	21.63	13.83	14.56	15.55	16.81	18.48	20.06	21.24
40	5.0	15.27	15.96	17.22	18.67	20.14	21.70	23.09	14.55	15.26	16.29	17.66	19.39	21.23	22.62
41	5.5	16.09	16.83	18.14	19.67	21.25	22.96	24.66	15.29	15.97	17.05	18.56	20.36	22.48	24.11
42	6.0	16.93	17.72	19.07	20.69	22.40	24.31	26.34	16.05	16.72	17.86	19.52	21.44	23.89	25.75
43	6.5	17.78	18.62	20.02	21.74	23.62	25.76	28.16	16.85	17.51	18.76	20.61	22.68	25.50	27.59
44	7.0	18.64	19.53	21.00	22.85	24.94	27.36	30.12	17.71	18.39	19.78	21.84	24.16	27.39	29.68
45	7.5	19.52	20.45	22.02	24.03	26.36	29.11	32.73	18.62	19.37	20.95	23.26	25.90	29.57	32.07
46	8.0	20.40	21.39	23.09	25.30	27.91	31.06	34.51	19.62	20.45	22.26	24.84	27.88	32.04	34.71
47	8.5	21.31	22.34	24.21	26.66	29.61	33.22	36.96	20.68	21.64	23.70	26.58	30.08	34.73	37.58
48	9.0	22.25	23.33	25.40	28.13	31.46	35.57	39.58	21.82	22.92	25.27	28.46	32.44	37.60	40.64
49	9.5	23.25	24.38	26.68	29.73	33.46	38.11	42.35	23.05	24.29	26.94	30.45	34.94	40.61	43.85
50	10.0	24.33	25.52	28.07	31.44	35.61	40.80	45.27	24.36	25.76	28.71	32.55	37.53	43.70	47.17
51	10.5	25.51	26.78	29.59	33.30	37.92	43.63	48.31	25.75	27.32	30.57	34.72	40.17	46.84	50.57
52	11.0	26.80	28.17	31.25	35.30	40.38	46.57	51.47	27.24	28.97	32.49	36.95	42.84	49.96	54.00
53	11.5	28.24	29.72	33.08	37.46	43.00	49.61	54.73	28.83	30.71	34.48	39.23	45.48	53.03	57.42
54	12.0	29.85	31.46	35.09	39.78	45.77	52.73	58.09	30.52	32.53	36.52	41.53	48.07	55.99	60.81
55	12.5	31.64	33.41	37.31	42.27	48.70	55.91	61.52	32.30	34.42	38.59	43.84	50.56	58.81	64.12
56	13.0	33.64	35.60	39.74	44.95	51.79	59.12	65.02	34.14	36.35	40.65	46.10	52.91	61.45	67.30
57	13.5	35.85	38.03	42.40	47.81	55.02	62.35	68.57	35.98	38.26	42.65	48.26	55.11	63.87	70.30
58	14.0	38.22	40.64	45.21	50.77	58.31	65.57	72.13	37.76	40.11	44.54	50.28	57.09	66.04	73.08
59	14.5	40.66	43.34	48.08	53.76	61.58	68.76	75.66	39.45	41.83	46.28	52.10	58.84	67.95	75.59
60	15.0	43.11	46.06	50.92	56.71	64.72	71.91	79.12	40.99	43.38	47.82	53.68	60.32	69.54	77.78
61	15.5	45.50	48.69	53.64	59.51	67.64	74.98	82.45	42.32	44.72	49.10	54.96	61.48	70.79	79.59
62	16.0	47.74	51.16	56.16	62.10	70.26	77.97	85.62	43.41	45.78	50.09	55.89	62.29	71.68	80.99
63	16.5	49.76	53.39	58.38	64.39	72.46	80.84	88.59	44.20	46.54	50.75	56.44	62.75	72.18	81.93
64	17.0	51.50	55.28	60.22	66.31	74.17	83.58	91.31	44.74	47.04	51.14	56.69	62.91	72.38	82.46
65	17.5	52.89	56.78	61.61	67.78	75.32	86.14	93.73	45.08	47.33	51.33	56.71	62.89	72.37	82.62
66	18.0	53.97	57.89	62.61	68.88	76.04	88.41	95.76	45.26	47.47	51.39	56.62	62.78	72.25	82.47

Contributor: Vaughan, Victor C., III

Reference: Hamill, P. V. V., et al. 1976. Mon. Vital Stat. Rep. 22(3):1-22.

127. SKELETAL OSSIFICATION AND FUSION

Part I. First Appearance of Ossification Centers Apparent in Roentgenograms

Bone or Epiphyseal Center: Standards for the foot are available (in appended reference), but normal variation is wide, including some familial variants, and therefore the information is of little clinical use. No standards are available for pisiform carpal bones. Plus/minus (±) values are standard deviations expressed to the nearest month.

	Bone or Epiphyseal Center ⟨Synonym⟩	Age at Appearance, mo[1]			Bone or Epiphyseal Center ⟨Synonym⟩	Age at Appearance, mo[1]	
		♂	♀			♂	♀
1	Humerus: head	3[2]	3[2]	3	Hamate	3 ± 2	2 ± 2
	Carpal bones[3]			4	Triangular ⟨triquetral⟩	30 ± 16	21 ± 14
2	Capitate	2 ± 2	2 ± 2	5	Lunate	42 ± 19	34 ± 13

[1] Unless otherwise indicated. [2] Weeks. [3] Except for the capitate and hamate bones, the variability of carpal centers is too great to make them very useful clinically.

continued

127. SKELETAL OSSIFICATION AND FUSION

Part I. First Appearance of Ossification Centers Apparent in Roentgenograms

	Bone or Epiphyseal Center ⟨Synonym⟩	Age at Appearance, mo[1]				Bone or Epiphyseal Center ⟨Synonym⟩	Age at Appearance, mo[1]	
		♂	♀				♂	♀
6	Trapezium ⟨greater multangular⟩	67 ± 19	47 ± 14	20	4th: middle phalanx	24 ± 6	15 ± 5
7	Trapezoid ⟨lesser multangular⟩	69 ± 15	49 ± 12	21	2nd: middle phalanx	26 ± 6	16 ± 5
8	Scaphoid ⟨navicular⟩	66 ± 15	51 ± 12	22	3rd: distal phalanx	28 ± 6	18 ± 4
	Metacarpal bones			23	4th: distal phalanx	28 ± 6	18 ± 5
9	II	18 ± 5	12 ± 3	24	1st: proximal phalanx	32 ± 7	20 ± 5
10	III	20 ± 5	13 ± 3	25	5th: distal phalanx	37 ± 9	23 ± 6
11	IV	23 ± 6	15 ± 4	26	2nd: distal phalanx	37 ± 8	23 ± 6
12	V	26 ± 7	16 ± 5	27	5th: middle phalanx	39 ± 10	22 ± 7
13	I	32 ± 9	18 ± 5	28	Sesamoid bone (of adductor pollux)	152 ± 18	121 ± 13
	Fingers (epiphyses)				Hip & knee		
14	3rd: proximal phalanx	16 ± 4	10 ± 3	29	Femur, distal	At birth[4]	At birth[4]
15	2nd: proximal phalanx	16 ± 4	11 ± 3	30	Tibia, proximal	At birth[4]	At birth[4]
16	4th: proximal phalanx	17 ± 5	11 ± 3	31	Femur: head	4 ± 2	4 ± 2
17	1st: distal phalanx	19 ± 7	12 ± 4	32	Patella	46 ± 11	29 ± 7
18	5th: proximal phalanx	21 ± 5	14 ± 4				
19	3rd: middle phalanx	24 ± 6	15 ± 5				

[1] Unless otherwise indicated. [4] Usually present in newborn.

Contributor: Vaughan, Victor C., III

Reference: Vaughan, V. C., III. 1975. In V. C. Vaughan, III, and R. J. McKay, ed. Nelson's Textbook of Pediatrics. Ed. 10. W. B. Saunders, Philadelphia. p. 34.

Part II. Modal Age at Onset and Completion of Fusion in Skeletal Areas

	Area of Skeletal Fusion	Modal Age, yr				Area of Skeletal Fusion	Modal Age, yr	
		♂	♀				♂	♀
	Elbow					Knee		
1	Onset in humerus	13.0-13.5	11.0-11.5	7	Onset in tibial tuberosity	15.0-15.5	13.5-14.0
2	Completion in ulna	15.0-15.5	12.5-13.0	8	Completion in fibula	17.5-18.0	16.0-16.5
	Foot & ankle					Hip & pelvis		
3	Onset in great toe	14.0-14.5	12.5-13.0	9	Onset in greater trochanter	15.5-16.0	14.0-14.5
4	Completion in tibia & fibula	15.5-16.0	14.0-14.5	10	Completion in symphysis pubis	After 18.0	17.5-18.0
	Hand & wrist					Shoulder & clavicle		
5	Onset in distal phalanges	15.0-15.5	13.0-13.5	11	Onset in greater tubercle of humerus	15.5-16.0	14.0-14.5
6	Completion in radius	17.5-18.0	16.0-16.5	12	Completion in clavicle	After 18.0	17.5-18.0

Contributor: Vaughan, Victor C., III

Reference: Vaughan, V. C., III. 1975. In V. C. Vaughan, III, and R. J. McKay, ed. Nelson's Textbook of Pediatrics. Ed. 10. W. B. Saunders, Philadelphia. p. 35.

128. SYNOVIAL FLUID COMPONENTS AND CHARACTERISTICS

Component or Characteristic: C3 is part of the protein complement system. Plus/minus (±) values are standard deviation unless otherwise indicated. Values in parentheses are ranges, estimate "c" unless otherwise specified (*see* Introduction).

	Condition	Component or Characteristic	Value	Reference
1	Normal	Intrinsic viscosity, dl/g	36.9 ± 0.9[1,2]; 38.0 ± 1.4[1,3]	3
2		Pyrophosphate, μM	3.6 ± 1.4	1
3		Cholesterol, mg/dl	22(21-23)[b]	11
4		Glucose difference, mg/dl	0(0-10)	5
5		Hyaluronic acid, mg/ml	3.74 ± 0.20[1,2]; 2.00 ± 0.25[1,3]	3
		Protein		
6		Total, g/dl	1.7(1.1-2.1)	10
7		Albumin, g/dl	0.9(0.4-1.65)	2
		Immunoglobulins, mg/dl		
8		IgG	290(50-410)	6
9		IgA	43(11-120)	6
10		IgM	4(1-10)	6
11		α_2-Macroglobulin, mg/dl	34(26-38)	6
		Leukocytes		
12		Total, no./μl	63(13-180)	10
13		Granulocytes, %	7(0-25)	10
14	Osteoarthritis	Intrinsic viscosity, dl/g	44.7 ± 7.7[1]	3
15		Pyrophosphate, μM	12.6 ± 7.0	1
16		Cholesterol, mg/dl	118(79-143)	4
17		Glucose difference, mg/dl	0(0-10)	10
18		Hyaluronic acid, mg/ml	1.90 ± 0.17[1]	3
		Protein		
19		Total, g/dl	3.1(1.3-4.9)	10
20		Albumin, g/dl	2.51(1.66-3.78)	10
21		C3, mg/dl	52(28-130)	7
		Immunoglobulins, mg/dl		
22		IgG	490(290-1200)	6
23		IgA	110(30-290)	6
24		IgM	43(6-110)	6
25		α_2-Macroglobulin, mg/dl	81(22-175)	9
26		Transferrin, mg/dl	107(44-202)	9
		Leukocytes		
27		Total, no./μl	720(70-3,600)	10
28		Granulocytes, %	7(0-58)	10
29	Rheumatoid arthritis	Intrinsic viscosity, dl/g	27.3 ± 3.3[1,4]; 31.6 ± 1.7[1,5]	3
30		Pyrophosphate, μM	4.6 ± 1.9	1
31		Cholesterol, mg/dl	119(79-143)	4
32		Glucose difference, mg/dl	24(0-87)	10
33		Hyaluronic acid, mg/ml	1.13 ± 0.10[1,4]; 1.29 ± 0.14[1,5]	3
		Protein		
34		Total, g/dl	5.0(3.30-8.89)	10
35		Albumin, g/dl	2.0(1.54-2.35)	2
36		C3, mg/dl	33(17-60)	7
		Immunoglobulins, mg/dl		
37		IgG	760(440-1350)	6
38		IgA	150(30-310)	6
39		IgM	115(40-270)	6
40		α_2-Macroglobulin, mg/dl	127(59-250)	9
41		Transferrin, mg/dl	135(56-189)	9

[1] Plus/minus (±) value is standard error. [2] Ages 21-42. [3] Ages 60-82. [4] Ages 18-43. [5] Ages 46-75.

continued

	Condition	Component or Characteristic	Value	Reference
42		Leukocytes Total, no./μl	14,000(450-62,000)	10
43		Granulocytes, %	65(0-96)	10
44	Gout	Pyrophosphate, μM	13.1 ± 8.5[1]	1
45		Glucose difference, mg/dl	10(0-50)	10
46		Hyaluronic acid, mg/ml	0.5	5
47		Protein Total, g/dl	4.2(2.8-5.0)	10
48		C3, mg/dl	50(37-74)	7
49		Leukocytes Total, no./μl	13,000(1,000-70,000)	10
50		Granulocytes, %	71(0-99)	10
51	Pseudogout	Pyrophosphate, μM	23.9 ± 10.5	1
52		Protein Total, g/dl	4.1	5
53		C3, mg/dl	45(22-65)	7
54		Leukocytes Total, no./μl	14,250(50-75,000)	5
55		Granulocytes, %	68(10-80)	5
56	Reiter's syndrome	Intrinsic viscosity, dl/g	22.6 ± 3.5[1]	3
57		Glucose difference, mg/dl	16(0-42)	12
58		Hyaluronic acid, mg/ml	0.86 ± 0.19[1]	3
59		Protein Total, g/dl	4.6(2.5-6.1)	12
60		Albumin, g/dl	2.83(2.00-3.68)[b]	10
61		C3, mg/dl	80(53-105)	7
62		Leukocytes Total, no./μl	18,500(1,000-53,000)	12
63		Granulocytes, %	66(0-96)	12
64	Systemic lupus	Glucose difference, mg/dl	22(−5 to +40)	10
65		Protein Total, g/dl	2.5(1.5-3.8)	10
66		Albumin, g/dl	1.41(1.11-2.10)	10
67		C3, mg/dl	30(16-44)[b]	7
68		Leukocytes Total, no./μl	2,860(100-18,200)	10
69		Granulocytes, %	5(0-32)	10
70	Pyogenic infections	Glucose difference, mg/dl	71(40-122)	10
71		Hyaluronic acid, mg/ml	0.4	5
72		Protein Total, g/dl	4.8(2.9-6.9)	10
73		Albumin, g/dl	2.68(1.52-3.81)	10
74		Leukocytes Total, no./μl	73,370(7,800-266,000)	10
75		Granulocytes, %	90(46-100)	10
76	Tuberculosis	Glucose difference, mg/dl	70(0-122)	10
77		Hyaluronic acid, mg/ml	1.72	5
78		Protein Total, g/dl	5.3(4.0-6.0)	10
79		Albumin, g/dl	3.31(2.78-4.27)	10
80		Leukocytes Total, no./μl	20,000(2,500-105,000)	10
81		Granulocytes, %	60(18-96)	10

[1] Plus/minus (±) value is standard error.

continued

Condition	Component or Characteristic	Value	Reference
82 Trauma	Intrinsic viscosity, dl/g	27.8 ± 2.9 [1]	3
83	Glucose difference, mg/dl	5(−5 to +25)	10
84	Hyaluronic acid, mg/ml	0.29(0.02-0.7)	8
	Protein		
85	Total, g/dl	3.85 ± 1.10	8
86	Albumin, g/dl	1.39 ± 0.22	8
	Immunoglobulins, mg/dl		
87	IgG	504 ± 115	8
88	IgA	120 ± 67	8
89	IgM	93 ± 37	8
90	α_2-Macroglobulin, mg/dl	124 ± 54	8
91	Transferrin, mg/dl	126 ± 63	8
	Leukocytes		
92	Total, no./μl	1,320(50-10,400)	10
93	Granulocytes, %	5(0-36)	10

[1] Plus/minus (±) value is standard error.

Contributor: McDuffie, Frederic C.

References

1. Altman, R. D., et al. 1973. Arthritis Rheum. 16:171-178.
2. Binette, J. P., and K. Schmid. 1965. Ibid. 8:14-28.
3. Castor, C. W., et al. 1966. Ibid. 9:783-794.
4. Chung, A. C., et al. 1962. Ibid. 5:176-182.
5. Cohen, A. S. 1975. Laboratory Diagnostic Procedures in the Rheumatic Diseases. Ed. 2. Little, Brown; Boston. pp. 1-64.
6. Hunder, G. G., and G. J. Gleich. 1974. Arthritis Rheum. 17:955-963.
7. Hunder, G. G., et al. 1977. J. Lab. Clin. Med. 89: 160-171.
8. Poortman, J. R., et al. 1974. Clin. Chim. Acta 55: 205-209.
9. Pruzanski, W., et al. 1973. Am. J. Med. Sci. 265:483-490.
10. Ropes, M. W., and W. Bauer. 1953. Synovial Fluid Changes in Joint Disease. Harvard Univ. Press, Cambridge.
11. Schur, P. H., and J. Sandson. 1963. Arthritis Rheum. 6:115-128.
12. Weinberger, H. J., et al. 1962. Medicine (Baltimore) 41:35-91.

V. NEUROLOGIC DISEASES

129. NEOPLASIA OF THE CENTRAL NERVOUS SYSTEM

Frequency: F = frequent, 20% or more in most series; C = common, 10-20%; U = uncommon, 1-10%; R = rare, <1%; VR = very rare (most individual cases reportable as such). **Sex Ratio:** All numerical ratios are male:female [ref. 22]. **Remarks:** CSF = cerebrospinal fluid; CNS = central nervous system. Figures in heavy brackets are reference numbers. Many of the references are general; they contain citations to a number of subjects which complement those specified in this table. Data in light brackets refer to the column heading in brackets.

	Tumor Type	Site	Fre-quency	Age, yr [Sex Ratio]	Growth Rate	Remarks
	Tumors of Neuroepithelial Origin					
	Primitive tumors capable of neuronal or glial differentiation					
1	Medulloblastoma	Cerebellum	U	0-10; second, though lower, peak at 18-30 [♂ > ♀]	Rapid	Frequently seeds via CSF. This & juvenile astrocytoma are the most common primary CNS tumors of children in most series. Subtypes: typical; desmoplastic; medullo-myoblastoma (very rare); pigmented papillary (very rare) (*see also* Remarks, entry 5). [17,18]
2	Medulloepithelioma [11]	Cerebrum	VR	<5, rarely older	Rapid	Can seed via CSF; may show mesenchymal differentiation in relationship to eye [10,21]
	Primitive tumors capable of neuronal differentiation					
3	Neuroblastoma	Cerebrum	VR [1]	<10 [1:1]	Rapid	Can seed via CSF. May have areas with marked mesenchymal response (i.e., desmoplasia) [17]. Common lesion in retroperitoneum of children. Very rarely occurs with glioblastoma multiforme (combination called "spongioneuroblastoma").
4	Retinoblastoma [10]	Eye	U to R	Children usually <2 [1:1]	Rapid	May seed via CSF or systemically. Bilateral in ∼25%. Thought to be congenital; probable dominant inheritance with variable penetrance.
5	Retinal anlage tumor [1]	Maxilla, mandible, anterior fontanelle	VR	Infancy	Slow	May rarely be malignant. Origin & "proper" nomenclature still a major controversy. Synonyms: Melanotic progonoma, melanotic neuroectodermal tumor of infancy, melanotic ameloblastoma, & others. Pigmented papillary subtype of medulloblastoma thought to be a related lesion.
6	Tumors with neuronal differentiation: gangliocytoma	Third ventricle & hypothalamus; temporal lobe	VR	<30	Slow	*See also* Ganglioglioma, entry 30.
	Tumors with glial differentiation					
7	Glioblastoma multiforme	Cerebrum; also brainstem & spinal cord	F [2]	Adults, especially 40-60 [3:2]	Rapid	May seed via CSF. Seeding of spinal subarachnoid space probably more common than generally recognized; >15% in one recent series [4]. Subtypes: the so-called Feigin tumor (entry 44), a glioblastoma with spindle cell sarcoma ("fibrosarcoma" or "angiosarcoma") [17], & the giant cell or monstrocellular glioblastoma (entry 43). Synonyms: spongioblastoma multiforme (archaic); astrocytoma grades 3 & 4; ? malignant astrocytoma; ? malignant oliogodenglioma; ? malignant ependymoma.

[1] In CNS. [2] Very rarely occurs in cerebellum.

continued

221

	Tumor Type	Site	Frequency	Age, yr [Sex Ratio]	Growth Rate	Remarks
8	Polar spongioblastoma	Midbrain, third & fourth ventricles	VR	<20	Rapid	May seed via CSF. The term "spongioblastoma" is used here in the narrow sense of Russell & Rubinstein [18]. Unfortunately, it has been applied by different authors to different tumors with different behaviors: benign cystic cerebellar tumors, infiltrating brainstem tumors, third ventricular tumors, & the usual "optic nerve glioma."
9	Gliomatosis cerebri	Diffuse	VR	Infants & young adults	Moderate to rapid	Almost certainly a diffuse or at least multifocal neoplasm from outset; may be associated with phakomatoses [17]

Tumors with astrocytic differentiation

Astrocytomas with tendency to infiltrate & undergo anaplasia

	Tumor Type	Site	Frequency	Age, yr [Sex Ratio]	Growth Rate	Remarks
10	Fibrillary astrocytoma	Cerebrum; also brainstem & spinal cord	C[3/]	Adults[3/] [7:5]	Variable	Usually infiltrates; often present well beyond apparent area of gross involvement. Has tendency to anaplasia, often terminating as glioblastoma multiforme.
11	Protoplasmic astrocytoma	Cerebrum	U	Adults	Variable	Infiltration common. Tendency to anaplasia, often terminating as glioblastoma multiforme.
12	Gemistocytic astrocytoma	Cerebrum	U[4/]	Adults	Moderate to rapid	Infiltration common. Tendency to anaplasia, often terminating as glioblastoma multiforme.
13	Astroblastoma [17,18]	Cerebrum	VR	Adults	Rapid	Disagreement on existence as a distinct entity [3]. Same term has been used for anaplastic infiltrative astrocytomas [12].

Astrocytomas tending to relative circumscription & only rarely showing anaplasia

	Tumor Type	Site	Frequency	Age, yr [Sex Ratio]	Growth Rate	Remarks
	Piloid astrocytoma					
14	Juvenile [3,17,18]	Cerebellum, optic nerve, brainstem, third ventricle	U; F in children	Most common in children [♂ > ♀]	Slow	Most common primary CNS tumor in children in some series. Rarely infiltrates significantly, and transition to rapidly growing tumor (e.g., glioblastoma multiforme) very rare. Long survival common when occuring in cerebellum or optic nerve. Classic "cystic cerebellar astrocytoma" & "optic nerve glioma."
15	Adult [17,18]	Cerebellum, optic nerve, brainstem, third ventricle	R	Most common in children [♂ > ♀]	Slow	Rarely infiltrates significantly or shows anaplasia
16	Subependymal giant cell astrocytoma [3,17, 18]	Lateral ventricle	R	Most common in children [♂ > ♀]	Slow	May infiltrate or be adjacent to infiltrating astrocytoma. Strong association with tuberous sclerosis which may be present with this tumor.
17	Subependymal glomerate astrocytoma [17,18]	....	....	....	....	*See* Subependymoma, entry 22

Tumors with ependymal differentiation

	Tumor Type	Site	Frequency	Age, yr [Sex Ratio]	Growth Rate	Remarks
	Ependymoma					
18	Typical	Fourth ventricle; also cerebrum & spinal cord	U	Children [3:2]	Slow	Rarely seed, despite reputation [19]. Most common glioma associated with syringomyelia [5].

[3/] Also seen in brainstem of children and young adults. [4/] Very rarely in other sites.

continued

	Tumor Type	Site	Frequency	Age, yr [Sex Ratio]	Growth Rate	Remarks
19	Malignant	Fourth ventricle	R	Children	Moderate to rapid	May seed via CSF. Major difference from typical ependymoma is presence of mitotic figures. [19]
20	Myxopapillary [17,18]	Conus medullaris & filum terminale	R	Young adults [♂ > ♀]	Slow	In CNS, seen only in noted sites; also reported in presacrum & subcutaneous tissue of lower back
21	Papillary	Fourth ventricle	R	Children	Probably slow	Rare tumor often confused with choroid plexus papilloma (entry 25)
22	Subependymoma	Fourth ventricle	R	Adults	Very slow	Most often "incidental" autopsy finding. Synonym: subependymal glomerate astrocytoma (entry 17)
23	Ependymoblastoma [16]	Any ventricle	VR	Children	Rapid	....
24	Cystic cerebral ependymoma of childhood [22]	Cerebral hemisphere	R	Children	Moderate to rapid	Tumors classified under this name may not be a homogeneous group. They are often massive lesions, and behave in a malignant manner.
25	Choroid plexus papilloma	Fourth ventricle; trigone of left lateral ventricle	R	Children	Slow growth	May seed via CSF; may be associated with increased CSF production. (*See* Remarks, entry 21).
26	Choroid plexus carcinoma	Fourth ventricle	R	Children	Moderate to rapid	May seed via CSF. May contain mucinous cells, making differential diagnosis with metastasis even more difficult.

Tumors with oligodendroglial differentiation

	Tumor Type	Site	Frequency	Age, yr [Sex Ratio]	Growth Rate	Remarks
27	Oligodendroglioma Typical [17,18]	Cerebrum	U	Adults	Slow to moderate	May seed via CSF. Most often infiltrative. Radiographic mineralization in ∿30% of cases. Long neurologic history quite common.
28	Malignant [17]	Cerebrum	VR	Adults	Rapid	May terminate as glioblastoma multiforme
29	Tumors of mixed glial elements: mixed glioma [8]	Cerebrum	U	Adults	Slow to rapid	Various mixes of astrocytic, oligodendroglial & (less commonly) ependymal elements. "Mix" may be diffuse, or different areas may show the distinct morphology of the dominant histologic cell type. Anaplasia is frequent. Those surviving longest tend to show more frequent transitions to glioblastoma multiforme.
30	Tumors with both neuronal & glial elements: ganglioglioma [17]	Cerebrum, cerebellum	R to VR	Adults	Slow	Unpredictable; histology may not reflect biologic behavior. Though many show a benign course, transitions to glioblastoma multiforme have been recorded. Synonyms: neuroastrocytoma; neuroglioma; Lhermitte-Duclos disease.

Tumors of Meninges & Related Structures

	Tumor Type	Site	Frequency	Age, yr [Sex Ratio]	Growth Rate	Remarks
31	Meningioma Routine	Meninges, especially convexity; also occurs within ventricles, especially trigone of left ventricle	C	20-60 [♀ > ♂]	Slow	Recurrence rate 11% with "complete" removal [20]; probably significantly higher with longer follow-up and with "incomplete" removal. Subtypes: meningothelial (endothelial); syncytial; fibroblastic (spindle cell); psammomatous; transitional. "Pure" forms are rare.

continued

	Tumor Type	Site	Fre- quency	Age, yr [Sex Ratio]	Growth Rate	Remarks
32	Angioblastic	Meninges of cere- brum	R	Adults	Slow	Includes "hemangioblastic" type, identical to hemangioblastoma of cerebellum (entry 42)
33	Hemangiopericytoma [13,17]	Meninges of cere- brum	VR	Adults	Moderate to rapid	Malignant behavior common, with early recurrence. Identical to pe- ripheral pericytoma.
34	Papillary [14]	Meninges of cere- brum	VR	Children & adults [♀ > ♂]	Moderate to rapid	Papillary pattern; frequent malig- nant features & behavior; 30% with distant metastases
35	Malignant [17]	Usually meninges of cerebrum	VR	Adults	Moderate to rapid	Cytologic features of malignancy; rapid recurrence
36	Meningiomatosis	Usually meninges of cerebrum	VR	Adults	Slow to rapid	Associated with Von Recklinghau- sen's disease
	Meningeal sarcoma					
37	Fibrosarcoma [17]	Meninges	R to VR	Adults	Moderate to rapid	May be seen in neurofibromatosis; recurrences common
38	Primary meningeal sar- comatosis [17,18]	Meninges	R to VR	Adults	Moderate to rapid	Diffuse involvement of meninges
39	Polymorphic cell sarcoma [17,18]	Meninges	R to VR	Children	Rapid	Commonly first recognized in pos- terior fossa; diffuse involvement usually seen at autopsy
	Primary melanotic tumors					
40	Melanoma [17]	Meninges	R to VR	Adults	Rapid	Presumption of metastasis until proven otherwise
41	Meningeal melanomatosis [7,17]	Meninges	R to VR	Adults	Rapid	Associated with neurocutaneous melanosis syndrome; multifocal or diffuse involvement of meninges often with invasion of adjacent brain
	Tumors of Blood Vessels [5]					
	Neoplasms					
42	Hemangioblastoma	Cerebellum	U	All ages	Slow	Morphological continuum with an- gioblastic meningioma (entry 32)
43	Monstrocellular sarcoma [17,22]	Cerebrum	R to VR	Adults	Rapid	Thought by many to be a variant of gliobastoma multiforme (entry 7)
44	Feigin tumor [17]	Cerebrum	R to VR	Adults	Rapid	A glioblastoma multiforme in which the "reactive" vascular-connective tissue component has become neoplastic, thus "glio- blastoma multiforme with fibrosarcoma (or angiosar- coma)." *See also* entry 7.
	Malformations [15]					
45	Capillary telangiectasia	Cerebrum, pons, cerebellum	*See* Re- marks	All ages [♂ > ♀]	Probably static	Common incidental autopsy find- ing. Rarely symptomatic; may be source of hemorrhage.
46	Cavernous angioma	Cerebrum	R	All ages [♂ > ♀]	Slow to moderate	May be multiple. Synonym: cav- ernous vascular malformation.
47	Arteriovenous malforma- tion	Cerebrum	R	All ages [♂ > ♀]	? Slow	Characteristically wedge-shaped in cerebrum, with apex toward ven- tricle
48	Venous malformation	Spinal leptome- ninges	R to VR	All ages [♂ > ♀]	? Slow	Known as Foix-Alajouanine disease when associated with intramedul- lary vascular malformation

[5] Includes malformations.

continued

	Tumor Type	Site	Fre-quency	Age, yr [Sex Ratio]	Growth Rate	Remarks
49	Sturge-Weber-Dimitri disease	Cerebrum	R to VR	Children or young adults	........:.....	Associated with first division trigeminal facial vascular malformation
	Tumors of Nerve Sheath Origin					
50	Schwannoma [6] Typical	Cranial nerve VIII & spinal nerves	U	Adults [♀ > ♂]	Slow	Multiple lesions associated with Von Recklinghausen's disease. Synonyms: neurinoma; neurilemoma.
51	Malignant	Peripheral nerve	VR	Adults	Moderate to rapid	Rarely metastasizes. Synonyms: malignant neurinoma; malignant neurilemoma.
52	Neurofibroma [6] Typical	Peripheral nerve, often plexuses	R	Adults	Slow	Associated with Von Recklinghausen's disease. Most often diffuse local involvement of nerve.
53	Malignant	Peripheral nerve	VR	Adults	Moderate to rapid	Local invasion is frequent, but metastases uncommon
	Primary Tumors of Reticuloendothelial Origin					
54	Primary malignant lymphoma [9]	Cerebrum	R	Adults [♂ > ♀]	Rapid	Often multiple lesions. Local infiltration is routine, and meninges may be involved. All histologic subtypes are seen. Usually not associated with systemic lymphoma. Seen with immunosuppressive therapy.
	Pineal Tumors[6]					
55	Teratoid Germinoma ("pure") [17]	Pineal	R to VR	Adults [♂ > ♀]	Moderate to rapid	May seed via CSF. "Ectopic" germinoma occurs, often in anterior third ventricle or suprasellar area; these often present with diabetes insipidus, visual field defects, & hypopituitarism [2]. Synonyms: dysgerminoma; seminoma; atypical teratoma.
56	Teratoma, adult [17]	Pineal	R to VR	[♂ > ♀]	Slow to moderate	May contain small or large areas of germinoma. Occasionally "ectopic."
57	Embryonal carcinoma [17]	Pineal	R to VR	Children & young adults	Moderate to rapid	....
58	Choriocarcinoma [17]	Pineal	VR	Children & young adults	Usually rapid	....
59	Epithelial cysts	Pineal	R to VR	....	Slow	Commonly ectodermal, but neuroepithelial types also occur
60	Neuroepithelial Pineoblastoma [17]	Pineal	R to VR	[♂ > ♀]	Moderate to rapid	May seed via CSF. Histologically indistinguishable from medulloblastoma (entry 1).
61	Pineocytoma [17]	Pineal	R to VR	[♂ > ♀]	Moderate to rapid	May seed via CSF. Usually histologically identical to neuroblastoma (entry 3).
62	Gliomas (*see* entries above)	Pineal	R to VR	[♂ > ♀]	Variable	Growth rate of primary pineal gliomas seems to parallel histology, i.e., they grow like their counterparts elsewhere

6/ Includes those ectopically located.

continued

	Tumor Type	Site	Fre-quency	Age, yr [Sex Ratio]	Growth Rate	Remarks
63	Lymphoma	Pineal	R to VR	....	Rapid	....
	Pituitary Tumors					
64	Neurohypophyseal Infundiculoma [17]	Pituitary & adjacent structures	U to VR	Children	Slow to moderate	Synonym: juvenile pilocytic astrocytoma (see entry 15)
65	Choristoma [17]	Pituitary & adjacent structures	U to VR	Adults	Slow to moderate	Probably identical to granular cell myoblastoma
66	Adenohypophyseal Pituitary adenoma	Pituitary & adjacent structures	U to VR	Adults [♂ > ♀]	Slow to moderate	Endocrine disturbances common. Classically divided into acidophilic, basophilic, & chromophobic types.
67	Pituitary carcinoma	Pituitary & adjacent structures	U to VR	Adults	....	Exquisitely rare tumor
68	Craniopharyngiomas	Pituitary & adjacent structures	U to VR	Adults [♂ > ♀]	Slow to moderate	Often extrasellar in origin; recurrences common
	Other Paraneoplastic & Malformative Mass Lesions					
69	Cyst Epidermoid	Cerebellopontile angle	R to VR	Usually adults	Static to slow	Synonyms "pearly tumor" & "cholesteatoma" are undesirable because of confusion with inflammatory lesions with same names
70	Dermoid	Often close to midline	R to VR	Adults	Static to slow	....
71	Colloid	Third ventricle	R to VR	Usually adults	Static to slow	Although presence in other than third ventricle is not accepted by some investigators, cysts apparently identical in histology occur in other ventricles; latter are rarely symptomatic. Synonym: colloid cyst of third ventricle.
72	Enterogenous	Ventral to spinal cord	R to VR	Adults	Static to slow	May be seen in Klippel-Feil syndrome
73	Arachnoid	Over cerebral hemispheres	R to VR	Children	Static to slow	May be grossly indistinguishable from neuroglial cyst
74	Neuroglial	Over cerebral hemispheres	R to VR	Children	Static to slow	May be grossly indistinguishable from arachnoidal cyst
75	Nasal glial heterotopia	Above nose or as intranasal polyps	R to VR	Often neonates	Static to slow	Synonym: nasal glioma

Contributor: Davis, Richard L.

References
1. Borello, E. D., and R. J. Gorlin. 1966. Cancer 19:196-206.
2. Camins, M. D., and L. A. Mount. 1974. Brain 97:447-456.
3. Davis, R. L. 1971. In J. Minckler, ed. Pathology of the Nervous System. McGraw-Hill, New York. v. 2, pp. 2007-2026.
4. Davis, R. L. Unpublished. Los Angeles County-Univ. Southern California Medical Center, Los Angeles, 1976.
5. Ferry, D. J., et al. 1969. Med. Ann. D. C. 38:363-365.
6. Harkin, J. C., and R. J. Reed. 1969. Atlas of Tumor Pathology. Armed Forces Institute of Pathology, Washington, D. C. Ser. 2, fasc. 3.
7. Harper, C. G., and D. G. T. Thomas. 1974. J. Neurol. Neurosurg. Psychiat. 37:760-763.
8. Hart, M. N., et al. 1974. Cancer 33:134-140.
9. Henry, J. M., et al. 1974. Ibid. 34:1293-1302.
10. Hogan, J. M., and L. E. Zimmerman. 1962. Ophthalmic Pathology: An Atlas and Textbook. Ed. 2. W. B. Saunders, Philadelphia.
11. Karch, S. B., and H. Urich. 1972. J. Neuropathol. Exp. Neurol. 31:27-53.
12. Kernohan, J. W., and G. P. Sayre. 1952. (Loc. cit. ref. 6). Sect. 10, fasc. 35 and 37.
13. Kruse, F., Jr. 1961. Neurology 11:771-777.

continued

129. NEOPLASIA OF THE CENTRAL NERVOUS SYSTEM

14. Ludwin, S. K., et al. 1975. Cancer 36:1363-1373.
15. McCormick, W. F., and S. S. Schochet, Jr. 1976. Atlas of Cerebrovascular Disease. W. B. Saunders, Philadelphia.
16. Rubinstein, L. J. 1970. Arch. Pathol. 90:35-45.
17. Rubinstein, L. J. 1972. (Loc. cit. ref. 6). Ser. 2, fasc. 6.
18. Russell, D. S., and L. J. Rubinstein. 1971. Pathology of Tumors of the Nervous System. Ed. 3. Williams and Wilkins, Baltimore.
19. Shuman, R. M., et al. 1975. Arch. Neurol. 32:731-739.
20. Simpson, D. 1957. J. Neurol. Neurosurg. Psychiat. 20:22-39.
21. Zimmerman, L. E., et al. 1972. Cancer 30:817-835.
22. Zulch, K. J. 1975. Atlas of Gross Neurosurgical Pathology. Springer-Verlag, New York.

130. EFFECTS OF TRAUMA ON CRANIUM, BRAIN, VERTEBRAL COLUMN, AND SPINAL CORD

Clinical Manifestations: CSF = cerebrospinal fluid. **Micropathology:** PMN = polymorphonuclear leukocyte. **Medico-** **Legal Problems:** DD = differential diagnosis. *Abbreviations:* C5 = fifth cervical vertebra; C6 = sixth cervical vertebra.

	Injury	Clinical Manifestations	Gross Pathology	Micropathology	Medico-Legal Problems	Reference
			Cranio-cerebral Trauma			
1	Skull fractures	Temporary unconsciousness common; headaches, nausea, etc. Symptoms due to damage of intracranial structures. Leak of CSF (rhinorrhea, otorrhea); ear bleeding in basilar fractures; "battle sign" (mastoid ecchymoses) in mid-fossae fractures; middle-ear injuries, with conduction deafness. Injury to cranial nerves. Impacted foreign body of skull, which has penetrated the brain, may be missed. Complicating pneumatocele rare.	Hair-line, comminuted, & depressed fractures. Entrance of gunshot wound has sharp edges, exit has bevelled edges. Presence of soot & powder on skin & bones indicates close range. Contrecoup fractures rare (only of orbital plates or with explosive gunshot wounds).	....	In trauma of head, X rays of skull must be made to avoid later charges of medical negligence. DD of "spectacle hematoma" (due to fractured orbital plates) from beating. In gunshot wounds, determination of entrance vs. exit, range, track, ricocheting injuries, etc. DD of destructive, close-range, explosive firearm injuries from crushing, blunt-force trauma.	1,5,6, 10,13- 15,18- 22,24- 26
			Trauma of Brain Membranes			
2	Epidural hematoma	May follow minor trauma. Rare in children (because of tightly adherent dura). Most are arterial hematomas. Lethal within hours. Syndrome of concussion, headache after symptoms-free interval, somnolence & coma. Neurological signs of ipsilateral compression of third cranial nerve & midbrain (Kernohan crus syndrome). Increased fever, falling pulse, increased blood pressure. Posterior & cerebellar location, with late & puzzling symptomatology.	Usually unilateral. In adults, almost always associated with skull fractures. More common on lateral convexity of brain, and of arterial origin (middle & anterior meningeal). Causes flattening of cerebral convolutions.	Organization of clot by outer dura; first capillary sprouting at 2-3 d, rich granulation tissue at 6-7 d	Artifactual hematomas in fire victims. Aging of injuries.	5-7,10, 12,14, 15,17, 18,20, 21,24- 26

continued

	Injury	Clinical Manifestations	Gross Pathology	Micropathology	Medico-Legal Problems	Reference
3	Traumatic dural thrombosis	Increased intracranial pressure & papilledema, without localizing signs or with motor & sensory deficit especially in lower extremities. May be complicated by carotid artery—cavernous sinus fistula.	Edema of brain, with or without cerebral softenings	Edema, focal encephalomalacia	Topical & temporal relationship to trauma	5,6,10, 14,15, 20,24-26
4	Subdural hematoma	More frequent than the epidural. May follow minor trauma more in ♂, in very young, in very old, & in chronic alcoholics. Acute, subacute, & chronic. (Function of rate of bleeding). Recurrent bleeding. Post-traumatic, symptom-free latent interval may be days or 1-2 wk. Chronic subdural more common in alcoholics. Headaches, disturbance of consciousness, & signs of ipsilateral compression of third cranial nerve.	Often bilateral. More common without fracture, or localized opposite a fracture site, from tears of bridging dural veins. Membranes formed by 6-10 d, rusty membrane by 6-8 wk. In newborn & infants, very delicate membranes. Occasionally may develop into "hygromas." Displacement of mid-line. Flattening of cerebral convolution only with "hygromas" or by rebleeding into old subdural sac. Blood adherent to dura by 4 d.	Organization only from dural side. Early reaction changes after 14-24 h. Significant number of WBC only after 1-2 d, fibroblasts & capillary sprouting by 4-5 d, rich granulation tissue by 10-20 d, dense connective tissue by 25 d.	Non-related to magnitude of trauma. Aging of injury. Mechanism of trauma. DD from rare, non-traumatic dural hematoma (? blood dyscrasia & severe dehydration in infants; rupture through arachnoid of intracerebral hemorrhage).	5-7,10, 12,14, 15,17, 18,20, 21,24-26
5	Subarachnoid hemorrhage	Most common bleeding sequel to head trauma. Meningeal irritation; cranial nerve palsies.	Seldom coagulated blood. At 1 wk, membranes brown, then rusty, then yellow for months; discoloration may disappear within 6-12 d, except with underlying contusions of brain, when membranes remain "rusty" for years.	WBC infiltration may appear within hours, or may be missing; intact RBC's may be seen even after 1 wk; mesothelial cell swelling starts at 12 h, obvious at 24-48 h; phagocytes appear from 2nd day on. Maximal proliferation of subarachnoid cells & phagocytes at 2-6 wk. Hemosiderin pigment in superficial glia of cortex may remain for years. Clearance of subarachnoid space in ∿6 wk	Relationship between minor trauma & ruptured berry aneurysm. Examination of arachnoid, after reflection of dura and before removal of brain, to prevent misinterpretation of artifactual subarachnoid hemorrhage caused by torn veins. DD: Recognition of natural basilar subarachnoid hemorrhage, without demonstrable aneurysm from traumatic basilar subarachnoid hemorrhage due to fracture of transverse process of atlas with laceration of vertebral artery.	5,6,10, 14,15, 17,20, 24-26

continued

	Injury	Clinical Manifestations	Gross Pathology	Micropathology	Medico-Legal Problems	Reference
			Blunt-Force Trauma of Brain [1/]			
6	Concussion	Transient loss of consciousness. Complications: post-concussion syndrome (headache, irritability, confusion, vertigo, tinnitus, retrograde amnesia). Loss of memory regarding accident.	....	Focal chromatolysis of neurons in brainstem within 24 h; petechial hemorrhages	DD from malingering	5-7,10, 12,14-18,20, 21,24-26
7	Contusion	Impaired consciousness or loss of consciousness. Shock in varying degrees. Headaches, vertigo, convulsions may occur. Focal or diffuse central neurological damage. Often bloody spinal fluid under increased pressure. Complications: cranial nerve palsy, epilepsy, mental retardation, traumatic aneurysm of cerebral arteries, arteriovenous fistulas, ischemic brain damage, "punch-drunk" syndrome in boxers, hydrocephalus, intracranial aerocele & pneumatocele, meningitis, & brain abscess. Post-traumatic syndrome (headache, vertigo, fatigue, insomnia).	Located on crest of convolutions. Common on undersurface of frontal & temporal lobes & on temporal poles. Contusion hemorrhages, contusion necroses, stretching necroses. Primary & secondary contusion; secondary brainstem hemorrhages. Edema of brain, with or without herniation of hippocampal unci & cerebellar tonsils. Old contusions: tissues brown-yellow, "moth-eaten"; rusty 6 wk. In "punch-drunk," lesions of corpus callosum.	Reactive astrocytic & microglial reaction starts at 24 h, obvious at 36 h. RBC disintegrated by 6 d. In contusion necrosis, necrosis completed by 48 h, and includes the glia of the first cortical layer.	DD: Blow vs. fall. Usually in blow, contusions larger at impact site (coup) than at 180° opposite to it (contre-coup); reverse holds true for falls. DD of old contusions from vascular encephalomalacia.	5-8,10, 12,14-18,20, 21,24-26
8	Intracerebral hematoma	Progressive intracranial pressure, headaches, blurred vision, lethargy. Unilateral motor disability with contralateral mydriasis.	Corresponds to location of contusions in the proximity of the horns of the lateral ventricles	....	DD from spontaneous intracerebral hemorrhage. DD of delayed traumatic apoplexy (of Bollinger) from natural disease.	5-7,10, 12,14-18,20, 21,24-26
			Trauma of Vertebral Column & Spinal Cord			
9	Fractures of spine	More in men. In cervical region mainly at C5-C6. Pain, rigidity of muscles, & limitation of movements. In neck fractures, dysphagia may be present. Symptoms related to cord injuries. Complications: scoliosis, kyphosis, lordosis, vascular insufficiency of vertebral arteries, hemorrhages into spinal canal.	In juveniles, severance of cartilaginous end plate of vertebral bodies, associated with epidural spinal hematoma; rupture of vertebral ligaments	In juveniles, fracture line involves almost exclusively the two layers of the growth-zone with opening of the bone marrow space	Diagnosis of neck trauma which often is left uncised at autopsy	2-7,9, 20

[1/] Lacerations of brain usually associated with fractures; in young infants, characteristic largely avascular tears of white matter, more fronto-temporal; edema of brain; post-hemorrhagic cyst.

continued

	Injury	Clinical Manifestations	Gross Pathology	Micropathology	Medico-Legal Problems	Reference
10	Concussion of spinal cord	Requires more trauma than for brain concussion. Temporary spinal cord dysfunction below level of injury. Loss of control of urinary & rectal sphincters.	Edema	Edema, small capillary hemorrhages, anemic softenings. Slight honeycomb appearance due to dilatation of perivascular spaces.	....	2-7,9, 20
11	Incised spinal cord injury	Brown-Sequard syndrome, with loss of proprioceptive function below lesion	Usually unilateral, with hemisection of cord common in stab wounds. Both dorsal ⟨posterior⟩ funiculi frequently severed.	Resembles contusions caused by fractures or dislocations. Ascending & descending degeneration in sensory & motor tracts.	....	2-7,9, 20
12	Blunt-force contusions/lacerations	Paralyses & anesthesia below level of injury. Loss of central control of autonomic regulation & temperature. Complications: spasticity, contractures, decubitus ulcers, osteoporosis, nephrolithiasis, ectopic muscle calcifications, thrombophlebitis, autonomic hyperreflexia (hypertension, bradycardia, headaches, diaphoresis).	Spinal cord swelling, degeneration of axons	Lesions appear early, more prominent centrally. Swelling & degeneration of axons. Torn axons with "terminal bulbs." Astrocytic gliosis.	....	2-7,9, 20
13	Traumatic hematomyelia	May follow indirect trauma to head & body. Loss of pain & temperature sensitivity below level of injury. At first, flaccid paralysis of extremities; later, spastic.	Rapidly clotting hemorrhagic softening of central gray matter, with resulting fusiform cavitation having smooth, yellow-stained walls	Fresh: perivascular infiltrates of RBC's, PMN's, & lymphocytes	....	2-7,9, 20

Trauma of Peripheral Nerves

	Injury	Clinical Manifestations	Gross Pathology	Micropathology	Medico-Legal Problems	Reference
14	Neurotmesis (transecting injury)	Flaccid paralyses	Wallerian degeneration, with changes in both distal & proximal stumps. In proximal stump regeneration, outgrowth may produce traumatic neuroma.		Relationship to injury. Aging of injury.	2,5,6, 11,15, 20
15	Axonotmesis (compression injury) & neurapraxia (contusion)	May follow compression during surgery, such as stretching of sciatic nerve, pressure on common peroneal nerve or its major branches by surgical foot supports, pressure by slight casts, or during narcotic coma. Palsies or paralyses may be reversible.	Nerve atrophy. Degeneration of axons with myelin changes. Regeneration of neurofibrils.		Burden of proof in legal suits for inadvertent surgical compression shifts to defendent physician who must provide evidence there was no negligence (res ipsa loquitur).	2,5,6, 11,15, 20

Birth Trauma: Cranio-cerebral

	Injury	Clinical Manifestations	Gross Pathology	Micropathology	Medico-Legal Problems	Reference
16	Skull fractures	Often with cephalhematoma	Subperiosteal hematoma. Permanent cranial deformation. Craniolacunia[2], with osseous necrosis; hyperostosis; complicating meningocele or meningoencephalocele.	....	DD from battered child & other postnatal trauma	5,7,16, 23

[2] Synonym: Lacunar skull.

continued

	Injury	Clinical Manifestations	Gross Pathology	Micropathology	Medico-Legal Problems	Reference
17	Growing skull fractures	Following forceps delivery	Persistent circular forceps holes, cephalhydrocele	....	....	5,7,16, 23
18	Tears of brain membranes	More in firstborn, prematures, monozygotic twins, cephalopelvic disparity	Subdural & subarachnoid hemorrhage; thrombosis of dural veins; encephalomalacia	....	....	5,7,16, 23
19	Parturitional chronic subdural hematoma	In some cases, associated with generalized hemorrhagic diathesis	Thin, brittle membranes; cicatricial polymicrogyria; sclerosis of white matter & basal ganglia	Granulation tissue in membranes; gliosis	....	5,7,16, 23
20	Traumatic porencephalia[3]	Cerebral palsy; mental deficiency	Cavitary defects of cerebellum & cerebrum; central & peripheral preservation of basal ganglia	Mantle sclerosis; cystic degeneration; diffuse patchy sclerosis; periventricular encephalomalacia; hemosiderin pigment	DD from infectious[4], toxic, & metabolic porencephalia[5]	5,7,16, 23
21	Parturitional internal hydrocephalus	Acute: death in 7-10 d postpartum, with rapid increase of head diameter. Subacute: fatal 1-3 yr. Chronic: mental deficiency to decerebrate; epilepsy.	Increase in brain volume; dilatation of cerebral ventricles; sclerotic polymicrogyria. Preservation of basal ganglia.	Gliosis; hemosiderin pigmentation; ependymal proliferation	DD from central porencephalia	5,7,16, 23
22	Parturitional status marmoratus	Hypermotility, athetosis, rigidity, speech disorders	Large, white, patchy lesions in putamen, often combined with sclerotic polymicrogyria	Glial scars, tangles of myelinated & non-myelinated nerve fibers, focal hypermyelination	....	5,7,16, 23
23	Parturitional status dysmyelinisatus	Mental deficiency, palsies, convulsions, rigidity	Cicatricial atrophy of globi pallidi & subthalmic nucleus[6], often combined with porencephalia or other parturitional injuries	Deficient myelinization, neuronal destruction, gliosis	....	5,7,16, 23
24	Parturitional lesions of cerebral cortex	Mental deficiency, palsies	Commonly underlying damage of meningeal hemorrhages. Fibromyelinic plaques; cortical status marmoratus; sclerotic schizogyria; sclerotic polymicrogyria (ulegyria); sclerotic platygyria; speleogyria.	Gliosis, focal hyper-myelinated nerve fibers, erratic nerve fibrils, neuron loss, hemosiderin & fat in glial cells	....	5,7,16, 23
25	Parturitional cerebral white matter sclerosis	Mental deficiency, motor paralysis	Irregular, patchy, gray-discolored, or spongy white matter; microcystic subcortical cavitation; selective sparing of gray matter	Demyelination, glial fibrosis	DD from diffuse sclerosis, progressive subcortical encephalopathy[7] or Pelizaeus-Merzbacher disease	5,7,16, 23
26	Akinesia algera[8]	Cranial nerve paralyses	Atrophy of pons, olives, & various associated nuclei of cranial nerves	Gliosis, demyelination	....	5,7,16, 23

[3] Synonym: Speleo-encephaly. [4] Such as toxoplasmosis. [5] As in gargoylism. [6] Synonym: Luy body. [7] Synonym: Schilder's disease. [8] Synonym: Mobius syndrome, a congenital motility disturbance of cerebral nerves.

continued

	Injury	Clinical Manifestations	Gross Pathology	Micropathology	Medico-Legal Problems	Refer-ence
			Birth Trauma: Spinal Cord & Peripheral Nerves			
27	Spinal cord contusions & lacerations	Palsy to quadriplegia	Hyperextension; luxation of vertebral column; separation-fracture of vertebrae; subdural & spinal hemorrhages; contusion to transection of cord	Edema & degenerative changes in early stages, with demyelination. End-bulb formation of interrupted nerve fibers.	DD from postnatal trauma	4-7,23
28	Syringo-myelia	More with breech delivery. Palsy to quadriplegia; vasomotor & trophic disturbances; muscular atrophy.	Cavitary cord lesion. More common at C5-C6.	Selective destruction of gray matter, with focally preserved columns of gray matter extending over several segments	....	4-7,23
29	Peripheral nerves: stretching &/or compressing injuries	Brachial plexus paralysis; Erb-Duchenne paralysis (upper plexus) common; Klumpke-Dejerine paralyses (lower plexus); Bell's palsy[2]	....	Nerve atrophy with axonal degeneration; hemorrhages in perineural tissues. In Bell's palsy[2], parotid gland hemorrhage.	....	4-7,23

[2] Synonyms: Facial nerve palsy, seventh nerve palsy.

Contributor: Perper, Joshua A.

References

1. Acosta, C., et al. 1972. J. Neurosurg. 36:531-536.
2. Aufdermauer, M. 1974. J. Bone Joint Surg. 56B: 513-519.
3. Bailey, F. W. 1971. In J. Minckler, ed. Pathology of the Nervous System. McGraw-Hill, New York. v. 2, pp. 1765-1774.
4. Boshes, B. 1973. In A. B. Baker and L. H. Baker, ed. Clinical Neurology. Rev. ed. 2. Harper and Row, Hagerstown, MD. v. 3, ch. 35, pp. 1-37.
5. Courville, C. B. 1964. Forensic Neuropathology. Callaghan, Chicago.
6. Feiring, E. H., ed. 1974. Brock's Injuries of the Brain and Spinal Cord. Ed. 5. Springer-Verlag, New York.
7. Ford, F. R. 1973. Disease of the Nervous System in Childhood and Adolescence. C. C. Thomas, Springfield, IL.
8. Graham, D. I., and J. H. Adams. 1971. Lancet 1:265-266.
9. Hardy, A. 1975. Spinal Cord Injuries. G. Thieme, Stuttgart.
10. Hooper, R. 1969. Patterns of Acute Head Injuries. E. Arnold, London.
11. Hughes, J. T. 1972. (Loc. cit. ref. 3). v. 3, pp. 2687-2695.
12. Jennett, B. 1972. Dev. Med. Child Neurol. 14:137-147.
13. Jongkees, L. B. W. 1965. Arch. Otolaryngol. 81:518-522.
14. Lindenberg, R. 1971. (Loc. cit. ref. 3). v. 2, pp. 1705-1765.
15. Lindenberg, R. 1972. (Loc. cit. ref. 3). v. 3, pp. 2726-2764.
16. Lindenberg, R., and E. Freytag. 1969. Arch. Pathol. 87:248-305.
17. Maloney, A. F. J., and W. J. Whatmore. 1969. Br. J. Surg. 56:23-31.
18. Meirowski, A. N. 1965. Neurological Surgery of Trauma. U.S. Government Printing Office, Washington, D.C. pp. 103-130.
19. Memon, M. X., and K. E. Paint. 1971. J. Neurosurg. 35:461-464.
20. Moritz, A. R. 1954. Pathology of Trauma. Lea and Febiger, Philadelphia.
21. Raimonds, A. J., and G. Samuelson. 1970. J. Neurosurg. 32:647-658.
22. Sammut, J. J. 1967. J. Laryngol. Otol. 81:137-142.
23. Schwartz, P. 1971. (Loc. cit. ref. 3). v. 2, pp. 1774-1806.
24. Vinken, P. J., and G. W. Bruyn, ed. 1975. Handb. Clin. Neurol. 23.
25. Vinken, P. J., and G. W. Bruyn, ed. 1977. Ibid. 24.
26. Voris, H. C. 1973. (Loc. cit. ref. 4). v. 2, ch. 23, pp. 1-43.

131. NON-VIRAL INFECTIONS OF THE NERVOUS SYSTEM

Bibliographic citations in Part II apply also to Part I. Data in brackets refer to the column heading in brackets.

Part I. Biologic and Epidemiologic Characteristics

Organism ⟨Synonym⟩	Biologic Characteristics	Epidemiologic Characteristics		Ref-er-ence
		Non-Primate Host [Vector]	Distribution	
Rickettsial				
1 *Rickettsia prowazekii; R. tsutsu-gamushi*	Coccobacillus; non-motile	Rodents [Tick; louse]	Worldwide	31
Bacterial				
2 *Treponema pallidum*	Spirochete; motile	....	Worldwide	8
3 *Borrelia recurrentis*	Spirochete; motile	Rodents; dog [Tick; louse]	Worldwide	11
4 *Leptospira interrogans* ⟨*L. ictero-hemorrhagiae*⟩	Spirochete (finely spiralled); motile	Rodents; domestic animals	Worldwide	17
5 *Pseudomonas aeruginosa*	Gram (−) pleomorphic bacillus; motile	....	Worldwide	9
6 *Brucella melitensis; B. suis*	Gram (−) coccobacillus; non-motile; no capsule	....	Worldwide	12
7 *Escherichia coli*	Gram (−) bacillus	....	Worldwide	29
8 *Salmonella cholerae-suis; S. enteri-tidis; S. havana; S. paratyphi-A; S. typhimurium*	Gram (−) bacillus; motile; no capsule	....	Worldwide	37
9 *Klebsiella pneumoniae*	Gram (−) bacillus; non-motile; large capsule	....	Worldwide	47
10 ⟨*Aerobacter aerogenes*⟩	Gram (−) bacillus	....	Worldwide	26
11 *Proteus mirabilis; P. vulgaris*	Gram (−) bacillus, often paired; motile	....	Worldwide	51
12 *Haemophilus influenzae*	Gram (−) pleomorphic coccus; non-motile	....	Worldwide	23
13 *Bacteroides fragilis; Fusobacteri-um necrophorum* ⟨*B. funduli-formis*⟩	Gram (−) bacillus; anaerobic; no spores	....	Worldwide	39, 43
14 *Neisseria gonorrhoeae*	Gram (−) paired cocci	....	Worldwide	15
15 *N. meningitidis*	Gram (−) paired cocci	....	Worldwide	28
16 *Mima polymorpha* var. *oxidans*	Gram (−) diplococcus; pleomor-phic	....	Worldwide	18
17 *Staphylococcus aureus*	Gram (+) coccus; non-motile	....	Worldwide	41
18 *Streptococcus* sp. ⟨*S. viridans*⟩	Gram (+) coccus, often in chains	....	Worldwide	42
19 *S. pneumoniae* ⟨*Diplococcus pneu-moniae*⟩	Gram (+) paired cocci	....	Worldwide	32
20 *S. pyogenes* ⟨*S. hemolyticus*⟩	Gram (+) coccus, often in chains	....	Worldwide	42
21 *Clostridium perfringens*	Gram (+) bacillus, anaerobic; non-motile; spores	....	Worldwide	35
22 *Listeria monocytogenes*	Gram (+) coccobacillus; motile	Sheep; horse	Worldwide	16
23 *Actinomyces bovis; A. israelii*	Gram (+) anaerobe	....	Worldwide	44
24 *Mycobacterium leprae*	Acid-fast bacillus; non-motile; no spores	....	Tropics; subtropics	33
25 *M. tuberculosis*	Acid-fast bacillus; non-motile; no spores	Cattle	Worldwide	3
26 *Nocardia asteroides*	Gram (+) acid-fast aerobe	Cattle	Worldwide	25

continued

Part I. Biologic and Epidemiologic Characteristics

Organism ⟨Synonym⟩	Biologic Characteristics	Epidemiologic Characteristics		Reference
		Non-Primate Host [Vector]	Distribution	
Fungal				
27	*Coccidioides immitis*	Dimorphic fungus	Cattle; dog; rodents	Southwestern U.S.; Latin America	13
28	*Paracoccidioides brasiliensis*	Dimorphic fungus	....	Latin America	24
29	*Rhizopus arrhizus; R. oryzae*	Phycomycete; non-septate	....	Worldwide	45
30	*Allescheria boydii*	Ascocarpic stage of *Monosporium apiospermum*	....	Tropics	1
31	*Blastomyces dermatitidis*	Dimorphic fungus	Dog; horse	North America	6
32	*Histoplasma capsulatum*	Intracellular; yeast-like	Numerous mammals	Worldwide	40
33	*Aspergillus amstelodami; A. flavus; A. fumigatus*	Pigmented fungus	Birds	Worldwide	48
34	*Candida albicans; C. tropicalis*	Yeast with no capsule	....	Worldwide	27
35	*Cladosporium trichoides*	Dimorphic fungus	Cattle	Tropics; subtropics	46
36	*Cryptococcus neoformans*	Yeast with polysaccharide capsule	Cattle; pigeon	Worldwide	52
37	*Sporotrichum schenckii*	Dimorphic fungus	....	Worldwide, especially South Africa	22
Protozoan				
38	*Trypanosoma gambiense*	Protozoan with flagellum	Swine; cattle [Tsetse-fly]	Africa	20
39	*Endolimax williamsi*	Enteric protozoan	Swine	Worldwide	21
40	*Entamoeba histolytica*	Enteric amoeba	....	Worldwide	4
41	*Naegleria gruberi*	Free-living amoeba	....	Temperate zones: Europe; U.S.	5
42	*Plasmodium falciparum; P. malariae; P. vivax*	Protozoan	[Mosquito]	Tropics; subtropics	7
43	*Toxoplasma gondii*	Intracellular protozoan	Cat; other mammals	Worldwide; more common in tropics	14
Helminthan				
44	*Fasciola hepatica*	Trematode (fluke)	Sheep; cattle	Sheep & cattle regions	34
45	*Paragonimus westermani*	Trematode (lung fluke)	Cat; dog; muskrat	Far east	50
46	*Schistosoma haematobium; S. japonicum; S. mansoni*	Trematode	Numerous mammals	Tropics; subtropics	2
47	*Echinococcus granulosus*	Eggs of canine tapeworm	Dog; wolf; sheep	Grazing regions	38
48	*Multiceps multiceps* ⟨*Coenurus cerebralis*⟩	Cestode	Dog; cat	Worldwide	49
49	*Taenia solium* ⟨*Cysticercus cellulosae*⟩	Eggs of swine tapeworm	Swine	Worldwide	10
50	*Setaria digitata*	Nematode	Cattle [Mosquito]	Tropics	19
51	*Toxocara canis*	Nematode	Dog; cat	Far east	36
52	*Trichinella spiralis*	Nematode	Swine; rodents; bear	Worldwide	30

Contributor: Aronson, Stanley M.

References: *See* Part II.

continued

Part II. Clinical Features and Pathological Characteristics

Age of Occurrence: I = infancy; **C** = childhood; **A** = adulthood; **S** = senium; **O** = opportunistic; − = uncommon; + = common; ++ = most common. **Organism Present in: Bl** = blood; **CSF** = cerebrospinal fluid; + = present; − = not present; ± = may or may not be present. **Local Changes: LM** = leptomeningitis; **PM** = pachymeningitis; **BA** = brain abscesses; **MA** = microabscesses; **Oth** = other; − = not present; + = present; ± = may or may not be present.

Organism ⟨Synonym⟩	Clinical Features						Organism Present in		Pathological Characteristics						Reference
	Age of Occurrence					Systemic Features [Modifying Factors]	Bl	CSF	Local Changes					Systemic Changes	
	I	C	A	S	O				LM	PM	BA	MA	Oth		
Rickettsial															
1 Rickettsia prowazekii; R. tsutsugamushi	−	+	+		−	Typhus	+	−	−	−	−	−	Fn[1/]	....	31
Bacterial															
2 Treponema pallidum	+	+	++	+	−	Syphilis	−	−	+	+	+	+	Fn[2/]	....	8
3 Borrelia recurrentis	−	+	+	−	−	Relapsing fever	+	−	−	−	−	−	Fn[3/]	....	11
4 Leptospira interrogans ⟨L. icterohemorrhagiae⟩	−	+	+	−	−	Weil's disease	+	±	+	−	−	−	Fn[3/]	Hepatitis; enteritis	17
5 Pseudomonas aeruginosa	+	−	−	+	+	....	−	+	+	−	+	+	....	....	9
6 Brucella melitensis; B. suis	−	+	+	−	−	Brucellosis	−	+	+	−	−	−	....	Brucellosis	12
7 Escherichia coli	+	−	−	+	+	[Prematurity]	−	+	+	−	+	+	....	Enteritis	29
8 Salmonella cholerae-suis; S. enteritidis; S. havana; S. paratyphi-A; S. typhimurium	+	−	−	−	+	[Septic abortion]	−	+	+	−	−	−	....	....	37
9 Klebsiella pneumoniae	+	+	−	+	+	[CNS abnormalities]	−	+	+	−	−	−	....	....	47
10 ⟨Aerobacter aerogenes⟩	+	−	−	−	+	[Hydrocephalus]	−	+	+	−	+	+	....	....	26
11 Proteus mirabilis; P. vulgaris	+	−	−	−	+	....	−	+	...	...	...	...	....	....	51
12 Haemophilus influenzae	−	++	−	−	−	....	±	+	+	−	+	−	....	Pyarthrosis	23
13 Bacteroides fragilis; Fusobacterium necrophorum ⟨B. funduliformis⟩	+	−	+	−	+	....	−	+	...	...	...	...	....	....	39, 43
14 Neisseria gonorrhoeae	−	+	+	−	−	....	+	+	+	−	−	−	....	Vaginitis; urethritis	15
15 N. meningitidis	−	++	++	+	−	Petechiae; consumptive coagulopathy	+	+	+	−	−	−	....	Adrenal hemorrhage; myocarditis	28
16 Mima polymorpha var. oxidans	−	−	+	−	−	Conjunctivitis	−	+	+	−	−	−	....	Conjunctivitis; urethritis; vaginitis	18
17 Staphylococcus aureus	+	+	+	+	+	[Diabetes mellitus; skull injury]	+	+	+	+	+	+	....	Otitis media; systemic abscesses	41
18 Streptococcus sp. ⟨S. viridans⟩	−	+	+	+	−	....	±	+	+	±	+	+	....	Endocarditis	42
19 S. pneumoniae ⟨Diplococcus pneumoniae⟩	−	+	+	+	−	....	±	+	+	±	+	+	....	Pneumonitis	32
20 S. pyogenes ⟨S. hemolyticus⟩	−	+	+	+	−	....	±	+	+	−	+	−	....	Endocarditis; pharyngitis	42

[1/] Neuropathy. [2/] Tabes dorsalis and general paresis. [3/] Encephalitis.

continued

Part II. Clinical Features and Pathological Characteristics

Organism (Synonym)	Age of Occurrence I	C	A	S	O	Systemic Features [Modifying Factors]	Organism Present in Bl	CSF	LM	PM	BA	MA	Oth	Systemic Changes	Reference
21 Clostridium perfringens	−	+	+	−	+	[Penetrating trauma; septic abortion]	−	+	−	−	+	+	....	....	35
22 Listeria monocytogenes	+	−	−	−	−	Monocytosis	+	+	+	...	±	...	Fn4/	Pneumonitis; conjunctivitis	16
23 Actinomyces bovis; A. israelii	−	+	+	+	−	Pneumonia	−	+	+	+	+	+	....	Osteomyelitis	44
24 Mycobacterium leprae	−	+	+	+	−	Leprosy	−	−	−	−	−	−	Fn1/	....	33
25 M. tuberculosis	−	++	++	+	−	Tuberculosis	−	+	+	+	+	+	....	Systemic tuberculosis	3
26 Nocardia asteroides	−	+	+	−	+	Pneumonia [Neoplasms; immunosuppression]	−	+	+	−	+	−	....	Pneumonitis	25

Fungal

Organism (Synonym)	I	C	A	S	O	Systemic Features [Modifying Factors]	Bl	CSF	LM	PM	BA	MA	Oth	Systemic Changes	Reference
27 Coccidioides immitis	−	+	+	−	−	Pneumonia	−	+	+	−	+	+	....	Pneumonitis	13
28 Paracoccidioides brasiliensis	−	−	+	−	−	Skin nodules	−	+	+	−	+	−	....	....	24
29 Rhizopus arrhizus; R. oryzae	−	+	+	+	+	Rhinitis [Diabetes mellitus acidosis]	−	+	...	...	...	...	Fn5/	Retro-orbital infection	45
30 Allescheria boydii	−	−	+	−	+	Dermatitis [Lumbar puncture]	−	+	+	+	+	−	....	....	1
31 Blastomyces dermatitidis	−	+	+	−	−	Dermatitis; pneumonia	−	+	+	−	+	−	....	....	6
32 Histoplasma capsulatum	−	+	+	−	+	Pneumonia [Leukemia; lymphoma]	−	+	+	−	+	−	....	....	40
33 Aspergillus amstelodami; A. flavus; A. fumigatus	+	+	+	+	+	Pneumonia [Neoplasms; debilitation; immunosuppression]	−	+	+	−	+	+	....	Pneumonitis	48
34 Candida albicans; C. tropicalis	+	+	+	+	+	Enteritis; vaginitis [Diabetes mellitus; pregnancy; neoplasm; immunosuppression]	−	+	+	−	−	+	....	Disseminated abscesses	27
35 Cladosporium trichoides	−	+	+	−	−	Dermatitis	−	−	−	−	+	−	....	Pneumonitis	46
36 Cryptococcus neoformans	−	+	+	+	+	Pneumonia [Leukemia; lymphoma; steroid therapy]	−	+	+	−	+	+	....	....	52
37 Sporotrichum schenckii	−	+	+	+	−	Dermatitis	−	−	−	+	−	−	....	....	22

Protozoan

Organism (Synonym)	I	C	A	S	O	Systemic Features [Modifying Factors]	Bl	CSF	LM	PM	BA	MA	Oth	Systemic Changes	Reference
38 Trypanosoma gambiense	−	+	+	−	−	Hepatosplenomegaly	+	+	+	−	−	−	Fn6/	Myocarditis	20
39 Endolimax williamsi	−	+	+	−	−	Dysentery	−	−	−	−	+	−	....	Enteritis	21
40 Entamoeba histolytica	−	+	+	−	−	Dysentery; hepatomegaly	−	−	−	−	+	−	....	Lung & liver abscesses	4

1/ Neuropathy. 4/ Rhomboencephalitis. 5/ Vasculitis. 6/ Hemorrhagic encephalitis.

continued

Part II. Clinical Features and Pathological Characteristics

Organism ⟨Synonym⟩	Clinical Features							Pathological Characteristics							Reference
	Age of Occurrence				Systemic Features [Modifying Factors]	Organism Present in		Local Changes					Systemic Changes	
	I	C	A	S	O		Bl	CSF	LM	PM	BA	MA	Oth		
41 Naegleria gruberi	−	+	+	−	−	....	−	+	+	−	−	−	....	....	5
42 Plasmodium falciparum; P. malariae; P. vivax	−	+	+	+	−	Hemolysis	+	−	−	−	−	−	Fn[3/]	....	7
43 Toxoplasma gondii	++	+	+	−	+	Lymphadenopathy [Immunosuppression [7/]	−	−	+	−	+	+	....	Retinitis	14

Helminthan

44 Fasciola hepatica	−	−	+	−	−	Dysentery; cirrhosis	−	−	−	−	+	−	....	Hepatitis	34
45 Paragonimus westermani	−	+	+	−	−	Pneumonia	−	−	+	−	+	−	....	Pneumonitis	50
46 Schistosoma haematobium; S. japonicum; S. mansoni	−	+	+	+	−	Diarrhea; hepatic failure	−	−	−	−	−	+	Fn[8/]	Cirrhosis	2
47 Echinococcus granulosus	−	−	+	−	−	Cysts; hypersensitivity	−	−	−	−	−	−	Fn[9/]	Disseminated cysts	38
48 Multiceps multiceps ⟨Coenurus cerebralis⟩	−	+	+	−	−	....	−	−	−	−	+	−	....	Myositis	49
49 Taenia solium ⟨Cysticercus cellulosae⟩	−	−	+	−	−	Disseminated cysts	−	−	−	−	...	...	Fn[9/]	Disseminated cysts	10
50 Setaria digitata	−	−	+	−	−	....	−	−	+	−	+	−	....	....	19
51 Toxocara canis	−	+	+	−	−	Visceral larval migrans	−	−	−	−	+	+	....	Disseminated granulomas	36
52 Trichinella spiralis	−	−	+	−	−	Myositis	−	−	−	−	+	−	....	Myositis; myocarditis	30

[3/] Encephalitis. [7/] In adults. [8/] Myelopathy. [9/] Cysts.

Contributor: Aronson, Stanley M.

References
1. Aronson, S. 1953. J. Neuropathol. Exp. Neurol. 12: 158-168.
2. Blankfein, R., and A. Chinco. 1965. Neurology 15: 957-967.
3. Boyd, G. 1956. AMA J. Dis. Child. 91:447-484.
4. Butt, C. G. 1966. N. Engl. J. Med. 274:1473-1476.
5. Callicott, J. 1968. Am. J. Clin. Pathol. 49:84-91.
6. Chick, E., et al. 1956. Am. J. Med. Sci. 231:253-262.
7. Coatney, G., et al. 1953. Am. J. Trop. Med. Hyg. 2: 958-988.
8. Cosco, N. 1941. N. Engl. J. Med. 225:450-451.
9. Curtin, J., et al. 1961. Ann. Intern. Med. 54:1077-1107.
10. Dolgopol, V., and M. Neustaedter. 1935. Arch. Neurol. Psychiatry 33:132-147.
11. Felsenfeld, O., et al. 1965. J. Immunol. 94:804-817.
12. Fincham, R., et al. 1963. J. Am. Med. Assoc. 184: 269-275.
13. Forbus, W., and A. M. Bestebreurtje. 1946. Mil. Surg. 99:653-719.
14. Frenkel, J. K. 1956. Ann. N.Y. Acad. Sci. 64:215-251.
15. Gisslen, L., et al. 1961. Bull. WHO 24:367-372.
16. Gray, M., and A. Killinger. 1966. Bacteriol. Rev. 30: 309-382.
17. Heath, C., et al. 1965. N. Engl. J. Med. 273:915-922.
18. Hermann, G., and T. Melnick. 1965. Am. J. Dis. Child. 110:315-318.
19. Innes, J. R. M., and C. Shoho. 1953. AMA Arch. Neurol. Psychiatry 70:325-349.
20. Janssen, P., et al. 1956. J. Neuropathol. Exp. Neurol. 15:269-281.
21. Kernohan, J., et al. 1960. Arch. Pathol. 70:576-580.
22. Klein, R., et al. 1966. Arch. Intern. Med. 118:145-149.
23. Koch, R., and M. Carson. 1955. J. Pediatr. 46:18-29.
24. Lacaz, C. 1953. Mycopathology 6:241-259.
25. Larsen, M. 1959. Arch. Intern. Med. 103:712-725.
26. Light, I. 1967. Postgrad. Med. 41:373-376.
27. Louria, D. B., et al. 1962. Medicine (Baltimore) 41: 307-337.
28. Macrae, J. 1955. Postgrad. Med. J. 31:92-96.
29. Manesis, J., and J. Stanosheck. 1965. Arch. Neurol. (Chicago) 13:214-217.
30. Most, H. 1965. J. Am. Med. Assoc. 193:871-873.
31. Noad, K., and W. Haymaker. 1953. Brain 76:113-131.
32. Olsson, R., et al. 1961. Ann. Intern. Med. 55:545-549.
33. Rosenberg, R., and R. Lovelace. 1968. Arch. Neurol. (Chicago) 19:310-314.
34. Ruggiero, F., et al. 1967. J. Neurosurg. 27:268-271.
35. Russell, J., and J. Taylor. 1963. Br. J. Surg. 50:434-437.
36. Sadun, E., et al. 1957. Am. J. Trop. Med. Hyg. 6:562-568.

continued

Part II.   Clinical Features and Pathological Characteristics

37. Saphra, I., and J. W. Winter. 1957. N. Engl. J. Med. 256:1128-1134.
38. Schantz, P., et al. 1970. Am. J. Trop. Med. Hyg. 19: 823-836.
39. Schoolman, A., et al. 1966. Arch. Intern. Med. 118: 150-153.
40. Schulz, D. 1953. Am. J. Clin. Pathol. 24:11-26.
41. Sher, J., et al. 1965. J. Neuropathol. Exp. Neurol. 24: 175-176.
42. Sherman, J. 1937. Bacteriol. Rev. 1:1-97.
43. Smith, W., et al. 1944. Ann. Intern. Med. 20:920-941.

44. Stevens, H. 1953. Neurology 3:761-772.
45. Straatsma, B. 1963. Lab. Invest. 11:963-985.
46. Symmers, W. 1960. Brain 83:37-51.
47. Thompson, A., et al. 1952. Arch. Intern. Med. 89: 405-420.
48. Tveten, L. 1965. Acta Neurol. Scand. 41:19-33.
49. Wainwright, J. 1957. J. Pathol. Bacteriol. 73:347-354.
50. Yokogawa, S., et al. 1960. Exp. Parasitol. 10:81-205.
51. Yu, J., and A. Grawaug. 1963. Arch. Dis. Child. 38: 391-396.
52. Zimmerman, L., and H. Rappaport. 1954. Am. J. Clin. Pathol. 24:1050-1072.

132.   VIRAL INFECTIONS OF THE CENTRAL NERVOUS SYSTEM

Last 4 columns: For ease of location, principal virus and disease names have been set in boldface, and laboratory findings and procedures have been underlined. **Laboratory Findings:** EEG = electroencephalogram; CF = complement-fixation antibodies; HI = hemagglutination-inhibition antibodies; Nt = neutralization antibodies. *Abbreviations:* CSF = cerebrospinal fluid; PMN = polymorphonuclear leukocytes. Figures in heavy brackets are reference numbers.

Part I.   Acute Infections

Laboratory Findings: IF = immunofluorescence antibodies

Virus ⟨Synonym⟩	Fre-quency	Clinical Manifestations ⟨Synonym⟩	Laboratory Findings	Pathology	Virus Isolation
			Meningitis		
1 Enteroviruses[1]	41% [9], 44% [5]	Headache, stiff neck, photophobia, fever. Onset usually acute. Derangements of consciousness or focal neurological signs rare. Course usually benign, of 7-10 d duration. **Echo:** May be rash; may be acute cerebellar ataxia in children [7]. **Mumps:** May become deaf, presumed due to labyrinthine damage. Parotitis may be absent. **LCM:** Upper respiratory symptoms may predominate. **Infectious mononucleosis:** May have sore throat, malaise, fever, cervical lymphadenopathy, splenomegaly.	CSF: Pressure—normal or mildly increased (rarely >250 mm H_2O). Cells—10-500 mononuclear leukocytes per μl (number varies with virus; may be 0; may be >2000 in **mumps; Coxsackie B5, or LCM**); may be 10-50% PMN early in infection. Protein—normal or up to 200 mg/100 ml. Glucose—normal; may be low in **mumps & LCM [11].** EEG: Usually normal. Serum antiviral antibodies[2]: 4-fold or greater rise in sera between acute & convalescent (3-6 wk later) stages. **Polioviruses**—CF, Nt; **Coxsackieviruses**—CF, Nt; **Echoviruses**—HI, Nt; **Mumps virus**—CF, HI; **LCM**—CF, Nt, indirect IF; **Arboviruses**—HI, Nt, CF. **Infectious mononucleosis**—IF antibodies to **Epstein-Barr virus,** serum heterophile agglutinin antibodies, & increased numbers of atypical lymphocytes in blood. Usually not helpful for **herpes simplex.**	Lymphocytic inflammatory infiltration in pia-arachnoid & adjacent structures. Arteritis & obstruction of CSF pathways quite uncommon.	**Enteroviruses:** Stool, throat washings, CSF, urine, blood; inoculate monkey kidney (MK) cells; most **Coxsackie A** require suckling mouse inoculation. May be multiple infection (in stool, throat). **Mumps virus:** CSF, saliva, urine, rarely blood; inoculate human (e.g., HeLa) or MK cells, or chick embryo amnion. **LCM:** CSF, blood; inoculate weanling or suckling mice, young guinea pigs, MK cells, baby hamster kidney (BHK) cells. **HSV:** Rarely can isolate from CSF; presence in skin lesions or saliva may be irrelevant to CNS infection. **Arboviruses:** Blood, CSF; difficult to isolate; inoculate suckling mice, suckling hamsters, cells (especially MK, BHK-21, HeLa, chick embryo).
2 Polioviruses	9% [9], 5% [5]				
Coxsackieviruses					
3 Group A	0% [9], 5% [5]				
4 Group B	19% [5,9]				
5 Echoviruses	13% [9], 15% [5]				
6 Mumps virus	17% [9], 8% [5]				
7 Lymphocytic choriomeningitis ⟨LCM⟩ virus	9% [9], 2% [5]				
8 Herpesvirus ⟨Herpes simplex virus; HSV⟩[3]	1% [9], <1% [5]				
9 Arboviruses	<1% [5, 9]				
10 Epstein-Barr virus ⟨Infectious mononucleosis virus⟩	Not established				
11 Unknown	31% [9], 45% [5]				

[1] Subgroup of picornaviruses.   [2] Antibodies to any of these viruses in CSF is strong presumptive evidence of recent infection.   [3] Herpesvirus type 2 is more common cause of meningitis than type 1.

continued

Part I. Acute Infections

Virus ⟨Synonym⟩	Frequency	Clinical Manifestations ⟨Synonym⟩	Laboratory Findings	Pathology	Virus Isolation
			Encephalitis		
12 Enteroviruses[1]	9% [9], 16% [5]	Acute generalized disturbance of cere-	CSF: Same as for men- ingitis. Pressure more	Gross: Usually minimal changes; severe cases	Same as for meningi- tis. Brain biopsy, IF,
13 Polioviruses	4% [9], 6% [5]	bral function—con- vulsions, confusion,	likely to be elevated. EEG: Usually abnor-	of **herpes simplex** or **eastern equine enceph-**	& culture may be required to establish
Coxsackieviruses		stupor, coma, apha-	mal; most commonly	**alitis** may show gross	diagnosis of **herpes**
14 Group A	2% [9], 1% [5]	sia, mutism, hemi- paresis, involuntary	diffusely slow; may be focal abnormalities	evidence of necrosis (hemorrhagic soften-	**simplex encephali- tis.**
15 Group B	2% [9], 5% [5]	movements, ataxia, cranial nerve defi-	(e.g., frontal & tempo- ral in **herpes simplex**	ing & swelling) of cerebral cortex & sub-	
16 Echoviruses	<1% [9], 4% [5]	cits; any or all may be present in vary-	**encephalitis**), or sei- zure activity. Periodic	cortical white matter acutely, & shrinkage	
17 Mumps virus	18% [9], 14% [5]	ing combinations. Aseptic meningitis	high voltage discharge in temporal lobe, espe-	& scarring later. Microscopic: Necrosis	
18 Lymphocytic chorio-	16% [9], 0% [5]	syndrome may be present, in addition.	cially when pattern changes rapidly over a	of nerve cells & neuro- nophagia (microglial	
meningitis ⟨LCM⟩		Illness varies with etiological virus.	few days, is highly sug- gestive of **HSV.** Radio-	nodules); perivascular cuffing (Virchow-	
virus		Usually lasts weeks,	isotope brain scan,	Robin spaces), & men-	
19 Herpesvirus ⟨Herpes	10% [9], 9% [5]	rarely months. Dif- ferent fatality rates	computerized tomog- raphy, angiography,	ingeal infiltration by lymphocytes & mono-	
simplex vi- rus; HSV⟩[4]		for different agents. 20% have residual	pneumoencephalogra- phy may show focal	nuclear leukocytes (later plasmocytes);	
20 Arboviruses[5]	16% [9], 6% [5]	mental deteriora- tion, memory loss,	damage (especially in **herpes simplex enceph-**	gray matter usually in- volved much more ex-	
21 Measles virus	0% [9], 4% [5]	personality change, hemiparesis, other	**alitis**). Serum antiviral anti-	tensively than white matter. In **herpes sim-**	
22 Epstein-Barr vi- rus ⟨Infec-	0% [9], 1% [5]	neurological defi- cits. In children, de-	bodies: Same as for meningitis	**plex encephalitis**, in- tranuclear eosinophilic	
tious mono- nucleosis		lay in mental devel- opment may not be apparent until years		(Cowdry type A) in- clusion bodies in neu- rons, oligodendroglia	
virus⟩		later.		& astrocytes.	
23 Influenza A2 virus	0% [9], 1% [5]	**Herpes simplex:** May present as acute delirium with auditory hallucinations,		Distribution of lesions: **Herpes simplex**—es-	
24 Unknown	31% [9], 49% [5]	or dementia with sucking & grasping re- flexes. May be clinical & pathological		pecially frontal (par- ticularly orbital sur- faces) & temporal	
		changes without fever or meningeal irritation. May mimic a space-		lobes. **Eastern equine**— greatest changes in	
		occupying lesion. Survivors may be left with an amnestic confabulatory syn-		brainstem & basal gan- glia. **Western equine**—	
		drome. Reported case fatality 20-60%, but milder cases probably often undiag-		greatest damage in basal ganglia & white	
		nosed. [10] **Eastern equine:** Very severe; 20-50% fa-		matter of cerebral hemispheres.	
		tal within a few days. Residual neuro- logical deficits in 80-90% of survivors.			

[1] Subgroup of picornaviruses. [4] Herpes simplex is probably the commonest sporadically occurring encephalitis. Herpes- virus type 1 causes almost all cases of HSV encephalitis in the adult. Herpesvirus type 2 causes most generalized herpes simplex infections in the newborn, including menin- goencephalitis. [3] [5] About 2400 cases in U.S. in past 10 years; incidence varies markedly from year to year. Order of frequency in U.S.: St. Louis > Western equine > Cali- fornia (almost never in adults) > Eastern equine (rare). Many more inapparent than clinically evident cases. Vene- zuelan equine has caused cases in Florida, although it oc- curs mainly in Central & South America. **Japanese B en- cephalitis** virus is important in Japan, and Murray Valley encephalitis virus in Australia & New Guinea.

continued

Part I. Acute Infections

	Virus (Synonym)	Fre-quency	Clinical Manifestations (Synonym)	Laboratory Findings	Pathology	Virus Isolation
			Myelitis: Poliomyelitis			
25	Enteroviruses [1]	81% [9], 64% [5]	**Poliomyelitis:** Incubation period of 5-35 d (average 17 d). In acute stages of viral infection of motor neurons, there may be tremor, fasciculations, resistance to passive movement; also usually fever and signs of meningeal inflammation. Later, flaccid asymmetric motor paralysis and arreflexia of cranial & spinal musculature (in 10-15%). The disease is more severe in adults than in children. Note: Most cases of poliomyelitis are abortive ("minor illness"), and indistinguishable from other cases of aseptic meningitis.	CSF: In **poliomyelitis**, changes are those of aseptic meningitis. Greatest changes are in preparalytic stage. Pressure—>150 mm H_2O in 2/3; >200 mm in 1/3; usually associated with respiratory insufficiency. Cells—(25-500)/μl; mainly PMN early, mainly lymphocytes by day 5. Protein—normal or increased; usually <100 mg/100 ml; may be slightly elevated early in the course, rising gradually to moderate levels by 2nd & 3rd wk, and returning to normal by 6th wk; especially increased for first 20-30 d in paralyzed patients, then gradual decrease. Glucose—normal. Other: In **poliomyelitis**, usually a polymorphonuclear leukocytosis in blood. Serum viral antibody studies are as for meningitis.	**Poliomyelitis:** Acutely—congestion of ventral (anterior) horns of spinal cord, with petechial hemorrhages, infiltrates of lymphocytes, histiocytes, & PMN; chromatolysis & necrosis of motor neurons, often with neuronophagia (especially at later stages). Later—loss of ventral (anterior) horn cells & of myelinated fibers in ventral horns & astrocytic gliosis. Surviving motor nerve cells may be pale & chromatolytic. Most severe lesions are in anterior two-thirds of spinal cord gray matter, usually sparing sacral segments. Lesser degrees of nerve cell destruction seen in brainstem tegmentum, Clarke's columns, dorsal root ganglia, hypothalamus, & motor cortex. [3] HSV has been reported as rare cause of progressive myelitis without encephalitis. [10]	Same as for meningitis.
26	Polioviruses [6]	78% [9], 62% [5]				
	Coxsackieviruses					
27	Group A	0% [5,9]				
28	Group B	<1% [5, 9]				
29	Echoviruses	<1% [5, 9]				
30	Mumps virus	<1% [5, 9]				
31	Unknown	19% [9], 36% [5]				
	Reference	4,8		4,6,8	2	1,6

[1] Subgroup of picornaviruses. [6] Since Salk (1953) and Sabin (1955) vaccines were introduced, there has been a sharp drop in incidence (50-60 cases annually vs. 10,000-25,000 previously). Cases now occurring in the U.S. are either vaccine-associated ($1/10^6$, mainly in adults), or unvaccinated cases.

Contributor: Lehrich, James R.

References
1. Andrewes, C., and H. G. Pereira. 1972. Viruses of Vertebrates. Ed. 3. Williams and Wilkins, Baltimore.
2. Blackwood, W., and J. A. N. Corsellis, ed. 1976. Greenfield's Neuropathology. Ed. 3. Year Book, Chicago.
3. Bodian, D. 1952. Poliomyelitis, Proc. 2nd Int. Poliomyelitis Conf. Univ. Copenhagen 1951, pp. 61-94, 402-407.
4. Brain, W. R., and J. N. Walton. 1969. Diseases of the Nervous System. Ed. 7. Oxford Univ. Press, London.
5. Buescher, E. L., et al. 1968. Res. Publ. Assoc. Res. Nerv. Ment. Dis. 44:147-163.
6. Lennette, E. H., and N. J. Schmidt, ed. 1969. Diagnostic Procedures for Viral and Rickettsial Infections. Ed. 4. American Public Health Association, New York.

continued

Part I. Acute Infections

7. McAllister, R. M., et al. 1959. N. Engl. J. Med. 261: 1159-1162.

8. Merritt, H. H., ed. 1973. A Textbook of Neurology. Ed. 5. Lea and Febiger, Philadelphia.

9. Meyer, H. M., Jr., et al. 1960. Am. J. Med. 29:334-347.

10. Rawls, W. E. 1973. In A. S. Kaplan, ed. The Herpesviruses. Academic Press, New York. pp. 291-325.

11. Wilfert, C. M. 1969. N. Engl. J. Med. 280:855-859.

Part II. Subacute and Chronic Infections

Pathology: PAS = periodic acid-Schiff. *Abbreviations:* EM = electron microscopy.

Virus ⟨Synonym⟩	Clinical Manifestations ⟨Synonym⟩	Laboratory Findings	Pathology	Virus Isolation
		Herpes zoster		
1 Varicella-zoster virus ⟨Herpesvirus varicellae⟩ [1]	**Ganglionitis-neuritis:** Sharp, stabbing pain (sometimes with pruritis) & hypalgesia in dermatomes of affected roots, followed in 3-4 d by vesicular eruption ⟨shingles⟩. Eruption may occur without preceding pain. In severe cases, there may be necrosis of sensory ganglia with permanent sensory loss; inflammation may spread to homolateral ventral ⟨anterior⟩ horns & motor roots, with resultant segmental motor weakness & muscle atrophy. Vesicles usually scab after 3-7 d, and usually gone by 2 wk. Almost always unilateral. Spinal dorsal root ganglia affected in 80% of cases, cranial ganglia in 20%. **Ophthalmic zoster:** In 20% of cases, trigeminal ⟨gasserian⟩ ganglion involvement, usually ophthalmic (first) division; may be temporary or permanent oculomotor palsy; may be panophthalmitis & keratitis (from involvement of nasociliary branch of ophthalmic nerve). **"Geniculate zoster"** ⟨Ramsay Hunt syndrome⟩: Vesicles in front of ear & mastoid region, sometimes loss of taste on anterior two-thirds of tongue, facial pa-	**CSF:** Cells—usually increased numbers of lymphocytes (up to $500/\mu l$); may appear before rash. Protein—usually normal; may be up to 110 mg/100 ml. Pressure and glucose normal. Vesicle scrapings (fixed and stained with hematoxylin & eosine): Balloon cells, multinucleate giant cells, occasional cells with intranuclear eosinophilic inclusions. Biopsies of early skin lesions more likely to show intranuclear inclusions. EM: Using phosphotungstic acid method, may see herpes nucleocapsids in vesicle fluid. Antibodies: CF or Nt rise within 6-7 d after onset of rash, and may persist for months; CF antibodies gone within 3 yr after recovery.	**Ganglionitis-neuritis:** Acute inflammation (mainly lymphocytes, a few PMNs, & plasmocytes) sometimes with hemorrhagic necrosis & swelling of one or more contiguous sensory ganglia & corresponding spinal or cranial nerves & nerve roots. Intranuclear eosinophilic inclusions may be seen in satellite & ganglion cells. Most commonly affected are C2, C3, C4, T2-T12, L1, & trigeminal ganglion (especially ophthalmic division). Motor nerves less commonly involved, but not rare. **Myelitis:** Lesions (microglial proliferation) usually seen in dorsal ⟨posterior⟩ columns at entry zone of involved root; Clarke's column, lateral & ventral horns also may be involved. Sometimes neuronophagia of dorsal & ventral horn neurons & central chromatolysis of ventral ⟨anterior⟩ horn cells. Necrosis of cord has been observed in a fatal case. **Encephalitis:** Involvement of brainstem, similar to that in myelitis often accompanies trigeminal or	Vesicle fluid is material of choice. Virus isolated from CSF with difficulty. Inoculate human fibroblasts (WI-38 or MRC), or epithelial (thyroid) cells.

[1] A DNA virus.

continued

Part II.   Subacute and Chronic Infections

Virus ⟨Synonym⟩	Clinical Manifestations ⟨Synonym⟩	Laboratory Findings	Pathology	Virus Isolation
	ralysis, & sometimes deafness or vestibular disturbances; many of these cases may be infection of brainstem rather than geniculate ganglion. **Post-herpetic neuralgia:** Especially in elderly. Usually in ophthalmic or intercostal nerve distribution. May persist years. **Encephalitis:** Rare; widespread in the distribution described in **Pathology** column, especially in debilitated or immunosuppressed patients. [12] "**Symptomatic zoster**": May be associated with intoxications (arsenic, bismuth, carbon monoxide), pneumonia, tuberculosis, uremia, lymphoma, Hodgkin's disease, or lesions of dorsal spinal roots (cutaneous eruptions may occur at same or different segmental level).		glossopharyngeal herpes. Rarely, there is widespread encephalitis, particularly involving medulla oblongata, cerebellar nuclei, thalamus, hypothalamus. [12]	
		Rabies		
2	Rhabdovirus group: rabiesvirus 2/	Usually transmitted by bite of rabid dog; can also be transmitted by cats, wolves, foxes, jackals, skunks, raccoons, vampire bats. Relatively long latent period after animal bite—usually 30-70 d; can be as short as 12 d, or as long as 1 yr (rarely); shorter if bites on face or neck. Virus travels to CNS via nerves & multiplies in neurons. **Classical type:** No symptoms during incubation period. Pain or numbness in region of bite, followed by depression, drowsiness, anxiety, sleep disturbance; then excitement, psychosis, twitching, seizures. Dysphagia, throat spasms, dysarthria, & facial numbness indicate medullary cranial nerve nuclei involvement. Most patients die in acute stages, and the later phase of generalized flaccid paralysis, caused by motor neuron destruction, is not evident. Usually fever, and there may be a terminal hyperpyrexia. Case fatality rate is high. **Paralytic type:** Rare. An ascending paralysis, beginning in legs and associated with sphincter incontinence. This is said to occur in patients bitten on toes by rabid vampire bats.	CSF: Cells—sometimes increased lymphocytes ((5-100)/ μl). Pressure—normal. Protein—may be increased. Glucose—normal. Blood: Peripheral leukocytosis, especially PMNs & large mononuclear cells. Urine: Slight albuminuria. Serology: Nt (in mice, in cell culture, or plaque reduction), indirect fluorescent rabies antibodies ⟨FRA⟩, HI, CF; useful primarily to assay immune status of individual or animal after pre-exposure or post-exposure vaccination, and for characterization of strains of rabiesvirus.	**Classical type:** Inflammatory lesions (perivascular infiltration with lymphocytes & some PMN & plasmocytes) in sensory ganglia, lower medulla oblongata, substantia nigra, hypothalamic & tuberal nuclei; sometimes peripheral nerves, spinal cord, cerebral & cerebellar cortex. There may be nodules of microglial & inflammatory cells (Babes nodules), degeneration & destruction of nerve cells (especially in medulla oblongata & spinal cord), neuronophagia. Eosinophilic Negri bodies, site of active virus replication, are seen within cytoplasm of nerve cells which appear relatively undamaged otherwise (pyramidal cells of hippocampus or cerebral cortex, Purkinje cells of cerebellum), & in areas of brain with minimal inflammation. If duration of disease is short, there may be little inflammation. Distribution of lesions is affected by site of wound. Fluorescent rabies antibodies ⟨FRA⟩ test may show viral antigen in smears of infected tissue. **Paralytic type:** Mainly affects lower spinal cord (dorsal horn neurons as severely as motor neurons), lower medulla oblongata, sciatic nerves, & lumbar sensory ganglia.	Sputum, saliva, nasal swab, throat swab, urine or CSF, CNS tissue (postmortem). Inoculate suckling mouse (1-2 d old), chick embryo (chorioallantoic membrane, allantoic sac, or yolk sac), or baby hamster kidney (BHK-21) cells.

2/ An RNA virus.

continued

Part II. Subacute and Chronic Infections

Virus ⟨Synonym⟩	Clinical Manifestations ⟨Synonym⟩	Laboratory Findings	Pathology	Virus Isolation
		Congenital Rubella Encephalomyelitis		
3 Rubella virus [2,3]	Occurs in infants born to mothers infected with rubella virus during pregnancy. Incidence of congenital defects is highest if infection occurs in first trimester. Infant is usually lethargic, hypotonic, inactive, at birth & up to several weeks. Over next several months may develop restlessness, head retraction, opisthotonus, rigidity, seizures, meningitis-like illness. Anterior fontanelle is usually large. Microcephaly is common. Other associated defects: deafness (cochlear), cardiac anomalies, congestive heart failure, cataracts, hepatitis, hyperpigmented skin areas. Some improvement may occur after age 6-12 mo.	CSF: Cells—lymphocytes increased. Pressure—normal. Protein—increased. Glucose—normal. Other: Nt & HI antibodies more sensitive than CF for congenital infection. IgM antirubella antibody at birth is diagnostic of congenital rubella infection. Thrombocytopenia may be present.	Chronic leptomeningitis (mononuclear cells, lymphocytes, plasmocytes). Small zones of necrosis and glial cell proliferation in basal ganglia, midbrain, pons, spinal cord. Sometimes vasculitis & perivascular calcification. Mild to moderate perivascular gliosis of white matter. Scattered basophilic deposits in vascular walls. Cortical neurons intact. Congenital anomalies in some cases (e.g., agenesis of corpus callosum, polymicrogyria, Dandy-Walker syndrome) [17].	Fetus persistently infected with rubella virus; may be shed for more than a year after birth—nasopharynx, eye, CSF (can recover virus from CSF in 25% of cases as long as 18 mo after birth). [7] Virus grows in many primary mammalian & ovine cell lines; growth detected by interference with superinfection by other viruses. Cytopathic effects & plaques produced in several continuous cell lines (e.g., BHK-21 hamster kidney, LLC-RK rabbit kidney, Vero monkey kidney).
		Chronic Progressive Rubella Panencephalitis [18,19]		
4 Rubella virus [2,3]	Quite rare. Children with congenital rubella who develop progressive neurological illness in second decade—spasticity, ataxia, intellectual deterioration, seizures, perimacular retinal pigmentation.	CSF: Cells—increased lymphocytes in some cases. Protein—increased; γ-globulin—increased. Antibodies to rubella increased. Glucose—normal. EEG: generalized slowing and periodic polyspikes or paroxysmal slow activity. Serum antibodies to rubella (HI and CF) quite high.	Widespread, progressive, subacute panencephalitis mainly affecting white matter, with atrophy, destruction, astrocytosis, diffuse infiltration of lymphocytes & plasmocytes, & scattered microglial nodules. Cerebellar sclerotic atrophy. No inclusions. EM & fluorescent antibody studies of brain tissue negative for virus.	Rubella virus isolated from brain in one case (co-cultivation with CV-1 monkey kidney cells).

[2] An RNA virus. [3] Acute encephalitis, myelitis, optic neuritis, & carotid artery thrombosis have also been reported to be associated with rubella, with serological & EM evidence of viral infection, but without isolation of virus from CNS [6].

continued

Part II. Subacute and Chronic Infections

Virus ⟨Synonym⟩	Clinical Manifestations ⟨Synonym⟩	Laboratory Findings	Pathology	Virus Isolation
		Cytomegalic Inclusion Disease ⟨CID⟩		
5	Herpesvirus group: cytomegalovirus ⟨CMV⟩[1]	Intrauterine infection may result in stillbirth or prematurity. Hydrocephalus, seizures, focal neurological deficits, & mental retardation are common in surviving infants. Pneumonitis, jaundice, hepatosplenomegaly, purpura, hemolytic anemia, chorioretinitis, optic atrophy may be seen. Congenital infection may occur without clinical symptoms. CNS involvement rare in infected adults.	Hemolytic anemia. Hyperbilirubinemia. Cytomegalic inclusion cells: In urine of 50% of infants with CID; also may be found in saliva, tracheal secretions, gastric washings, milk. CF & Nt antibodies: Titers ⩾1:8 considered evidence of previous CMV infection; <1% of normal infants (age 6 mo-1 yr) have CF titers, compared to 100% of infected infants. Rising titers beyond time of decline of maternal antibody also help in diagnosis. Indirect, immunofluorescence test for CMV IgM antibody indicates active infection. [2]	Periventricular lesions: Thickening & granularity of ependyma, areas of calcification, deposition of iron- & calcium-containing granules, & subependymal swelling of astrocytes, & gliosis. Cytomegalic inclusions may be found in astrocytes & small vessel endothelium. Slight perivascular infiltration with lymphocytes & plasmocytes. Hydrocephalus may result from these lesions. EM shows viral particles in nucleus & cytoplasm, & cytomegalic inclusion cells in affected tissues.	Only in human fibroblasts; best accomplished in human diploid cell lines (e.g., WI-38). Virus may be isolated from urine, mouth swabs, biopsy or autopsy tissue suspensions, or peripheral blood leukocytes. Cell cultures, derived from trypsinized tissue or blood leukocytes, may help in demonstrating small quantities of virus.
		Subacute Sclerosing Panencephalitis ⟨SSPE⟩ [14]		
6	Paramyxovirus group: measles virus[2]	A progressive disease of children & young adults. Onset is insidious, with psychological & intellectual deterioration, poor school performance, & abnormal behavior. After weeks to months, patient may suddenly develop seizures, myoclonic jerks, apraxia, visual impairment. There may be cranial nerve palsies & chorioretinitis. Fever is rare in early stages. In the terminal stage, patient is in a decorticate state, often with multifocal myoclonus. Death, usually a result of intercurrent infection, comes after a period of months (in children) to years (in adolescents). In occasional cases, the course fluctuates and may stabilize or improve without treatment.	CSF: Cell count, pressure, total protein, & glucose may be normal. Increased IgG γ-globulin; first zone colloidal gold curve. Increased measles antibodies: CF, HI, Nt, hemolysis-inhibiting, & other assays. Oligoclonal M components of IgG, some with measles antibody activity. EEG: Slow, early in the disease; later, a synchronous burst-suppression pattern, with biphasic periodic slow-wave ((2-4)/ s) discharges, which may or may not be synchronous with myoclonic jerks. Measles antibodies (CF, HI, Nt, hemolysis-inhibiting, & other assays) elevated in serum (levels are much higher than ordinarily seen during or after measles or measles vaccination).	A subacute encephalitis involving white & gray matter; either may predominate. Perivascular & diffusely infiltrating lymphocytes & plasmocytes. Diffuse proliferation of microglia & astrocytes, & destruction of myelin (not selectively destroyed, however) & of neurons, in more chronic cases. Intranuclear eosinophilic inclusion bodies (type A) in oligodendrocytes, astrocytes, & neurons. There may be intracytoplasmic inclusions in late stages of the disease. Histochemical and cytochemical studies: Inclusions are composed of RNA & ribonucleoprotein. EM: Tubular paramyxovirus-like nucleocapsids (170-190 Å diameter) within intranuclear inclusions in neurons & glial cells. Immunofluorescence: Measles antigen in nuclei & cytoplasm of neurons & glial cells.	Requires explant cell culture of brain tissue (biopsy or recent autopsy), & subsequent cell fusion or co-cultivation (with monkey kidney cells). Isolation not common.

[1] A DNA virus. [2] An RNA virus.

continued

Part II. Subacute and Chronic Infections

Virus ⟨Synonym⟩	Clinical Manifestations ⟨Synonym⟩	Laboratory Findings	Pathology	Virus Isolation
		Progressive Multifocal Leukoencephalopathy ⟨PML⟩		
7 Papovavirus group: JC-PML virus 1,4/; SV40 1,5/	Rare. Most cases occur in anergic adults, often as a late complication of a systemic disease (lymphoproliferative, myeloproliferative, carcinomatous, granulomatous), and/or immunosuppressive therapy. Rapid course, typically 2-4 mo from first neurological symptom until death; rare cases reported with remissions or long courses. Clinical symptoms & signs are diverse, reflecting multiple CNS lesions. Early, there may be monoparesis, hemiparesis, personality change, mental impairment; later, severe dementia & paralysis. Headache & seizures rare.	CSF: Normal; no evidence of increased intracranial pressure. Other: As with underlying disease. HI antibodies to JC-PML virus found with increasing incidence in normals with increasing age: 0-4 yr, 17%; 10-14 yr, 60%; 50-59 yr, 75% [20]. SV40 antibodies rare unless individuals have been exposed to monkeys or to contaminated vaccines. One PML patient, from whom SV40 was isolated, had 8-fold increase in antibodies to SV40 during last 8 mo of life. [21]	Multiple discrete foci of demyelination (destruction of myelin with relative preservation of axons). Foci tend to become confluent, producing large plaques. Asymmetrical involvement, anywhere in CNS, although lesions rare in spinal cord. Oligodendrocytes in & around lesions show characteristic nuclear enlargement; eosinophilic intranuclear inclusion bodies often found. Giant astrocytes, with pleomorphic & hyperchromatic nuclei, found in most cases, and may be indistinguishable from malignant astrocytes seen in glioblastomas. Inflammatory cells sparse or absent in lesions. EM: Papovavirus-like particles (28-40 nm) in oligodendrocytes & around lesions. [22] Immunofluorescence: JC-PML virus antigen identified in lesions. [15].	From brain tissue (autopsy or biopsy), by inoculation of primary cultures of human fetal glial cells with homogenized brain tissue (JC-PML virus) [16], or in explant brain cell cultures fused to monkey kidney cells (SV40) [21]. JC-PML can be identified under EM by agglutination of negatively stained virions with antiserum to JC-PML virus [15].
		Transmissible Spongiform Encephalopathies: Kuru; Creutzfeldt-Jakob ⟨C-J⟩ Disease [9]		
8 Agents not well characterized and probably not appropriately termed virus(es); difficult to separate from diseased tissue; resistant to X-irradiation, ultraviolet light, & chemical inactivation; have passed through 200 nm filters, but not 100 nm 6/	Kuru: Found only among primitive Fore tribes of New Guinea highlands. Once was commonest cause of death. Probably transmitted by handling cannibalized brain tissue. Insidious onset, without fever or systemic illness, of cerebellar ataxia (head, trunk, & legs more than arms) becoming progressively more severe, with patient unable to walk or move without ataxic tremors. Dysphagia develops, and patients die of inanition or infection 4-24 mo after onset. C-J disease: Relatively uncommon cerebral disease of rapid evolution, in which profound dementia is combined with ataxia & diffuse myoclonic jerking. Early, there are changes in behavior, emotional responses, memory, & reasoning, together with visual distortions or impaired acuity. Progression is rapid, with	CSF: Normal. EEG, in C-J disease: Non-specific slowing early in illness, evolving to distinctive slow sharp periodic complexes on increasingly flat background. No antibodies to agents detected in serum or CSF.	Kuru: Severe loss of neurons, vacuolization of neuronal cytoplasm, marked astrocytosis, spongiform degeneration of cortex in some cases. PAS-positive plaques may be present. Little inflammation. Pathology diffuse, most marked in cerebellum & pons, and to a lesser extent in basal ganglia & hypothalamus. C-J disease: Gray matter may be affected at all levels, but principally cerebral & cerebellar cortex. Widespread neuronal destruction & loss. Intense astrocytic proliferation & fibrous gliosis. Severely affected regions show spongy loos-	Agents have not been isolated. Spongiform encephalopathy transmitted to chimpanzees, other primates, & some other mammals by intracerebral inoculation of affected brain tissue [9]. One case of person-to-person transmission of C-J disease by corneal transplantation has been reported [8].

1/ A DNA virus. 4/ Isolated from all but 2 cases thus far.
5/ Isolated from 2 cases. 6/ The agent of scrapie, a disease of sheep which appears to be related to Kuru & C-J diseases,
has been estimated at <45-50 nm by membrane filtration; isolation of 14-nm, virus-like particles from scrapie-infected mouse brain has been reported [5,10].

continued

Part II. Subacute and Chronic Infections

Virus ⟨Synonym⟩	Clinical Manifestations ⟨Synonym⟩	Laboratory Findings	Pathology	Virus Isolation
	deterioration obvious from week to week. Myoclonic jerks appear eventually and can be triggered by sudden stimuli (noise, bright lights) or occur spontaneously. Ataxia, dysarthria, & delirium progress to eventual coma. Death, usually in less than a year, usually results from intercurrent infection.		ening of tissue texture, shown by EM to be result of vacuoles within cytoplasmic processes of glial cells. No inflammation. In some cases, occipito-parietal cerebral cortex involved almost exclusively (Heidenhain type).	
Reference	4,13	4,11,13	3	1,11

Contributor: Lehrich, James R.

References

1. Andrewes, C., and H. G. Pereira. 1972. Viruses of Vertebrates. Ed. 3. Williams and Wilkins, Baltimore.
2. Benyesh-Melnick, M. 1969. (Loc. cit. ref. 11). pp. 701-732.
3. Blackwood, W., and J. A. N. Corsellis, ed. 1976. Greenfield's Neuropathology. Ed. 3. Year Book, Chicago.
4. Brain, W. R., and J. N. Walton. 1969. Diseases of the Nervous System. Ed. 7. Oxford Univ. Press, London.
5. Cho, H. J., and A. S. Greig. 1975. Nature (London) 257:685-686.
6. Connolly, J. H., et al. 1975. Brain 98:583-594.
7. Desmond, M. M., et al. 1967. J. Pediatr. 71:311-331.
8. Duffy, P., et al. 1974. N. Engl. J. Med. 290:692-693.
9. Gibbs, C. J., Jr., and D. C. Gajdusek. 1971. Res. Publ. Assoc. Res. Nerv. Ment. Dis. 49:383-410.
10. Hunter, G. D. 1974. Prog. Med. Virol. 18:289-306.
11. Lennette, E. H., and N. J. Schmidt, ed. 1969. Diagnostic Procedures for Viral and Rickettsial Infections. Ed. 4. American Public Health Association, New York.
12. McCormick, W. F., et al. 1969. Arch. Neurol. (Chicago) 21:559-570.
13. Merritt, H. H., ed. 1973. A Textbook of Neurology. Ed. 5. Lea and Febiger, Philadelphia.
14. Meulen, V. ter, et al. 1972. Curr. Top. Microbiol. Immunol. 57:1-38.
15. Narayan, O., et al. 1973. N. Engl. J. Med. 289:1278-1282.
16. Padgett, B. L., et al. 1971. Lancet 1:1257-1260.
17. Rorke, L. B., and A. J. Spiro. 1967. J. Pediatr. 70:243-255.
18. Townsend, J. J., et al. 1975. N. Engl. J. Med. 292(19):990-993.
19. Weil, M. L., et al. 1975. Ibid. 292(19):994-998.
20. Weiner, L. P., and O. Narayan. 1974. Prog. Med. Virol. 18:229-240.
21. Weiner, L. P., et al. 1972. N. Engl. J. Med. 286:385-390.
22. Zu Rhein, G. M. 1969. Prog. Med. Virol. 11:185-247.

133. DISORDERS OF MYELIN

Abbreviations: CNS = central nervous system; PNS = peripheral nervous system.

	Disorder ⟨Synonym⟩	Clinical Data	Gross Pathology	Microscopic Pathology	Etiology	Reference
			Acquired Allergic [1] & Infectious Diseases [2]			
1	Multiple sclerosis ⟨MS⟩	Mainly 18- to 40-yr age group. Chronic. Relapsing & remitting.	CNS involved. Grossly visible periventricular & disseminated gray plaques in cerebral & spinal cord white matter.	Lesions devoid of myelin & oligodendrocytes. Perivascular inflammation & intense gliosis. Relative sparing of axons.	Unknown. ? Viral.	2,21, 22,24-26

[1] Inflammatory. [2] The demyelinating diseases.

continued

	Disorder ⟨Synonym⟩	Clinical Data	Gross Pathology	Microscopic Pathology	Etiology	Reference
	Variants of MS					
2	Acute multiple sclerosis	Age group similar to that for MS. Acute. Signs similar to those for MS, but more severe & fatal.	CNS involved. Grossly visible, pink, periventricular plaques.	Multiple lesions rich in perivascular infiltrates. Sparing of axons.	Unknown. ? Viral.	2,21, 22,24, 25
3	Balo's concentric sclerosis	Age group similar to that for MS. Progressive. Signs similar to those for MS.	CNS involved. Grossly visible, periventricular plaques.	Concentric zones of demyelination separated by myelinated areas. Sparing of axons.	Unknown. ? Viral.	2,21, 22,24, 25
4	Devic's disease ⟨Neuromyelitis optica⟩	Age group similar to that for MS. Acute and/or progressive. Para- or quadriplegia.	CNS involved. Grossly visible optic nerve & spinal cord plaques.	Lesions show severe demyelination & sometimes necrosis. Some sparing of axons.	Unknown. ? Viral.	2,21, 22,24, 25
5	Acute disseminated encephalomyelitis ⟨Postinfectious or post-vaccination encephalomyelitis⟩	Most age groups. Acute. Signs same as those for acute MS.	CNS involved. Lesions often microscopic; related to subpial areas.	Intense inflammation & patchy perivascular demyelination throughout CNS. Subpial inflammation & demyelination. Some sparing of axons.	Virus (post-infectious). Iatrogenic (post-rabies immunization), or unknown.	2,11, 21,22, 24-26
6	Acute hemorrhagic leukoencephalopathy ⟨Weston Hurst disease⟩	Most age groups. Acute. Fulminant onset, with seizure, coma, & death.	CNS involved. Widespread, grossly visible, hemorrhagic lesions.	Acute hemorrhage; lymphocytic & polymorphonucleocytic infiltrates. Often necrosis of vessels.	? Virus	2,11, 21,22, 24-26
7	Progressive multifocal leukoencephalopathy	Most age groups. Subacute course, with motor & sensory findings. Often associated with abnormalities of the reticuloendothelial system.	CNS involved. Grossly visible "snowball" plaques.	Demyelination, with little inflammation. Bizarre glial changes & viral inclusions. Sparing of axons.	Papovavirus	11
8	Idiopathic polyneuritis	Most age groups. Acute & chronic. Usually monophasic. Progressive weakness.	PNS involved. Microscopic lesions prominent in radicular regions.	Intense PNS inflammation accompanied by demyelination. Sparing of axons.	? Virus	4,23
9	Diphtheritic neuropathy	Most age groups. Acute. Fulminant onset of quadriparesis.	PNS involved. Microscopic lesions scattered throughout PNS, more prominent in radicular regions.	Demyelination, no inflammation. Remarkable sparing of axons.	*Corynebacterium diphtheriae*	2
			Hereditary Metabolic Diseases			
10	Metachromatic leukodystrophy	Infantile, juvenile, or adult forms. Subacute. Dementia, spasticity, blindness, & signs of peripheral nerve disease.	CNS & PNS involved. Grossly visible, symmetrical lesions of white matter. Sometimes hydrocephalus.	Widespread devastation of myelin & axons. Nerve cells & Schwann cells contain specific inclusions.	Arylsulfatase A deficiency	15,18

continued

	Disorder ⟨Synonym⟩	Clinical Data	Gross Pathology	Microscopic Pathology	Etiology	Reference
11	Krabbe's disease ⟨Globoid cell leukodystrophy⟩	Infantile, or rarely juvenile. Subacute. Dementia, spasticity, & signs of peripheral nerve disease.	CNS & PNS involved. Grossly visible CNS lesions. Large-scale reduction of white matter.	Widespread loss of myelin & axons. Globoid cells & specific inclusions pathognomonic. Nerve cells may be spared.	Galactocerebroside-β-galactosidase deficiency	29,30, 33
12	Adrenoleukodystrophy	Juvenile & adult forms. Sex-linked recessive (males). Subacute. Dementia, spasticity, & blindness.	CNS & PNS involved. Grossly visible, large, symmetrical CNS lesions in white matter.	Extensive loss of myelin & axons. Inflammation & macrophages containing specific inclusions. Same inclusions present in adrenals & PNS.	Unknown; may be related to synthesis of a long-chain fatty acid	5,9,27
13	Refsum's disease	Juvenile or adult. Subacute. Night blindness, deafness, ataxia, & signs of peripheral nerve disease.	PNS mainly. Nerves show hypertrophic changes.	Schwann cell proliferation. Onion bulbs. Demyelination. Remyelination. Some axonal loss.	Phytanic acid α-oxidase deficiency	7,28
14	Pelizaeus-Merzbacher disease ⟨Sudanophilic leukodystrophy⟩	Congenital or infantile. Subacute. Sex-linked recessive. Spasticity, dementia, abnormal eye movements.	CNS involved. Congenital form shows complete lack of CNS myelin. Infantile form: tigroid or patchy depletion of white matter.	Total depletion of myelin or hypomyelination. Sudanophilic inclusions.	? Disorder of cholesterol esters	31,32
15	Spongy degeneration of white matter ⟨Canavan's disease⟩	Infantile. Familial. Subacute. Megalencephaly. Failure to meet developmental milestones.	PNS involved. Hydrocephalus. Widespread loss of white matter.	Vacuolation of myelin. Fiber loss. Hypertrophic astrocytes containing bizarre mitochondria. Alzheimer type II astrocytes.	Biochemical defect unknown	1,6
16	Alexander's disease ⟨Dysmyelinogenetic leukodystrophy⟩	Infantile. Subacute. Megalencephaly. Failure to meet developmental milestones.	CNS involved. Diffuse loss of white matter.	Poor myelination. Hypomyelination. Rosenthal fibers. Axonal sparing.	Biochemical defect unknown	8
17	Phenylketonuria	Infantile & late onset. Subacute. Intellectual retardation, seizures. Treatment may prevent development of neurologic disease.	CNS involved. Brain macrocephalic.	Myelin pallor. Spongy changes in white matter.	? Defect in phenylalanine 4-monooxygenase[3]	10,12, 13
		Acquired Toxic Metabolic Disorders				
18	Hexachlorophene neuropathy	Newborn. Flaccid paraparesis. Usually epidemic in nurseries.	CNS mainly involved. White matter diffusely involved.	Myelin edema, with spongiform changes in white matter.	Topical application of hexachlorophene	20
19	Hypoxic encephalopathy: anoxic anoxia & anemic anoxia (carbon dioxide poisoning)	All ages. Intellectual loss, ataxia, & extrapyramidal signs of varying intensity.	CNS involved. Grossly visible lesions. Laminar necrosis.	Loss of nerve cells. Myelin destruction. Axons relatively spared.	Decrease in arterial oxygen content & tension	19

[3] Synonym: Phenylalanine hydroxylase.

continued

	Disorder ⟨Synonym⟩	Clinical Data	Gross Pathology	Microscopic Pathology	Etiology	Reference
			Nutritional Diseases			
20	Vitamin B_{12} deficiency	Predominantly adults. Spasticity, proprioceptive sensory loss, peripheral neuropathy. Rarely, blindness & dementia.	CNS usually, & PNS occasionally, involved. Grossly visible lesions. Spinal cord shrinkage in thoracic region.	Myelin & axonal loss in corticospinal tracts. Punctate myelin loss in centrum semiovale.	Vitamin B_{12} deficiency	17
21	Central pontine myelinolysis	Abrupt onset, quadriparesis, stupor. Commonly associated with alcoholism, malnutrition, & liver disease.	CNS involved. Lesions grossly visible & restricted to midpons & telencephalon.	Myelin loss with axonal sparing. No inflammation.	Nutritional deprivation	3
22	Marchiafava-Bignami disease	Gradual onset of dementia, aphasia, seizures, & spasticity. Associated with malnutrition & alcoholism.	CNS involved. Lesions grossly visible in corpus callosum & anterior commissure.	Diffuse loss of myelin in affected regions	Alcoholism	14
			Traumatic Diseases			
23	Edema	All ages. Nature of neurologic findings depends on site of trauma.	CNS involved. Lesions usually microscopic. Sometimes seen as yellow areas in white matter.	Myelin pallor	Injury secondary to tumors, trauma, circulatory disorders, etc.	2,25
24	Compression	All ages. Nature of neurologic findings depends on site of trauma.	CNS & PNS involved. Lesions microscopic.	Myelin loss from affected areas. Remyelination.	Injury due to tourniquet, carpal tunnel syndrome, etc.	16

Contributor: Raine, Cedric S.

References

1. Adachi, M., et al. 1973. Hum. Pathol. 4:331-347.
2. Adams, R. D., and R. L. Sidman. 1968. Introduction to Neuropathology. McGraw-Hill, Blakiston Division, New York.
3. Adams, R. D., et al. 1959. Arch. Neurol. Psychiatry. 81:154-172.
4. Asbury, A. K., et al. 1969. Medicine (Baltimore) 48:173-215.
5. Blaw, M. E. 1970. Handb. Clin. Neurol. 10:128-133.
6. Bogaert, L. van. 1970. Ibid. 10:203-211.
7. Fardeau, M., and W. K. Engel. 1969. J. Neuropathol. Exp. Neurol. 28:278-294.
8. Herndon, R. M., et al. 1970. Ibid. 29:524-551.
9. Igarashi, M., et al. 1976. J. Neurochem. 26:851-860.
10. Jervis, G. A. 1963. In F. L. Lyman, ed. Phenylketonuria. C. C. Thomas, Springfield, IL. pp. 96-100.
11. Johnson, R. T., and L. P. Weiner. 1972. Multiple Sclerosis UCLA Forum Med. Sci. 16:245-264.
12. Knox, W. E. 1972. In J. B. Stanbury, ed. The Metabolic Basis of Inherited Disease. Ed. 3. McGraw-Hill, New York. pp. 266-295.
13. Malamud, N. 1966. J. Neuropathol. Exp. Neurol. 25:254-268.
14. Merritt, H. H., and A. D. Weisman. 1945. Ibid. 4:155-163.
15. Moser, H. W. 1972. (Loc. cit. ref. 12). pp. 688-729.
16. Ochoa, J., et al. 1972. J. Anat. 113:433-455.
17. Pant, S. S., et al. 1968. Acta Neurol. Scand. 44(Suppl. 35).
18. Peiffer, J. 1970. Handb. Clin. Neurol. 10:43-66.
19. Plum, F., et al. 1962. Arch. Intern. Med. 110:18-25.
20. Powell, H., et al. 1973. J. Pediatr. 82:976-981.
21. Prineas, J. 1975. Hum. Pathol. 6:531-554.
22. Prineas, J. W. 1970. Handb. Clin. Neurol. 9:107-160.
23. Prineas, J. W., and J. M. McLeod. 1976. J. Neurol. Sci. 27:427-458.

continued

133. DISORDERS OF MYELIN

24. Raine, C. S. 1976. Prog. Neuropath. 3:225-251.
25. Raine, C. S., and H. H. Schaumburg. 1977. In P. Morell, ed. Myelin. Plenum, New York. pp. 271-323.
26. Schaumburg, H. H., and C. S. Raine. 1977. (Loc. cit. ref. 25). pp. 325-351.
27. Schaumburg, H. H., et al. 1975. Arch. Neurol. 32: 577-591.
28. Steinberg, D. 1972. (Loc. cit. ref. 12). pp. 833-853.

29. Suzuki, Y., and K. Suzuki. 1971. Science 171:73-75.
30. Volk, B. W., and M. Adachi. 1970. Handb. Clin. Neurol. 10:67-93.
31. Watanabe, I., et al. 1969. J. Neuropathol. Exp. Neurol. 28:243-256.
32. Watanabe, I., et al. 1972. Ibid. 32:313-333.
33. Yunis, E. J., and R. E. Lee. 1969. Lab. Invest. 21: 415-419.

134. AGE-RELATED CHANGES IN THE CENTRAL NERVOUS SYSTEM

This table does not represent a complete bibliographic search; instead, it presents data that are more likely to be reliable. It does not include the diverse results of postmortem examinations of patients with senile dementias which could reflect degenerative diseases and not aging.

	Property Measured	Structure	Age Range from	to	Change	Reference
		Gross Anatomy				
1	Weight	Whole brain	18-20 mo[1]	60-70 yr	Decreased	3,21
2			20-30 yr[2]	70-80 yr	Decreased	3,21
3			21-30 yr	81-90 yr	Decreased	12
4			30-34 yr	85-96 yr	Decreased	2
5			12-19 yr	90 yr	Decreased	4
6	Volume	Whole brain	20-29 yr	80-89 yr	Decreased	5
7		Dentate nucleus	24 yr	99 yr	Decreased	4
8		Ventral cochlear nucleus	50 yr	90 yr	Decreased	17
9		Cerebral hemispheres: ventricles	20-29.9 yr	80-89.9 yr	Increased	4
10	Dimensions	Cerebellum, cerebrum	20-30 yr	80-90 yr	Decreased	4
11		Brain ventricles	Adult	Senium	Increased	3
12	Width	Brain gyri	Adult	>75 yr	Increased	5
13	Width & length	Pons	21-30 yr	60-90 yr	No change	4
14	Width, length, & height	Cerebellum	21-30 yr	60-100 yr	Decreased	4
15	Thickness	Tunica intima of brain arteries	1 yr	90 yr	Increased	15
		Histology & Cytology				
16	Number of neurons	Cerebral cortex: superior temporal gyrus; superior frontal gyrus	41 yr	87 yr	Decreased	6
17		Cerebellum: Purkinje cells	60 yr	100 yr	Decreased	10
18		Cerebral cortex	15-54 yr	65-89 yr	No change	8
19		Inferior olivary nucleus	Birth	89 yr	No change	20
20		Locus coeruleus	Birth	86 yr	Decreased	7
21		Facial nucleus	Birth	75 yr	No change	26
22		Ventral cochlear nucleus	0.3 yr	90 yr	No change	16
23		Trochlear & abducens nuclei	Birth	89 yr	No change	7
24	Number of neuroglia	Cerebral cortex: superior frontal gyrus	25 yr	72 yr	Increased	4
25		Cranial nerve nuclei; inferior olive; locus coeruleus; reticular formation	26-27 yr	61-82 yr	Increased	4
26	Integrity of dendrites	Cerebral cortex: horizontal dendrites of pyramidal cells	58 yr	96 yr	Decreased	23
27	Number of synapses	Cerebral cortex	15-54 yr	65-89 yr	No change	8
28		Olfactory bulb glomeruli	16-30 yr	76-91 yr	Increased	24

[1] Female. [2] Male.

continued

	Property Measured	Structure	Age Range from	Age Range to	Change	Reference
29	Numbers of neurofibrillary tangles & senile plaques	Cerebral cortex	7th decade	9th decade	Increased	25
30	Cytoplasmic basophilia[3]	Cerebellum: Purkinje cells	9 wk	>50 yr	Decreased	1
31		Inferior olivary nucleus	11 d	91 yr	Decreased	18
32	Lipofuscin content	Inferior olivary nucleus	11 d	91 yr	Increased	18
33			3 mo	70 yr	Increased	7
34	Melanin content	Substantia nigra	Birth	60 yr	Increased	19
		Biochemistry				
35	Water content	Whole brain	31-40 yr	81-90 yr	Increased	9
36	Lipid content Total fatty acids	Whole brain	33 yr	98 yr	Decreased	28
37			21-30 yr	85-90 yr	Decreased	11
38	Cholesterol, cerebrosides, phospholipids	Whole brain	20 yr	100 yr	Decreased	13
39	Protein content Total protein	Whole brain	31-40 yr	71-80 yr	Decreased	9
40	Protein nitrogen	Whole brain	16-20 yr	81-90 yr	Decreased	9
41	RNA content	Ventral ⟨anterior⟩ horn cells	40 yr	>60 yr	Decreased	14
42	Enzyme activity Monoamine oxidase[4]	Hindbrain	45 yr	65 yr	Increased	22
43	Acetylserotonin methyltransferase[5], monoamine oxidase, histamine methyltransferase	Pineal body	40-55 yr	55-70 yr	No change	27

[3] Relative amount of cytoplasmic RNA, estimated in sections. [4] Synonym: Amine oxidase (flavin-containing). [5] Synonym: Hydroxyindole-O-methyltransferase.

Contributor: Bondareff, William

References
1. Andrew, W. 1939. Am. J. Anat. 64:351-375.
2. Appel, F. W., and E. M. Appel. 1942. Hum. Biol. 14: 48-68.
3. Arendt, A. 1972. In G. Holle, ed. Handbuch der Allgemeinen Pathologie. Springer-Verlag, Berlin. v. 6, pt. 4, pp. 490-542.
4. Blinkov, S. M., and I. I. Glezer. 1968. The Human Brain in Figures and Tables. Plenum Press, New York.
5. Brizzee, K. R. 1975. In J. M. Ordy and K. R. Brizzee, ed. The Neurobiology of Aging. Plenum Press, New York. pp. 401-423.
6. Brody, H. 1955. J. Comp. Neurol. 102:511-556.
7. Brody, H. 1973. In M. Rockstein, ed. Development and Aging in the Nervous System. Academic Press, New York. pp. 121-133.
8. Cragg, B. G. 1975. Brain 98:81-90.
9. Davis, J. M., and W. A. Himwich. 1975. (Loc. cit. ref. 5). pp. 329-357.
10. Hall, T. C., et al. 1976. Neuropathol. Appl. Neurobiol. 1:267-292.
11. Himwich, W. A. 1973. (Loc. cit. ref. 7). pp. 151-169.
12. Himwich, W. A., and H. E. Himwich. 1959. In J. E. Birren, ed. Handbook of Aging and the Individual. Univ. Chicago Press, Chicago. pp. 187-215.
13. Horrocks, L. A., et al. 1975. (Loc. cit. ref. 5). pp. 359-367.
14. Hydén, H. 1967. In H. Hydén, ed. The Neuron. Elsevier, Amsterdam. pp. 179-219.
15. Klassen, A. C., et al. 1968. J. Neuropathol. 27:607-624.
16. Konigsmark, B. W., and E. A. Murphy. 1970. Nature (London) 228:1335-1336.
17. Konigsmark, B. W., and E. A. Murphy. 1972. J. Neuropathol. Exp. Neurol. 31:304-316.
18. Mann, D. M. A., and P. O. Yates. 1974. Brain 97:481-488.
19. Mann, D. M. A., and P. O. Yates. 1974. Ibid. 97:489-498.
20. Monagle, R. D., and H. Brody. 1974. J. Comp. Neurol. 155:61-66.
21. Peress, N. S., et al. 1973. Prog. Brain Res. 40:473-484.
22. Robinson, A. J., et al. 1972. Lancet 1:290-291.
23. Scheibel, M. E., et al. 1975. Exp. Neurol. 47:392-403.
24. Smith, C. B. 1942. J. Comp. Neurol. 77:589-596.
25. Terry, R. D., and H. M. Wisniewski. 1972. In C. M. Gaitz, ed. Aging and the Brain. Plenum Press, New York. pp. 89-116.

continued

26. Van Buskirk, C. 1945. J. Comp. Neurol. 82:303-333.
27. Wurtman, R. J., et al. 1964. J. Clin. Endocrinol. 24: 299-301.
28. Yamamoto, A., and G. Rouser. 1973. J. Gerontol. 28: 140-142.

135. EFFECTS OF INTRAUTERINE PATHOGENS ON THE CENTRAL NERVOUS SYSTEM

Probable route of infection was transplacental unless otherwise indicated. **Maternal Infection:** Either = either asymptomatic or symptomatic. **Clinical Disorders:** EEG = electroencephalogram. **Laboratory Diagnosis—Method:** C = culture; S = serology; VI = virus isolation. **Pathology:** CNS = central nervous system.

	Agent ⟨Synonym⟩	Maternal Infection	Clinical Disorders	Laboratory Diagnosis		Pathology	Reference
				Method	Reference		
			Viruses				
1	Herpesvirus ⟨Herpes simplex⟩[1,2]	Either	? Mental & motor deficits	VI; S	1,18,20	Microcephaly, intracranial calcification, focal necrosis	8,14,24
2	Cytomegalovirus (Cytomegalic inclusion disease)	Asymptomatic	Mental & motor deficits, seizures	VI; S	1,18,20	Microcephaly, periventricular calcification, focal necrosis, polymicrogyria[3]	3
3	Varicella-zoster virus	Symptomatic	Seizures, abnormal EEG	VI; S	1,18,20	Dilated ventricles, necrosis	9,17
4	Variola virus	Symptomatic	....	VI; S	1,18,20	Focal necrosis	18
5	Polioviruses (Poliomyelitis)	Symptomatic	Poliomyelitis	VI; S	1,18,20	Encephalomyelitis	7
6	Coxsackieviruses, group B	Symptomatic	? Motor deficits	VI; S	1,18,20	Meningoencephalitis	12,13,19
7	? Echoviruses	....	....	S	1,18,20	Dysraphia	15
8	Rubella virus	Either	Mental retardation, dystonia, seizures, perceptual deficits	VI; S	1,18,20	Vasculopathy, focal ischemic necrosis, microcephaly, chronic meningoencephalitis, ? hydrocephalus	1,21,22
9	Western equine encephalitis virus	Symptomatic	Spasticity, motor deficits, or may recover without sequelae	S	1	? Encephalomyelitis	6,23
10	? Influenza virus[4]	....	....	S	14,16	Anencephalia, spina bifida, cephalocele	14,16
11	? Mumps virus[4]	....	....	.....	....	Aqueductal stenosis with hydrocephalus	11
			Bacteria				
12	*Treponema pallidum*	Usually latent stage	Neurological symptoms develop during juvenile period; resemble adult forms	S	1	Usually CNS lesions do not develop until juvenile period; resemble adult forms. Rarely, fulminant meningoencephalitis & fetal death. ? Mental retardation.	26
13	*Campylobacter fetus* ⟨Vibrio fetus⟩[5]	Asymptomatic	Neonatal meningitis	C	1	Meningoencephalitis; parenchymal hemorrhage	4

[1] Usually type 2.   [2] For information on transplacental route of infection, consult reference 25.   [3] Synonym: Micropolygyria.   [4] Route of infection undetermined.   [5] Route of infection uncertain but presumed to be transplacental.

continued

Agent ⟨Synonym⟩	Maternal Infection	Clinical Disorders	Laboratory Diagnosis		Pathology	Reference
			Method	Reference		
14 *Escherichia coli* [6]	Either	Neonatal meningitis. May have permanent neurological sequelae.	C	1	Purulent meningitis with vasculitis & infarction, ± hydrocephalus	2
15 *Listeria monocytogenes* [7]	Asymptomatic	....	C	1	Granulomatous meningoencephalitis	26
16 *Mycobacterium tuberculosis*	Usually symptomatic	Meningitis. May have permanent neurological sequelae.	C	1	Granulomatous meningoencephalitis	10
Protozoa						
17 *Toxoplasma gondii*	Asymptomatic	Mental retardation, abnormalities of head size	S; C	1	Necrotizing, granulomatous meningoencephalitis; intracranial calcification	26

[6] Infection ascends from maternal genital tract. Other bacterial organisms associated with ascending infection from maternal genital tract and possible neonatal meningitis are *Streptococcus faecalis*, *Proteus*, *Klebsiella*, *Pseudomonas*, *Staphylococcus*, alpha- and beta-hemolytic *Streptococcus*, Pneumococcus, *Listeria*, and *Candida* [ref. 5]. [7] Other bacterial organisms associated with transplacental infection and possible meningoencephalitis include *Staphylococcus*, *Streptococcus*, Pneumococcus, *Vibrio cholerae*, *Salmonella typhi*, *Borrelia*, and *Leptospira* [ref. 5].

Contributor: Nelson, James S.

References

1. Bell, W. E., and W. F. McCormick. 1975. Neurologic Infections in Children. W. B. Saunders, Philadelphia.
2. Berman, P. H., and B. Q. Banker. 1966. Pediatrics 38:6-24.
3. Bignami, A., and L. Appiciutoli. 1964. Acta Neuropathol. 4:127-137.
4. Burgert, W., Jr., and J. W. C. Hagstrom. 1964. Arch. Neurol. (Chicago) 10:196-199.
5. Ciba Foundation. 1973. Intrauterine Infect. Ciba Found. Symp. 10(n.s.).
6. Copps, S. C., and L. E. Giddings. 1959. Pediatrics 24:31-33.
7. Elliot, G. B., and J. E. McAllister. 1956. Am. J. Obstet. Gynecol. 72:896-902.
8. Florman, A. L., et al. 1973. J. Am. Med. Assoc. 225:129-132.
9. Garcia, A. G. P. 1963. Pediatrics 32:895-901.
10. Hughesdon, M. R. 1946. Arch. Dis. Child. 21:121-138.
11. Johnson, R. T. 1972. N. Engl. J. Med. 287:599-604.
12. Kibrick, S., and K. Benirschke. 1956. Ibid. 255:883-889,
13. Kibrick, S., and K. Benirschke. 1958. Pediatrics 22:857-875.
14. Krugman, S., and A. A. Gershon, ed. 1975. Infect. Fetus Newborn Infant Proc. Symp. (Prog. Clin. Biol. Res. 3).
15. Lapinleimu, K., et al. 1972. Teratology 5:345-351.
16. Leck, I. 1963. Ibid. 17:70-80.
17. McKendry, J. B. J., and J. D. Bailey. 1973. Can. Med. Assoc. J. 108:66-68.
18. Monif, G. R. G. 1969. Viral Infections of the Human Fetus. Macmillan, London.
19. O'Shaughnessey, W. J., and H. A. Buechner. 1962. J. Am. Med. Assoc. 179:71-72.
20. Overall, J. C., and L. A. Glasgow. 1970. J. Pediatr. 77:315-333.
21. Rorke, L. B. 1973. Arch. Otolaryngol. 98:249-251.
22. Rorke, L. B., and A. J. Spiro. 1967. J. Pediatr. 70:243-255.
23. Shinefield, H. R., and T. E. Townsend. 1953. Ibid. 43:21-25.
24. South, M. A., et al. 1969. Ibid. 75:13-18.
25. Witzleben, C. L., and S. G. Driscoll. 1965. Pediatrics 36:192-199.
26. Wolf, A., and D. Cowen. 1959. J. Neuropathol. Exp. Neurol. 18:191-243.

Diseases of the spine encompass many of the known human ailments, since any structural or biochemical bony or neurologic abnormality must necessarily affect the spinal column and its contents. Efforts, therefore, have been made to confine the content of these tables to pathology which is usually unique to the spine. Consequently, the exceedingly extensive material on vascular, inflammatory, infectious, and metabolic afflictions has been excluded. For information on these disorders, consult reference 16 in Part I.

Part I. Congenital Anomalies

In the early development, segmentation is first visualized along the neural tube. Each segment or somite forms—by migration of cells—portions of the spine, integument, muscle, and nervous tissue. The membranous vertebral column thus formed is transformed into a cartilaginous vertebral column, and then into the ossified skeletal column by endochondral ossification. Failure of the orderly sequence results in congenital spinal anomalies.

Definition: L5 = fifth lumbar vertebra; S1 = first sacral vertebra.

	Disorder	Definition	Symptoms	Classification	Reference
1, 2	Basilar impression	Spine pressed or assimilated into base of skull	Disturbance of spinal cord, brainstem, & cerebellum	Primary: Atlantooccipital fusion; atlantoaxial dislocation; bifid posterior arch of atlas; Klippel-Feil syndrome; Morquio's syndrome; cleidocranial dysostosis Secondary: Soft skull base; rickets; osteomalacia; Paget's disease; hyperparathyroidism; renal osteodystrophy	9,14, 19,20
3	Atlantoaxial abnormalities	Structural abnormalities between vertebrae 1 & 2	None, or as severe as medullary compression & quadriplegia	Laxity of transverse atlantal ligament; congenital agenesis of dens; os odontoideum; hypoplasia of dens; occipitalization (assimilation) of atlas	12,24, 25
4	Klippel-Feil syndrome	Failure of segmentation at 3rd -8th wk, with short neck, decreased motion, total cervical fusion, & with decreased total number of vertebrae & craniovertebral anomalies	Joint & spinal nerve root irritation	....	15,23
5, 6, 7, 8, 9	Myelodysplasia	Failure of neural tube closure with resultant adjacent mesodermal abnormalities	Depend on degree & level of involvement; vary from no neurologic abnormality to being incompatible with life	Spina bifida occulta: Bony posterior defect without meningeal herniation Dermal sinus: Sinus composed of stratified squamous epithelium, extending from skin to dura Meningocele: Posterior spinal defect, with wide spinal canal & herniation of meninges Myelomeningocele: Posterior spinal defect, with wide spinal canal & herniation of meninges & neural tissue Myeloschisis: Extensive dysrhaphia, with exposure of spinal cord	2-4,13
10	Diastematomyelia	Osseous or cartilaginous spicule between dura & vertebral body	Tethering of spinal cord, with vascular, mechanical, and metabolic compromise	....	17
11	Congenital spondylolisthesis	Deficiency of posterior elements, inferior facet of L5 or superior facet of S1	Pain, weakness of legs	....	7,26

continued

Part I. Congenital Anomalies

	Disorder	Definition	Symptoms	Classification	Reference
12	Lumbar & sacrococcygeal agenesis	Failure in development of lower somites	Varies from asymptomatic to complete paraplegia	....	6
13	Spondyloepiphyseal dysplasia	Congenital chondrodystrophy of large bones, and spinal epiphyseal ossification	Mainly mechanical	Spondyloepiphyseal dysplasia congenita (autosomal dominant); pseudoachondroplasia (dominant & recessive forms); spondyloepiphyseal dysplasia tarda (sex-linked recessive)	11
14	Scoliosis & kyphosis	Pathological curvature of the spine	Mechanical problems, leading to pain & movement limitation, & infrequently neurologic deficit unless the latter is the primary cause	Abnormal bone development: Failure of formation or segmentation (hemivertebra, bloc vertebra, etc.)	8
15				Abnormal neurologic development: Myelodysplasia, poliomyelitis, cerebral palsy, etc.	
16				Abnormal muscle development: Marfan's syndrome, Morquio's syndrome, arthrogryposis, etc.	
17	Spinal stenosis	Narrow spinal canal less than the acceptable limits of normal, especially in the critical lateral recess area of the lumbar region of the canal	Usually asymptomatic until degenerative spinal diseases are superimposed—hypertrophied facets & ligamentum flavum, narrowed, degenerated disks, etc.	Primary: Achondroplasia; narrow canal without dwarfism or other skeletal anomalies	1,5,10, 18,21, 22
18				Secondary: Acquired secondarily to spinal degeneration	

Contributor: Rouhe, Stanley A.

References
1. Alexander, E., Jr. 1969. J. Neurosurg. 31:513-519.
2. Amador, L. M. 1955. J. Pediatr. 47:300-310.
3. American Academy of Orthopaedic Surgeons. 1972. Symp. Myelomeningocele 1970 (St. Luois).
4. Anderson, F. M. 1968. J. Pediatr. 73:163-177.
5. Bailey, J. A., II, et al. 1970. J. Bone Joint Surg. 52A:1285-1301.
6. Banta, J. V., and O. Nichols. 1969. Ibid. 51A:693-703.
7. Borkow, S. E., and B. Kleiger. 1971. Clin. Orthop. 81:73-76.
8. Bradford, D. S., et al. 1975. In R. H. Rothman and F. A. Simeone, ed. The Spine. W. B. Saunders, Philadelphia. v. 1, pp. 271-1385.
9. Chamberlain, W. E. 1939. Yale J. Biol. Med. 11:487-496.
10. Cohen, M. E., et al. 1967. J. Pediatr. 71:367-376.
11. Diamond, L. S. 1970. J. Bone Joint Surg. 52A:1587-1594.
12. Garber, J. N. 1964. Ibid. 46A:1782-1791.
13. Gardner, W. J. 1960. Cleveland Clin. Q. 27:88-100.
14. Gardner, W. J. 1973. In J. R. Youmans, ed. Neurological Surgery. W. B. Saunders, Philadelphia. v. 1, pp. 628-644.
15. Gunderson, C. H., et al. 1967. Medicine (Baltimore) 46:491-512.
16. Jaffe, H. L. 1972. Metabolic, Degenerative, and Inflammatory Diseases of the Bones and Joints. Lea and Febiger, Philadelphia.
17. James, C. C., and L. P. Lassman. 1964. Arch. Dis. Child. 39:125-130.
18. Kessler, J. T. 1975. J. Neurol. Neurosurg. Psychiatry 38(12):1218-1224.
19. McGregor, M. 1948. Br. J. Radiol. 21:171-187.
20. McRae, D. L. 1960. Am. J. Roentgenol. 84:3-25.
21. Murone, I. 1974. J. Bone Joint Surg. 56B:30-36.
22. Roth, M., et al. 1976. Neuroradiology 10:277-286.
23. Shoul, M. I., and M. Ritvo. 1952. Am. J. Roentgenol. 68:369-385.
24. Spillane, D., et al. 1957. Brain 80:11-48.
25. Wadia, N. H. 1967. Brain 90:449-472.
26. Wiltse, L. L. 1961. Clin. Orthop. 21:156-163.

continued

Part II. Neoplasms of the Spine

In addition to the neoplasms listed below, metastatic tumors from mammary gland, lung, kidney, prostate, etc. occur in the spine. *Symbol*: ± = with or without.

	Neoplasm	X-Ray Appearance	Signs & Symptoms	Treatment
	Primary Benign			
1	Osteochondroma	In spine when multiple	Usually no symptoms	None
2	Osteoid osteoma	Has nidus in facet	Symptoms relieved by acetylsalicylic acid (Aspirin)	Surgery
3	Aneurysmal bone cyst	"Blow out" of body	Pain	Radiation
4	Osteoblastoma	"Giant osteoid osteoma"	Pain	Surgery
5	Giant cell tumor	May be totally destructive of a vertebra	Pain	Radiation
6	Hemangioma	In vertebral body with vertical striations	Mild pain	Surgery
7	Eosinophilic granuloma	Solitary lesion in spine, lytic vertebral body	Constant pain	Radiation
	Primary Malignant			
8	Multiple myeloma	Lytic lesions, solitary or generalized	Unrelenting pain ± neurodeficit	Radiation, chemotherapy
9	Ewing's sarcoma	Moth-eaten body	Pain ± neurodeficit	Radiation, chemotherapy
10	Primary reticulum cell sarcoma	Destruction of body	Pain ± neurodeficit	Surgery
11	Chondrosarcoma	Calcific stippling	Pain ± neurodeficit	Surgery
12	Osteogenic sarcoma	Lytic lesions, with or without osteoblastic lesions	Pain ± neurodeficit	Surgery ± radiation
13	Paget's disease	Destruction	Pain ± neurodeficit	Radiation
14	Chondroma	Lytic vertebrae	Pain ± neurodeficit from displacement	Surgery
	Intraspinal			
15	Extradural tumors	Usually metastatic, usually bony involvement	Pain ± neurodeficit (in bone, nerve, or cord)	Surgery, radiation, & chemotherapy
16	Intradural extramedullary tumors: Meningiomas; neurofibromas; sarcomas	With or without erosion, scalloping, or foraminal enlargement	Pain & neurodeficit (in nerve, cord, or bone)	Surgery
17	Intramedullary tumors: gliomas	With or without erosion or scalloping	Canal enlargement	Surgery, radiation, & chemotherapy

Contributor: Rouhe, Stanley A.

General References

1. Austin, G. 1972. In G. Austin, ed. The Spinal Cord. Ed. 2. C. C. Thomas, Springfield, IL. pp. 281-346.
2. Baker, G. S., and D. W. Mulder. 1973. In A. B. Baker and L. H. Baker, ed. Clinical Neurology. Harper and Row, Hagerstown, MD. v. 2, ch. 33, pp. 1-15.
3. Francis, K. C. 1975. In R. H. Rothman and F. A. Simeone, ed. The Spine. W. B. Saunders, Philadelphia. v. 2, pp. 811-822.
4. Simeone, F. A. 1975. (Loc. cit. ref. 3). v. 2, pp. 823-835.

continued

Part III. Degenerative Disk Disease

Symbols: C = cervical; T = thoracic; L = lumbar; S = sacral; ± = with or without.

	Spinal Disk	Spinal Nerve Root	Location of Pain or Paresthesia	Sensory Loss	Motor Loss	Reflex Loss
1	C2	C3	Neck, suboccipital	± suboccipital	None	None
2	C3	C4	Neck, suboccipital	± neck	Trapezius	None
3	C4	C5	Base of neck, shoulder, upper arm	Over deltoideus	Deltoideus	Biceps
4	C5	C6	Neck, shoulder, scapula, arm, thumb	Lateral arm, thumb	Biceps	Biceps
5	C6	C7	Neck, shoulder, scapula, sternum, index finger	Lateral arm, middle finger	Triceps	Triceps
6	C7	C8	Ulnar aspect of hand or forearm	Little finger	Hand intrinsics, wrist extensors	None
7	T1	T2	Axilla, forearm, chest	Axilla	Not detectable	None
8	T2-T8	T2-T8	Spine, across chest or abdomen	Radicular	Not detectable	None
9	T8-L1	T8-L1	Abdomen	Abdomen	Rectus abdominis	None
10	L1	L1	Inguinal region, hip	Iliac crest, inguinal region	Iliopsoas, hip flexion	None
11	L2 ± L1	L2	Anterior lateral thigh	Anterior thigh	Iliopsoas, adductors of thigh	None
12	L3 ± L2	L3	Anterior thigh	Across knee	Adductors of thigh, or quadriceps	None
13	L4 ± L3	L4	Anterior thigh to knee, medial calf	Posterior lateral thigh, medial calf	Quadriceps	Patellar
14	L5 ± L4	L5	Posterior thigh, leg, great toe	Posterior lateral thigh, lateral calf, great toe	Dorsiflexion of foot or toes; atrophy of anterior aspect of leg	None
15	S1 ± L5	S1	Posterior thigh, leg, small toe	Posterior thigh, posterior calf, lateral toes	Plantar flexion of foot or toes; atrophy of posterior aspect of leg	Achilles tendon
16	S2 ± S1	S2	Posterior medial thigh	Posterior thigh, posterior calf	Foot intrinsics	None

Contributor: Rouhe, Stanley A.

General References

1. Austin, G. 1972. In G. Austin, ed. The Spinal Cord. Ed. 2. C. C. Thomas, Springfield, IL. pp. 349-440.
2. Francis, K. C. 1975. In R. H. Rothman and F. A. Simeone, ed. The Spine. W. B. Saunders, Philadelphia. v. 1, pp. 387-442.
3. Simeone, F. A. 1975. (Loc. cit. ref. 2). v. 2, pp. 443-513.

Part IV. Trauma

Symptoms: S = soft tissue—skin, muscle, or ligaments, with pain, ache, spasm, or "soreness" being the major symptom; V = vascular—intermittent ischemia with dizziness, or vascular compression with stroke (paralysis, etc.); R = radicular—nerve root pain, weakness, or numbness, etc.; M = myelopathy—spinal cord involvement, with long track signs (weakness, autonomic abnormalities, sensory loss, etc.). **Treatment**: Sg = surgery, decompress, and fuse. *Symbol*: ± = with or without.

	Spinal Region	Structure Involved or Condition	Symptoms	Work-Up	Treatment
1	Craniocervical	Ligaments	S, intermittent; V (vertebral vessels); R; M	X ray, tomogram	Immobilize
2		Arch of atlas ⟨C1⟩: "Hangman's fracture"	Often only S, ± neurovascular	X ray, tomogram	Immobilize

continued

Part IV. Trauma

	Spinal Region	Structure Involved or Condition	Symptoms	Work-Up	Treatment
3		Lateral mass of atlas ⟨C1⟩	Often V + S	X ray, tomogram, angiogram	Immobilize
4		Dens of axis ⟨C2⟩; axis ⟨C2⟩ lamina	None, M, or S	X ray, tomogram	Immobilize
5	Cervical	Muscle or ligaments: "Whip-lash injury"	Multiple: Pain, dizziness, tinnitus, etc.	X ray	Symptomatic
6		Spinous process or lamina	Pain, stiffness, etc.	X ray	Symptomatic + brace
7		Pedicle or facet	R	X ray, tomogram, myelogram	Traction ± Sg
8		Body compression	R + M	X ray ± myelogram	Traction ± Sg
9		Tear drop	Often asymptomatic	X ray ± myelogram	Traction ± brace, Sg
10		Fracture-dislocation	S, R, ± M	X ray ± myelogram	Traction ± Sg
11	Thoracic	Spinous process or lamina	S ± M	X ray	Symptomatic
12		Pedicle or ribs	S + chest + R	X ray, myelogram	Symptomatic ± Sg
13		Body	R ± M	X ray, myelogram	Symptomatic ± Sg
14		Fracture-dislocation	R + M	X ray, myelogram	Symptomatic ± Sg
15	Lumbar	Spinous process or lamina	S	X ray	Symptomatic
16		Pedicle or transverse process	R ± urologic	X ray, myelogram, i.v. pyelogram	Symptomatic ± Sg
17		Body	R ± gastrointestinal	X ray, myelogram	Traction + symptomatic ± Sg
18		Fracture-dislocation	R ± genitourinary ± gastrointestinal	X ray, myelogram	Traction + symptomatic ± Sg

Contributor: Rouhe, Stanley A.

General References

1. Austin, G. 1972. In G. Austin, ed. The Spinal Cord. Ed. 2. C. C. Thomas, Springfield, IL. pp. 227-280.
2. Clark, K. 1973. In J. R. Youmans, ed. Neurological Surgery. W. B. Saunders, Philadelphia. v. 2, pp. 1067-1074.
3. Dohn, D. F. 1973. (Loc. cit. ref. 2). pp. 1075-1084.
4. Macnab, I. 1975. In R. H. Rothman and F. A. Simeone, ed. The Spine. W. B. Saunders, Philadelphia. v. 2, pp. 515-528.
5. Norrell, H. A. 1975. (Loc. cit. ref. 4). v. 2, pp. 529-566.
6. White, R. J., and D. Yashon. 1973. (Loc. cit. ref. 2). pp. 1049-1066.
7. White, R. J., and D. Yashon. 1973. (Loc. cit. ref. 2). pp. 1085-1088.

137. CRANIAL NEUROMUSCULAR DISORDERS

For general information on most disorders, consult reference 259. Data in broken brackets are synonyms.

	Disorder	Reference
	Cranial Nerve I ⟨Olfactory⟩	
1	Neoplastic	263
2	Anosmia & stellar distension	83
3	Esthesioneuroblastoma ⟨Olfactory neuroblastoma⟩	118,141,232
4	Esthesioneuroepithelioma, olfactory	32
5	Malignant tumors of ethmoid bone	197
6	Demyelinating: Olfaction in multiple sclerosis	17
	Hereditary	
7	Anosmia & olfactory genetics	14
8	Anosmia & hypogonadotropic hypogonadism	62
9	Anosmia & hypogonadism with ovarian mosaicism	164
	Traumatic	
10	Anosmia, post-traumatic	246
11	Smell defects after head injury	178

continued

	Disorder	Reference
	Miscellaneous	
12	Cranial manifestations of fibrous dysplasia of bone	269
13	Smell abnormalities	98
	Cranial Nerve II ⟨Optic⟩	
14	Neoplastic	67
15	Arachnoid cysts involving portion of intraorbital optic nerve	190
16	Carcinomatous optic neuropathy	248
17	Chromophobe adenoma	234
18	Ganglioneuroma of optic chiasma	182
19	Gliomas of anterior visual pathways	189
20	Gliomas of optic nerve	24
21	Gliomas in children, optic	64
22	Gliomas in adults, optic	151
23	Hemangiomas of optic disk	229
24	Intracanalicular meningioma with chronic optic disk edema	169
25	Malignant teratoid medulloepithelioma of optic nerve	137
26	Meningeal carcinomatosis & blindness	10
27	Meningioma of optic foramen	74
28	Metastatic carcinoma in both optic nerves	252
29	Metastatic disease of optic nerve	265
30	Metastatic squamous cell carcinoma	93
31	Ocular involvement in leukemia & allied disorders	8
32	Optic nerve compression	186
33	Papilledema & spinal cord tumors	12
34	Primary optic atrophy in Von Recklinghausen's disease ⟨Multiple neurofibromatosis⟩	101
35	Tumors of eye & adnexa	210
36	Tumors of optic nerve, primary	44
37	Visual field changes following anterior temporal lobectomy	112
38	Visual field defects due to optic nerve compression by mass lesions	57
39	Visual field distortions in cases of brain tumor	84
40	Infectious/inflammatory	67
41	Bilateral optic atrophy after vaccination against common cold	102
42	Multiple sclerosis & optic-chiasmatic arachnitis	200
43	Neuromyelitis optica following infectious mononucleosis	267
44	Optic atrophy after smallpox	184
45	Optic neuritis	153,181,195
46	Optic atrophy in herpes zoster ophthalmicus	202
47	Subacute neuromyelitis with optic neuritis after iodochlorhydroxyquin ⟨Chloroiodoquine⟩	260
48	Demyelinating	67
49	Acute optic neuritis	41
50	Acute unilateral retrobulbar neuritis	71
51	Bitemporal visual field defects in presumed multiple sclerosis	222
52	Ocular manifestations of multiple sclerosis	75
53	Optic & olfactory involvement in multiple sclerosis	17
54	Optic neuritis	153,195
55	Optic-chiasmatic arachnitis in multiple sclerosis	31
56	Pituitary adenomas	148
57	Slowly progressive & acute visual impairment in multiple sclerosis	165
58	Hereditary	67,262
59	Charcot-Marie-Tooth disease with primary optic dystrophy	231
60	Leber's disease with symptoms resembling disseminated sclerosis	176
61	Ocular dominance & amblyopia	73
62	Olivopontocerebellar degeneration with macular dystrophy	194
63	Optic atrophy	72,242

continued

	Disorder	Reference
64	Optic nerve drusen	166
65	Sex-linked heredodegenerative neurological disorder associated with Leber's optic atrophy	48
66	Tay-Sachs & Sandhoff's diseases	127
67	Toxic/deficient	67
68	Blindness during streptomycin & chloramphenicol therapy	261
69	Diabetic ophthalmoplegia	132
70	Irreversible bilateral optic damage after ethambutol therapy	36
71	Tobacco amblyopia	206
72	Tobacco-alcohol amblyopia	257
73	Toxic ocular manifestation of chloramphenicol therapy	70
74	Toxic optic neuropathies	119
75	Traumatic	67
76	Indirect injury of optic nerves & chiasma	152
77	Lesions of optic chiasma	16
78	Optic atrophy after seemingly trivial trauma	245
79	Transitory cortical blindness in head injury	128
80	Visual field defects after penetrating missile wounds of brain	253
81	Visual lesions in closed head injury	76
82	Vascular	67
83	Blood circulation disorders of optic nerve & chiasma	42
84	Fundus oculi in transient monocular blindness	117
85	Infarction in optic nerve	107
86	Ischemic optic neuropathy	78
87	Miscellaneous	67
88	Acute optic neuropathy in older patients	106
89	Visual field changes following anterior temporal lobectomy	112
	Cranial Nerves III ⟨Oculomotor⟩, IV ⟨Trochlear⟩, and VI ⟨Abducens⟩	
90	Neoplastic	66
91	Chronic abducens nerve palsy as sign of basisphenoid tumors	223
92	Eye signs in pineal tumors	204
93	Ocular palsy occurring with pituitary tumors	213
94	Pinealomas & tumors of posterior portion of third ventricle	203
95	Infectious/inflammatory	66
96	Delayed trochlear nerve palsy	167
97	Ophthalmoplegia in acute polyneuritis	126
98	Superior orbital fissure syndrome	174
99	Demyelinating	66
100	Neuro-ophthalmologic evaluation of abducens paralysis	235
101	Ocular findings in multiple sclerosis	228
102	Unilateral internuclear ophthalmoplegia	173
103	Hereditary	66
104	Hereditary ptosis	2
105	Ophthalmoplegia in myotonic dystrophy	179
106	Progressive external ophthalmoplegia	95,100
107	Progressive ophthalmoplegia	94
108	Toxic/deficient: Abducens nerve palsy in diphenylhydantoin ⟨Dilantin⟩ intoxication	183
109	Traumatic	66
110	Acquired lesions of trochlear nerve	49
111	Bilateral aberrant regeneration of oculomotor nerve following trauma	168
112	Delayed traumatic bilateral abducens paralysis	214
113	Direct injury of oculomotor nerve in craniocerebral trauma	187
114	Divergence paralysis & head trauma	227
115	Ocular motility following head trauma	111
116	Ocular sequelae of head injuries	77
117	Oculomotor palsy from minor head trauma	110

continued

	Disorder	Reference
118	Vascular	66
119	Carotid-cavernous aneurysms ⟨Pulsating exophthalmos⟩	87
120	Disturbances of oculomotor functions accompanying extradural hemorrhage	247
121	Isolated oculomotor palsy caused by intracranial aneurysm	162
122	Oculomotor palsy due to supraclinoid internal carotid-artery berry aneurysm	39
123	Pulseless disease presenting with isolated abducens nerve palsy & recurrent cutaneous angiitis	13
124	Strangulation of abducens nerve by lateral branches of basilar artery	82
125	Miscellaneous	66
126	Oculomotor palsy in children	63
127	Paralysis of cranial nerves III, IV, & VI	220
128	Painful ophthalmoplegia	216
129	Progressive external ophthalmoplegia	53,88
	Cranial Nerve V ⟨Trigeminal⟩	
	Neoplastic	
130	Intracranial tumor	104
131	Malignant neurilemoma of supraorbital nerve	138
132	Neurilemoma ⟨Neurinoma⟩ of trigeminal ⟨Gasserian⟩ ganglion	134
133	Tic douloureux & its relationship to tumors of posterior fossa	211
134	Trigeminal neurilemomas ⟨Neurinomas⟩	114
	Infectious/inflammatory	
135	Primary amyloidosis of trigeminal ⟨Gasserian⟩ ganglion	37
136	Trigeminal neuralgia	38
	Demyelinating	
137	Atypical trigeminal neuralgia in patients with multiple sclerosis	121
138	Rare forms of paroxysmal trigeminal neuralgia & their relations to disseminated sclerosis	143
139	Trigeminal neuralgia associated with multiple sclerosis	56,116,199,221
140	Hereditary: Inherited tic douloureux	85
141	Traumatic: Paratrigeminal epidermoid tumors	30
142	Vascular: Trigeminal neuralgia	86,105,157
	Miscellaneous	
143	Raeder's paratrigeminal syndrome	68
144	Trigeminal neuralgia	52,157,170,180,244, 250
145	Trigeminal sensory neuropathy & Bell's palsy	61
	Cranial Nerve VII ⟨Facial⟩	
	Neoplastic	
146	Facial nerve tumors	208
147	Facial nerve tumors & progressive facial palsy	230
148	Facial palsy & tumor, recurrent	243
149	Neurilemoma, intraparotid	20
150	Neurilemoma with intracranial extension	81
151	Neurilemomas ⟨Neurinomas⟩	155,192
	Infectious/inflammatory	
152	Bell's palsy	3,264
153	Bell's palsy & infectious mononucleosis	240
154	Bell's palsy associated with acute herpetic gingival stomatitis	225
155	Facial paralysis due to malignant external otitis	59
156	Herpesvirus ⟨Herpes simplex virus⟩ in Bell's palsy ⟨Idiopathic facial paralysis⟩	4
157	Herpes zoster oticus & facial paralysis ⟨Ramsay Hunt's syndrome⟩	6
	Demyelinating	
158	Facial myokymia	92
159	Facial myokymia in multiple sclerosis	15

continued

Disorder	Reference
Hereditary	
160 Inherited Bell's palsy	266
161 Peripheral facial paralysis	237
Traumatic	
162 Facial palsy following head injury	205
163 Injuries to facial nerve	185
164 Temporal bone fractures & facial nerve injury	142
165 Vascular: Hemifacial spasm	51,159,160,219
Miscellaneous	
166 Behcet's disease with recurrent facial paralysis	5
167 Bell's palsy	40,145
168 Bell's palsy & trigeminal sensory neuropathy	61
169 Facial nerve surgery	188
170 Hemifacial spasm	159
171 Peripheral facial nerve paralysis in diabetes	172
172 Vestibular symptoms in Bell's palsy ⟨Idiopathic facial palsy⟩	175
Cranial Nerve VIII ⟨Vestibulocochlear⟩	
Neoplastic	
173 Acoustic nerve tumors	150
174 Acoustic neurilemoma ⟨Neurinomas⟩	109,149
175 Acoustic neurofibromas, bilateral	124
176 Acoustic neurofibromas	103
Infectious/inflammatory	
177 Allergy as a cause of fluctuant hearing loss	65
178 Antigenic excitation in Meniere's disease	268
179 Hearing loss after *Haemophilus influenzae* meningitis	123
Demyelinating	
180 Auditory & vestibular aberrations in multiple sclerosis	196
181 Neuro-otologic effects of multiple sclerosis	89
Hereditary	
182 Bilateral acoustic neurofibromas	124
183 Familial bilateral acoustic neuroma	193
184 Genetically determined deafness	9
185 Hereditary deafness	97,171
186 Hereditary nephropathy with hearing loss	156
187 Hereditary progressive perceptive deafness	251
188 Hereditary renal dysfunction & deafness	54
189 Heredity as factor in labyrinthine deafness & paroxysmal vertigo ⟨Meniere's syndrome⟩	46
190 Inherited congenital profound deafness	19
Toxic/deficient	
191 Gentamicin progressive-cochlear toxicity	90
192 Hydroxychloroquine-induced vertigo	207
193 Neomycin ototoxicity	47
194 Nitrous oxide & irreversible hearing loss	91
195 Permanent deafness associated with furosemide administration	209
Traumatic	
196 Audiological & vestibular effects of head injury	27
197 Cochlear & vestibular function in skull injury without fracture of petrosal bone	23
198 Post-traumatic conduction deafness	254
199 Post-traumatic dizziness	255
200 Transverse fracture of temporal bone	120
Vascular	
201 Neurovascular cross-compression	158
202 Unilateral nerve deafness in childhood	239

continued

137. CRANIAL NEUROMUSCULAR DISORDERS

	Disorder	Reference
	Miscellaneous	
203	Metabolic errors & sudden deafness	80
204	Perilymphatic fistula	18
205	Positional vertigo	144
206	Vestibular nerve function in myxedema	28
	Cranial Nerve IX ⟨Glossopharyngeal⟩	
207	Vascular: Glossopharyngeal neuralgia	11,43
	Miscellaneous	
208	Glossopharyngeal neuralgia	35
209	Glossopharyngeal neuralgia & ossification of stylohyoid ligament	136
210	Glossopharyngeal neuralgia with asystole & seizures	125
	Cranial Nerve X ⟨Vagus⟩	
	Neoplastic	
211	Intrathoracic neurofibroma of vagus nerve	226
212	Neurilemoma of vagus nerve in neck	55
213	Toxic/deficient: Alcoholic polyneuropathy	198
214	Traumatic: Palsy of recurrent nerve following mediastinoscopy	270
215	Vascular: Glossopharyngeal neuralgia	11,43
	Miscellaneous	
216	Neuropathology of esophagus in diabetes mellitus	238
217	Pharyngoesophageal dysphagia & recurrent nerve ⟨Recurrent laryngeal nerve⟩ palsy	147
	Cranial Nerve XI ⟨Accessory⟩	
218	Neoplastic: Tumors in region of foramen magnum	69
	Traumatic	
219	Accessory nerve injury	271
220	Iatrogenic accessory nerve injury	256
	Cranial Nerve XII ⟨Hypoglossal⟩	
	Neoplastic	
221	Chemodectoma	218
222	Dumb-bell neurilemoma ⟨Neurinoma⟩ of hypoglossal nerve	29
223	Hypoglossal neurilemoma ⟨Neurinoma⟩	139
224	Hypoglossal neurofibroma	122
225	Infectious/inflammatory: Hypoglossal nerve palsy complication in infectious mononucleosis	236
226	Toxic/deficient: Isolated hypoglossal nerve paralysis following influenza vaccination	115
227	Traumatic: Bilateral hypoglossal nerve palsy following a second carotid endarterectomy	22
228	Vascular: Transient hemilingual paralysis due to compression by a saccular carotid aneurysm	113
229	Miscellaneous: Unilateral hypoglossal nerve atrophy	60
	Mixed Cranial Nerves	
	Neoplastic	
230	Cranial nerve syndromes associated with nasopharyngeal malignancy	212
231	Neurological complications of Wegener's granulomatosis	99
232	Ophthalmo-neurologic symptoms in malignant nasopharyngeal tumors	129
233	Solitary plasmacytoma producing cranial neuropathy	7
234	Temporal bone lesions causing multiple nerve damage	34
235	Tumors of glomus jugulare	33,256
	Infectious/inflammatory	
236	Cranial nerve palsy in tetanus	201
237	Malignant external otitis	58
238	Neurologic manifestations of sarcoidosis	133
239	Special syndrome of endocranial otitic complications	135

continued

	Disorder	Reference
240	Demyelinating: Multiple sclerosis	177,249
	Hereditary	
241	Ataxia-telangiectasia	154
242	Familial oculomotor palsy with Bell's palsy	79
243	Hereditary late-onset ptosis & dysphagia	26
244	Oculopharyngeal muscular dystrophy	1,258
245	Progressive facial hemiatrophy ⟨Romberg's disease⟩	217
246	Toxic/deficient: Cranial nerve paralysis after spinal anesthesia	215
	Traumatic	
247	Carotid-cavernous fistula	140,146
248	Cranial nerve injuries	163,191
249	Neurological damage after cannulation of internal jugular vein	45
250	Transverse fracture of clivus	224
	Vascular	
251	Carotid-cavernous aneurysms ⟨Pulsating exophthalmos⟩	87
252	Carotid-cavernous fistula	140
253	Saccular aneurysms of internal carotid artery in cavernous sinus	161
254	Superior orbital fissure syndrome	50
	Miscellaneous	
255	Cavernous sinus syndrome	130,131
256	Garcin's syndrome	241
257	Neurologic complications of Sjögren's syndrome	21
258	Ocular manifestations of carotid-cavernous fistulas	108
259	Progressive supranuclear palsy	96
260	Superior orbital fissure syndrome	25

Contributors: Jannetta, Peter J.; Zorub, David S.; and Bissonette, David J.

References

1. Aarli, J. A. 1969. Acta Neurol. Scand. 45:484-492.
2. Aberfeld, D. C. 1971. Birth Defects Orig. Artic. Ser. 7(2):63-65.
3. Adour, K. K., et al. 1974. Arch. Otolaryngol. 99:114-117.
4. Adour, K. K., et al. 1975. J. Am. Med. Assoc. 233:527-530.
5. Aggarwal, J. L. 1973. Br. J. Ophthalmol. 57:704-705.
6. Aleksic, S. N., et al. 1973. J. Neurol. Sci. 20:149-159.
7. Alexander, M. P., et al. 1975. Arch. Neurol. (Chicago) 32:777-778.
8. Allen, R. A., and B. R. Straatsma. 1961. Arch. Ophthalmol. 66:490-508.
9. Altmann, F. 1964. Acta Oto-Laryngol., Suppl. 187:1-39.
10. Altrocchi, P. H., et al. 1973. J. Neurol. Neurosurg. Psychiatry 36:206-210.
11. Al-Ubaidy, S. S., et al. 1974. Br. J. Oral Surg. 11:243-245.
12. Ammerman, B. J., et al. 1975. Surg. Neurol. 3:55-57.
13. Amnuellaph, P., et al. 1973. Br. Med. J. 3:27-28.
14. Amoore, J. E. 1971. In H. Autrum, et al., ed. Handbook of Sensory Physiology. Springer-Verlag, New York. v. 4, pt. 1, pp. 245-256.
15. Andermann, F., et al. 1961. Brain 84:31-44.
16. Anderson, D. L., and L. A. Lloyd. 1964. Can. Med. Assoc. J. 90:110-115.
17. Ansari, K. A. 1976. Eur. Neurol. 14:138-145.
18. Arenberg, K., et al. 1972. Laryngoscope 82:243-246.
19. Arias, S. 1974. Birth Defects Orig. Artic. Ser. 10(10):230-243.
20. Aston, S. J., and F. C. Sparks. 1975. Arch. Surg. (Chicago) 110:757-758.
21. Attwood, W., and C. M. Poser. 1961. Neurology 11:1034-1041.
22. Bageant, T. E., et al. 1975. Anesthesiology 43:595-596.
23. Bandini, A. 1963. Inf. Med. (Genoa) 18:15-16, 226-227.
24. Bane, W. M., and J. C. Long. 1964. Am. J. Ophthalmol. 57:649-654.
25. Banks, P. 1967. Oral Surg. Oral Med. Oral Pathol. 24:455-458.
26. Barbeau, A. 1966. Symp. Prog. Muskeldystrophie Myotonie Myasthenie (Heidelberg) 1965, pp. 102-109.
27. Barber, H. O. 1969. Ann. Otol. Rhinol. Laryngol. 78:239-252.
28. Barlow, R. A. 1922. Am. J. Med. Sci. 164:402-409.
29. Bartal, A. D., et al. 1973. J. Neurol. Neurosurg. Psychiatry 36:592-595.
30. Bauman, C. H. H., and P. C. Bucy. 1956. J. Neurosurg. 13:455-468.
31. Bell, R. A., et al. 1975. Arch. Ophthalmol. 93:191-193.

continued

32. Berger, L., and H. Coutard. 1926. Bull. Assoc. Fr. Etude Cancer 15:404-414.

33. Bickerstaff, E. R., and J. S. Howell. 1953. Brain 75: 576-593.

34. Binns, P. M., and H. D. Fairman. 1966. J. Laryngol. Otol. 80:125-137.

35. Bohm, E., and R. R. Strang. 1962. Brain 85:371-388.

36. Boman, G., et al. 1974. Scand. J. Respir. Dis. 55:176-180.

37. Borghi, G., and G. Tagliabue. 1961. Acta Neurol. Scand. 37:105-110.

38. Borne, G. 1968. J. Neurosurg. 28:480-482.

39. Botterell, E. H., et al. 1962. Am. J. Ophthalmol. 54: 609-616.

40. Brackmann, D. E. 1974. Otolaryngol. Clin. North Am. 7:357-368.

41. Bradley, W. G., and C. W. M. Whitty. 1968. J. Neurol. Neurosurg. Psychiatry 31:10-18.

42. Bregat, P. 1974. Rev. Oto-Neuro-Ophthalmol. (Paris) 46:189-190.

43. Brihaye, J., et al. 1956. J. Neurosurg. 13:299-302.

44. Brihaye-van Greetruyden, M. 1966. Ophthalmologica 151:627-628.

45. Briscoe, C. E., et al. 1974. Br. Med. J. 1:314.

46. Brown, M. R. 1949. Ann. Otol. Rhinol. Laryngol. 58: 665-670.

47. Brown, R. D., et al. 1973. Acta Oto-Laryngol. 76: 128-135.

48. Bruyn, G. W., and L. N. Went. 1964. J. Neurol. Sci. 1:59-80.

49. Burger, L. J., et al. 1970. Brain 93:567-574.

50. Calliauw, L., and K. Deberdt. 1966. Psychiatr. Neurol. Neurochir. 69:149-154.

51. Campbell, E., and C. Keedy. 1947. J. Neurosurg. 4: 342-347.

52. Carney, L. R. 1967. Neurology 17:1143-1151.

53. Caroff, R. B. 1969. Arch. Ophthalmol. 82:845-850.

54. Cassady, G., et al. 1965. Pediatrics 35:967-979.

55. Catteno, D. M. 1973. Ohio State Med. J. 69:381-384.

56. Chakravorty, B. G. 1966. Arch. Neurol. (Chicago) 14:95-99.

57. Chamlin, M. 1957. Arch. Ophthalmol. 58:37-58.

58. Chandler, J. R. 1968. Laryngoscope 78:1257-1294.

59. Chandler, J. R. 1972. Ann. Otol. Rhinol. Laryngol. 81:648-658.

60. Chang, V. S., et al. 1975. Cancer (Philadelphia) 35(6): 1537-1544.

61. Ch'ien, L. T., and J. H. Halsey, Jr. 1970. N. Engl. J. Med. 282:224-225.

62. Christian, J. C., et al. 1971. Birth Defects Orig. Artic Ser. 7(6):166-171.

63. Chutorian, A., and A. P. Gold. 1974. Trans. Am. Neurol. Assoc. 99:199-200.

64. Chutorian, A. M., et al. 1964. Neurology 14:83-95.

65. Clemis, J. 1975. Otolaryngol. Clin. North. Am. 8: 374-383.

66. Cogan, D. G. 1956. Neurology of the Ocular Muscles. Ed. 2. C. C. Thomas, Springfield, IL. pp. 84-117.

67. Cogan, D. C. 1966. Neurology of the Visual System. C. C. Thomas, Springfield, IL.

68. Cohen, D. M., et al. 1975. Am. J. Ophthalmol. 79: 1044-1049.

69. Cohen, L., and D. Macrae. 1962. J. Neurosurg. 19: 462-469.

70. Cole, J. G., et al. 1956. Am. J. Ophthalmol. 44:18-20.

71. Collins, W. J. 1965. Arch. Neurol. (Chicago) 13:409-412.

72. Cordes, F. C. 1952. Am. J. Ophthalmol. 35:1272-1284.

73. Coren, S., et al. 1975. Am. J. Optom. Physiol. Opt. 52:47-50.

74. Craig, W. M., and L. J. Gogela. 1950. J. Neurosurg. 7: 44-48.

75. Croll, M. 1965. Am. J. Ophthalmol. 60:822-829.

76. Crompton, M. R. 1970. Brain 93:785-792.

77. Cross, A. G. 1948. Ann. R. Coll. Surg. Engl. 2:233-240.

78. Cullen, J. F. 1968. Trans. Ophthalmol. Soc. U.K. 87: 759-774.

79. Currie, S. 1970. Brain 93:193-198.

80. Currier, W. D. 1975. Otolaryngol. Clin. North Am. 8:501-505.

81. Curtin, J. M., and J. P. Lanigan. 1964. J. Laryngol. Otol. 78:212-219.

82. Cushing, H. 1910. Brain 33:204-235.

83. Cushing, H. 1917. J. Nerv. Ment. Dis. 44:415-423.

84. Cushing, H. 1922. Brain 44:341-396.

85. Daly, R. F., et al. 1973. Neurology 23:937-939.

86. Dandy, W. C. 1934. Am. J. Surg. 24:447-455.

87. Dandy, W. E. 1937. Zentralbl. Neurochir. 2:165-206.

88. Danta, G., et al. 1974. Trans. Am. Neurol. Assoc. 99: 28-34.

89. Dayal, U. S., et al. 1966. Laryngoscope 76:1798-1809.

90. Dayal, U. S., et al. 1975. Can. J. Otolaryngol. 4:348-351.

91. Delaruelle, J., et al. 1974. Acta Oto-Rhino-Laryngol. Belg. 28:586-591.

92. De Silva, K. L., et al. 1972. Postgrad. Med. J. 48:657-662.

93. Deutsch, A. R., et al. 1973. Ann. Ophthalmol. 5:1317-1321.

94. Dimauro, S., et al. 1973. Arch. Neurol. (Chicago) 29: 170-179.

95. Direkze, M., et al. 1975. Acta Neurol. Scand. 51:245-248.

96. Dix, M. R., et al. 1971. J. Neurol. Sci. 13:237-256.

97. Dolowitz, D. A., and F. E. Stephens. 1961. Ann. Otol. Rhinol. Laryngol. 70:851-860.

98. Douek, E. 1974. The Sense of Smell and Its Abnormalities. Churchill-Livingstone, Edinburgh.

continued

99. Drachman, D. A. 1963. Arch. Neurol. (Chicago) 8: 145-155.

100. Drachman, D. A. 1968. Ibid. 18:654-674.

101. Dresner, E., and D. A. D. Montgomery. 1949. Q. J. Med. 18:93-103.

102. Edmund, J., and E. Godtfredsen. 1965. Br. J. Ophthalmol. 49:46-48.

103. Edwards, C. H., and J. H. Patterson. 1951. Brain 74: 144-190.

104. Ehni, G. 1950. Arch. Neurol. Psychiatry 64:692-698.

105. Eisenbrey, A. B., and W. M. Hegarty. 1956. J. Neurosurg. 13:647-649.

106. Ellenberger, C., Jr., et al. 1973. Arch. Neurol. (Chicago) 28:182-185.

107. Ellenberger, C., Jr., and M. G. Netsky. 1968. J. Neurol. Neurosurg. Psychiatry 31:606-611.

108. Elliot, A. J. 1954. Postgrad. Med. 15:191-196.

109. Erickson, L. S., et al. 1965. Laryngoscope 75:601-627.

110. Eyster, E. F., et al. 1972. J. Am. Med. Assoc. 220: 1083-1086.

111. Falbe-Hansen, I., and E. Gregersen. 1959. Acta Ophthalmol. 37:359-370.

112. Falconer, M. A., and J. L. Wilson. 1958. Brain 81: 1-14.

113. Farrell, F. W., Jr., et al. 1972. Neurology 22:106-114.

114. Fee, W. E., Jr., et al. 1975. Laryngoscope 85:371-376.

115. Felix, J. K., et al. 1976. Am. J. Dis. Child. 130:82-83.

116. Finesilver, B. 1939. J. Nerv. Ment. Dis. 90:757-764.

117. Fisher, C. M. 1959. Neurology 9:333-347.

118. Fitz-Hugh, G. S., et al. 1965. Arch. Otolaryngol. 81: 161-168.

119. Foulds, W. S., et al. 1974. Br. J. Ophthalmol. 58: 386-390.

120. Frederickson, J. M., et al. 1962. Arch. Otolaryngol. 78:770-784.

121. Friedlander, A. H., et al. 1974. J. Oral Surg. 32:301-303.

122. Friedman, L., and A. A. Eisenberg. 1935. Ann. Surg. 101:834-838.

123. Gamstorp, I., and I. Klockhoff. 1974. Dev. Med. Child Neurol. 16:678-679.

124. Gardner, W. J., and O. Turner. 1940. Arch. Neurol. Psychiatry 44:76-99.

125. Garretson, H. D., and A. R. Elvidge. 1963. Arch. Neurol. (Chicago) 8:26-31.

126. Gibberd, F. B. 1970. Ibid. 23:161-164.

127. Gilbert, F., et al. 1975. Proc. Natl. Acad. Sci. USA 72:263-267.

128. Gjerris, F., and L. Mellemgaard. 1969. Acta Neurol. Scand. 45:623-633.

129. Godtfredsen, E. 1944. Acta Psychiatr. Neurol. Scand. Suppl. 34.

130. Godtfredsen, E. 1964. Acta Neurol. Scand. 40:69-75.

131. Godtfredsen, E. 1965. Ibid. 41:43-51.

132. Goldstein, J. E., and D. G. Cogan. 1960. Arch. Ophthalmol. 64:592-600.

133. Goodson, J. N. 1960. South. Med. J. 53:1111-1116.

134. Gordy, P. D. 1965. J. Neurosurg. 22:90-94.

135. Gradenigo, G. 1904. Ann. Otol. Rhinol. Laryngol. 13:637.

136. Graf, C. J. 1959. J. Neurosurg. 16:448-453.

137. Green, W. R., et al. 1974. Arch. Opthalmol. 91:451-454.

138. Grinberg, M. A., et al. 1974. Am. J. Ophthalmol. 78:489-492.

139. Haase, E. 1946. J. Neuropathol. Exp. Neurol. 5:66-71.

140. Hamby, W. B. 1966. Carotid-cavernous Fistula. C. C. Thomas, Springfield, IL.

141. Hamilton, A. E., et al. 1973. J. Neurosurg. 38:548-556.

142. Harker, L. A., and B. F. McCabe. 1974. Otolaryngol. Clin. North Am. 7:425-431.

143. Harris, W. 1950. Br. Med. J. 2:1015-1019.

144. Harrison, M. S., et al. 1972. Brain 95:369-372.

145. Hauser, W. A., et al. 1971. Mayo Clin. Proc. 46:258-264.

146. Henderson, J. W., and R. C. Schneider. 1959. Am. J. Ophthalmol. 48:585-597.

147. Henderson, R. D., et al. 1974. J. Thorac. Cardiovasc. Surg. 68:507-512.

148. Henderson, W. R. 1939. Br. J. Surg. 26:811-921.

149. Higgs, W. A. 1973. Arch. Otolaryngol. 98:73-76.

150. House, W. F., ed. 1968. Ibid. 88(6).

151. Hoyt, W. F., et al. 1973. Brain 96:121-132.

152. Hughes, B. 1962. Bull. Johns Hopkins Hosp. 111: 98-126.

153. Hutchinson, W. M., et al. 1976. Br. Med. J. 1:64-66.

154. Hyams, S. W., et al. 1966. Am. J. Ophthalmol. 62: 1118-1127.

155. Isamat, F., et al. 1975. J. Neurosurg. 43:608-612.

156. Iversen, U. M. 1974. Acta Paediatr. Scand., Suppl. 245:1-23.

157. Jannetta, P. J. 1967. J. Neurosurg. 26(Suppl.):159-162.

158. Jannetta, P. J. 1975. Surg. Forum 26:467-468.

159. Jannetta, P. J. 1975. Trans. Am. Acad. Ophthalmol. Otolaryngol. 80:319-322.

160. Jannetta, P. J. 1976. In T. P. Morley, ed. Current Controversies in Neurosurgery. W. B. Saunders, Philadelphia. pp. 435-442.

161. Jefferson, G. 1938. Br. J. Surg. 26:267-302.

162. Jefferson, G. 1947. Proc. R. Soc. Med. 40:419-432.

163. Jennett, W. B. 1974. In E. H. Feiring, ed. Brock's Injuries of the Brain and Spinal Cord and Their Coverings. Ed. 5. Springer, New York. pp. 162-166.

164. Jones, J. R., et al. 1975. Am. J. Obstet. Gynecol. 121:991-994.

continued

165. Kahana, E., et al. 1973. Neurology 23:729-733.
166. Kamin, D. F., et al. 1973. Arch. Ophthalmol. 89: 359-372.
167. Keane, J. R. 1975. Ibid. 93:382-383.
168. Keane, J. R. 1975. J. Neurosurg. 43:95-97.
169. Kennerdell, J. S., et al. 1975. Ann. Ophthalmol. 7: 507-512.
170. Kerr, F. W. L., and R. H. Miller. 1966. Arch. Neurol. (Chicago) 15:308-319.
171. Konigsmark, B. W. 1969. N. Engl. J. Med. 281:713-720, 774-778, 827-832.
172. Kruk-Zagajewska, A., et al. 1974. Otolaryngol. Pol. 28:535-539.
173. Kupfer, C., and D. G. Cogan. 1966. Arch. Ophthalmol. 75:484-489.
174. Lakke, J. P. 1962. Arch. Neurol. (Chicago) 7:289-300.
175. Lammli, K., et al. 1974. Acta Otolaryngol. 78:15-18.
176. Lees, F., et al. 1964. J. Neurol. Neurosurg. Psychiatry 27:415-421.
177. Lehmann, H. J., et al. 1972. Eur. Neurol. 8:257-269.
178. Leigh, A. D. 1943. Lancet 1:38-40.
179. Lessell, S., et al. 1971. Am. J. Ophthalmol. 71:1231-1235.
180. Lewy, F. H., and F. Grant. 1938. Arch. Neurol. Psychiatry 40:1126-1134.
181. Lock, S., ed. 1975. Br. Med. J. 3:265-266.
182. Love, J. G., and J. W. Kernohan. 1937. Proc. Staff Meet. Mayo Clin. 12:300-304.
183. Manlapaz, J. S. 1959. J. Pediatr. 55:73-77.
184. Mathur, S. P., and P. B. Mathur. 1959. Br. J. Ophthalmol. 43:378-379.
185. McCabe, B. R. 1972. Laryngoscope 82:1891-1896.
186. Meadows, S. P. 1949. Proc. R. Soc. Med. 42:1017-1034.
187. Memon, M. Y., and K. W. E. Paine. 1971. J. Neurosurg. 35:461-464.
188. Miehlke, A. 1973. Facial Nerve Surgery. W. B. Saunders, Philadelphia.
189. Miller, N. R., et al. 1974. Brain 97:743-754.
190. Miller, N. R., et al. 1975. Arch. Ophthalmol. 93(11): 1117-1121.
191. Mohanty, S. K., et al. 1973. J. Neurosurg. 38:86-88.
192. Money, R. A., and G. C. Halliday. 1965. Ibid. 23: 539-541.
193. Moyes, P. D. 1968. Ibid. 29:78-82.
194. Murdoch, J. L., and J. Nissim. 1971. Birth Defects Orig. Artic. Ser. 7(1):246.
195. Nikoskelainen, E., et al. 1974. Acta Neurol. Scand. 50:690-718.
196. Noffsinger, D., et al. 1972. Acta Oto-Laryngol., Suppl. 303:1-63.
197. Noordenbos, W. 1950. Folia Psychiatr. Neurol. Jpn. 53:342-348.
198. Noval, D. J., et al. 1974. Arch. Neurol. (Chicago) 30: 273-284.
199. Olafson, R. A., et al. 1966. J. Neurosurg. 24:755-759.
200. Palleske, H. 1975. Acta Neurochir. 31:293.
201. Patel, R. P., et al. 1973. Br. Med. J. 1:681.
202. Pemberton, J. W. 1964. Am. J. Ophthalmol. 58:852-854.
203. Poppne, J., and R. Marino, Jr. 1968. J. Neurosurg. 28:356-364.
204. Posner, M., and H. Horrax. 1946. Ibid. 3:15-24.
205. Potter, J. M. 1964. J. Laryngol. Otol. 78:654-657.
206. Potts, A. M. 1973. Surv. Ophthalmol. 17:313-339.
207. Prince, D. S., and J. G. Hardin. 1975. J. Am. Med. Assoc. 233:984.
208. Pulec, J. L. 1969. Ann. Otol. Rhinol. Laryngol. 78: 962-968.
209. Quick, C. A., et al. 1975. Ibid. 84:94-101.
210. Reese, A. B. 1956. Atlas of Tumor Pathology. Armed Forces Institute of Pathology, Washington, D.C. Sect. 10, fasc. 38.
211. Revilla, A. G. 1974. J. Neurosurg. 4:233-239.
212. Riggs, H. E., et al. 1957. Arch. Neurol. Psychiatry 77:473-482.
213. Robert, C. M., Jr., et al. 1973. J. Neurosurg. 38:17-19.
214. Roberts, M., and G. Owens. 1972. J. Trauma 12: 254-257.
215. Robles, R. 1968. Northwest Med. 67:845-847.
216. Roca, P. D. 1975. Ann. Ophthalmol. 7:823-834.
217. Rogers, B. O. 1963. Excerpta Med. Int. Congr. Ser. 66:681-689.
218. Ross, D. E., and S. C. Jackson. 1962. Am. J. Surg. 103:628-631.
219. Ruby, J. R., and P. J. Jannetta. 1975. Surg. Neurol. 4:369-370.
220. Rucker, C. W. 1966. Am. J. Ophthalmol. 61:1293-1298.
221. Rushton, J. G., and R. A. Olafson. 1965. Arch. Neurol. (Chicago) 13:383-386.
222. Sacks, J. G., et al. 1975. J. Am. Med. Assoc. 234:69-72.
223. Sakalas, R., et al. 1975. Arch. Ophthalmol. 93:186-190.
224. Sanders, B. B., et al. 1973. J. Neurosurg. 39:610-614.
225. Sapiro, S. M. 1975. Oral Surg. Oral Med. Oral Pathol. 39:403-408.
226. Sarin, C. L., et al. 1974. Br. J. Dis. Chest 68:46-50.
227. Savitsky, N., and M. J. Madonick. 1945. Arch. Neurol. Psychiatry 53:135-137.
228. Savitsky, N., and L. Rangell. 1950. Assoc. Res. Nerv. Ment. Dis. Proc. 28:403-413.
229. Schindler, R. F., et al. 1975. Can. J. Ophthalmol. 10:305-318.
230. Schneck, S. A., et al. 1960. Arch. Neurol. (Chicago) 2:452-457.
231. Schneider, D. E., and M. M. Abeles. 1937. J. Nerv. Ment. Dis. 85:541-547.

continued

232. Schochet, S. S., Jr., et al. 1975. Acta Neuropathol. 31:181-189.
233. Seikert, R. G. 1956. Arch. Neurol. Psychiatry 76: 1-13.
234. Senelick, R. C., and H. J. L. Van Dyk. 1974. Am. J. Ophthalmol. 78:485-488.
235. Shrader, E. C., and N. S. Schlezinger. 1960. Arch. Ophthalmol. 63:84-91.
236. Sibert, J. R. 1972. Postgrad. Med. J. 48:691-692.
237. Singhh, S. 1973. J. Assoc. Physicians India 21:905-907.
238. Smith, B. 1974. J. Neurol. Neurosurg. Psychiatry 37:1151-1154.
239. Snead, O. C., III, et al. 1975. Dev. Med. Child Neurol. 17:84-88.
240. Snyder, R. D. 1973. Lancet 2:917-918.
241. Spiegel, L. A. 1943. Ann. Otol. Rhinol. Laryngol. 52:706-712.
242. Stansbury, J. R. 1948. Am. J. Ophthalmol. 31:1153-1163.
243. Stewart, B. M. 1966. Arch. Otolaryngol. 83:543-546.
244. Stookey, B., and J. Ransohoff. 1959. Trigeminal Neuralgia, Its History and Treatment. C. C. Thomas, Springfield, IL.
245. Sullivan, G., and E. M. Helveston. 1969. Arch. Ophthalmol. 81:159-161.
246. Sumner, D. 1964. Brain 87:107-120.
247. Sunderland, S., and K. C. Bradley. 1953. J. Neurol. Neurosurg. Psychiatry 16:35-46.
248. Susac, J. O., et al. 1973. Am. J. Ophthalmol. 76: 672-679.
249. Sutherland, J. M. 1975. Proc. Aust. Assoc. Neurol. 12:17-21.
250. Taarnhφj, P. 1952. J. Neurosurg. 9:288-290.
251. Teig, E. 1968. Acta Oto-Laryngol. 65:365-372.
252. Terry, T. L., and E. B. Dunphy. 1933. Arch. Ophthalmol. 10:611-614.
253. Teuber, H.-L., et al. 1960. Visual Field Defects After Penetrating Missile Wounds of the Brain. Harvard Univ. Press, Cambridge.
254. Thorburn, I. B. 1957. J. Laryngol. Otol. 71:542-545.
255. Toglia, J. U., et al. 1970. Arch. Otolaryngol. 92: 485-492.
256. Valtonen, E. J., et al. 1974. Acta Chir. Scand. 140: 453-455.
257. Victor, M., and P. M. Dreyfus. 1965. Arch. Ophthalmol. 74:649-657.
258. Victor, M., et al. 1962. N. Engl. J. Med. 267:1267-1292.
259. Vinken, P. J., and G. W. Bruyn, ed. 1975. Handbook of Clinical Neurology. American Elsevier, New York. v. 23.
260. Vitale, C., et al. 1974. Ann. Med. Interne 125:941-944.
261. Walker, G. F. 1961. Br. J. Ophthalmol. 45:555-559.
262. Walsh, F. B., and W. F. Hoyt. 1969. Clinical Neuro-ophthalmology. Ed. 3. Williams and Wilkins, Baltimore. v. 1.
263. Walsh, F. B., and W. F. Hoyt. 1969. Ibid. v. 3.
264. Ware, M., and T. D. V. Swinscow, ed. 1971. Br. Med. J. 4:2-3.
265. Weizenblatt, S. 1959. Am. J. Ophthalmol. 47:77-83.
266. Willbrand, J. W., et al. 1974. Ann. Otol. Rhinol. Laryngol. 83:343-346.
267. Williamson, P. M. 1975. Proc. Aust. Assoc. Neurol. 12:153-155.
268. Wilson, W. H. 1972. Laryngoscope 82:1726-1735.
269. Windholz, F. 1947. Am. J. Roentgenol. 58:51-63.
270. Windstrom, A. 1975. Chest 67:365-366.
271. Wright, T. A. 1975. Clin. Orthop. Relat. Res. 108: 15-18.

138. PERIPHERAL NERVES

Part I. Normal Values

The distribution of **Fiber Diameter** of myelinated fibers falls into a bimodal pattern. The mean diameter for each peak is given, with the values of the two peaks separated by a slash. **Internode Length** varies as a function of fiber diameter, and is also bimodally distributed; mean internode length is given for each peak (the values in this column are related to the corresponding values in column two). Data in brackets refer to the column heading in brackets. Values in parentheses are ranges, estimate "c" (*see* Introduction).

	Nerve	Fiber Diameter μm	Internode Length mm	Myelinated Fibers[1] no./mm²	Schwann Cell Nuclei no./mm²	Conduction Velocity, m/s [Compound Action Potential, μV]	Reference
1	Great auricular	....	....	7230(4400-9650)	....	....	2
2	Radial	3-6/9	....	7,160(3,480-11,000)	....	....	8
3	Splanchnic	3-5/15	....	9,460(4,900-13,330)	....	....	1,6

[1] Unless otherwise indicated.

continued

Part I. Normal Values

	Nerve	Fiber Diameter μm	Internode Length mm	Myelinated Fibers[1] no./mm^2	Schwann Cell Nuclei no./mm^2	Conduction Velocity, m/s [Compound Action Potential, μV]	Reference
4	Common peroneal	5.1/10.8	0.34/0.96	....	....	45(38-55)	5
5						51(41-59)	9
6						[4.0(1-18)]	12
7	Deep peroneal[2]	5/10.0	0.55/0.85	4310(1810-7560)	....	....	10,11
8	Sural	4-5/11; 3-6/9-13	0.5/1.0	....	....	[9.5(4-26)]	2
9				4370(3810-6420)	3200	....	13
10				5560(2040-8990)	....	....	8
11				8,135(7,000-10,000)	2300	....	7
12				10,000	(1753-2920)	....	3
13				10,130(7,150-14,300)	(1458-6000)	[19(6-47)]	4
14		....	....	28,896(19,500-68,800)[3]	....	....	7
15				39,800[3]	....	....	13
16				47,000[3]	....	....	8
17				47,180(19,440-68,810)[3]	....	....	4

[1] Unless otherwise indicated. [2] Synonym: Anterior tibial. [3] Unmyelinated fibers.

Contributor: Verity, M. Anthony

References

1. Appenzeller, O., and G. Ogin. 1973. J. Neurol. Neurosurg. Psychiatry 36:777-785.
2. Dyck, P. J., et al. 1967. Proc. 6th Int. Congr. Electroencephalogr. Clin. Neurophysiol. (Vienna) 1965, p. 673.
3. Dyck, P. J., et al. 1970. Mayo Clin. Proc. 45:286-327.
4. Dyck, P. J., et al. 1971. Ibid. 46:400-431.
5. Dyck, P. J., et al. 1971. Ibid. 46:433-436.
6. Low, P. A., et al. 1975. Brain 98:341-356.
7. Ochoa, J., and W. G. P. Mair. 1969. Acta Neuropathol. 13:197-216.
8. O'Sullivan, D. J., and M. Swallow. 1968. J. Neurol. Neurosurg. Psychiatry 31:464-470.
9. Stevens, J. C., et al. 1973. Brain Res. 52:37-59.
10. Swallow, M. 1966. J. Neurol. Neurosurg. Psychiatry 29:205-213.
11. Vizoso, A. D. 1950. J. Anat. 84:342-353.
12. Walsh, J. C. 1971. Arch. Neurol. (Chicago) 25:404-414.
13. Walsh, J. C. 1971. J. Neurol. Neurosurg. Psychiatry 34:42-50.

Part II. Pathology

ABBREVIATIONS & SYMBOLS

AD = axonal degeneration
CAP = compound action potential
CSF = cerebrospinal fluid
CV = conduction velocity
IgA = immunoglobulin A
IP = inheritance pattern
SD = segmental demyelination
← = a leftward shift in fiber diameter spectrum as compared to normal, i.e., a significant preferential loss of large fibers with small fibers still present

→ = a rightward shift in fiber diameter spectrum, i.e., a preferential loss of small fibers with large fibers still remaining
± = equivocal single fiber involvement usually associated with inadequate investigative technique
+ = rare scattered single fiber involvement
++ = approximately 10-50% fiber involvement
+++ = greater than 50% fiber involvement
↓ = decrease(d)
↑ = increase(d)

continued

Part II. Pathology

Figures in heavy brackets are reference numbers. Data in light brackets refer to the column heading in brackets.

	Condition ⟨Synonym⟩	Clinical Comment	Myelinated Fibers [Intact Fibers, no./mm²]	Unmyelinated Fibers [Intact Fibers, no./mm²]	Other Changes [Schwann Cell Nuclei Density, no./mm²]	Conduction Parameters	Refer-ence
			Infections				
1	Acute idiopathic post-infec-tious poly-neuropathy	Guillain-Barré-Strohl syndrome. Progres-sive polyradiculopa-thy; motor involve-ment >sensory. Al-bumino-cytologic dissociation in CSF.	SD. Myelin ovoid formation. AD, ++. ←.	....	Lymphocyte infil-tration	CV ↓ 50%	7,22,41
2		With hyponatremia, due to inappro-priate vasopres-sin 1/ secretion	Same as entry 1	....	Radiculopathy	....	75
3	Diphtheritic neuropathy	Due to Corynebacte-rium diphtheriae	SD & paranodal demyelination, +++	Minimal ↓ in fiber no.	Dorsal root ganglia loss. Schwann cell degeneration.	CV ↓ 50-100%	47
4	Leprosy	Lepromatous type: mononeuritic or dis-tal sensory neuropa-thy	SD, ++. AD, +.	....	Schwann cell pro-liferation. Fibro-sis.	....	79
5		Tuberculoid type: mononeuritis	AD, +++	....	Nodular fibrosis. Schwann cell pro-liferation, +++.	....	79
			Exogenous Toxins				
6	Inorganic Arsenic	Sensory neuropathy; pain	Distal SD & AD, +	....	....	....	16
7	Lead	Motor involvement >>sensory	SD, +++	....	....	....	16
8	Mercury	Proximal neuropathy >distal; sensory in-volvement >motor	AD, ++	....	....	....	25,45
9	Gold	Distal, mixed neuro-pathy	....	....	....	....	101
10	Organic Isoniazid	Induced pyridoxine deficiency	....	....	....	CV ↓	73
11	Nitrofurantoin	Renal failure. Mixed sensorimotor neuro-pathy.	AD, ++	....	....	....	96
12	Vincristine	Leukemia. Distal, mixed polyneuro-pathy.	SD, +. AD, +, with neuro-filament ag-gregates.	....	....	....	18
13	Organophos-phate	Distal sensorimotor neuropathy	AD, ++. Nerve fi-ber loss. Myelin irregularities.	....	Endoneural hyper-plasia	....	5

1/ Synonym: ADH.

continued

Part II. Pathology

	Condition ⟨Synonym⟩	Clinical Comment	Myelinated Fibers [Intact Fibers, no./mm²]	Unmyelinated Fibers [Intact Fibers, no./mm²]	Other Changes [Schwann Cell Nuclei Density, no./mm²]	Conduction Parameters	Reference
14	Acrylamide	Distal sensorimotor neuropathy	AD. ←. Neurofilament accumulation. [4370]	....	....	CV ↓; CAP ↓	48
15	Solvents: *n*-Hexane, toluene	"Glue-sniffing" neuropathy. Motor involvement >sensory	Paranodal demyelination, +. Axon loss with neurofilament aggregation. ←. Büngner band formation. [6851;7441]	Normal	....	....	9,97
16	Alcohol: Chronic alcoholism	Distal sensorimotor neuropathy; acrodystrophic	AD, ++2/ [(1000-3900)2/; (7,320-11,800)3/]	Normal	....	CV ↓ 5-10%	67,90, 104
			Hepatic Failure				
17	Cholemia	....	SD, ++. AD, +.	....	....	CV ↓ 10%; CAP ↓	84
18		Biliary cirrhosis. Distal sensory neuropathy.	SD, +	....	Foam cell4/ infiltration	....	97
			Renal Failure				
19	Uremia	Chronic distal neuropathy, predominantly sensory	SD, +. AD, +. [6345]	Normal	Schwann cell loss	CV ↓ 10%	6,39
			Congenital & Hereditary Disorders				
20	Hypertrophic Hereditary motor & sensory neuropathy type I	Charcot-Marie-Tooth disease. High arch. Adult onset. IP, dominant.	SD, ++. AD, +. ←. [2820]	Normal [46,888]	Schwann cell hyperplasia, +. "Onion-bulb" formation, +.	CV, slow; CAP, abnormal	37,38, 63,71, 80
21	Hereditary motor & sensory neuropathy type III	Dejerine-Sottas disease. ↑ CSF protein. Onset in infancy. IP, recessive.	SD, +++ [192]	Normal [63,750]	Schwann cell hyperplasia, ++. "Onion-bulb" formation, +++.	CV, absent; CAP, abnormal	38,49
22	Hyperimmunoglobulinemia A	Excess IgA synthesis in jejunum. Sensory neuropathy.	No myelinated fibers	....	....	....	107
23	Sensory radicular neuropathy of Denny-Brown ⟨Hereditary sensory neuropathy type I⟩	Penetrating ulcers. Adult onset.	→ [950]	Severe loss	Dorsal root ganglion & dorsal column loss	CAP ↓	34,88

2/ Sural nerve. 3/ Splanchnic nerve. 4/ Synonym: Xanthoma cell.

continued

Part II. Pathology

	Condition ⟨Synonym⟩	Clinical Comment	Myelinated Fibers [Intact Fibers, no./mm²]	Unmyelinated Fibers [Intact Fibers, no./mm²]	Other Changes [Schwann Cell Nuclei Density, no./mm²]	Conduction Parameters	Reference
24	Congenital sensory neuropathy	Insensitivity to pain. Type A: ± anhidrosis; type B: hyperplastic myelinopathy. IP, recessive.	Severe loss. SD.	Partial loss	....	CV, very slow; CAP, absent	28,74, 100, 109
25	Familial dysautonomia ⟨Riley-Day syndrome⟩	Absent lacrimation. Postural hypotension. Jewish children.	[8810]	Greatly ↓ fiber no. [3617]	....	CV, slow; CAP ↓	1,20,78, 86
26	Chronic polyradiculoneuropathy of infancy	↑ CSF protein. ↓ spinal & cranial nerve root myelination.	....	....	....	....	59
			Ischemic & Collagen Vascular Diseases				
27	Arteriopathy	Distal, asymmetric. Vascular obstruction and/or thrombosis. Perivascular connective tissue proliferation.	SD, ++. AD, ++.	....	....	....	26,42
28	Subacute bacterial endocarditis	Acute, asymmetric mononeuropathy. Embolization.	Segmental infarction. AD, ++.	Segmental infarction & degeneration	....	....	57
29	Polyarteritis nodosa	Acute & chronic mononeuropathy. Vasculitis, thrombosis, & recanalization.	Segmental infarction. AD, ++.	....	....	....	17
30	Systemic lupus erythematosus	Acute mononeuropathy. Guillain-Barré-like syndrome	....	....	....	....	56
31	Dermatomyositis; polymyositis	Proximal neuropathy	Patchy demyelination. SD. Axon no. ↓.	Focal loss	Perineural & endoneural connective tissue proliferation	....	60,70
32	Rheumatoid arthritis	Entrapment syndrome (40%). Distal motor sensory neuropathy (30%). Distal sensory motor neuropathy (10%).	AD, ±. Patchy demyelination.	Focal loss	Vasculitis with microinfarcts	CV, focal delay or ↓ (30-50%)	40,106
33	Entrapment neuropathy	Median nerve in carpal tunnel; ulnar nerve; posterior tibial nerve; common peroneal nerve[5]; lateral femoral cutaneous nerve[6]; sciatic nerve; obturator nerve; suprascapular nerve	↓ in no. of large myelinated fibers	....	Endoneural connective tissue proliferation	CV ↓	36,56,92

[5] Synonym: Lateral popliteal nerve. [6] Synonym: Lateral cutaneous nerve of thigh.

continued

Part II. Pathology

No.	Condition ⟨Synonym⟩	Clinical Comment	Myelinated Fibers [Intact Fibers, no./mm²]	Unmyelinated Fibers [Intact Fibers, no./mm²]	Other Changes [Schwann Cell Nuclei Density, no./mm²]	Conduction Parameters	Reference
34	Familial pressure neuropathy	....	Fiber loss variable. SD, +. Tomaculous change (sausage-body neuropathy). [(5,500-12,300)²/]	Normal	Endoneural connective tissue proliferation	CV ↓ (28 m/s); CAP ↓ (3.5 μV)	12,43,68
35	Amyloidosis⁷/ Familial	Andrade type ⟨Portuguese⟩	AD, +. →. Büngner band formation. [2250; 4587]	Fiber no. ↓ [(10,000-11,000)]	Endoneural amyloid masses	CV ↓ 10%; CAP ↓	2,27,35
36		Swiss type. Carpal tunnel syndrome. Vitreous opacities.	AD, +. ←.	Significant ↓ in fiber no.	Epineural deposits	CV ↓ 10%	81
37		Van Allen type. Distal sensorimotor neuropathy. Nephropathy. Peptic ulceration. IP, autosomal dominant.	AD, ±.	Fiber no. ↓	Nerve root & blood vessel involvement	....	99
38	Sporadic	Dissociated sensory loss (pain, temp). Distal sensory & autonomic involvement.	Depletion. →. [2250]	Severe loss	Epineural deposits. Vascular amyloid. Intraneural infiltration. Schwann cell inclusions.	....	93
	Dysglobulinemia Syndromes						
39	Multiple myeloma [32,65]	....	SD, ++. Widening of myelin lamellae. AD, +. [(2120-3370)]	AD, ++. [14,900; 19,300]	Lymphocyte infiltration. Amyloidosis. Vascular microemboli. Schwann cell inclusions. [(1410; 2755)]	....	11,13, 32,65, 76,102, 107
40	Waldenström's macroglobulinemia [76, 102]	....	Same as entry 39	....			
41	Lymphoproliferative disorders [13, 32]	....	....	....			
42	Chronic infection [11]	....	....	....			
43	μ-Chain disease [13]	....	....	....			
44	Hyperimmunoglobulinemia A (see also entry 22) [107]	....	....	....			

²/ Sural nerve. ⁷/ For information on B-cell dyscrasia, consult references 13 and 55; see also entries 39, 40, and 43.

continued

Part II. Pathology

	Condition ⟨Synonym⟩	Clinical Comment	Myelinated Fibers [Intact Fibers, no./mm²]	Unmyelinated Fibers [Intact Fibers, no./mm²]	Other Changes [Schwann Cell Nuclei Density, no./mm²]	Conduction Parameters	Reference
45	Chediak-Higashi syndrome	....	....	....	Same as entries 39-44	CV ↓ 20%	64
			Metabolic Diseases				
46	Acute porphyria	Acute onset. Proximal neuropathy. Motor involvement >sensory. δ-Aminolevulinate synthase induction.	SD, ±. AD, ++.	Fiber no. ↓, +	....	....	24,89,91
47	Metachromatic leukodystrophy	Arylsulfatase A deficiency	SD, +++, with myelin irregularities	....	Schwann cell metachromatic inclusions. Myelin bodies.	CV ↓ 50%	29,46, 105
48	Krabbe's disease ⟨Globoid cell leukodystrophy⟩	....	SD, ++. 50% ↓ in no. of fibers. ←. AD minimal.	Normal	Prismatic inclusions. Cholesterol & acid phosphatase increase in Schwann cell cytoplasm.	....	82
49	Tangier disease	Recurrent sensorimotor neuropathy. ↓ plasma cholesterol. Absent serum α-lipoprotein. Cholesterol ester storage in reticuloendothelial system.	Demyelination, +. AD, +.	Minimal ↓ in fiber no.	....	....	44,62
50	Niemann-Pick disease	....	AD, +. Axon no. ↓	....	Schwann cell hyperplasia, +. Cytoplasmic granular bodies; foam cells.	CV ↓ 50%	52
51	Glycogenosis type II ⟨Pompé's disease⟩	Deficient α-glucosidase[8]	Normal	Normal	Schwann cell & pericyte glycogen accumulation	....	4
52	Fabry's disease ⟨Angiokeratoma corporis diffusum⟩	....	Unimodal distribution: diameter, 6-8 μm. Small fibers. [3630]	Normal	Xanthomatous deposits in perineurium	....	61
			Endocrine Disorders				
53	Diabetes mellitus	Distal, symmetric, predominantly sensory neuropathy	SD, ++ (AD, +, when severe)[2] [(1800-3170)[2]]	Fiber no. ↓	Schwann cell hyperplasia, +. Onion-bulb formation ±, when severe.	CV ↓	10,51, 58,66, 94

[2] Sural nerve. [8] Synonym: α-1,4-Glycosidase.

continued

Part II. Pathology

	Condition ⟨Synonym⟩	Clinical Comment	Myelinated Fibers [Intact Fibers, no./mm²]	Unmyelinated Fibers [Intact Fibers, no./mm²]	Other Changes [Schwann Cell Nuclei Density, no./mm²]	Conduction Parameters	Reference
54		Proximal, acute mononeuropathy 9/. Subacute proximal neuropathy (amyotrophy).	SD, +++; AD, +. 9/ SD, +; paranodal demyelination. 3/ [4270 (2580-7130)3/]	....	Endothelial proliferation. Arterial narrowing. Ischemic infarcts.	....	3,50,108
55		Autonomic neuropathy	....	Fiber no. ↓. Degeneration of autonomic ganglia.	....	....	66
56	Hypothyroidism	Sensory polyneuropathy. Entrapment syndrome (carpal tunnel).	SD, +	Normal	....	CV ↓ 30%; CAP ↓	36,72

Hypertrophy or Hyperplasia 10,11/

57	Dejerine-Sottas disease	See entry 21					38,49
58	Multiple mucosal neuroma syndrome	Autonomic disturbance. Marfanoid features. Pheochromocytoma. Medullary thyroid carcinoma.	Minimal SD or AD. Axoplasmic glycogen. Fiber no. ↓. [3450]	Axon swelling. ←. [25,000]	Schwann cell hyperplasia, +++. No onion-bulb formation. Metachromasia.	....	58,83
59	Localized hypertrophic neurofibrosis	....	Axon no. ↓. AD, +.	....	Isomorphic endoneural fibrosis	CV ↓ >50%	31,85
60	Refsum's syndrome	Relapsing polyneuropathy. Cerebellar dysfunction. ↑ serum phytanic acid.	Fiber no. ↓	Normal	Onion-bulb formation, ++. Endoneural collagen proliferation. Schwann cell inclusions (osmophilic, crystalloid).	....	21,46,77
61	Giant axonal neuropathy	Hair change. Distal sensorimotor neuropathy.	Segmental axon enlargement: 15-25 μm. Fiber no. normal or ↓, +. Neurofilament aggregation.	Normal	Onion-bulb formation, +	....	8,15,23, 54

Carcinoma

62	Remote involvement of nerve 12/	Mixed sensorimotor (80%)	SD, +. AD, ++. Fiber no. ↓.	....	Lymphocyte infiltration. Dorsal column degeneration.	....	19,30, 33,53, 102
63		Sensory radiculopathy					
64		Motor neuron variant					
65	Malignant lymphoma	Often asymptomatic	SD, ++. AD, +. [(1550-6070)]	....	[(1880-4470)]	CV ↓; CAP ↓	103

3/ Splanchnic nerve. 9/ Femoral nerve. 10/ For information on hypertrophic neuropathy of acromegaly, consult reference 87. 11/ For information on neuroaxonal dystrophy, consult references 14, 69, and 98. 12/ There can also be direct or metastatic involvement of nerve.

continued

138. PERIPHERAL NERVES

Part II. Pathology

Contributor: Verity, M. Anthony

References

1. Aguayo, A. J., et al. 1971. Arch. Neurol. (Chicago) 24:106-116.
2. Andrade, C. 1952. Brain 75:408-427.
3. Appenzeller, O., and E. P. Richardson. 1966. Neurology 16:1205-1209.
4. Araoz, C., et al. 1974. Ibid. 24:739-742.
5. Aring, C. D. 1942. Brain 65:34-47.
6. Asbury, A. K., et al. 1963. Arch. Neurol. (Chicago) 8:413-428.
7. Asbury, A. K., et al. 1969. Medicine (Baltimore) 48:173-215.
8. Asbury, A. K., et al. 1972. Acta Neuropathol. 20:237-247.
9. Asbury, A. K., et al. 1973. Annu. Meet. Am. Assoc. Neuropathol. (Freeport, Grand Bahama) 49th.
10. Ballin, R. H. M., and P. K. Thomas. 1968. Acta Neuropathol. 11:93-102.
11. Barron, K. D., et al. 1960. J. Nerv. Ment. Dis. 131:10-31.
12. Behse, F., et al. 1972. Brain 95:777-794.
13. Benson, M. D., et al. 1975. Lancet 1:10-12.
14. Berard-Badier, M., et al. 1971. Acta Neuropathol., Suppl. 5:30-39.
15. Berg, B. O., et al. 1972. Pediatrics 49:894-899.
16. Blackwood, W., and J. A. N. Corsellis, ed. 1976. Greenfield's Neuropathology. Ed. 3. E. Arnold, London.
17. Bleehen, H. S., et al. 1963. Q. J. Med. 32:193-209.
18. Bradley, W. G., et al. 1970. J. Neurol. Sci. 10:107-131.
19. Brain, W. R., et al. 1965. Brain 88:479-500.
20. Brown, W. J., et al. 1964. J. Neurol. Neurosurg. Psychiatry 27:131-139.
21. Cammermeyer, J. 1956. J. Neuropathol. Exp. Neurol. 15:340-361.
22. Carpenter, S. 1972. J. Neurol. Sci. 15:125-140.
23. Carpenter, S., et al. 1974. Arch. Neurol. (Chicago) 31:312-316.
24. Cavanagh, J. V., and R. S. Mellick. 1965. J. Neurol. Neurosurg. Psychiatry 28:320-327.
25. Chang, L. W., and H. A. Hartmann. 1972. Acta Neuropathol. 20:316-334.
26. Chopra, J. S., and L. J. Hurwitz. 1967. J. Neurol. Neurosurg. Psychiatry 30:207-214.
27. Coimbra, A., and C. Andrade. 1971. Brain 94:199-206.
28. Comings, D. E., and T. D. Amromin. 1974. Neurology 24:838-848.
29. Cravioto, H., et al. 1966. Acta Neuropathol. 7:111-124.
30. Croft, P. B., et al. 1967. Brain 90:31-66.
31. Da Gama Imaginario, J., et al. 1964. J. Neurol. Sci. 1:340-347.
32. Dayan, A. D., and T. D. Lewis. 1966. Neurology 16:1141-1144.
33. Denny-Brown, D. 1948. J. Neurol. Neurosurg. Psychiatry 11:73-87.
34. Denny-Brown, D. 1951. Ibid. 14:237-252.
35. Dyck, P. J., and E. H. Lambert. 1969. Arch. Neurol. (Chicago) 20:490-507.
36. Dyck, P. J., and E. H. Lambert. 1970. J. Neuropathol. Exp. Neurol. 29:631-658.
37. Dyck, P. J., et al. 1967. Proc. 6th Int. Congr. Electroencephalogr. Clin. Neurophysiol. (Vienna) 1965, p. 673.
38. Dyck, P. J., et al. 1970. Mayo Clin. Proc. 45:286-327.
39. Dyck, P. J., et al. 1971. Ibid. 46:400-431.
40. Dyck, P. J., et al. 1972. Ibid. 47:461-475.
41. Dyck, P. J., et al. 1975. Ibid. 50:621-637.
42. Eames, R. A., and L. S. Lang. 1967. J. Neurol. Neurosurg. Psychiatry 30:215-226.
43. Earl, C. J., et al. 1964. Q. J. Med. 33:481-498.
44. Engel, W. K., et al. 1967. Arch. Neurol. (Chicago) 17:1-9.
45. Etoh, K. 1971. Shinkei Kenkyu No Shimpo 15:606-618.
46. Fardeau, M., and W. K. Engel. 1969. J. Neuropathol. Exp. Neurol. 28:278-294.
47. Fisher, C. M., and R. D. Adams. 1956. Ibid. 15:243-268.
48. Fullerton, P. 1969. J. Neurol. Neurosurg. Psychiatry 32:186-192.
49. Gilroy, J., et al. 1966. Am. J. Med. 40:368-383.
50. Goodman, J. I. 1954. Diabetes 3:266-271.
51. Gregersen, G. 1968. Acta Med. Scand. 183:55-60.
52. Gumbinas, M., et al. 1975. Neurology 25:107-113.
53. Henson, R. A., and H. Urich. 1970. In P. J. Vinken and G. W. Bruyn, ed. Handbook of Clinical Neurology. North-Holland, Amsterdam. v. 8, pp. 131-148.
54. Igisu, H., et al. 1975. Neurology 25:717-721.
55. Isobe, T., and E. F. Osserman. 1974. N. Engl. J. Med. 290:473-477.
56. Johnson, R. T., and E. P. Richardson. 1968. Medicine (Baltimore) 47:337-369.
57. Jones, H. R., Jr., and R. G. Siekert. 1968. Arch. Neurol. (Chicago) 19:535-537.
58. Joosten, E., et al. 1974. Acta Neuropathol. 30:251-261.
59. Kasman, M., et al. 1976. Neurology 26:565-573.
60. Kibler, R. F., and F. C. Rose. 1960. Br. Med. J. 1:1781-1784.
61. Kocen, R. S., and P. K. Thomas. 1970. Arch. Neurol. (Chicago) 22:81-88.
62. Kocen, R. S., et al. 1967. Lancet 1:1341-1345.
63. Kriel, R. L., et al. 1974. Neurology 24:801-809.

continued

Part II. Pathology

64. Lockman, L. A., et al. 1967. J. Pediatr. 70:942-951.
65. Logothetis, J., et al. 1968. Arch. Neurol. (Chicago) 19:389-397.
66. Low, P. A., et al. 1975. Brain 98:341-356.
67. Low, P. A., et al. 1975. Ibid. 98:357-364.
68. Madrid, R., and W. G. Bradley. 1975. J. Neurol. Sci. 25:415-448.
69. Martin, J. J., and L. Martin. 1972. Eur. Neurol. 8:239-250.
70. McEntee, W. J., and E. L. Mancall. 1965. Neurology 15:69-75.
71. Meier, C., et al. 1976. J. Neurol. 211:111-124.
72. Murray, I. P. C., and J. A. Simpson. 1958. Lancet 1:1360-1363.
73. Ochoa, J. 1970. Brain 93:831-850.
74. Ogden, T. E., et al. 1959. J. Neurol. Neurosurg. Psychiatry 22:267-276.
75. Posner, J. B., et al. 1967. Arch. Neurol. (Chicago) 17:530-541.
76. Propp, R. P., et al. 1975. Neurology 25:980-988.
77. Refsum, S. 1946. Acta Psychiatr. Neurol., Suppl. 38.
78. Riley, C. M., et al. 1949. Pediatrics 3:468-478.
79. Rosenberg, R. N., and R. E. Lovelace. 1968. Arch. Neurol. (Chicago) 19:310-314.
80. Roussy, G., and G. Levy. 1926. Rev. Neurol. 1:427-450.
81. Rukavina, J. G., et al. 1956. Medicine (Baltimore) 35:239-334.
82. Schlaepfer, W. W., and A. L. Prensky. 1972. Acta Neuropathol. 20:55-66.
83. Schmike, R. N., et al. 1968. N. Engl. J. Med. 279:1-7.
84. Seneviratne, K. N., and O. A. Peiris. 1970. J. Neurol. Neurosurg. Psychiatry 33:609-614.
85. Simpson, D. A., and M. Fowler. 1966. Ibid. 29:80-84.
86. Solitare, G. B., and G. S. Cohen. 1965. Neurology 15:321-327.
87. Stewart, B. M. 1966. Arch. Neurol. (Chicago) 14:107-110.
88. Swanson, A. G., et al. 1965. Ibid. 12:12-18.
89. Sweeney, V. P., et al. 1970. Brain 93:369-380.
90. Thevanard, A. 1942. Rev. Neurol. 74:193-212.
91. Thomas, P. K. 1971. Proc. R. Soc. Med. 64:295-298.
92. Thomas, P. K., and P. M. Fullerton. 1963. J. Neurol. Neurosurg. Psychiatry 26:520-527.
93. Thomas, P. K., and R. H. M. King. 1974. Brain 97:395-406.
94. Thomas, P. K., and R. G. Lascelles. 1966. Q. J. Med. 35:489-509.
95. Thomas, P. K., and J. T. Walker. 1965. Brain 88:1079-1088.
96. Toole, J. F., et al. 1968. Arch. Neurol. (Chicago) 18:680-687.
97. Towfighi, J., et al. 1976. Neurology 26:238-243.
98. Ule, G. 1972. Acta Neuropathol. 21:332-339.
99. Van Allen, M. W., et al. 1969. Neurology 19:10-25.
100. Vassella, F., et al. 1968. Arch. Dis. Child. 43:124-130.
101. Walsh, J. C. 1970. Neurology 20:455-458.
102. Walsh, J. C. 1971. Arch. Neurol. (Chicago) 25:404-414.
103. Walsh, J. C. 1971. J. Neurol. Neurosurg. Psychiatry 34:42-50.
104. Walsh, J. C., and J. G. McLeod. 1970. J. Neurol. Sci. 10:457-469.
105. Webster, H. D. 1962. J. Neuropathol. Exp. Neurol. 21:534-541.
106. Weller, R. O., et al. 1970. J. Neurol. Neurosurg. Psychiatry 33:592-604.
107. Whitaker, A., et al. 1974. Arch. Neurol. (Chicago) 30:359-371.
108. Williams, I. R., and R. F. Mayer. 1976. Neurology 26:108-116.
109. Winkelmann, R. K., et al. 1962. Arch. Dermatol. 85:325-339.

139. CLINICAL ASSESSMENT OF THE AUTONOMIC NERVOUS SYSTEM

To obtain uncontaminated and meaningful results, patients should be off the autonomic and allied drugs, e.g., antihypertensives, diuretics (especially when hyponatremia occurs), phenothiazines, antidepressants, etc. [ref. 7]. Localization of lesions is achieved by the process of elimination of afferent or efferent pathway dysfunction. The only test for direct assessment of central pathways is the hyperventilation test for vasomotor center function. Central pathways of the autonomic nervous system, especially cephalic to the brainstem, are ill understood. The term brainstem may imply all the higher centers until further elucidation. Some of the tests are potentially dangerous, e.g., the tyramine test; investigators should use them cautiously. *Abbreviations*: b.p. = blood pressure; GI = gastrointestinal; i.v. = intravenous; S2 (S3, S4) = second (third, fourth) sacral segment of spinal cord; wt = weight.

	Test	Technique	Pathways	Normal Response & Remarks	Reference
			Pupillary Tests		
1	Light reflex	Expose pupil to bright light; observe ipsilateral & contralateral pupils for direct & consensual constriction responses, respectively	Retinal receptors → optic nerve → pretectal region & Edinger-Westphal nucleus → cranial nerve III → ciliary ganglion → postganglionic fibers in short ciliary nerves to the sphincter pupillae	Normal response consists of constriction of pupils. Parasympathetic-cranial nerve III involvement will produce dilated non-responsive pupil. Involvement of ciliary ganglion would result in Adie's pupil.	12

continued

	Test	Technique	Pathways	Normal Response & Remarks	Reference
2	Ciliospinal reflex	Patient asked to focus on distant object. A firm pinch then applied to neck or upper chest for 5 s. Pupillary dilatation occurs ipsilaterally & contralaterally.	Sensory afferents → brainstem & hypothalamus → sympathetic efferents → iris	Normal response: 1-2 mm pupillary dilatation. Onset of pupillary dilatation described as brisk (less than 0.5 s latent period) or slow. Normal response indicates integrity of spinal cord below midcervical region and of thoracocervicocephalic sympathetic chain.	37
3	Drug tests Pilocarpine	0.0625% pilocarpine, 2 drops 5 min apart, in conjunctival sac of each eye. Record change in pupil size after 20 min.	Parasympathetic end-organ response	None or minimal response in normals. Marked pupillary constriction in cases of parasympathetic denervation supersensitivity (Adie's pupil). This test replaces the methacholine chloride (Mecholyl) test, as methacholine chloride is difficult to obtain.	6
4	Hydroxyamphetamine	1% hydroxyamphetamine solution, 2 drops in each conjunctival sac. Observe change in pupil size after 10 min.	Sympathetic end-organ response	Normal pupil dilates. No dilatation indicates postganglionic lesion. This is a very reliable test in distinguishing preganglionic from postganglionic lesion.	41,42
5	Cocaine	1-2 drops of 5% cocaine instilled in each conjunctival sac. Observe pupillary response after 10 min.	Sympathetic end-organ response	Normal response is mydriasis. Preganglionic lesion will impair dilatation, and postganglionic lesion will produce no dilatation.	41
6	Epinephrine	3 drops of 1:1000 epinephrine instilled in each conjunctival sac, 3 times within 3 min. Check pupil size after 15 min.	Sympathetic end-organ response	Prominent dilatation indicates end-organ hypersensitivity	41,44
			Skin & Mucous Membrane Function Tests		
7	Lacrimation	A strip of filter paper, 35 × 5 mm, is hooked into inferior fornix of eye. Measure extent of soaking after 5 min.	Trigeminal afferents → lacrimal nucleus → nerve of pterygoid canal[1] → pterygopalatine ganglion[2] → lacrimal gland	Normal soaking: >15 mm in 5 min. <10 mm soaking or a bilateral difference, when the lesser value does not exceed 27% of the larger one, are considered significant	4,13, 19
8	Salivation	Cannulate parotid duct. Collect secretions with slow, continuous suction, with and without stimulation with lemon juice.	Inferior salivatory nucleus → cranial nerve IX → lesser petrosal nerve → otic ganglion → parotid gland	Normal secretion: ∼1 ml/min	25
9	Sweat	Quinizarin compound applied to whole body or its appropriate portion. Patient exposed to 43.3°C heat in a cradle for 15-35 min to raise core temperature by 1°C.	Increased blood temperature → hypothalamus → sympathetic efferent pathways → postganglionic cholinergic nerve endings	Onset of sweating turns quinizarin compound into a dark blue-violet color. Sweat disturbance indicates central or efferent dysfunction.	18
10	Acetylcholine	1% solution of acetylcholine perchlorate applied to sweat glands by electrophoresis; local sweating observed with use of iodine paper	Postganglionic nerve endings & end-organ response	Absence of sweating indicates postganglionic lesion. Not routinely used.	34

[1] Synonym: Vidian nerve. [2] Synonym: Sphenopalatine ganglion.

continued

	Test	Technique	Pathways	Normal Response & Remarks	Reference
11	Intradermal histamine	Inject intradermally 0.1 ml of 1:1000 histamine phosphate. Note size of flare after 5, 10, 15, & 20 min.	This axon reflex involves dorsal root ganglia & afferent fibers	Size of flare varies normally between 6 & 24 cm. Same as triple response of Lewis, and can also be obtained by a mechanical stimulus.	3,35
			Cardiovascular & Vasomotor System Tests		
12	Orthostatic adaptation	Pulse rate, systolic & diastolic b.p. are measured when patient in prone position and immediately upon standing. Repeated after 3, 5, & 10 min, and again when recumbent. Use of tilt table may accentuate failure in orthostatic adaptation.	Aortic & carotid baroreceptor afferents → vasomotor center → sympathetic & parasympathetic efferent responses	Pulse rate increases normally by 8-16 beats/min, and systolic b.p. decreases by 10-15 mm Hg. In autonomic dysfunction, pulse rate may be fixed and postural hypotension marked.	2,26, 35
13	Valsalva's maneuver	Subject, in semirecumbent position, breathes through a mouthpiece attached by a connecting tubing to an anaeroid manometer, and maintains expiratory strain of 40 mm Hg for 10-12 s; b.p. & heart rate recorded	Strain → baroreceptor afferents → brainstem & vasomotor center → sympathetic efferents → end-organ. Release → baroreceptor afferents → vasomotor center → parasympathetic efferents → end-organ	One of the most important tests of baroreceptor function. Normal response consists of 4 phases. Phase II shows tachycardia in response to decreased b.p., and phase IV is indicated by bradycardia in response to systolic overshoot phenomenon. Abnormal responses: (i) absence of systolic b.p. overshoot in phase IV, (ii) lower heart rate in phase II than in phase IV, (iii) fall in mean b.p. in phase II below 50% of previous resting mean pressure.	24,27, 29,30
14	Lobeline	Give rapid antecubital i.v. injection of 0.5 ml of 1% solution of α-lobeline hydrochloride. Onset of cough indicates response.	Carotid body → respiratory center → vagus nerve	No direct test for integrity of baroreceptor fibers from carotid sinus. However, chemoreceptor fibers from the carotid body can be tested, thus providing indirectly the status of afferent fibers from the baroreceptors.	5,26
15	Hyperventilation	Patient, in supine position, breathes as fast and as deeply as possible for 15 s; arterial b.p. recorded	Alkalosis & vasoconstriction → depressed vasomotor center responsiveness	Normally, b.p. reduced from 16-55 mm Hg, with an average change of 32 mm Hg. One of the few tests available for testing the higher centers of the autonomic nervous system.	23
16	Mental arithmetic	Patient performs random-number addition or subtraction under noisy conditions for 1-10 min; b.p. is recorded	Cerebrum → brainstem → sympathetic efferents	Mean arterial b.p. elevated ∿15%. Provides an indirect means of testing the efferent system with a different afferent pathway.	33
17	Cold pressor	Record baseline b.p. Immerse one hand up to wrist in ice water (1-4°C) for 1 min. Record b.p. change at 30 s & 60 s.	Sensory afferents → spinothalamic tracts → suprapontine, infrathalamic relays → sympathetic efferent pathways & end-organs	Normal response is rise in systolic & diastolic b.p. of ∿10-20 mm Hg. Diastolic pressure more reliable index.	21,31, 43

continued

	Test	Technique	Pathways	Normal Response & Remarks	Reference
18	Hand grip	Patient grips hand dynamometer 3 times, as hard as possible. Mean value taken as maximum voluntary contraction (MVC). Asked to maintain sustained grip at 30% of MVC for up to 5 min. Baseline heart rate & b.p. recorded initially, and then once per min during grip.	Afferents from activated muscle & neurons from motor cortex → vasomotor center → sympathetic efferents	Rise in diastolic b.p. of more than 16 mm Hg considered normal; below 10 mm Hg considered abnormal. Test still of experimental value only. Abnormal results found in 2 patients with Shy-Drager syndrome. A safe & non-invasive test for integrity of autonomic function.	14-16
			Tests for Altered Biochemical Responses		
19	Plasma norepinephrine response	Measure plasma norepinephrine levels 2 min & 5 min after patient attains upright posture	Not definite. Probably baroreceptors → brainstem → sympathetic efferents.	Mean increment of norepinephrine levels much below normal range	8
20	Plasma renin	Patient lies supine for 2 h and, then in tilt-up position (45-85° to horizontal adjusted to prevent syncope) for 2 h. Venous blood taken for measuring renin levels at 1-h intervals.	Not fully understood. Baroreceptors → brainstem, thalamus, & hypothalamus → sympathetic efferents to juxtaglomerular apparatus.	Normal values by technique of Brown, et al.: 4-20 units/liter. Levels increase 2-4 times when patient tilted up or standing. Response absent in patients with lesions of efferent sympathetic pathways.	11,32
21	Atropine	Administration of atropine, 0.03 mg/kg body wt, i.v. Record basal heart rate initially, then at 5, 10, & 15 min after injection.	Parasympathetic blockade at end-organ	Anticipated increase in normal individuals: 38 ± 5 beats	9,20
22	Norepinephrine infusion	Infusion of 0.1-0.13 μg·kg^{-1}·min^{-1} i.v. for 15-20 min	End-organ response	Normally systolic b.p. increased by 22 mm Hg. Response exaggerated in cases of denervation supersensitivity.	17,39
23	Phenylephrine	Bolus of 50 μg of phenylephrine injected i.v.; b.p. recorded	Acts on arterial smooth muscle receptors	Normal range of increase in b.p. is 10-63 mm Hg. This increase may produce reflex slowing of heart rate, indicating baroreceptor function.	23
24	Tyramine	Bolus of tyramine administered i.v. in increasing doses of 250, 500, 1000, 1500, & 2000 μg. Higher doses given in 1000 μg increments up to a limit of 6000 μg. After each dose, b.p. response measured with a 10-15 min interval between doses.	Tyramine releases catecholamine stores at efferent endings & end-organs	A rise in systolic b.p. greater than 20 mm Hg after injection of 1000 μg is an exaggerated response. Absence of b.p. rise after 6000 μg may be considered a depressed response. Particularly used in patients who have been on antihypertensive agents.	23,43
			Gastrointestinal Function Tests		
25	Clinical evaluation	With patient in supine position & relaxed, listen for bowel sounds with stethoscope. Rectal examination may be performed in supine or lateral decubitus position.	Parasympathetic efferent pathways via vagus & sacral parasympathetic nerves	Decreased bowel sounds & sphincter tone may indicate parasympathetic dysfunction	43,44

continued

	Test	Technique	Pathways	Normal Response & Remarks	Reference
26	Radiological evaluation	Cineoesophagogram & barium enema employed to test GI motility. Intraluminal manometry can also be used.	Parasympathetic efferent pathways via vagus & sacral parasympathetic nerves	Diminished motility occurs in cases of autonomic dysfunction. Patient can respond to 1.5 mg methacholine chloride ⟨Mecholyl⟩ administration with excessive motility, as in cardiac achalasia.	28
27	Hollander's	Performed in morning after 12-h fast & no smoking. Nasogastric tube passed into stomach, and patient instructed not to swallow saliva. 2 basal samples of 15 min each taken. Insulin, 0.2 units/kg, administered i.v.; 8 separate samples, representing successive 15 min periods, collected and acidity measured.	Hypothalamus, thalamus, & brainstem → vagus nerve → gastric parietal cells	Anacid (non-acid) basal sample: rise of 10 meq/liter considered positive response. Acid basal sample: rise of 20 meq/liter over basal level in 2 successive samples considered positive response.	36
28	Pentagastrin	Inject pentagastrin, 6 mg/kg body wt, subcutaneously; aspirate gastric secretion for 60 min	Acts on parietal cell mass directly	Output reflects total output of parietal cell mass, while Hollander's test (entry 27) reflects acid output stimulated by vagus nerve. Peak acid output after insulin expressed as percentage of peak acid output after pentagastrin quantitatively indicates vagal intactness. Normal range is 45-165%.	22
			Genitourinary Function Tests		
29	Bladder functions	Measurement of residual urine and cystometrogram to determine bladder tonus, rhythmic contraction waves, sensation of fullness & urgency, & micturition contractions	Supranuclear control exerted by limbic system, including hypothalamus, frontal lobe, & paracentral lobule. Fibers descend in lateral columns of spinal cord. Efferent parasympathetic supply is from S2, S3, & S4 → bladder wall → postganglionic fibers to muscle, except trigone.	Cystometrogram helpful in localizing lesions in afferent, efferent, or central pathways. Of great importance in diagnosing & treating autonomic hyperreflexia which occurs as a result of spinal cord injury above midthoracic level.	1,43
30	Sexual functions Bulbocavernosus reflex	Pinch dorsum of glans penis. Palpate perineum behind scrotum for contraction of bulbocavernosus muscle.	Sensory afferents → spinal cord → efferents via anterior sacral roots	Reflex indicates integrity of pelvic (S3 & S4) parasympathetic reflex arc	10
31	Penile erection	Evaluate history of loss of erection in ♂, non-response in ♀	Sensory efferents → parasympathetic efferents → end-organs	Impotence may be an early feature of idiopathic orthostatic hypotension	38,40
32	Ejaculation	Evaluate history of premature ejaculation, ejaculatory incompetence in ♂, and failure to reach climax in ♀	Sensory afferents → sympathetic efferents → end-organs	Premature ejaculation in ♂ and failure to reach climax in ♀ are more frequently due to psychological difficulties	38,40

continued

139. CLINICAL ASSESSMENT OF THE AUTONOMIC NERVOUS SYSTEM

Contributor: Khurana, Ramesh K.

References

1. Abramson, A. S., et al. 1973. Bull. N.Y. Acad. Med. 49:775-785.
2. Allen, S. C., et al. 1945. Am. J. Physiol. 143:11-20.
3. Appenzeller, O., and E. J. McAndrews. 1966. J. Nerv. Ment. Dis. 143:190-194.
4. Baum, J. L. 1973. Int. Ophthalmol. Clin. 13:157-184.
5. Berliner, K. 1940. Arch. Intern. Med. 65:896-901.
6. Cohen, D. N., and Z. N. Zakov. 1975. Am. J. Ophthalmol. 79:883-885.
7. Corbett, J. L. 1976. Curr. Ther. 17(7):53-64.
8. Cryer, P. E., and S. Weiss. 1976. Arch. Neurol. (Chicago) 33:275-277.
9. Das, G., et al. 1975. Am. J. Cardiol. 36:281-285.
10. DeJong, R. N. 1967. The Neurologic Examination. Harper and Row, New York. pp. 700-701.
11. Dobkin, B. H., and N. P. Rosenthal. 1975. Bull. Los Angeles Neurol. Soc. 40:101-110.
12. Duke-Elder, S. 1971. Neuro-Ophthalmology. C. V. Mosby, St. Louis. v. 12, pp. 640-654.
13. Duke-Elder, S. 1971. (Loc. cit. ref. 12). v. 12, pp. 957-969.
14. Ewing, D. J., et al. 1973. Lancet 2:1354-1356.
15. Ewing, D. J., et al. 1974. Clin. Sci. Mol. Med. 46:295-306.
16. Freyschuss, U. 1970. Acta Physiol. Scand., Suppl. 342.
17. Goldenberg, M., et al. 1948. Am. J. Med. 5:792-806.
18. Guttmann, L. 1947. Postgrad. Med. J. 23:353-366.
19. Hanson, J., et al. 1975. Arch. Otolaryngol. 101:293-295.
20. Heimbach, D. M., and J. R. Crout. 1972. Arch. Intern Med. 192:430-432.
21. Hines, E. A., Jr., and G. E. Brown. 1939. Proc. Staff Meet. Mayo Clin. 14:185-187.
22. Hosking, D. J., et al. 1975. Br. Med. J. 2:588-590.
23. Ibrahim, M. M. 1975. Br. Heart J. 37:868-872.
24. Johnson, R. H., and J. M. K. Spalding. 1974. Contemp. Neurol. Ser. 11:45-49.
25. Johnson, R. H., and J. M. K. Spalding. 1974. Ibid. 11:248-265.
26. Johnson, R. H., et al. 1965. Lancet 1:731-733.
27. Korner, P. I., et al. 1976. J. Appl. Physiol. 40:434-440.
28. Kramer, P., and F. J. Ingelfinger. 1951. Gastroenterology 19:242-251.
29. Leon, D., et al. 1970. Am. Heart J. 80:729-739.
30. Levin, A. B. 1966. Am. J. Cardiol. 18:90-99.
31. Lovallo, W. 1975. Psychophysiology 12:268-282.
32. Love, D. R., et al. 1971. Clin. Sci. 41:289-299.
33. Ludbrook, J., et al. 1975. Clin. Exp. Pharmacol. Physiol., Suppl. 2:67-70.
34. MacMillan, A. L., and J. M. K. Spalding. 1969. J. Neurol. Neurosurg. Psychiatry 32:155-160.
35. Monnier, M. 1968. Functions of the Nervous System. Elsevier, Amsterdam. v. 1, pp. 638-644.
36. Read, R. C., and J. E. Doherty. 1970. Am. J. Surg. 119:155-162.
37. Reeves, A. G., and J. B. Posner. 1969. Neurology 19:1145-1152.
38. Sarrel, R. M. 1975. Postgrad. Med. 58:67-72.
39. Schneider, P. B. 1962. Arch. Intern. Med. 110:240-248.
40. Silver, J. R. 1975. Br. Med. J. 3:480-482.
41. Thompson, H. S. 1975. In American Academy of Ophthalmology and Otolaryngology. Companion Source Manual. Rochester, MN. Sec 5, pp. 196-207.
42. Thompson, H. S., and J. H. Mensher. 1971. Am. J. Opthalmol. 72:472-480.
43. Thompson, P. D., and K. L. Melmon. 1968. Anesthesiology 29:724-731.
44. Wichser, J., and N. Vijayan. 1972. Calif. Med. 117:28-37.

140. CIRCULATORY DISORDERS OF THE CENTRAL NERVOUS SYSTEM

Part I. Angiopathies

	Disease	Classification	Reference		Disease	Classification	Reference
1	Amyloidosis	....	45	8		Traumatic	42
2	Aneurysms	Arteriovenous	38		Angiitis		
3		Dissecting	1,29		Infectious	Viral diseases	
4		Fusiform	47	9		Herpes simplex	51
5		Inflammatory	20	10		Rubella	3,7
6		Miliary	13	11		Subacute sclerosing panencephalitis	19
7		Saccular	25	12		Rabies	37

continued

Part I. Angiopathies

	Disease	Classification	Reference		Disease	Classification	Reference
		Rickettsial diseases		32	Arteriolone-	....	11
13		Epidemic[1] & scrub typhus	49		crosis, fi-		
14		Rocky Mountain spotted fever	49		brinoid		
		Bacterial diseases		33	Arteriolo-	....	12
15		Purulent	2		sclerosis		
16		Syphilitic	26	34	Atheroscle-	Extracranial	14,43
17		Tuberculous	4	35	rosis	Intracranial	23
		Mycoses		36		Spinal	18
18		Aspergillosis	55	37	Congenital	Arteriovenous malformations	16
19		Candidiasis	10	38	anomalies	Cavernous angiomas	52
20		Mucormycosis	48	39		Telangiectasis	53
21		Nematode parasites: *Angiostrongylus cantonensis*	31	40		Varices	35
22	Non-infec-	Aorto-cervical arteritis	44	41	Mineraliza-	Idiopathic calcification	30
23	tious	Focal aseptic necrosis of cerebral arteries	21	42	tion	Siderosis	28
24		Granulomatous angiitis of CNS & cranium	17,22, 34	43	Neoplasms	Hemangioblastoma	46
				44		Hemangiopericytoma	36
25		Polyarteritis nodosa	15			Vascular changes associated with:	
26		Rheumatic fever	5	45		Angioblastoma[2]	40
27		Rheumatoid arteritis	41	46		Gliomas	32
28		Scleroderma	24	47		Metastases	9
29		Systemic lupus erythematosus	39	48	Miscella-	Drug-induced angiopathy	27
30		Thromboangiitis obliterans	54	49	neous	Fibromuscular dysplasia	33
31		Wegener's granulomatosis	8	50		Postradiation angiopathy	6
				51		Thrombotic thrombocytopenic purpura	50

[1] Synonym: European typhus. [2] Synonym: Angioblastic meningioma.

Contributors: Garcia, Julio H., and Mena, H.

References

1. Chang, V., et al. 1975. Neurology 25:573-579.
2. Chernick, N. L., et al. 1973. Medicine (Baltimore) 52: 563-581.
3. Connolly, J. H., et al. 1975. Brain 98:583-594.
4. Dastur, D. K., and V. S. Lalitha. 1973. Prog. Neuropathol. 2:351-408.
5. Denst, J., and K. T. Neuberger. 1948. Arch. Pathol. 46:191-201.
6. De Reuck, J., and H. vander Eecken. 1975. Eur. Neurol. 13:481-494.
7. Desmond, M. M., et al. 1967. J. Pediatr. 71:311-331.
8. Drachman, D. A. 1963. Arch. Neurol. (Chicago) 8: 145-155.
9. Earle, K. M. 1954. J. Neuropathol. Exp. Neurol. 13: 448-454.
10. Edelson, R. N., et al. 1975. N.Y. State J. Med. 75: 900-904.
11. Feigin, I., and P. Prose. 1959. Arch. Neurol. (Chicago) 1:98-110.
12. Fisher, C. M. 1969. Acta Neuropathol. 12:1-15.

13. Fisher, C. M. 1972. Am. J. Pathol. 66:313-330.
14. Fisher, C. M., et al. 1965. J. Neuropathol. Exp. Neurol. 24:455-476.
15. Ford, R. G., and R. G. Siekert. 1965. Neurology 15: 114-122.
16. Glasauer, F. E. 1974. N.Y. State J. Med. 74:1787-1991.
17. Hughes, J. T., and B. Brownell. 1966. Neurology 16: 293-298.
18. Jellinger, K. 1967. J. Neurol. Neurosurg. Psychiatry 30:195-206.
19. Johnson, K. P., et al. 1974. Adv. Neurol. 6:77-86.
20. Jones, H. R., Jr., et al. 1969. Ann. Intern. Med. 71: 21-28.
21. Kernohan, J. W., and H. W. Woltman. 1943. J. Am. Med. Assoc. 122:1173-1177.
22. Kolodny, E. H., et al. 1968. Arch. Neurol. (Chicago) 19:510-524.
23. Lascelles, R. G., and E. H. Burrows. 1965. Brain 88: 85-96.

continued

Part I. Angiopathies

24. Lee, J. E., and J. M. Haynes. 1967. Neurology 17:18-22.

25. McCormick, W. F., and J. D. Nofzinger. 1965. J. Neurosurg. 22:155-159.

26. Merritt, H. H., et al. 1946. Neurosyphilis. Oxford Univ. Press, New York.

27. Moossy, J. 1970. In R. G. Siekert, ed. Cerebrovascular Survey Report. Whiting Press, Rochester, MN. pp. 9-26.

28. Neumann, M. A. 1962. J. Neuropathol. Exp. Neurol. 21:302-303.

29. Norman, R. M., and H. Urich. 1957. J. Pathol. Bacteriol. 73:580-582.

30. Norman, R. M., and H. Urich. 1960. J. Neurol. Neurosurg. Psychiatry 23:142-147.

31. Nye, S. W., et al. 1970. Arch. Pathol. 89:9-19.

32. Nyström, S. 1960. Acta Pathol. Microbiol. Scand., Suppl. 137.

33. Palubinskas, A. J., et al. 1966. Am. J. Roentgenol. Radium Ther. Nucl. Med. 98:907-913.

34. Parker, F., et al. 1975. Am. J. Pathol. 79:57-80.

35. Paterson, J. H., and W. McKissock. 1956. Brain 79:233-266.

36. Peña, C. E. 1975. Acta Neuropathol. 33:279-284.

37. Perl, D. P. 1975. In G. M. Baer, ed. The Natural History of Rabies. Academic Press, New York. v. 1, pp. 235-272.

38. Perret, G., and H. Nishioka. 1966. J. Neurosurg. 25:467-490.

39. Piper, P. G. 1953. J. Am. Med. Assoc. 153:215-217.

40. Pitkethly, D. T., et al. 1970. J. Neurosurg. 32:539-544.

41. Ramos, M., and T. I. Mandybur. 1975. Arch. Neurol. (Chicago) 32:271-275.

42. Rumbaugh, C. L., et al. 1970. Radiology 96:49-54.

43. Samuel, K. C. 1956. J. Pathol. Bacteriol. 71:391-401.

44. Schrire, V. 1967. Aust. Ann. Med. 16:33-40.

45. Schwartz, P. 1967. Trans. N.Y. Acad. Sci. 30:22-46.

46. Spence, A. M., and L. J. Rubinstein. 1975. Cancer (Philadelphia) 35:326-341.

47. Stehbens, W. E. 1963. Arch. Pathol. 75:45-64.

48. Stehbens, W. E. 1965. Med. J. Aust. 1:765-766.

49. Stehbens, W. E. 1972. Pathology of the Cerebral Blood Vessels. C. V. Mosby, St. Louis. p. 612.

50. Symmers, W. St. C. 1956. Brain 79:511-521.

51. Viloria, J. E., and J. H. Garcia. 1976. Beitr. Pathol. 157:14-22.

52. Voigt, K., and M. G. Yasargil. 1976. Neuro-Chir. 19:59-68.

53. White, R. J., et al. 1958. J. Neuropathol. Exp. Neurol. 17:392-398.

54. Wolman, L. 1958. J. Clin. Pathol. 11:133-138.

55. Young, R. C., et al. 1970. Medicine (Baltimore) 49:147-173.

Part II. Hemorrhages

	Type of Hemorrhage ⟨Synonym⟩	Associated Conditions or Etiological Factors	Reference		Type of Hemorrhage ⟨Synonym⟩	Associated Conditions or Etiological Factors	Reference
1	Extradural	Blood dyscrasias	28		Subarachnoid	Angiitis, non-infectious	
2	⟨Epidural⟩	Infections of neighboring structures	31	16		Anaphylactoid purpura	19
				17		Polyarteritis nodosa	12
3		Trauma	16,17	18		Rheumatic fever	13
4		Vascular malformations	20	19		Systemic lupus erythematosus	69
5		Unknown	40			Blood dyscrasias	
6	Intradural	Blood dyscrasias	55			Anemia	
7	⟨Subdural⟩	Chemotherapy	73	20		Aplastic	4
8		Epilepsy	14	21		Pernicious	37
9		Hemodialysis	41	22		Sickle cell	25
10		Infections of neighboring structures	6	23		Anticoagulant therapy	54
				24		Hemophilia	60
11		Metastatic neoplasms	56	25		Leukemia	45
12		Nutritional deficiencies	29	26		Polycythemia vera	30
13		Ruptured aneurysm, arteriovenous malformations	9,64	27		Thrombocytopenic purpura	5
						Drugs	
14		Trauma	1,22, 32,75	28		Insulin	49
				29		Pentylenetetrazole	51
15		Unknown	44	30		Hypernatremia	70

continued

Part II.   Hemorrhages

Type of Hemorrhage ⟨Synonym⟩	Associated Conditions or Etiological Factors	Reference	Type of Hemorrhage ⟨Synonym⟩	Associated Conditions or Etiological Factors	Reference
	Infections, leptomeningeal		52	Leukemia	45
31	Viral	37	53	Macroglobulinemia	38
32	Purulent	71	54	Polycythemia	61
33	Syphilitic	57	55	Thrombocytopenic purpura	8
34	Tuberculous	24	56	Decompression sickness[1]	27
35	Fungal	43,65	57	Demyelinating conditions	26
	Neoplasms		58	Drugs	72
36	Adenoma, pituitary	76	59	Eclampsia	52
37	Carcinoma, metastatic	67	60	Extrinsic compression of arteries or veins, secondary brainstem hemorrhage	10
38	Chordoma	59			
39	Glioma	23			
40	Meningioma	2	61	Heat stroke	62
41	Osteochondroma	33	62	Hypernatremia	58
42	Papilloma, choroid plexus	15	63	Hypoxemia	68
43	Occlusive cerebrovascular disease	3	64	Infections[2]	7,77
44	Ruptured arterial aneurysm & arteriovenous malformations	36,50	65	Inflammatory & necrotizing lesions of small blood vessels	34
45	Trauma	46	66	Intraparenchymal neoplasms[3]	48
46	Unknown	11,63	67	Open-heart surgery	47
47 Intracerebral	Arterial embolism	21	68	Ruptured intracranial arterial aneurysms & arteriovenous malformations	39,53
48	Arteriolosclerosis	18			
	Blood dyscrasias				
49	Afibrinogenemia	8	69	Trauma	18,35
50	Anemia, sickle cell	74	70	Unknown	42,55
51	Hypoprothrombinemia	66			

[1] Synonym: Caisson disease.   [2] Tuberculosis and other bacterial infections.   [3] Primary and metastatic.

Contributors: Garcia, Julio H., and Mena, H.

References

1. Anderson, F. M. 1952. Pediatrics 10:11-18.
2. Askenasy, H. M., and A. D. Behmoaram. 1960. Neurology 10:484-489.
3. Askenasy, H. M., et al. 1962. Ibid. 12:288-292.
4. Boon, T. H., and J. N. Walton. 1951. Q. J. Med. 20:75-92.
5. Brodie, G. N., et al. 1970. Br. Med. J. 1:540-541.
6. Browder, J. 1943. Bull. N.Y. Acad. Med. 19:168-176.
7. Cammermeyer, J. 1953. Arch. Neurol. Psychiatry 70:54-63.
8. Chalgren, W. S. 1953. Neurology 3:126-136.
9. Clarke, E., and J. N. Walton. 1953. Brain 76:378-404.
10. Cohen, S. I., and S. M. Aronson. 1968. Arch. Neurol. (Chicago) 19:257-263.
11. Dekaban, A., and D. McEachern. 1952. Arch. Neurol. Psychiatry 67:641-649.
12. Diaz-Rivera, R. S. and A. J. Miller. 1946. Ann. Intern. Med. 24:420-443.
13. Easby, M. H. 1934. Med. Clin. North Am. 18:307-310.
14. Echlin, F. A., et al. 1956. J. Am. Med. Assoc. 161:1345-1350.
15. Ernsting, J. 1955. J. Neurol. Neurosurg. Psychiatry 18:134-136.
16. Frera, C. 1969. Acta Neurochir. 20:31-35.
17. Freytag, E. 1963. Arch. Pathol. 75:402-413.
18. Freytag, E. 1968. J. Neurol. Neurosurg. Psychiatry 31:616-620.
19. Gairdner, D. 1948. Q. J. Med. 17:95-122.
20. Gallagher, J. P., and E. J. Browder. 1968. J. Neurosurg. 29:1-12.
21. Ghatak, N. R. 1975. Hum. Pathol. 6:599-610.
22. Gilmartin, D. 1964. Lancet 1:1061-1062.
23. Glass, B., and K. H. Abbott. 1955. Arch. Neurol. Psychiatry 73:369-379.
24. Goldzieher, J. W., and J. R. Lisa. 1947. Am. J. Pathol. 23:133-145.
25. Greer, M., and D. Schotland. 1962. Neurology 12:114-123.
26. Hart, M. N., and K. M. Earle. 1975. J. Neurol. Neurosurg. Psychiatry 38:585-591.

continued

Part II. Hemorrhages

27. Haymaker, W., and C. Davison. 1950. J. Neuropathol. Exp. Neurol. 9:29-59.
28. Hooper, R. 1959. Br. J. Surg. 47:71-87.
29. Ingraham, F. D., and D. D. Matson. 1944. J. Pediatr. 24:1-37.
30. Johnson, D. R., and W. S. Chalgren. 1951. Neurology 1:53-67.
31. Kelly, D. L., and J. M. Smith. 1968. J. Neurosurg. 28:67-69.
32. Kempe, C. H., et al. 1962. J. Am. Med. Assoc. 181:17-24.
33. King, L. S., and J. Butcher. 1944. Arch. Pathol. 37:282-285.
34. Lewis, I. C., and M. G. Philpott. 1956. Arch. Dis. Child. 31:369-371.
35. Lindenberg, R., and E. Freytag. 1969. Arch. Pathol. 87:298-305.
36. Locksley, H. B. 1966. J. Neurosurg. 25:219-239.
37. Locksley, H. B., et al. 1966. Ibid. 24:1034-1056.
38. Logothetis, J., et al. 1960. Arch. Neurol. (Chicago) 3:564-573.
39. MacKenzie, I. 1953. Brain 76:184-214.
40. Markham, J. W., et al. 1967. J. Neurosurg. 26:334-342.
41. Marshall, S., and F. Hinman, Jr. 1962. J. Am. Med. Assoc. 182:813-814.
42. McCormick, W. F., and D. B. Rosenfield. 1973. Stroke 4:946-954.
43. McKee, E. E. 1950. Am. J. Clin. Pathol. 20:381-384.
44. McKissock, W., et al. 1960. Lancet 1:1365-1369.
45. Moore, E. W., et al. 1960. Arch. Intern. Med. 105:451-468.
46. Nathanson, M., et al. 1953. Neurology 3:721-724.
47. Nelson, J. S., et al. 1973. Acta Neuropathol. 25:163-165.
48. Oldberg, E. 1933. Arch. Neurol. Psychiatry 30:1061-1073.
49. Pedersen, A. L. 1944. Acta Psychiat. Neurol. Scand. 19:483-494.
50. Quickel, K. E., and R. J. Whaley. 1967. Neurology 17:716-719.
51. Roback, H. N., and C. W. Miller, Jr. 1940. Arch. Neurol. Psychiatry 44:627-635.
52. Robb, J. P. 1955. Neurology 5:679-690.
53. Robertson, E. G. 1949. Brain 72:150-185.
54. Russek, H. I., and B. L. Zohman. 1953. Am. J. Med. Sci. 225:8-13.
55. Russell, D. S. 1954. Proc. R. Soc. Med. 47:689-693.
56. Russell, D. S., and H. Cairns. 1934. Brain 57:32-48.
57. Sands, I. J. 1930. Arch. Neurol. Psychiatry 24:85-93.
58. Simmons, M. A., et al. 1974. N. Engl. J. Med. 291:6-10.
59. Simonsen, J. 1963. Acta Pathol. Microbiol. Scand. 59:13-20.
60. Singer, R. P., and R. L. Schneider. 1962. Neurology 12:293-294.
61. Sloan, L. H. 1933. Arch. Neurol. Psychiatry 30:154-165.
62. Sohal, R. S., et al. 1968. Arch. Intern. Med. 122:43-47.
63. Spatz, E. L., and J. W. D. Bull. 1957. J. Neurosurg. 14:543-547.
64. Stehbens, W. E. 1963. Arch. Pathol. 75:45-64.
65. Stehbens, W. E. 1965. Med. J. Aust. 1:765-766.
66. Stephens, C. A. L., Jr. 1954. Circulation 9:682-686.
67. Strang, R. R., and T. I. Ljungdahl. 1962. Med. J. Aust. 1:90-91.
68. Towbin, A. 1969. Arch. Neurol. (Chicago) 20:35-43.
69. Tremaine, M. J. 1934. N. Engl. J. Med. 211:754-759.
70. Volpe, J. 1974. Ibid. 291:43-45.
71. Walton, J. N. 1953. Neurology 3:517-543.
72. Weiss, S. R., et al. 1970. Int. Surg. 53(1):123-127.
73. Wells, C. E., and D. Urrea. 1960. Arch. Neurol. (Chicago) 3:553-558.
74. Wertham, F., et al. 1942. Arch. Neurol. Psychiatry 47:752-767.
75. Whittier, J. R. 1951. Ibid. 65:463-471.
76. Wright, R. L., et al. 1965. Arch. Neurol. (Chicago) 12:326-331.
77. Yarnell, P. R., and J. Stears. 1974. Neurology 24:870-873.

Part III. Mechanisms of Edema

	Etiological Factors	Reference		Etiological Factors	Reference
1	Diabetic ketoacidosis	27		Encephalopathies	
2	Drugs	12,26	5	Lead	19
3	Eclampsia	8	6	Spongiform	11
4	Encephalomalacia, ischemic	18	7	Hemodialysis	13

continued

Part III. Mechanisms of Edema

	Etiological Factors	Reference		Etiological Factors	Reference
	Hemorrhage		18	Hypoxemic states	24
8	Extradural[1]	22	19	Inappropriate secretion of vasopressin[3]	7
9	Intracerebral	17		Infections	
10	Intradural[2]	20	20	Cerebral abscess	10
11	Subarachnoid	25	21	Purulent meningitis	3
12	Hepatic failure	21	22	Neoplasia	1,6
13	Hydrocephalus	9	23	Pseudotumor cerebri	5
14	Hypertension, systemic	16	24	Trauma to head or spine	14
15	Hyponatremia	5	25	Venous return, impaired	2
16	Hypotension, systemic	23	26	Water intoxication	15
17	Hypothermia	4			

[1] Synonym: Epidural. [2] Synonym: Subdural. [3] Synonym: Antidiuretic hormone.

Contributors: Garcia, Julio H., and Mena, H.

References
1. Aleu, F., et al. 1966. Am. J. Pathol. 48:1043-1061.
2. Boettner, R., and C. R. Sachatello. 1974. Anesth. Analg. (Cleveland) 53:254-257.
3. Dodge, P. R., and M. N. Swartz. 1965. N. Engl. J. Med. 272:954-960.
4. Englund, G. 1968. In J. Minckler, ed. Pathology of the Nervous System. McGraw-Hill, New York. v. 1, pp. 997-1004.
5. Fishman, R. A. 1975. N. Engl. J. Med. 293:706-711.
6. Hirano, A., and T. Matsui. 1975. Hum. Pathol. 6:611-621.
7. Ivy, H. K. 1968. Med. Clin. North Am. 52(4):817-826.
8. Jewett, J. F. 1973. N. Engl. J. Med. 289:976-977.
9. Klosovsky, B. N. 1968. (Loc. cit. ref. 4). v. 1, pp. 456-462.
10. Krayenbühl, H. A. 1966. Clin. Neurosurg. 14:1-24.
11. Lampert, P. W., et al. 1972. Am. J. Pathol. 68:626-652.
12. Lampert, P., et al. 1973. Acta Neuropathol. 23:326-333.
13. Leonard, A., and F. L. Shapiro. 1975. Ann. Intern. Med. 82:650-658.
14. Lindenberg, R. 1966. Clin. Neurosurg. 12:129-142.
15. Manz, H. J. 1974. Hum. Pathol. 5:291-313.
16. Marshall, W. J. S., et al. 1969. Arch. Neurol. (Chicago) 21:545-553.
17. Mutlu, N., et al. 1963. Ibid. 8:644-661.
18. Ng, L. K. Y., and J. Nimmannitya. 1970. Stroke 1: 158-163.
19. Pentschew, A. 1965. Acta Neuropathol. 5:133-160.
20. Rabe, E. F., et al. 1968. Neurology 18:559-570.
21. Record, C. O., et al. 1975. Br. Med. J. 2:540.
22. Rothman, J., and M. Gershowitz. 1974. Am. J. Roentgenol. Radium Ther. Nucl. Med. 122:531-537.
23. Steegmann, A. T. 1968. (Loc. cit. ref. 4). v. 1, pp. 1005-1029.
24. Steinbereithner, K. 1967. In L. Klatzo and F. Seitelberger, ed. Brain Edema. Springer-Verlag, New York. pp. 67-78.
25. Stornelli, S. A., and J. D. French. 1964. J. Neurosurg. 21:769-780.
26. Torack, R. M., et al. 1960. Am. J. Pathol. 36:273-287.
27. Young, E., and R. F. Bradley. 1967. N. Engl. J. Med. 276:665-669.

Part IV. Ischemic Disturbances

	Classification or Etiological Factor	Reference		Classification or Etiological Factor	Reference
	Occlusive		7	Strangulation	4,13
1	Arteries	7,9,10		Non-occlusive	
2	Cervical	2	8	Cardiac arrest	16
3	Intracranial	3,17	9	Cardiac dysrhythmias	18,19
	Veins & sinuses		10	Hypertension, intracranial	14
4	With inflammation	12,20	11	Hypotension	1
5	Without inflammation	8	12	Shock	15
	Simultaneous occlusion of arteries & veins		13	Trauma to head	11
6	Hanging	6	14	Vasospasm	5

continued

140. CIRCULATORY DISORDERS OF THE CENTRAL NERVOUS SYSTEM

Part IV. Ischemic Disturbances

Contributors: Garcia, Julio H., and Mena, H.

References

1. Adams, J. H., et al. 1966. Brain 89:235-268.
2. Castaigne, P., et al. 1970. Ibid. 93:231-258.
3. Castaigne, P., et al. 1973. Ibid. 96:133-154.
4. Dooling, E. C., and E. P. Richardson, Jr. 1976. Arch. Neurol. (Chicago) 33:196-199.
5. Fein, J. M., and R. Boulos. 1973. J. Neurosurg. 39:337-347.
6. Garcia, J. H. 1975. Hum. Pathol. 6:583-598.
7. Garcia, J. H. 1976. In R. G. Siekert, ed. Cerebrovascular Survey Report. Whiting Press, Rochester, MN. pp. 20-32.
8. Garcia, J. H., et al. 1975. Stroke 6:164-171.
9. Gore, I., and D. P. Collins. 1960. Am. J. Clin. Pathol. 33:416-426.
10. Greenlee, J. E., and G. L. Mandell. 1973. Stroke 4:958-963.
11. Gurdjian, E. S., and E. S. Gurdjian. 1976. J. Trauma 16:35-51.
12. Kaufman, D. M., et al. 1975. Medicine (Baltimore) 54:485-498.
13. Kowada, M., et al. 1968. J. Neurosurg. 28:150-157.
14. Marshall, L. F., et al. 1975. Ibid. 43:318-322.
15. McGovern, V. J. 1971. Pathol. Annu. 6:279-298.
16. Romanul, F. C. A., and A. Abramowicz. 1964. Arch. Neurol. (Chicago) 11:40-65.
17. Sindermann, F., et al. 1970. Brain 93:199-210.
18. Terplan, K. L. 1973. Am. J. Dis. Child. 125:175-185.
19. Vost, A., et al. 1964. J. Pathol. Bacteriol. 88:463-470.
20. Young, R. C., et al. 1970. Medicine (Baltimore) 49:147-173.

141. NEURO-OPHTHALMIC DISORDERS

Symbols: + = usually or often; ± = sometimes or rarely; ? = variable or questionable.

	Type of Disorder	Classification	Ocular Signs & Symptoms	Non-ocular Correlates	Etiology & Pathogenesis
			Ocular Motor System		
1	Muscular	Extra-ocular Dysthyroid orbitopathy	Exophthalmos; ophthalmoplegia & diplopia; congestion; positive forced duction	Hyper-, hypo-, or euthyroid	Unknown
2		Myasthenia	Ptosis, ophthalmoplegia, & diplopia; edrophonium-responsive; diurnal variation; eyelid twitch	Skeletal muscle weakness: +	Myoneural block
3		Dystrophies	Ptosis & ophthalmoplegia; pigmentary retinal degeneration	Skeletal, pharyngeal, & cardiac myopathies	Genetic. Mitochondrial abnormalities: ?
4		Intra-ocular Pupil Horner's syndrome	Unilateral ptosis & miosis. Hyporesponsive: cocaine. Hyperresponsive: epinephrine [1]/, hydroxyamphetamine.	Facial anhidrosis of affected side	Sympathetic nerve paralysis
5		Adie's syndrome	Semimydriatic; myotonic reactivity; anisocoria; cholinergic hypersensitivity	Absent patellar & Achilles tendon reflexes	Ciliary ganglion lesion: ?
6		Argyll-Robertson	Pupils irregular. Miosis: +. Hyporeactive to light: +. Hyporeactive to near objects: ±.	Tabes dorsalis	Neurosyphilis: +
7		Accommodation Presbyopia	Decreased near focusing	Onset at middle age	Physiologic sclerosis of lens
8		Paralysis	Inability to near focus	None	Cranial nerve III ⟨Oculomotor nerve⟩ or ciliary paralysis

[1]/ Synonym: Adrenalin.

continued

141. NEURO-OPHTHALMIC DISORDERS

	Type of Disorder	Classification	Ocular Signs & Symptoms	Non-ocular Correlates	Etiology & Pathogenesis
9	Oculomotor nerves	Cranial nerve III (Oculomotor nerve)	Ptosis; ophthalmoplegia; exotropia; mydriasis	....	Aneurysm; vascular accident; trauma; tumor
10		Diabetes	Pupil spared: +. Orbital pain: +. Diabetic retinopathy.	Peripheral neuropathy; systemic diabetic manifestations	Ischemic neuropathy: ?
11		Aneurysms	Mydriasis; orbital pain; papilledema; intra-ocular hemorrhage	Sudden headache: +. Collapse & coma: +. Subarachnoid hemorrhage: +.	Congenital weakness of circle of Willis: ?
12		Miscellaneous syndromes Benedikt's	Cranial nerve III (Oculomotor nerve) paralysis	Dyskinesia; intention tremor of contralateral arm	Lesion in red nucleus
13		Weber's	Cranial nerve III (Oculomotor nerve) paralysis	Contralateral hemiplegia	Lesion adjacent to interpeduncular fossa
14		Aberrant regeneration	Anomalous ocular & pupillary movements	None	Trauma; aneurysm; syphilis
15		Cranial nerve IV (Trochlear nerve)	Diplopia on down-gaze (reading, walking); inability to depress eye in adducted position; head tilt to contralateral side	None	Trauma; vascular accidents
16		Cranial nerve VI (Abducens nerve)	Esotropia; diplopia; inability to abduct eye; compensatory head turn toward side of lesion	Facial pain with petrositis	Elevated intracranial pressure; tumor; aneurysm; diabetes; petrositis; dural shunt; multiple sclerosis
17		All ocular motor nerves	Ptosis; total ophthalmoplegia; mydriasis	Bruit: ±. Facial hypoesthesia.	Cavernous sinus syndrome; orbital apex lesions
18	Conjugate gaze disturbances	Horizontal Cerebral Irritative	Clonic deviation of eyes to side opposite lesion	Convulsive seizure	Epileptogenic focus
19		Paralytic	Transient deviation of eyes to side of lesion during stupor or coma	Contralateral hemiplegia	Cerebrovascular accident
20		Pontine	Persistent paralysis of gaze toward side of lesion; gaze nystagmus. Ocular bobbing: ±.	Contralateral hemiplegia; facial paralysis on side of lesion	Vascular accident; tumor; demyelination; remote neuroblastoma
21		Cerebellar	Paresis of gaze toward side of lesion: ±. Nystagmus, horizontal or vertical; saccadic pursuit; dysmetria; flutter; loss of vestibular suppression	Ataxia; adiadochokinesia; titubation; dysarthria	Tumor; demyelination; vascular accident; degeneration
22		Vertical Basal ganglia & extrapyramidal nuclei	Preferential paralysis of vertical gaze; downward gaze paralysis in progressive supranuclear palsy; intact vestibular response; slow saccades	Chorea: ±. Parkinsonoid features; dementia	Hereditary: Huntington's disease. Idiopathic: progressive supranuclear palsy.

continued

289

	Type of Disorder	Classification	Ocular Signs & Symptoms	Non-ocular Correlates	Etiology & Pathogenesis
23		Anterior midbrain (para-tectal)	Inability to look upward (pre-tectal) or downward (infra-aqueductal); convergence nystagmus; pupillary & convergence paralysis (Parinaud's syndrome)	Aqueductal obstruction: ±	Pineal body & third ventricle tumors; vascular accident; multiple sclerosis
24		Posterior medulla oblongata	Downbeat nystagmus	Various pyramidal & other brainstem signs	Herniation through foramen magnum; Arnold-Chiari malformation
25		Cerebellum & cerebellar tracts	Vertical gaze nystagmus; ocular bobbing; opsoclonus	Same as for entry 21	Same as for entry 21
26	Dissociated eye movements	Internuclear ophthalmoplegia	Paresis of medial rectus muscle on attempted conjugate gaze; nystagmus of abducting eye	Other symptoms of multiple sclerosis	Bilateral internuclear ophthalmoplegia: multiple sclerosis. Unilateral internuclear ophthalmoplegia: vascular occlusion; tumor.
27		Skew deviation	Diplopia; hypertropia, concomitant or variable	Other brainstem signs	Lateralized brainstem lesions: vascular, neoplastic, or demyelinative
28	Nystagmus	Congenital Sensory type	Horizontal; predominantly pendular; varies with attention; poor vision dating from infancy	Compensatory head oscillations: +	Poor visual acuity in infancy; albinism; macular aplasia; opaque media [2]
29		Motor type	Horizontal; predominantly jerk-like; varies with direction of gaze (least at neutral point); good vision at neutral point	Head turn to position of least nystagmus	Hereditary, recessive: ±
30		Latent nystagmus	Horizontal; jerk-type; elicited by covering either eye; slow drift to side of occlusion. Esotropia: ±.	None	Unknown
31		Acquired Oculomotor hypotonia	Horizontal or vertical in direction of gaze; jerk-type	Cerebellar hypotonia	Incomplete paralysis of gaze; drugs (diphenyl-hydantoin [3], barbiturates)
32		Vestibular	Jerk-type	Vertigo; nausea & vomiting	Inflammatory or destructive lesion of labyrinth or CNS nuclei
33		Spasmus nutans	Horizontal, fine movements; usually unilateral; self-limited	Head nodding; head turn	Unknown
34		Periodic alternating nystagmus	Horizontal; jerk pattern, regular cycle in one direction, then in other	Cerebellar or brainstem signs: +. Congenital: ±	Unknown

[2] Includes any or all of the following: cornea, lens, aqueous humor, or vitreous humor. [3] Synonym: Dilantin.

continued

	Type of Disorder	Classification	Ocular Signs & Symptoms	Non-ocular Correlates	Etiology & Pathogenesis
			Ocular Sensory System		
35	Retinal disease	Photoreceptors Congenital Stationary night blindness	Poor dark adaptation; extinguished electroretinogram	None	Hereditary, dominant; presumed metabolic defect in rods
36		Leber's amaurosis	Total blindness; extinguished electroretinogram; keratoconus; cataract	None	Absence of rods & cones; X-linked inheritance
37		Albinism	Poor vision; photophobia; horizontal nystagmus	With or without cutaneous albinism	Recessive or X-linked inheritance
38		Hereditary pigmentary retinopathies Retinitis pigmentosa	Poor dark adaptation, progressing to blindness; extinguished electroretinogram; pigmentation of retina; ophthalmoplegia (Kearn-Sayre's syndrome)	Deafness (Usher's syndrome); abetalipoproteinemia & acanthocytosis (Bassen-Kornzweig syndrome); dementia (Vogt-Spielmeyer's syndrome); ichthyosis & polyneuropathy; skeletal myopathy & heart block (Kearn-Sayre's syndrome)	Progressive degeneration of rods, then of cones; migration of pigment into retina
39		Macular degeneration	Central scotoma; reduced visual acuity; various types of central pigmentary retinopathy; ceroid lipofuscinosis	None	Degeneration of central retina; hereditary, dominant or recessive
40		Senile macular degeneration	Central scotoma; reduced visual acuity; central pigmentary retinopathy; metamorphopsia	None	Hereditary, ?
41		Poisons & solar retinopathy	Loss of central vision; pigmentation of macula; corneal & lenticular deposits (chloroquine)	None	Chloroquine; gazing at sun or eclipse
42		Ganglion cells Hereditary Sphingolipidosis	Blindness; opacification of retina & cherry-red spot (Tay-Sachs & Niemann-Pick diseases); optic atrophy	Dementia	Hereditary, recessive
43		Optic atrophy	Blindness; optic atrophy	None	Hereditary, dominant
44		Secondary Glaucoma	Elevated intraocular pressure; cupping of optic disk; field defects; blindness	None	Strangulation of nerve fibers
45		Tumors & trauma	Optic atrophy	None; or hamartoma ±	Neoplasia; trauma to optic nerve
46		Vascular Retinal artery occlusion	Amaurosis fugax: ±. Blindness: +. Cherry-red spot; optic atrophy. Low retinal arterial pressure: ±.	Brain involvement, with embolus or ischemia	Embolus; carotid artery occlusion; glaucoma

continued

	Type of Disorder	Classification	Ocular Signs & Symptoms	Non-ocular Correlates	Etiology & Pathogenesis
47		Retinal vein occlusion	Reduced visual acuity; hemorrhagic retinopathy	Hyperviscosity: ±. Diabetes: ±.	Endothelial proliferation; thrombosis; optic nerve tumor
48		Tumor: retinoblastoma	Blindness; white mass in fundus ("amaurotic cat's eye")	None	Hereditary, dominant; mutation
49	Optic nerve	Demyelinative Retrobulbar neuritis	Central scotoma; pain with eye movement. Internuclear ophthalmoplegia: ±.	Systemic manifestations of multiple sclerosis: 20%	Idiopathic; multiple sclerosis
50		Devic's disease	Bilateral central scotoma	Transverse myelitis	Demyelination in childhood
51		Schilder's disease [4]	Optic atrophy	Leukoencephalopathy; hypoadrenalism	Hereditary, X-linked
52		Vascular Ischemic neuropathy	Blindness in one or both eyes. Altitudinal hemianopia: ±. Pale, swollen optic disk.	None	Presumably arteriosclerotic
53		Temporal arteritis	Same as for entry 52	Headaches; scalp tenderness; pain on chewing; polymyalgia rheumatica; elevated erythrocyte sedimentation rate	Giant cell arteritis
54		Poisons Toxic amblyopia	Cecocentral scotoma; preferential loss of color discrimination	Malnutrition	Alcoholism ("spree drinkers")
55		Methanol	Acute blindness; optic atrophy	Debauchment	Methanol
56		Tumors Glioma	Optic atrophy; exophthalmos	Childhood. Neurofibromatosis: ±.	Hereditary, dominant
57		Meningioma	Same as for entry 56	Intracranial extension	Neoplasia
58	Optic chiasma	Demyelination	Decreased visual acuity; irregular field constriction. Bitemporal: ?.	Other manifestations of multiple sclerosis; transverse myelitis	Multiple sclerosis; Devic's disease
59		Chiasmatic arachnoiditis	Same as for entry 58	None	Trauma; idiopathic
60		Tumors Pituitary	Bitemporal hemianopia or other field defect; progressive loss of vision	Enlarged sella turcica visualized by X ray; endocrinopathy	Neoplasia
61		Craniopharyngioma	Same as for entry 60	Suprasellar calcification; erosion of clinoids visualized by X ray; retarded growth	Congenital rests
62		Meningioma (suprasellar)	Same as for entry 60	Erosion of clinoids visualized by X ray	Neoplasia
63		Aneurysms	Same as for entry 60	Curvilinear calcification visualized by X ray	....
64	Geniculo-calcarine [5] tract	Dominant hemisphere	Right homonymous hemianopia: ±	....	....
65		Occipital lobe	Symmetric optokinetic nystagmus	None. Migraine: ±.	Vascular
66		Parietal lobe	Asymmetric optokinetic nystagmus	Aphasia; alexia; agraphia	Neoplasia; vascular; degenerative

[4] Synonym: Adrenoleukodystrophy. [5] Synonym: Geniculostriate.

continued

	Type of Disorder	Classification	Ocular Signs & Symptoms	Non-ocular Correlates	Etiology & Pathogenesis
67		Non-dominant hemisphere	Left homonymous hemianopia: ±	....	....
68		Occipital lobe	Symmetric optokinetic nystagmus	None. migraine: ±.	Vascular
69		Parietal lobe	Asymmetric optokinetic nystagmus	Topographic agnosia; constructional apraxia	Neoplasia; vascular; degenerative
70		Both hemispheres Occipital lobe	Bilateral field loss or blindness; hallucinations	None	Vascular; trauma; congenital
71		Parietal lobe	Bilateral field loss; ocular motor apraxia	Balint's syndrome; dementia	Vascular; degenerative; neoplasia

Contributors: Cogan, David G., and Robins, Stephen M.

General References

1. Bach-y-Rita, P., and G. C. Collins, ed. 1971. Symp. Control Eye Mov. San Francisco, 1969.
2. Cogan, D. G. 1974. Neurology of the Visual System. C. C. Thomas, Springfield, IL.
3. Cogan, D. G. 1975. Neurology of the Ocular Muscles. Ed. 2. C. C. Thomas, Springfield, IL.
4. Duke-Elder, S., and G. I. Scott. 1971. In S. Duke-Elder, ed. System of Ophthalmology. C. V. Mosby, St. Louis. v. 12.
5. Gay, A. J., et al. 1974. Eye Movement Disorders. C. V. Mosby, St. Louis.
6. Lennerstrand, G., and P. Bach-y-Rita, ed. 1975. Basic Mechanisms of Ocular Motility and Their Clinical Implications. Pergamon Press, Oxford.
7. Walsh, F. B., and W. F. Hoyt. 1969. Clinical Neuro-Ophthalmology. Ed. 3. Williams and Wilkins, Baltimore. v. 1-3.

142. AUDITORY AND VESTIBULAR DISORDERS

Part I. Audiometry

Standard terminology and reference data are listed in references 1 and 2. Hearing threshold level ⟨HL⟩ equals the sound pressure level, in decibels, by which the threshold of audibility for that ear exceeds the standard audiometric threshold. Hearing loss ⟨hearing level⟩ for speech equals the difference, in decibels, between speech levels at which the average normal ear and the defective ear reach the same degree of intelligibility, often set at 50%. **Pure tone threshold shift** is the average hearing threshold level for 500, 1000, and 2000 Hz in the better ear. The **Stenger test** is a method for confirmation of a unilateral, non-organic hearing loss: A subject will always detect a binaurally presented, minimally suprathreshold sound of the same frequency in the better hearing ear only. There are two speech tests generally performed during routine screening audiometry: **speech reception threshold** ⟨SRT⟩, and speech discrimination ability. **Discrimination for speech** equals the percent of items in an appropriate form of test, usually phonetically balanced ⟨PB⟩ monosyllabic words, that is correctly repeated, written down, or checked by the listener. (For further information, consult reference 7.) **Acoustic impedance** is the complex ratio of sound pressure on a surface to the flux through that surface. **Tympanometry curve** refers to the tympanic membrane compliance curves, which can usually be classified into types A, B, and C. Type A curve yields a peak sound transmission at a pressure in the external audi- tory canal of 0 mm Hg (relative to middle-ear pressure), and indicates normal membrane compliance. Type B curve (flat) indicates that the tympanic membrane compliance is reduced and does not change significantly with changes in the external auditory canal pressure. Type C curve indicates that maximal membrane compliance, and therefore peak sound transmission, occurs with negative pressure in the external auditory canal. [ref. 11] The **acoustic reflex threshold** is the threshold (HL) at which a compliance change is detected as a consequence of stapedial muscle contraction in the test ear; this response is usually elicited by a probe tone presented to the opposite ear. **Tone decay** refers to the rapidity of adaptation to a tone presented near audiometric threshold. **Békésy audiometry** refers to the threshold for pulsed versus continuous sweep-frequency pure tones. Type I curve indicates that both the pulsed and the continuous pure tone traces superimpose around the subjects' auditory sensitivity thresholds. In type II curve, the pulsed and continuous tones are superimposed below 1000 Hz. Above 1000 Hz, the continuous trace separates from, and shows higher thresholds than, the pulsed trace. Type III curve shows a complete adaptation of the continuous tone (the continuous tone separates from the pulsed tone trace at frequencies below 1000 Hz). Type IV curve shows a complete separation throughout all the frequencies between the pulsed and the continuous tone. Type

continued

Part I. Audiometry

V curve shows wide, inconsistent variations of the traces, and is typical of subjects having non-organic hearing loss. **Binaural loudness balance** is a test of recruitment, and is performed by comparing the sensation for loudness in an abnormal ear relative to a normal ear. Recruitment is defined as an abnormal gain in loudness function [ref. 9]. **Conductive** and **Sensorineural** hearing losses may occur in various combinations. *Abbreviations:* PTT = pure tone threshold; th = threshold; th_a = threshold for conduction in air; th_b = threshold for bone conduction.

	Type of Measurement	Normal Condition	Type of Hearing Loss					Reference
			PTT	Conductive	Sensorineural	Central	Non-Organic	
1	Pure tone threshold shift, dB [1]	0 < th < 25	25 < th < 40 [2]; 40 < th < 55 [3]; 55 < th < 70 [4]; 70 < th < 90 [5]; th > 90 [6]	$th_b - th_a > 10$ [7]	$th_b - th_a < 10$ [7]	Normal	....	3,5
2	Stenger test (pure tone or speech)	....	....	....	Negative	Negative	Positive	9
	Speech							
3	Spondaic word reception threshold ⟨Air SRT⟩	Averaged threshold of 2 better speech-range frequencies (out of 500, 1000, or 2000 Hz)	....	....	Should correspond to average of 2 better pure tone responses in speech range frequencies, within the range of hearing loss recorded for a given subject [8]	Normal	Should be ± 6 dB from PTT	8
4	Discrimination with 50-word list (W-22)	90-100%	Varies with type & severity of loss	....	Predictably related to threshold loss [9]; poor relationship to threshold loss [10]	Variable response —consistent	Variable response— inconsistent	7,12
5	Acoustic impedance	1,000-3,000 Ω [11]	....	....	....	Normal	....	11
6	Tympanometry curve	Type A	....	Type A, B, or C [12]	Type A	Type A	....	11
7	Acoustic reflex threshold	85 ± 40 dB [13]	Sums linearly with threshold shift (entry 1)	....	....	Absent	....	11
	Special tests							
8	Tone decay, dB	0	....	0	(0-25) [9]; (7-25) [10]	Variable	....	13
9	Békésy curve	Type I	....	....	Type II [9]; type III or IV [10]	Type I	Type V	10
10	Binaural loudness balance	Recruitment absent	....	Recruitment absent	Recruitment present [9]; recruitment absent [10]	Decruitment	Recruitment absent	6

[1] If level for poorer ear minus level for better ear > 25 dB, add 5 dB to better ear threshold [ref. 1,2]. [2] Slight handicap. [3] Mild handicap. [4] Marked handicap. [5] Severe handicap. [6] Profound handicap. [7] Test-retest reliability = ± 5 dB in most clinical situations [ref. 4]. [8] In classification of sensorineural hearing loss, same criteria hold for both PTT & SRT. [9] Cochlear. [10] Retrocochlear. [11] Interquartile range. [12] May occur in various combinations. [13] High incidence of absent reflex threshold in children aged 2-5 yr with a probe tone of ≥ 110 dB may correlate with known high incidence of conductive middle ear problems in this age group.

Contributor: Black, F. Owen

References

1. American National Standards Institute, Inc. 1960. Acoust. Terminol. ANSI S1. 1-1960 (R-1971).

2. American National Standards Institute, Inc. 1969. Specif. Audiometers ANSI S3. 6-1969 (R-1973).

continued

Part I. Audiometry

3. Carhart, R. 1965. Arch. Otolaryngol. 82:253-260.
4. Carhart, R., and J. F. Jerger. 1959. J. Speech Hear. Disord. 24:330-345.
5. Davis, H. 1965. Trans. Am. Acad. Ophthalmol. Otolaryngol. 69:740-751.
6. Dix, M. R. 1968. Ann. Otol. Rhinol. Laryngol. 77: 1131-1151.
7. Goetzinger, C. P. 1972. In J. Katz, ed. Handbook of Clinical Audiology. Williams and Wilkins, Baltimore. pp. 157-179.

8. Hirsh, I. J., et al. 1952. J. Speech Hear. Disord. 17: 321-337.
9. Hopkinson, N. T. 1974. In J. Jerger, ed. Modern Developments in Audiology. Academic Press, New York. pp. 194-197.
10. Jerger, J. 1960. J. Speech Hear. Res. 3:275-287.
11. Jerger, J. 1970. Arch. Otolaryngol. 92:311-324.
12. Liden, G. 1967. Sensorineural Hearing Processes and Disorders. Little, Brown; Boston. pp. 339-357.
13. Owens, E. 1964. J. Speech Hear. Disord. 29:14-22.

Part II. Vestibular Tests

The **caloric test** consists of a thermal stimulus (usually air or water irrigations) to the external auditory canal which creates a differential density in the horizontal semicircular canal endolymph. In responsive subjects, this stimulus yields nystagmus which is usually recorded electro-oculographically and analyzed as a steady state response. The **Hallpike test** is a particular caloric test in which temperatures of 44°C and 30°C are given sequentially at intervals to each ear and the nystagmus velocity recorded, yielding four separate nystagmus responses. The combined cold and warm responses are compared for symmetry between ears, and the directional responses are determined (cold response from one ear, warm from the other) for directional preponderance. Some laboratories compare warm vs. cold temperature responses. The **ocular counter-rolling index** is defined as one-half the average maximum ocular roll in minutes of arc, for right and left tilt. For gain phase curves (impulsive stimuli) from rotary tests of semicircular canal function, consult reference 5. For ataxia test battery data (age- and sex-weighted) of vestibulo-spinal function, consult references 2 and 3. Values are expressed as means plus or minus standard deviations, unless otherwise indicated. Data in brackets refer to the column heading in brackets.

	Type of Measurement	Specification [No. of Subjects]	Value		Reference
			Right Ear	Left Ear	
	Semicircular Canal Function				
1	Caloric test	Normal threshold for nystagmus, °C [14] Cold	36.24 ± 0.50	36.12 ± 0.74	6
2		Hot	38.27 ± 0.37	38.09 ± 0.36	
3	Hallpike test (water irrigation)	Steady state maximum slow-phase nystagmus velocity, degrees of visual field angle/s Cold, 30°C [47]	21 ± 6.3	21 ± 6.9	4
4		Hot, 40°C [47]	23 ± 9.2	23 ± 13.3	
5		Ear difference [20]	−7.09[L]	11.59[L]	1
6		Temperature difference [20]	−13.29[L]	13.29[L]	
7		Interaction: temperature vs. ear [20]	−10.45[L]	10.45[L]	
	Otolithic Function				
8	Ocular counter-rolling index	Maximum ocular roll, minutes of arc [550] Normal	344		7
9		Abnormal	<120		

[L] 95% confidence limits.

Contributor: Black, F. Owen

References
1. Black, F. O., et al. 1973. Ann. Otol. Rhinol. Laryngol., Suppl. 6.
2. Black, F. O., et al. 1977. Trans. Am. Acad. Ophthalmol. Otolaryngol., v. 84.
3. Fregly, A. R. 1974. In H. H. Kornhuber, ed. Handbook of Sensory Physiology. Springer-Verlag, New York. v. 6, pt. 2, pp. 321-360.
4. Hammersma, H. 1957. Thesis. Univ. Amsterdam, Netherlands.

5. Kornhuber, H. H. 1974. (Loc. cit. ref. 3). v. 6, pt. 1, pp. 3-14.
6. McLeod, M. E., and J. C. Meek. 1962. Natl. Tech. Inf. Serv. Ord. N65-36425.
7. Miller, E. F., II. 1970. In J. Stahle, ed. Vestibular Function on Earth and in Space. Pergamon Press, New York. pp. 97-113.

143. ELECTROENCEPHALOGRAPHIC CHANGES DURING ALERTNESS, RELAXATION, AND SLEEP

The electroencephalogram ⟨EEG⟩ is very sensitive to changes in alertness of the subject; drowsiness and sleep, therefore, have been classified by EEG pattern [ref. 3]. Stage 0 (or W) corresponds to the waking stage, both while relaxed and alert. Stage 1 depicts relatively low-voltage activity with mixed frequencies usually recorded during the transition from waking to sleep or after movements during sleep. Stage 2 is characterized by the occurrence of sleep spindles (12-14 Hz) and K complexes. Stage 3 is defined by slow activity (2 Hz or slower), occurring 20-50% of the time. Stage 4 is defined by the occurrence of the 2-Hz or slower activity more than 50% of the time. Stage REM ⟨rapid eye movement⟩ is characterized by low-voltage, mixed-frequency EEG interspersed with eye movements and a general lack of muscle tone or activity. Movement time ⟨MT⟩ represents muscle artifact or general body movement of the subject, which obscures the EEG tracing. Data are for a normal adult. Figures in heavy brackets are reference numbers.

SLEEP STAGES

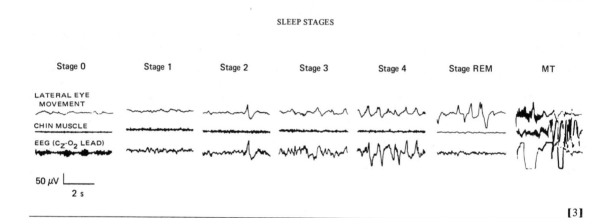

[3]

INTEGRATED EEG ACTIVITY DURING SLEEP

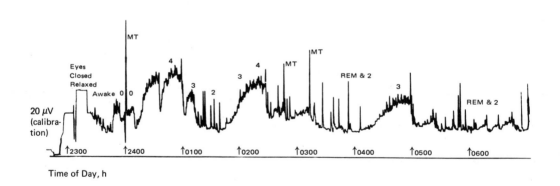

[1,2,4]

Contributor: Bickford, Reginald G.

References

1. Agnew, H. W., Jr. 1968. Psychophysiology 5(2):214.
2. Maynard, D., et al. 1969. Electroencephalogr. Clin. Neurophysiol. 27:672-673.
3. Rechtschaffen, A., and A. Kales, ed. 1968. Natl. Inst. Neurol. Dis. Blindness Publ. 204.
4. Sims, J. K., et al. 1972. San Diego Symp. Biomed. Eng. Proc. 11:87.

144. CLASSIFICATION OF ELECTROENCEPHALOGRAPHIC PATTERNS

Single-channel recordings, such as those shown below, provide only minimum samples of the variety and complexity of patterns that develop and spread over the cerebral hemispheres. Multiple-channel recordings are needed to bring out the details and complexity of the electroencephalogram. Compression amplification is advantageous for revealing in a single tracing both high-voltage and low-voltage components. The instrumental characteristic of the amplification and recording system used here is shown at the right.

Figures in heavy brackets are reference numbers.

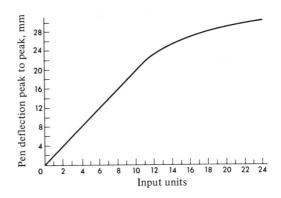

Part I. Normal Resting, Wakeful Activity During Childhood

Occipital resting activity (eyes closed) was recorded with monopolar leads with the common reference electrode on the earlobe [3]. Activity from the anterior areas usually show less alpha activity and a greater admixture of low-voltage fast activity (beta waves).

	Age	Pattern[1]	Voltage Level & Dominant Frequency
1	3 days		Low-voltage irregular activity, no dominant frequency [1,3]
2	3 months		Low voltage, 1½-3 cycles/s [1,3]
3	5 months		Moderately high voltage, 1½-4 cycles/s [1,3]
4	6 months		High voltage, 4 cycles/s [1,3]
5	11 months		Moderate voltage, 4-5 cycles/s [1,3]
6	20 months		High voltage, 4 cycles/s, mixed with moderate voltage, 8 cycles/s alpha waves [1,3]
7	4 years		High voltage, 7-8 cycles/s alpha waves [1,3]

[1] 50 μV |_____| = voltage X time scale for pattern.
     1 s

continued

297

144. CLASSIFICATION OF ELECTROENCEPHALOGRAPHIC PATTERNS

Part I. Normal Resting, Wakeful Activity During Childhood

Age		Pattern [1]	Voltage Level & Dominant Frequency
8	8 years		Moderate voltage, 9-10 cycles/s alpha waves [1,3]
9	12 years		High voltage, 9 cycles/s alpha waves [1,3]
10	14 years		Low voltage, 9 cycles/s alpha waves [1,3]
11	16 years		9-10 cycles/s alpha waves [1,3]
12	>16 years		9-10 cycles/s, M-shaped alpha waves [2] [1,2]
13			9-10 cycles/s, U-shaped alpha waves [2] [1,2]
14			11 cycles/s, spindling alpha waves [1,3]
15			Low-voltage, fast activity [3] [1,3]

[1] 50 µV ⌐_____⌐ = voltage × time scale for
                1 s
pattern. [2] Unusual, but normal, activity. [3] Low-voltage, fast background activity occurs in some persons with eyes closed. It also appears as a nonspecific attention response in persons with well-developed alpha waves, i.e., the alpha waves drop out with attention, leaving a background of low-voltage fast activity.

Contributors: Gibbs, Frederic A., and Gibbs, Erna L.

References
  1. Chatrian, G. E., et al. 1959. Electroencephalogr. Clin. Neurophysiol. 11:497-510.
  2. Gastaut, H., et al. 1952. Marseille Med. 89:296-310.
  3. Gibbs, F. A., and E. L. Gibbs. 1950. Atlas of Electroencephalography. Ed. 2. Addison-Wesley, Cambridge, MA. v. 1.

Part II. Normal Drowsiness and Sleep

Depth of Sleep		Pattern [1]	Description
1	Infantile drowsiness		Long runs of slow activity [1]
2	Juvenile drowsiness		Paroxysmal slow activity (short runs) [1]

[1] 50 µV ⌐_____⌐ = voltage × time scale for pattern.
                1 s

continued

Part II. Normal Drowsiness and Sleep

	Depth of Sleep	Pattern[1/]	Description
3	Adult drowsiness		Flattening [2]
4	Sudden, brief arousal		K-Complex [3]
5	Light sleep (most marked in childhood)		Biparietal humps [1]
6	Any phase of sleep		Occipital positive sharp waves [1]
7	Deeper sleep		14 cycles/s, spindles [2]
8	Moderately deep sleep		Spindles mixed with slow activity [2]
9	Very deep sleep		2 cycles/s, slow waves [2]
10	Exceedingly deep sleep (common in childhood, rare in old age)		1 cycle/s, slow waves [2]

[1/] 50 µV $\llcorner$_____$\lrcorner$ = voltage X time scale for pattern.

1 s

Contributors: Gibbs, Frederic A., and Gibbs, Erna L.

References

1. Gibbs, F. A., and E. L. Gibbs. 1950. Atlas of Electro-encephalography. Ed. 2. Addison-Wesley, Cambridge, MA. v. 1.

2. Loomis, A. L., et al. 1936. J. Exp. Psychol. 19:249-279.

3. Loomis, A. L., et al. 1938. J. Neurophysiol. 1:413-430.

continued

Part III. Nonparoxysmal Abnormalities

Electroencephalographic abnormalities are nonspecific with regard to etiology; they can be produced by anything that can injure the brain, e.g., trauma, encephalitis, vascular disease, hypoxia, hypoglycemia, metabolic disorders, toxic substances, and drugs. Light anesthesia produced by most anesthetics is associated with fast activity. Abnormal fast activity usually increases in drowsiness and light sleep.

Moderately slow activity is commonly associated with a slightly obtunded state or light stupor. Very slow activity is commonly associated with coma. A recording that appears to be flat, i.e., isoelectric, at double the usual amplification (in the absence of drugs or infection), creates a presumption of irreversible coma [3].

For additional information, consult reference 1. **Abnormality:** + signs indicate degree of severity, from mild (+) to very severe (++++).

	Abnormality	Pattern [1]	Description
1	Irritation (+) & depression	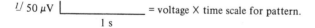	Slightly fast [1]
2	Irritation (++) & depression		Moderately fast [1]
3	Irritation (+++) & depression		Exceedingly fast [1,2]
4	Depression (+)		Slightly slow [1]
5	Depression (++)		Moderately slow [1]
6	Depression (+++)		Very slow [1]
7	Depression (++++)		Flattening & exceedingly slow [1,3]

[1] 50 μV └─────────┘ = voltage × time scale for pattern.
         1 s

Contributors: Gibbs, Frederic A., and Gibbs, Erna L.

References

1. Gibbs, F. A., and E. L. Gibbs. 1964. Atlas of Electroencephalography. Addison-Wesley, Reading, MA. v. 3.

2. Gibbs, E. L., et al. 1950. Dis. Nerv. Syst. 11(11):323-326.

3. Silverman, D., et al. 1970. Neurology 20:525-533.

continued

Part IV. Seizure Discharges

Hypsarrhythmia, the 2- and 3-cycles/s spike and wave discharges, commonly appears in the awake recording and also during sleep. The grand mal type of discharge almost never appears in the awake, interseizure recording; it is seen in status epilepticus and in sleep, most often in children with petit mal variant and petit mal epilepsy. The last three "controversial" patterns most commonly appear in sleep recordings and are relatively rare in awake recordings. For additional information, consult reference 2.

Abnormality	Pattern [1/]	Description
1	Infantile spasms		Hypsarrhythmia [5]
2	Petit mal variant		2 cycles/s, spike & wave [4]
3	Petit mal		3 cycles/s, spike & wave [3]
4	Grand mal		Crescendo spiking [3]
5	Diencephalic epilepsy		14 & 6 cycles/s, positive spikes [1,8]
6			6 cycles/s, spike & wave [7,10]
7	Psychomotor variant		Mid-temporal rhythmic discharge [6,9]

[1/] 50 μV ⌊_____⌋ = voltage X time scale for pattern.
      1 s

Contributors: Gibbs, Frederic A., and Gibbs, Erna L.

continued

144. CLASSIFICATION OF ELECTROENCEPHALOGRAPHIC PATTERNS

Part IV. Seizure Discharges

References

1. Gibbs, E. L., and F. A. Gibbs. 1951. Neurology 1: 136.
2. Gibbs, F. A., and E. L. Gibbs. 1952. Atlas of Electroencephalography. Addison-Wesley, Cambridge, MA. v. 2.
3. Gibbs, F. A., et al. 1935. Arch. Neurol. Psychiatry 34:1133-1148.
4. Gibbs, F. A., et al. 1939. Ibid. 41:1111-1116.
5. Gibbs, E. L., et al. 1954. Pediatrics 13:66-73.
6. Gibbs, F. A., et al. 1963. Neurology 13:991-998.
7. Hill, J. D. N., and G. Parr, ed. 1963. Electroencephalography. Ed. 2. MacDonald, London.
8. Holbrook, T. J. 1970. Clin. Electroencephalogr. 1(1): 36-40.
9. Lipman, I. J., and J. R. Hughes. 1969. Electroencephalogr. Clin. Neurophysiol. 27:43-47.
10. Thomas, J. 1957. Neurology 7:438-442.

Part V. Spikes

All types of spiking are most evident in sleep, all can be focal or generalized, and all are commonly followed by one or more slow waves. Frontoparietal single spike and wave discharges are a common paroxysmal dysrhythmia [3] which is not shown below. It does not correlate with petit mal, but does correlate with convulsive disorder. Slow waves with sharp component and spike-like waves are epileptiform, but unlike the patterns below, they are not clearly epileptic. For additional information, consult reference 3.

	Occurrence	Pattern [1]	Description & Location
1	Common in premature children (associated with visual difficulties); rare in adults		Needles; usually occipital, sometimes midtemporal [2,3]
2	Often asymptomatic, but commonly associated with convulsions or psychomotor seizures; usually found in adults		Small, sharp spikes; usually diffuse or arising from multiple foci, but particularly common in the anterior temporal area [3]
3	When focal in the anterior temporal area, usually associated with psychomotor seizures		Moderate-voltage spikes; can be focal in any area [1]
4	Convulsions, either focal or generalized; occasionally found in the anterior temporal area in association with psychomotor seizures; usually seen in children		High-voltage slow spikes; can be focal in any area [3]

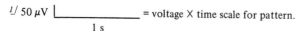

[1] 50 μV ⌊_____⌋ = voltage X time scale for pattern.
     1 s

Contributors: Gibbs, Frederic A., and Gibbs, Erna L.

References

1. Gibbs, E. L., et al. 1948. Arch. Neurol. Psychiatry 60:95.
2. Gibbs, F. A., et al. 1968. Johns Hopkins Med. J. 122: 343-349.
3. Gibbs, F. A., and E. L. Gibbs. 1952. Atlas of Electroencephalography. Addison-Wesley, Cambridge, MA. v. 2.

continued

144. CLASSIFICATION OF ELECTROENCEPHALOGRAPHIC PATTERNS

Part VI. Additional Patterns with Specific Clinical Correlates

	Occurrence	Pattern[1/]	Description
1	Common in infants with mental retardation due to brain damage		Extreme spindles; very high voltage, almost continuous sleep spindles [2]
2	Common in older adolescents & adults with psychiatric disorders		Mitten patterns; slow spike & wave in frontal areas during deep sleep [3,4]
3	Common in patients with severe hepatic insufficiency, markedly elevated blood ammonia, precoma or coma		Triphasic waves, chiefly in frontal areas, present awake & during sleep [1]

[1/] 50 μV L_____ = voltage X time scale for pattern.
1 s

Contributors: Gibbs, Frederic A., and Gibbs, Erna L.

References

1. Adams, R. D., and J. M. Foley. 1953. Res. Publ. Assoc. Res. Nerv. Ment. Dis. 32:198-237.
2. Gibbs, E. L., and F. A. Gibbs. 1962. Science 138: 1106-1107.
3. Gibbs, F. A., and E. L. Gibbs. 1963. J. Neuropsychiatry 5:6-13.
4. Lyketsos, G., et al. 1953. Arch. Neurol. Psychiatry 69:707-712.

VI. ENDOCRINOLOGY AND ENDOCRINOPATHIES

145. ANTERIOR PITUITARY HORMONES

Abbreviations: cAMP = cyclic adenosine 3′,5′-monophosphate; DNA = deoxyribonucleic acid; GFR = glomerular filtration rate; mol wt = molecular weight; RNA = ribonucleic acid. Figures in heavy brackets are reference numbers. Data in light brackets refer to the column heading in brackets.

	Structure & Properties	Source [Targets]	Assay Methods	Principal Actions	Effects of Deficiency (−) & Excess (+)	Control of Secretion: Stimulated by (S), Inhibited by (I), Modification (M)
	Adrenocorticotropic Hormone ⟨Corticotropin; ACTH⟩ [2,3,7,8,11,15,17,27,29,30,38,40]					
1	Polypeptide, 39 amino acids. Mol wt = 4941. Soluble in aqueous solvents at all pH's. Inactivated by treatment with trypsin, chymotrypsin, by oxidation of methionine, and by acetylation or succinylation of amino groups. Activity retained after limited pepsin A digestion.	Basophil cells of pituitary. Ectopically from malignant tumors, particularly lung. [Adrenal cortex]	In vivo: Corticosterone production by hypophysectomized rat after intravenous injection of ACTH. Depletion of rat adrenal ascorbic acid content. In vitro: cAMP production by isolated adrenal cortical cells. Reducing activity of isolated cortical cells, measured by ferricyanide reaction in cytochemical system. For receptor binding, competition of labeled & unlabeled ACTH for binding sites on isolated cortical cells. Radioimmunoassay: Guinea pig or rabbit antiserum. ^{125}I-labeled ACTH as tracer. Normal ACTH secretion shows diurnal rhythm, reaching peak output & plasma levels in early morning hours (0400-0800), 10-80 pg/ml; <10 pg/ml in evening.	Stimulates growth of adrenal cortex & production of glucocorticoids by cells of zona fasciculata. Increases levels of adrenal cortical cAMP.	(−): Insufficient glucocorticoid production, with lowered plasma levels of hydrocortisone [1] & decreased urinary 17-hydroxycorticosteroids (see Adrenal hormones, table 154) (+): Elevated plasma hydrocortisone [1] & urinary 17-hydroxycorticosteroid levels. Loss of normal diurnal rhythm. Cushing's syndrome, with hypertension, truncal obesity, impaired glucose tolerance, pigmentation.	(S): Decreased plasma hydrocortisone [1] levels. Via the hypothalamus, increased pituitary levels of corticotropin-releasing hormone ⟨CRH⟩. Stress (e.g., pain, fear, fever, hypoglycemia) through elevation of CRH. (I): Increased plasma hydrocortisone [1] levels (direct feedback on pituitary). Decreased hypothalamic release of CRH. (M): In certain tumors (especially ectopic), fragments of the ACTH molecule may also be elaborated.
	Follicle-stimulating Hormone ⟨Follitropin; FSH⟩ [1-3,18,19,28,38]					
2	Glycopeptide, with chemical features similar to those of LH (entry 4). Alpha (common) subunit, 89 amino acids, identical in sequence to LH-alpha. Beta subunit, 115 amino acids, differs in	Basophil cells of anterior pituitary. [Ovary: granulosa cells of maturing follicles. Testis: supporting cells [2] of seminiferous tubules]	In vivo: Ovarian weight increase in rats pretreated with human chorionic gonadotropin ⟨HCG⟩. In vitro: Estrogen production or promotion of growth & maturation in cultured ovarian granulosa cells.	♂: Promotes spermatocyte maturation (in presence of testosterone) through action on supporting cells [2]. Increases cAMP production & synthesis of androgen-binding protein by sup-	(−): Usually accompanied by deficiency in LH. Failure of ovarian follicular maturation, oocyte development, & ovulation. Ovarian atrophy, amenorrhea. Decreased plasma levels of estrogen. Testicular atrophy with fail-	(S): Low plasma estrogen or testosterone levels (e.g., post-menopausal or castration). Via hypothalamic-pituitary axis, increase in luteinizing hormone-releasing hormone ⟨LH-RH⟩ (less potent for FSH release than

[1] Synonym: Cortisol. [2] Synonym: Sertoli cells.

continued

Structure & Properties	Source [Targets]	Assay Methods	Principal Actions	Effects of Deficiency (−) & Excess (+)	Control of Secretion: Stimulated by (S), Inhibited by (I), Modification (M)
sequence from LH-beta, conferring biological & immunological specificity to hormone. Contains 18-20% carbohydrate. Mol wt, ∿32,000.	cell[2]—enriched rats. cAMP production by ovarian granulosa cells or testicular tissue in culture. For receptor binding, specific displacement of labeled FSH from isolated granulosa cells. Radioimmunoassay: Rabbit, guinea pig antiserum. ^{125}I-labeled purified FSH as tracer. Specific assays for alpha subunit (cross-reacts with alpha from other gonadotropins) & beta subunits as well as for native FSH.	porting cells[2]. Stimulates estrogen production (through aromatization of testosterone) by supporting cells[2]. ?: Stimulates cAMP & estradiol production in follicular granulosa cells. Together with LH, promotes follicular growth & maturation preparatory to ovulation.	ure of spermatogenesis. (+): Naturally occurring isolated FSH excess unknown. Exogenously (usually combined with LH) may produce ovarian hypertrophy & increased estrogen secretion.	for LH release, but same releasing factor probably acts on both hormones). (I): Increase in plasma estrogens, ? progesterone, ? testosterone. Decrease in LH-RH from hypothalamus. (M): In addition to FSH & LH, alpha subunit secreted in response to administration of LH-RH.

Growth Hormone ⟨Somatotropin; GH⟩ [2,3,8,14,17,20,22,24,31,34,35,38-40]

Structure & Properties	Source [Targets]	Assay Methods	Principal Actions	Effects of Deficiency (−) & Excess (+)	Control of Secretion
3	Polypeptide, single-chain, 191 amino acids. Mol wt, ∿22,000. Soluble & stable in aqueous solutions over wide pH range, including strong acetic acid. Insoluble in acetone & ethanol. Dimeric forms (mol wt, ∿45,000) commonly found, often stable to denaturants. Biological activity retained after reduction of disulfide bridges, tryptophan modification (nitrophenylsulfenyl chloride), methionine oxidation, limited tyrosine nitration, or limited digestion by plasmin or tryp-	Acidophil cells[3] of anterior pituitary. In rare instances, ectopically from lung malignancies. Human placental lactogen[4], a peptide from placenta, resembles GH in chemical properties & certain biological actions (see Prolactin, entry 5). [Most mammalian connective tissue, muscle, & visceral organs]	In vivo: Weight gain, increased width of tibial epiphyseal cartilage, or activity of renal ornithine decarboxylase after injection into hypophysectomized rats. For lactogenic activity, stimulation of crop sac in pigeons or mammary gland growth & milk production in mice. In vitro: Lipolysis of epididymal fat pad; casein production by mouse mammary tissue in culture. For receptor binding, competition with labeled GH for binding to rabbit liver cells (specific for somatotropic activity), to lym-	Wide-ranging general anabolic & growth promoting effects. Increases protein, DNA, & RNA synthesis and decreases protein catabolism. Increases lipolysis & free fatty acid production. Antagonizes action of insulin, decreasing glucose utilization, and increasing gluconeogenesis. Stimulates secretion of insulin (directly, and indirectly through effect on glucose metabolism). Acts on kidney to increase GFR, and promotes retention of phosphate, sodium, & potassium. In-	(−): May occur as isolated deficiency, or accompanying deficiencies of other pituitary hormones, e.g., FSH (entry 2) & LH (entry 4). Dwarfism with short, but proportionate, stature & delayed epiphyseal closure. Increased sensitivity to insulin. Delayed onset of otherwise normal puberty. (+): Gigantism (before puberty) or acromegaly (after puberty). General proliferation & hypertrophy of bony & soft tissues. Before epiphyseal closure, proportionate long-bone growth. Impaired glucose tolerance or outright diabetic state. Osteoporosis. In-	(S): Acute hypoglycemia. Fasting. Administration of amino acids (e.g., arginine). Increased plasma estrogens. Decreased plasma GH ("short loop" feedback). Stress (pain, fear, pyrexia, surgery), probably through action of growth hormone—releasing hormone ⟨GRH⟩ from hypothalamus. Normal diurnal variation found in GH secretion, with maximum output after onset of sleep. (I): Glucose loading. Elevated plasma GH levels ("short loop" feedback). Somatostatin (exogenously or via hypothalamic-pituitary axis).

[2] Synonym: Sertoli cells.　[3] Synonym: Eosinophil cells.　[4] Synonyms: Human chorionic somatomammotropin; HCS.

continued

Structure & Properties	Source [Targets]	Assay Methods	Principal Actions	Effects of Deficiency (−) & Excess (+)	Control of Secretion: Stimulated by (S), Inhibited by (I), Modification (M)
sin. Inactivated by acetylation or succinylation of amino groups or by complete tyrosine nitration. Activity probably resides in one or more active cores within peptide chain.		phocytes, rat liver or mammary cells (for lactogenic & somatotropic activity). Radioimmunoassay: ^{125}I-labeled GH as tracer, antisera from several species.	creases cartilage & collagen synthesis, hence augmenting bone growth. May stimulate hepatic production of peptide intermediate, somatomedin. Moderate lactogenic effect (see Prolactin, entry 5).	creased renal blood flow & extracellular volume.	

Luteinizing Hormone ⟨Interstitial-cell-stimulating hormone; Lutropin; LH; ICSH⟩ [2,3,17,19,25,28,36-38]

	Structure & Properties	Source [Targets]	Assay Methods	Principal Actions	Effects of Deficiency (−) & Excess (+)	Control of Secretion: Stimulated by (S), Inhibited by (I), Modification (M)
4	Glycopeptide. Two dissimilar subunits: alpha (common), 89 amino acids; beta (hormone-specific), 115 amino acids. Non-covalently associated, separable by denaturing agents (urea, guanidine, propionic acid) or countercurrent distribution. Extensive disulfide linkages within subunits. 15% carbohydrate, linked to asparagine residues. Mol wt, ∿29,000. Soluble in aqueous solutions, optimally above pH 7. Inactivated by reduction of disulfides, oxidation of methionine, esterification, methylation, or treatment with common proteolytic enzymes. Separate subunits biologically inactive.	Basophil cells of anterior pituitary. Rare instances of alpha subunit produced ectopically by malignant tumors (lung, intestinal tract). [Testis: interstitial cells [5]. Ovary: granulosa & luteal cells.]	In vivo: Depletion of ovarian ascorbic acid in pseudopregnant rats. Increase in ventral prostate weight in hypophysectomized rats. In vitro: Stimulation of testosterone production by interstitial cells [5] of rat testis or mouse interstitial cell [5] tumors. Stimulation of morphological luteinization or progesterone secretion by ovarian granulosa cells in culture. Progesterone or cAMP production by isolated luteal tissue. For receptor binding: displacement of labeled LH or human chorionic gonadotropin ⟨HCG⟩ from luteal or granulosa cells. Radioimmunoassay: Rabbit, guinea pig antiserum, ^{125}I-labeled purified LH as tracer. Specific assays for separate subunits as well as for intact LH.	♂: Stimulates production of testosterone by interstitial cells [5] of testis. Increases interstitial cell [5] cAMP. ♀: Maturation of ovarian follicular cells & stimulation of estrogen secretion after "priming" by FSH (entry 2). Induction of ovulation (midcycle LH surge). Maintenance of corpus luteum & progesterone production during later stages of menstrual cycle or early pregnancy. Increases luteal cell cAMP.	(−): Failure of oocyte maturation, ovulation, & luteinization. Low plasma progesterone & estrogen levels. Atrophy & failure of testosterone production by interstitial cells [5] of testis. Decreased libido, hair growth, & secondary sex characteristics. (+): Hypertrophy of interstitial cells [5], with excessive testosterone production. Accelerated ovulation & luteinization, elevated plasma estrogen & progesterone.	(S): Low plasma levels of estrogens, progesterone, testosterone (e.g., post-menopausal or castration). Rise in plasma estrogen (at time of midcycle LH surge only). Increase in pituitary levels of luteinizing hormone—releasing hormone ⟨LH-RH⟩ via hypothalamic-pituitary axis or exogenous administration. (I): Elevated plasma levels of estrogens, progesterone, testosterone. Decrease in LH-RH from hypothalamus. Adrenergic blocking agents or serotonin at pharmacological levels (through decrease in hypothalamic LH-RH release).

[5] Synonym: Leydig cells.

continued

	Structure & Properties	Source [Targets]	Assay Methods	Principal Actions	Effects of Deficiency (−) & Excess (+)	Control of Secretion: Stimulated by (S), Inhibited by (I), Modification (M)
	Prolactin ⟨Lactogenic hormone; LTH; PRL⟩ [2,3,5,6,10,12,13,16,20,32,38,39]					
5	Polypeptide. Mol wt, ∼22,000. Partially sequenced. Chemical properties & amino acid sequences closely resemble GH (entry 3).	Acidophil cells[3] of anterior pituitary. Accumulates in large concentrations in amniotic fluid during pregnancy. Isolated cases of ectopic prolactin production by lung malignancies. Human placental lactogen[4], from placenta during pregnancy, is chemically & immunologically similar to GH & PRL, with marked lactogenic & moderate somatotropic activity. [Mammary gland]	In vivo: Growth of crop sac in pigeons. Stimulation of mammary gland growth in estrogen-primed rabbits, mice, rats. In vitro: Cellular development & alveolar secretion in mouse or rabbit mammary tissue in culture. ^{32}P incorporation into casein, or N-acetyl-lactosamine synthetase induction in mouse mammary tissue. For receptor activity, competition with labeled PRL for binding to rat liver, rat or rabbit mammary cells. Radioimmunoassay: Guinea pig, rabbit, or rat antisera; [^{125}I]PRL as tracer. Extensive cross-reactivity among species. Normal plasma levels under 5 ng/ml (slightly higher in ♀), but vary due to normal diurnal rhythm.	Growth & differentiation of mammary gland tissue and stimulation of milk production. Also shows all major actions of GH, but potency weak and physiological significance questionable.	(−): No known conditions or consequences of isolated prolactin deficiency. (+): Galactorrhea, gynecomastia in ♂ or non-puerperal ♀.	(S): Thyrotropin-releasing hormone ⟨TRH⟩[6] (exogenously administered; ? from hypothalamus under normal conditions); probably also a separate hypothalamic prolactin-releasing hormone ⟨PRH⟩[7]. Suckling or mammary gland stimulation (via reflex pathway, probably stimulating release of PRH). Stress (e.g., surgery, fear, strenuous exercise). Coitus in females. Hypothyroidism (? via increase in TRH). Increased plasma estrogens. Hypoglycemia. Pyrocatechol[8] depletion (e.g., by reserpine, phenothiazines), through reduction in hypothalamic production of prolactin-release inhibiting hormone ⟨PRIH⟩[9]. Sleep (basis for normal diurnal rhythm of prolactin output). (I): PRIH from hypothalamus, exerts potent tonic control. Catecholamine administration (especially dopamine), stimulates increase in PRIH release.
	Thyrotropin ⟨Thyroid-stimulating hormone; TSH⟩ [2-4,9,21,23,26,33,38]					
6	Glycopeptide. Properties similar to LH (entry 4) & FSH (entry 2). Alpha (common) subunit, 89 amino acids, identical in sequence to LH-alpha. Beta subunit, 115 amino acids, differs in sequence from LH- & FSH-beta,	Thyrotropic (basophilic) cells of anterior pituitary. Free alpha subunit also secreted in certain pituitary tumors or after stimulation by thyrotropin-releasing hormone ⟨TRH⟩[6]. Human chorionic thyrotropin ⟨HCT⟩, from placenta, has	In vivo: Release into plasma of labeled thyroid hormone by mice pretreated with radioiodine. In vitro: Increase in weight & morphological change in thyroid slices in culture. Release of ^{131}I from thyroid slices in culture. Endocytosis of	Increases iodine uptake & thyroid-gland size. Increases synthesis of thyroid hormones—L-3,5,3′-triiodothyronine ⟨T$_3$⟩ & thyroxine ⟨T$_4$⟩ from 3-iodotyrosine precursors. Accelerates release of thyroid hormone from	(−): Decreased plasma levels of thyroid hormone (measured as T$_3$, T$_4$, or protein-bound iodine) with signs & symptoms of hypothyroidism ⟨myxedema⟩. Isolated TSH deficiency rare; usually accompanies deficiency of other pituitary hormones.	(S): Decrease in plasma thyroid hormone (direct feedback to pituitary). Chronically low iodine intake. Via the hypothalamic-pituitary axis, increase in pituitary levels of thyrotropin-releasing hormone ⟨TRH⟩[6]. Exposure to cold tem-

[3] Synonym: Eosinophil cells. [4] Synonyms: Human chorionic somatomammotropin; HCS. [6] Synonyms: Thyrotropin-releasing factor; TRF. [7] Synonyms: Prolactin-releasing factor; PRF. [8] Synonym: Catechol. [9] Synonyms: Prolactin-inhibiting factor; PIF.

continued

Structure & Properties	Source [Targets]	Assay Methods	Principal Actions	Effects of Deficiency (−) & Excess (+)	Control of Secretion: Stimulated by (S), Inhibited by (I), Modification (M)
conferring biological & immunological specificity to hormone. Contains 15-18% carbohydrate, linked to asparagine residues. Mol wt ~28,000.	comparable biological action & chemical features but differing immunological properties. [Thyroid gland (follicular cells)]	colloid, with lysozyme formation, by thyroid cells in culture. For receptor binding: specific displacement of labeled TSH from isolated thyroid cells. Radioimmunoassay: Purified TSH as tracer, guinea pig or rabbit antibody. Normal plasma levels: 3-10 microunits/ml. Specific assays for alpha subunit (cross-reacts with alpha from FSH & LH) & beta subunit as well as native TSH.	thyroglobulin and, hence, release from gland into circulation. Increases thyroid gland cAMP.	(+): Increased plasma levels of thyroid hormone. Isolated TSH excess seen only in rare instances of pituitary thyrotropic tumors.	peratures (via TRH release). (I): Increase in plasma thyroid hormones (direct feedback to pituitary). Decrease in TRH reaching pituitary from hypothalamus. Increase in circulating corticosteroids or estrogens (via decreased TRH). (M): In addition to TSH, alpha subunit secreted in response to TRH administration or in certain pituitary tumors.

Contributor: Keutmann, Henry T.

References

1. Baker, H. W. G., et al. 1976. Recent Prog. Horm. Res. 32:429-476.
2. Bayliss, R. I. S., ed. 1974. Clin. Endocrinol. Metab. 3(3).
3. Bondy, P. K., and L. E. Rosenberg, ed. 1974. Duncan's Diseases of Metabolism. Ed. 7. W. B. Saunders, Philadelphia. v. 2, pp. 951-1679.
4. Dumont, J. E. 1971. Vitam. Horm. (NY) 29:287-412.
5. Frantz, A. G. 1976. In J. A. Parsons, ed. Peptide Hormones. Macmillan, London. pp. 199-230.
6. Frantz, A. G., et al. 1972. Recent Prog. Horm. Res. 28:527-590.
7. Garren, L. D., et al. 1971. Ibid. 27:433-478.
8. Greep, R. O., and E. B. Astwood, ed. 1974. Handb. Physiol., Sect. 7 Endocrinol. 4.
9. Hershman, J. M., and J. A. Pittman, Jr. 1971. N. Engl. J. Med. 285:997-1006.
10. Horrobin, D. F. 1973. Prolactin: Physiology and Clinical Significance. Medical and Technical, Ltd., Lancaster, England.
11. Irvine, W. J., and E. W. Barnes. 1972. Clin. Endocrinol. Metab. 1(2):549-594.
12. Jacobs, L. S., et al. 1973. J. Clin. Endocrinol. Metab. 33:996-1004.
13. Josimovich, J. B., ed. 1974. Lactogenic Hormones, Fetal Nutrition, and Lactation. J. Wiley, New York.
14. Knobil, E., and J. Hotchkiss. 1964. Annu. Rev. Physiol. 26:47-74.
15. Lefkowitz, R. J., et al. 1970. Proc. Natl. Acad. Sci. USA 65:745-752.
16. Li, C. H., et al. 1970. Arch. Biochem. Biophys. 141: 705-712.
17. Loraine, J. A., and E. T. Bell. 1971. Hormone Assays and Their Clinical Applications. Ed. 3. Williams and Wilkins, Baltimore.
18. Means, A. R., et al. 1976. Recent Prog. Horm. Res. 32:477-527.
19. Moudgal, N. R., ed. 1974. Gonadotropins and Gonadal Function. Academic Press, New York.
20. Niall, H. D., et al. 1973. Recent Prog. Horm. Res. 29: 387-416.
21. Odell, W. D., et al. 1965. J. Clin. Endocrinol. Metab. 25:1179-1188.
22. Pecile, A., and E. E. Müller, ed. 1968. Growth Hormone. Excerpta Medica, Amsterdam.
23. Pierce, J. G. 1971. Endocrinology 89:1331-1344.
24. Raiti, S., ed. 1973. U.S. Dep. HEW Publ. (NIH) 74: 612.
25. Reichert, L. E., Jr., et al. 1973. Recent Prog. Horm. Res. 29:497-532.
26. Reichlin, S., et al. 1971. Ibid. 28:229-286.
27. Riniker, B. 1972. In M. Margoulies and F. C. Greenwood, ed. Structure-Activity Relationships of Protein and Polypeptide Hormones. Excerpta Medica, Amsterdam. pp. 519-520.
28. Saxena, B. B., et al. 1972. Gonadotropins. Wiley-Interscience, New York.
29. Sayers, G., and N. D. Giordano. 1973. In S. A. Berson and R. S. Yalow, ed. Peptide Hormones. North-Holland, Amsterdam. pp. 359-363.

continued

30. Scott, A. P., et al. 1976. (Loc. cit. ref. 5). pp. 247-271.
31. Singh, R. N. P., et al. 1974. Endocrinology 94:883-891.
32. Sinha, Y. N., et al. 1973. J. Clin. Endocrinol. Metab. 36:509-516.
33. Smith, B. R., and R. Hall. 1976. (Loc. cit. ref. 5). pp. 233-246.
34. Sönksen, P. H. 1975. Proc. R. Soc. Med. 68:707-709.
35. Tsushima, T., and H. G. Friesen. 1973. J. Clin. Endocrinol. Metab. 37:334-337.

36. Vaitukaitis, J. L., et al. 1976. Recent Prog. Horm. Res. 32:289-331.
37. Ward, D. N., et al. 1973. Ibid. 29:533-561.
38. Williams, R. H. 1974. Textbook of Endocrinology. Ed. 5. W. B. Saunders, Philadelphia.
39. Wolstenholme, G. E. W., and J. Knight, ed. 1972. Lactogenic Hormones. Churchill-Livingstone, Edinburgh.
40. Yalow, R. S. 1974. Recent Prog. Horm. Res. 30:597-633.

146. DISORDERS OF ANTERIOR PITUITARY FUNCTION

Figures in heavy brackets are reference numbers.

Principal Signs & Symptoms	Pathophysiology	Diagnosis	Treatment
Acromegaly [1,3-7,9-11,14]			

1 | Prepubertal. Excessive statural growth, leading to gigantism if untreated. In some cases: headaches, visual loss, diabetes mellitus, anterior pituitary insufficiency. **Adult.** Acute: overgrowth of hands, feet, facial bones, mandible (prognathism); increased perspiration & salivation. Chronic: enlargement of tongue, thickening of skin, enlargement of salivary glands & sweat gland pores; increased pigmentation; epithelial outgrowths. In some cases: osteoarthritis, hypertension, cardiac failure, cardiac arrhythmia, diabetes mellitus, headaches, visual loss, anterior pituitary insufficiency. Serum phosphorus frequently elevated. Enlargement of visceral organs: liver, spleen, & intestinal tract. Hirsutism, infertility, galactorrhea, or amenorrhea may occur in ♀. | Growth hormone ⟨GH⟩ excess. Basal fasting serum levels variably increased, >5 ng/ml. Oral or i.v. administration of glucose fails to suppress within 1 h serum levels <5 ng/ml. In early cases only night-time sleeping serum levels may be elevated. Functional derangement of normal GH regulating system may be occasionally at fault, but predominant cause is development of GH-producing tumors of the pituitary gland. In prepubertal subjects, skeletal epiphyses fail to close, and gigantism is produced. | Clinical features. Rate of somatic growth, disproportionate growth, & sequellae of GH excess. Laboratory features. Elevation of resting basal serum GH level >5 ng/ml & failure to be suppressed <5 ng/ml during the first 2 h of an oral or i.v. glucose tolerance test. Frequent elevation of fasting serum phosphorus level & impairment of glucose tolerance. Enlargement of the sella turcica in ∿90% of cases. Skeletal X rays may show tufting of distal phalanges of fingers with "spade-like" deformity, enlarged clavicles, expanded rib cage, large bones, developed sesamoid bone of the thumb, osteoarthritis of proximal joints, cardiac enlargement, or enlarged liver & spleen. Thickened heel pad or increased skin thickness may be demonstrated. | Medical. Estrogens: control somatic changes; do not lower GH level or alleviate hypertension. Menstrual disturbance in women & gynecomastia in men are side effects at high dosage required, 5 mg diethylstilbestrol ⟨stilbestrol⟩, or equivalent, daily. Medroxyprogesterone: lowering of GH & clinical remission are temporary in most cases, but can achieve control in a few patients. Ergobromocryptine: a potentially useful drug for sustained lowering of GH level by oral dosage; clinical trials in process; no known benefit for control of pituitary tumor growth. Radiation therapy. Local implantation of radioactive substance, yttrium-90, in pituitary fossa: associated with high rates of destruction of normal pituitary functions; potential hazards to optic chiasma & oculomotor nerves by displacement of implanted radiation sources. Conventional X-ray therapy: primarily limited in effectiveness to radiosensitive tumors; associated with depilation of scalp hair & significant radiation to temporal lobes; results are slow in evolution over 3- to 6-yr interval. Alpha-particle therapy: |

shows favorable results. Proton-beam therapy: clinical & laboratory remissions are associated with a favorable result in 85% of cases; anterior pituitary insufficiency is ∿10% with proton therapy alone.

Surgical therapy. Sublabial, transsphenoidal, microsurgical approach: the preferred method of surgery; not indicated for initial therapy if tumor is localized to sella, since proton beam-therapy can accomplish similar results without anesthesia or surgical risks; incidence of anterior pituitary insufficiency is ∿50%; diabetes insipidus is absent or temporary. Transethmoidal & transnasal approach: limited exposure of sella; allows decompression of a recurrent or invasive tumor, but is unlikely to

continued

Principal Signs & Symptoms	Pathophysiology	Diagnosis	Treatment
	benefit the clinical disorder; low incidence of anterior pituitary insufficiency experienced. Transfrontal approach: reserved for acute visual impairment by chiasmal compression, or for failure of other forms of treatment; high incidence of anterior pituitary insufficiency & moderate incidence of diabetes insipidus are associated with this procedure.		

Growth Hormone Deficiency [2,8,12,13]

Principal Signs & Symptoms	Pathophysiology	Diagnosis	Treatment
2 <u>Intra-uterine.</u> Acute: hypoglycemia & seizures in neonatal period. Chronic: growth failure. <u>Prepubertal.</u> Acute: delayed statural growth. Chronic: slow maturation of epiphyses; dwarfism. <u>Adult.</u> Acute: reactive hypoglycemia. Chronic: mild hypoglycemia.	Damage to hypothalamic region results in loss of growth hormone—releasing hormone ⟨GH-RH⟩, decrease of GH release from pituitary gland, & lack of GH effect which supports glucose formation by the liver. Destructive lesions, trauma, surgery, localized hemorrhage, or spontaneous atrophy may be causative. Hypoglycemia develops, especially after glucose challenge due to normal insulin release & exaggerated response to insulin. Adaptation occurs by decreasing output of insulin, lessening the degree of hypoglycemia.	<u>Clinical features.</u> Short stature, diminished growth rate. Symptoms of hypoglycemia—episodes of hunger & weakness. <u>Laboratory features.</u> X rays of wrist & hand show retardation of bone age. Fasting serum GH level: below 5 ng/ml. Response of serum GH to arginine infusion or insulin-induced hypoglycemia does not exceed 7 ng/ml.	In childhood, or if epiphyses remain open in presence of short stature: intramuscular injections of purified human GH 2-3/wk. Adults: should not receive GH; hypoglycemia treated with a high-protein diet, with frequent feedings. In unresponsive cases, cortisone therapy may be used, but is associated with risks of side effects unless hypopituitarism is present.

Contributor: Kliman, Bernard

References
1. Davidoff, L. M. 1926. Endocrinology 10:461-483.
2. Frantz, A. G., and M. T. Rabkin. 1964. N. Engl. J. Med. 271:1375-1381.
3. Hardy, J. 1974. Excerpta Med. Int. Congr. Ser. 303: 180-194.
4. Hartog, M., et al. 1965. Br. Med. J. 2:396-398.
5. Jackson, I. M. D., and B. J. Ormston. 1972. J. Clin. Endocrinol. Metab. 35:413-415.
6. Kjellberg, R. M., and B. Kliman. 1974. Excerpta Med. Int. Congr. Ser. 303:234-252.
7. Lawrence, J. H., et al. 1970. J. Clin. Endocrinol. Metab. 31:180-198.
8. Merimee, T. J., et al. 1965. Lancet 2:668-670.
9. Rand, R. W. 1966. Ann. Surg. 164:587-592.
10. Ray, B. S., and M. Horwith. 1964. Clin. Neurosurg. 10:31-59.
11. Roth, J., et al. 1970. N. Engl. J. Med. 282:1385-1391.
12. Soyka, L. F., et al. 1970. J. Clin. Endocrinol. Metab. 30:1-14.
13. Stiel, J. N., et al. 1970. Metabolism 19:158-164.
14. Zervas, N. T. 1969. N. Engl. J. Med. 280:429-437.

147. POSTERIOR PITUITARY HORMONES

Abbreviation: cAMP = cyclic adenosine 3′,5′-monophosphate. Figures in heavy brackets are reference numbers. Data in light brackets refer to the column heading in brackets.

Structure & Properties	Source [Targets]	Assay Methods	Principal Actions	Effects of Deficiency (−) & Excess (+)	Control of Secretion: Stimulated (S), Inhibited (I)
		Vasopressin [1] ⟨Arginine vasopressin; Antidiuretic hormone⟩			
1 Octa-pep-	Synthesized in supra-optic & paraventric-	Bioassay: Antidiuresis in rats [35].	Conservation of water through production	(−): Diabetes insipidus—polyuria,	(S): Direct effect on hypothalamic osmorecep-

[1] Release is independent of oxytocin release [11].

continued

Structure & Properties	Source [Targets]	Assay Methods	Principal Actions	Effects of Deficiency (−) & Excess (+)	Control of Secretion: Stimulated (S), Inhibited (I)
tide [1]	ular nuclei of hypothalamus. Bound to a specific neurophysin in storage form [20,36]. Circulates unbound, distributed in extracellular fluid volume, with half-life in plasma of 17-35 min [25]. Clearance by liver & kidneys [23]. [Receptors on surface of cells of renal collecting tubule [18]]	Radioimmunoassay: [29,30] Human plasma level, pg/ml: Normal hydration (recumbent), 1.6 ± 0.5[2/]; (upright), 2.1 ± 0.2. 20 h dehydration (recumbent), 3.7 ± 0.6; (upright), 4.7 ± 0.6. 3% saline infusion (recumbent), 5.0 ± 0.6. Up to 40 pg/ml or higher with volume depletion. [16, 28]	of concentrated urine. Binds with receptors on cell surfaces, activating adenylate cyclase, producing cAMP which leads to phosphorylation of specific protein and, ultimately, to increased permeability of nephron to water & urea and increased water reabsorption. [13,15,18, 19,22]	hyposthenuria, dehydration, thirst; may be idiopathic, familial, or resulting from hypothalamic or pituitary damage [12]. (+): Syndrome of inappropriate antidiuretic hormone—water retention with hypoosmolality of blood, hyponatremia, & sodium loss in urine [3].	tors increased by hypertonicity of blood[3/] [28,29]. Effect mediated by arterial or atrial baroreceptors—increased by hypotension, hypovolemia, upright posture, β-adrenergic drugs, nicotine, positive pressure ventilation [4, 6,14,31,32]. Pathway not well demonstrated; increased by glucocorticoid deficiency, administration of clofibrate, anti-neoplastic drugs, ? chlorpropamide [7].

Renal effect increased by chlorpropamide [27].
(I): Direct effect on hypothalamic osmoreceptors decreased by hypotonicity of blood[3/] [28,29]. Effect mediated by arterial or atrial baroreceptors—decreased by hypertension, hypervolemia, recumbent posture, atrial tachycardias, left atrial distention, α-adrenergic drugs [4,6,14,31,32]. Pathway not well demonstrated; decreased by ethanol, glucocorticoids [26]. Renal effect decreased by prostaglandins [2].

Oxytocin[4/]

Structure & Properties	Source [Targets]	Assay Methods	Principal Actions	Effects of Deficiency (−) & Excess (+)	Control of Secretion: Stimulated (S), Inhibited (I)
2 Octapeptide	Synthesized in supraoptic & paraventricular nuclei of hypothalamus [9,33]. Bound to a specific neurophysin in storage form [20]. Clearance by liver & kidneys [23]. [Myoepithelial cells of mammary gland ducts, pregnant uterus (probable), uterine ⟨Fallopian⟩ tubes (possible) [5, 11]].	Bioassay: Rat uterus contraction, guinea pig or rabbit milk ejection, human mammary gland duct pressure. Radioimmunoassay: [8,10,17] Human plasma level, pg/ml: Basal level, <3 [9,10,30]; stimulated level (controversial), up to 300 [10,21,30][5/].	Milk ejection, uterine contraction, assists sperm transport in ♀ reproductive tract (possible) [5,11,24]	Unknown	(S): By suckling, genital stimulation during parturition or copulation (possible) [5,9,11,21, 30,34]

[2/] Plus/minus (±) value is standard error. [3/] Less than 1% change is an effective blood stimulator. [4/] Release is independent of vasopressin release. [5/] Fetus has high plasma levels at term.

Contributor: Coggins, Cecil H.

continued

References

1. Acher, R. 1974. Handb. Physiol., Sect. 7 Endocrinol. 4(1):119-130.
2. Anderson, R. J., et al. 1975. J. Clin. Invest. 56:420-426.
3. Bartter, F. C., and W. B. Schwartz. 1967. Am. J. Med. 42:790-806.
4. Berl, T., et al. 1974. Kidney Int. 6:247-253.
5. Bissett, G. W. 1974. Handb. Physiol., Sect. 7 Endocrinol. 4(1):493-520.
6. Boykin, J., et al. 1975. Am. J. Physiol. 229:1486-1491.
7. Boykin, J., et al. 1976. Clin. Res. 24:269A.
8. Chard, T. 1973. J. Endocrinol. 58:143-160.
9. Chard, T. 1975. Clin. Endocrinol. 4:89-106.
10. Chard, T., et al. 1970. J. Endocrinol. 48:223-234.
11. Cobo, E. 1969. Am. J. Obstet. Gynecol. 105:877-887.
12. Coggins, C. H., and A. Leaf. 1967. Am. J. Med. 42:807-813.
13. DeLorenzo, R. J., et al. 1973. Proc. Natl. Acad. Sci. USA 70:880-884.
14. de Torrente, A., et al. 1975. Kidney Int. 8:355-361.
15. Dousa, T. P. 1974. Mayo Clin. Proc. 49:188-199.
16. Dunn, F. L., et al. 1973. J. Clin. Invest. 52:3212-3219.
17. Fabian, M., et al. 1969. J. Endocrinol. 43:175-189.
18. Handler, J. S., and J. Orloff. 1973. Handb. Physiol. Sect. 8 Renal Physiol., pp. 791-814.
19. Hays, M., and S. D. Levine. 1974. Kidney Int. 6:307-322.
20. Hope, D. B., and J. C. Pickup. 1974. Handb. Physiol. Sect. 7 Endocrinol. 4(1):173-190.
21. Kumaresan, P., et al. 1975. Obstet. Gynecol. 46:272-274.
22. Kurtzman, N. A., and S. Boonjarern. 1975. Nephron 15:167-185.
23. Lauson, H. D. 1974. Handb. Physiol., Sect. 7 Endocrinol. 4(1):287-393.
24. Marshall, J. M. 1974. Ibid. 4(1):469-492.
25. Maxwell, D., et al. 1976. Clin. Res. 24:407A.
26. Millerschoen, N., and D. S. Riggs. 1969. Am. J. Physiol. 217:431-437.
27. Moses, A. M., and M. Miller. 1974. N. Engl. J. Med. 291:1232-1239.
28. Robertson, G. L., and S. Athar. 1974. J. Clin. Endocrinol. Metab. 42:613-620.
29. Robertson, G. L., et al. 1973. J. Clin. Invest. 52:2340-2352.
30. Robinson, A. G., and A. G. Frantz. 1973. Metabolism 22:1047-1057.
31. Schrier, R. W., and T. Berl. 1975. N. Engl. J. Med. 292:81-88, 141-145.
32. Share, L. 1974. Handb. Physiol., Sect. 7 Endocrinol. 4(1):243-255.
33. Swaab, D. F., et al. 1975. J. Endocrinol. 67:461-462.
34. Tindal, J. S. 1974. Handb. Physiol., Sect. 7 Endocrinol. 4(1):257-268.
35. Weinstein, H., et al. 1960. Endocrinology 66:712-718.
36. Zimmerman, E. A., et al. 1974. Ibid. 95:931-936.

148. DISORDERS OF POSTERIOR PITUITARY FUNCTION

Figures in heavy brackets are reference numbers.

	Principal Signs & Symptoms	Pathophysiology	Diagnosis	Treatment
		Diabetes Insipidus ⟨Vasopressin Deficiency⟩ [4]		
1	Polyuria, hyposthenuria, thirst. Dehydration if access to water is impaired.	Failure of kidneys to concentrate urine in absence of vasopressin. Idiopathic, familial, or associated with damage to hypothalamus or posterior pituitary from trauma, surgery, primary or metastatic tumors, infections, etc. Complete or partial deficiency. Rare variants in which vasopressin is released in response to hypovolemia but not hyperosmolality of blood.	By controlled dehydration test. Hypertonic saline infusion or nicotine stimulation less valuable. [2, 4,5,7]	Reduction of salt & protein intake; thiazide diuretics; chlorpropamide; replacement of vasopressin with long-acting preparations or analogs (vasopressin tannate, subcutaneously, or desamino-D-arginine vasopressin as nasal spray) [6]

continued

Principal Signs & Symptoms	Pathophysiology	Diagnosis	Treatment
	Vasopressin Excess [1]		
2 Impaired excretion of water load; hypotonicity of blood & hyponatremia, leading to lethargy, confusion, seizures, with inappropriately large quantities of urinary sodium & normal circulation	Leads to excessive retention of water, expanding total body water, increasing cardiac output & (slightly) blood pressure, which in turn lead to increased sodium excretion & hyponatremia. Syndrome of inappropriate antidiuretic hormone occurring with: malignant tumors, especially of lung, producing vasopressin-like material; central nervous system tumors, trauma, hemorrhage, infection, etc.; infections of lung; some anti-neoplastic drugs; acute intermittent porphyria; adrenal glucocorticoid insufficiency. Rare variant "reset osmostat" at lower than normal osmolality [3].	Hyponatremia, with normal circulation, no edema, & prompt excretion of all administered sodium	Restriction of fluid intake; treatment of underlying disease

Contributor: Coggins, Cecil H.

References

1. Bartter, F. C., and W. B. Schwartz. 1967. Am. J. Med. 42:790-806.
2. Coggins, C. H., and A. Leaf. 1967. Ibid. 42:807-813.
3. DeFronzo, R., et al. 1976. Ann. Intern. Med. 84:538-542.
4. Miller, M., et al. 1970. Ibid. 73:721-729.
5. Moses, A. M., and D. H. P. Streeten. 1967. Am. J. Med. 42:368-377.
6. Robinson, A. G. 1976. N. Engl. J. Med. 294:507-511.
7. Schrier, R. W., and T. Berl. 1975. Ibid. 292:81-88, 141-145.

149.   HORMONES OF THE HYPOTHALAMUS

Abbreviations: ACTH = adrenocorticotropic hormone; CNS = central nervous system; GI = gastrointestinal; mol wt = molecular weight; MSH = melanocyte-stimulating hormone; sol. = soluble. Figures in heavy brackets are reference numbers. Data in light brackets refer to the column heading in brackets.

Structure & Properties	Source [Targets]	Assay Methods	Principal Actions	Effects of Deficiency (−) & Excess (+)	Control of Secretion: Stimulated by (S), Inhibited by (I)
		Corticotropin-Releasing Hormone ⟨Adrenocorticotropin-releasing hormone; CRH; CRF⟩ [2-5,8,10,11,14-16,18,20]			
1 Basic peptide, with NH_2-terminal structure like that of α-MSH, and COOH-terminal structure like that of lysine vasopressin; at least 2 structures, α & β Inactivated by oxidation, reduction, peptic & tryptic proteolysis, disulfide linkages	Hypothalamus & neurohypophysis [ACTH-secreting cells of anterior pituitary]	In vivo: Release of ACTH (i) into peripheral circulation by injection of sample into rats pretreated with cortisone monoacetate, dexamethasone, or chlorpromazine, morphine, & pentobarbital Na; (ii) measured by ascorbic acid	Stimulates release of ACTH from basophils of anterior pituitary into blood; also increases rate of synthesis of ACTH by basophilic cells	(−): Insufficient release of ACTH into circulation (+): Not definitely known; presumably excessive secretion of ACTH & therefore of glucocorticoids	(S): Neural impulses from CNS—neurosecretory cells function as transducers; low blood levels of corticosteroids & ACTH; cyclic nyctohemeral control through hypothalamus; stress (I): High blood levels of corticosteroids (long-term)

continued

Structure & Properties	Source [Targets]	Assay Methods	Principal Actions	Effects of Deficiency (−) & Excess (+)	Control of Secretion: Stimulated by (S), Inhibited by (I)
		depletion from adrenal cortex in rats with stereotaxic hypothalamic lesions. In vitro: Release of ACTH into medium from one-half of anterior pituitary, as compared to release from other untreated half			& of ACTH (short-term)—negative feedback from adrenal cortex normally controls secretion of CRH; final target organ probably more important

Growth Hormone—Releasing Hormone [1] [2-5,8,10,11,14-18,20]

Structure & Properties	Source [Targets]	Assay Methods	Principal Actions	Effects of Deficiency (−) & Excess (+)	Control of Secretion: Stimulated by (S), Inhibited by (I)
2. Probably a peptide; acidic. Mol wt = 2500; stable in boiling 0.1 N HCl; inactivated by proteolysis; not activated by thioglycollate	Hypothalamus [Growth hormone-⟨GH-⟩ synthesizing acidophils (alpha cells) of anterior pituitary]	Elevation of plasma GH in monkey. In vivo or in vitro depletion of GH from rat hypophysis	Stimulates: Release of GH from anterior pituitary into blood	(−): Decreased release of GH; consequent decreased rate of growth (+): Excessive release of GH (self-limiting)	(S): CNS stimulation; decreased blood levels of GH (depletion of GH in pituitary) (I): High blood levels of GH (negative feedback) & glucose

Luteinizing Hormone—Releasing Hormone [2] [2-6,8-11,14-18,20]

Structure & Properties	Source [Targets]	Assay Methods	Principal Actions	Effects of Deficiency (−) & Excess (+)	Control of Secretion: Stimulated by (S), Inhibited by (I)
3. Amino acid sequence: (pyro)-Glu·His·Trp·Ser·Tyr·Gly·Leu·Arg·Pro·Gly·NH₂ Sol. in 0.1 N HCl; stable to heat	Hypothalamus [Follicle-stimulating hormone-⟨FSH-⟩ & luteinizing hormone-⟨LH-⟩ secreting basophils (delta cells) of anterior pituitary]	In vivo: Increase in plasma FSH in oophorectomized rats pretreated with estrogen & progesterone; increase in plasma LH in castrated ♂ rats pretreated with testosterone, or oophorectomized ♀ rats pretreated with estradiol & progesterone; depletion of pituitary FSH in ♂ rats, normal or castrated; depletion of ovarian ascorbic acid in pseudopregnant rats. In vitro: Release of LH from anterior pituitary from oophorectomized ♀ rats pretreated with estrogen & progesterone. In vivo or in vitro release of FSH from rat anterior pituitary	Stimulates: Release of FSH & LH into peripheral blood; ovulation. Decreases: Ovarian ascorbic acid	(−): Excessive storage & decreased release of FSH in cells of pituitary; absence of ovulation; presumably, decreased release of LH from anterior pituitary, with consequent decreased levels of estrogen & progesterone (+): Stimulation of ovulation (more frequent or multiple) through increased release of FSH into blood; excessive release of LH (to a maximum); premature ovulation	(S): Neural stimulation from CNS; constant exposure to light; low levels of FSH or of estrogens; dopamine; proestrus, puberty (I): High levels of FSH, estrogens, or progesterone in blood (negative feedback); suckling stimulus

Thyrotropin-Releasing Hormone ⟨TRH⟩[3] [2-6,8-11,14-18,20]

Structure & Properties	Source [Targets]	Assay Methods	Principal Actions	Effects of Deficiency (−) & Excess (+)	Control of Secretion: Stimulated by (S), Inhibited by (I)
4. Bovine, ovine, porcine sources: L-	Hypothalamus & neurohypophysis	In vivo: Release of ¹³¹I in iodine-de-	Stimulates: Release of TSH from baso-	(−): Presumably inadequate release	(S): Neural impulses from CNS;

[1] Synonyms: Growth hormone—releasing factor; Somatotropin-releasing hormone; GRH, GRF, SRH, SRF. [2] Synonyms: Luteinizing hormone—releasing factor; LH-RH; LRH; LH-RF; LRF. Follicle-stimulating hormone—releasing hormone ⟨Gonadotropin-releasing hormone; GN-RH; FSH-RH⟩ is identical to LH-RH. [3] Other synonyms: Thyrotropin-releasing factor; Thyroid-stimulating hormone—releasing hormone.

continued

Structure & Properties	Source [Targets]	Assay Methods	Principal Actions	Effects of Deficiency (−) & Excess (+)	Control of Secretion: Stimulated by (S), Inhibited by (I)
(pyro)Glu·His· Pro·NH$_2$ (synthetic tripeptide has activity) Sol. in dilute acetic acid; destroyed by boiling in 6 N HCl; not inactivated by proteolysis	[Thyrotropin-⟨TSH-⟩ secreting cells of anterior pituitary]	ficient mice pretreated with codeine & thyroxine ⟨T$_4$⟩ In vitro: Release of TSH from incubated rat anterior pituitary (0.01 ng TRH releases 200-2000 ng TSH)	phils of anterior pituitary; secretory phase of thyroid gland	of TSH & thyroid hormone (+): Excessive release of TSH into peripheral circulation	low blood levels of thyroid hormones & TSH (I): High blood levels of TSH & thyroid hormones (negative feedback)

MSH Release-inhibiting Hormone [4] ⟨MSH release-inhibiting factor; MRIH; MIF⟩ [2-5,8,10,11,14-16,18,20]

Structure & Properties	Source [Targets]	Assay Methods	Principal Actions	Effects of Deficiency (−) & Excess (+)	Control of Secretion: Stimulated by (S), Inhibited by (I)
5 Structure unknown, not a polypeptide Mol wt, <1000; stable to heat	Hypothalamus [MSH-secreting cells of pars intermedia of pituitary]	Inhibition of release of MSH from hypothalamus of rat; increase of hypothalamic & decrease in plasma concentrations of MSH	Inhibits: Release of MSH from pituitary into circulation	(−): Not specifically known; possibly allows excessive pigmentation (+): Probably blanching of skin	(S): Exposure to dark background; neural stimulation from CNS (I): High blood levels of MSH (negative feedback)

Prolactin Release-inhibiting Hormone ⟨PRIH; PIF⟩ [2-5,8,10,11,14-16,18,20]

Structure & Properties	Source [Targets]	Assay Methods	Principal Actions	Effects of Deficiency (−) & Excess (+)	Control of Secretion: Stimulated by (S), Inhibited by (I)
6 Polypeptide of low mol wt; different from epinephrine, oxytocin, & vasopressin, or any kinin Sol. in 0.1 N HCl; stable to boiling	Same part of hypothalamus that secretes luteinizing hormone of cattle, rat, sheep & swine [Prolactin-⟨LTH⟩ secreting basophils of anterior pituitary]	Inhibition of depletion of anterior pituitary LTH after stimulation of cervix of rat in estrus; inhibition of release of LTH from anterior pituitary of rat in vitro	Inhibits: Release of LTH from anterior pituitary of ♂ & ♀	(−): Unknown; probably permits release of LTH in greater than normal amounts (+): Unknown; presumably prevents release of LTH, thereby inhibiting milk release or reaccumulation of milk after suckling-induced depletion	(S): Unknown; presumably excessive lactation (I): Lactation; high blood levels of PRIH (negative feedback); increased blood levels of gonadal steroids

Somatostatin ⟨Growth hormone—inhibiting factor; GHIF; SRIF⟩ [1,7,12,13,19]

Structure & Properties	Source [Targets]	Assay Methods	Principal Actions	Effects of Deficiency (−) & Excess (+)	Control of Secretion: Stimulated by (S), Inhibited by (I)
7 First sequenced from extracts of sheep hypothalamus. Occurs in both cyclic & linear forms, which have equivalent biological activity. Has been synthesized by solid	Found in almost all parts of the CNS. Greatest amount is in hypothalamus, particularly in median eminence & arcuate nucleus. Present in delta cells of pancreatic islets	Bioassay measures inhibition of growth hormone ⟨GH⟩ from pituitary cells in tissue culture Radioimmunoassay, using [^{125}I]-Tyr$_1$ somatostatin	Can inhibit secretion of GH, thyrotropin ⟨TSH⟩, prolactin, ACTH, insulin, glucagon, gastrin, & secretin. Also inhibits gastric acid secretion, gall bladder contraction, & pancreatic exocrine	Unknown. Passive immunization experiments with somatostatin antiserum indicate that somatostatin deficiency leads to increased GH & TSH secretion. Increased delta cell	Unknown

[4] There is a possibility of an MSH-releasing hormone ⟨MSH-releasing factor; MRH; MRF⟩.

continued

Structure & Properties	Source [Targets]	Assay Methods	Principal Actions	Effects of Deficiency (−) & Excess (+)	Control of Secretion: Stimulated by (S), Inhibited by (I)
phase methodology.	of Langerhans; also in GI tract, with highest amounts in stomach, duodenum, & upper jejunum. [Pituitary, possibly several cell types of CNS, beta & alpha cells of pancreatic islets of Langerhans, gastrin- & secretin-producing cells of GI tract, gastric parietal cells, pancreatic exocrine cells, & gall bladder]	Immunohistochemical techniques used to identify location of somatostatin in tissues	secretion. Physiological role unknown, but passive immunization experiments indicate somatostatin influences GH & TSH secretion. Somatostatin presumably acts locally, and secretion into plasma probably inconsequential except in hypothalamic-pituitary portal circulation.	number & increased pancreatic somatostatin content found in human & several types of experimental diabetes, but the importance of this is unclear.	

Contributors: Pritham, Gordon H.; Kliman, Bernard; Weir, Gordon

References
1. Arimura, A., and A. V. Schally. 1976. Endocrinology 98:1069-1072.
2. Burgus, R., and R. Guillemin. 1970. Annu. Rev. Biochem. 39:499-526.
3. Escamilla, R. F., ed. 1971. Laboratory Tests in Diagnosis and Investigation of Endocrine Functions. Ed. 2. F. A. Davis, Philadelphia
4. Frieden, E., and H. Lipner. 1971. Biochemical Endocrinology of the Vertebrates. Prentice-Hall, Englewood Cliffs, NJ.
5. Gray, C. H., and A. L. Bacharach, ed. 1967. Hormones in Blood. Ed. 2. Academic Press, New York. v. 1.
6. Gual, C., et al. 1972. Recent Prog. Horm. Res. 28: 173-200.
7. Guillemin, R., and J. E. Gerich. 1976. Annu. Rev. Med. 27:379-388.
8. James, V. H. T., ed. 1968. Recent Advances in Endocrinology. Ed. 8. Little, Brown; Boston.
9. Kastin, A. J., et al. 1973. Recent Prog. Horm. Res. 28:201-227.
10. Martini, L., and W. F. Ganong, ed. 1967. Neuroendocrinology 2.
11. McCann, S. M., and J. C. Porter. 1969. Physiol. Rev. 49:240-284.
12. Orci, L., et al. 1976. Proc. Natl. Acad. Sci. USA 73: 1338-1342.
13. Patel, Y. C., and G. C. Weir. 1976. Clin. Endocrinol. 5:191-194.
14. Prunty, F. T. G., and H. Gardiner-Hill, ed. 1972. Mod. Trends Endocrinol. 4.
15. Schwartz, T. B., ed. 1968. Yearb. Endocrinol. 1967/ 1968.
16. Schwartz, T. B., ed. 1971. Ibid. 1971.
17. Schwartz, T. B., ed. 1972. Ibid. 1972.
18. Sunderman, F. W., and F. W. Sunderman, Jr. 1971. Laboratory Diagnosis of Endocrine Disease. W. H. Green, St. Louis.
19. Terry, L. C., et al. 1976. Science 192:565-567.
20. Turner, C. D., and J. T. Bagnara. 1971. General Endocrinology. Ed. 5. W. B. Saunders, Philadelphia.

150. THYROID AND PARATHYROID HORMONES

Abbreviations: ACTH = adrenocorticotropic hormone; cAMP = cyclic adenosine 3′,5′-monophosphate; GI = gastrointestinal; i.v. = intravenous; mol wt = molecular weight; P = phosphate; TSH = thyrotropin. Figures in heavy brackets are reference numbers. Data in light brackets refer to the column heading in brackets.

Structure & Properties	Source [Targets]	Assay Methods	Principal Actions	Effects of Deficiency (−) & Excess (+)	Control of Secretion: Stimulated by (S), Inhibited by (I)
L-Thyroxine ⟨L-Tetraiodothyronine; T₄⟩ [9,21]					
1	Two benzene rings, with ether link-	Thyroid gland [Many different	Protein-bound iodide ⟨PBI⟩, buta-	Generally stimulates O_2 consumption &	(−): Results in decreased metabolic	(S): Increased pituitary TSH secre-

continued

Structure & Properties	Source [Targets]	Assay Methods	Principal Actions	Effects of Deficiency (−) & Excess (+)	Control of Secretion: Stimulated by (S), Inhibited by (I)
age forming 110° angulation; four iodine substitutes at 3′, 5′, 3, 5 positions; 4′-hydroxy substitution, & alanine side chain at 1 position. Thyroxine tightly bound to plasma proteins (thyroxine-binding globulin, 75%; prealbumin[L/], 15%; albumin, 10%). Approximately 99.98% bound, 0.02% free in serum. Extraction from precipitated plasma proteins by ethanol, acetone, butanol. Inactivation by many tissues involves deiodination. Production rate = 80-100 μg/d, half-life = 7 days, volume of distribution = 11.7 liters. Serum concentration normally 4-11 μg/100 ml.	cell types & organs are sensitive to and bind thyroid hormones. A few (spleen, lymph nodes, thymus, testes) appear resistant to the calorigenic & chromatin-binding properties of thyroid hormones.]	nol-extractable iodide ⟨BEI⟩, thyroxine by column chromatography (T_4 I) Competitive protein-binding displacement assay (Murphy-Pattee T_4) Radioimmunoassay	metabolic activity of organ or tissue by unknown mechanism. Decreases O_2 consumption of the pituitary. RNA & protein synthesis increased, amino acid incorporation increased, diverse enzymatic activities increased. Alterations in mitochondrial structure & function, cell-membrane-bound ATPase, Na^+- and K^+-activated, increased. (+): Results in increased metabolic activity of intact organism & many organ functions. Metabolic activity & all functions of skin, heart, liver, brain, & bone increased. TSH secretion markedly reduced; prolactin secretion slightly reduced.	rate of intact organism & reduction of many organ functions. Metabolic activity of skin, skeletal & cardiac muscle, liver, brain, & bone decreased. ACTH & growth hormone ⟨GH⟩ secretion from pituitary decreased. Thyrotropin ⟨TSH⟩ secretion from pituitary increased. Pituitary prolactin secretion sometimes increased.	tion. Excessive iodide ingestion in susceptible individuals (i.e., multinodular goiter or hyperfunctioning thyroid nodule). (I): Decreased pituitary TSH secretion. Excessive iodide ingestion in susceptible individuals (i.e., Hashimoto's thyroiditis or treated Graves' disease); goitrogens, such as lithium; thiourea drugs, thiocyanate, sodium perchlorate.

L-Triiodothyronine ⟨T_3⟩ [7,11,19,21]

2	Similar to entry 1, except that structure contains only three iodine substitutions at 3,5,-3′ positions. (3, 3′,5′-triiodothyronine probably inactive; T_4 → RT_3 molecule termed "reverse T_3".) Triiodothyronine bound less tightly to serum proteins (thyroxine-binding globulin, 90%; albumin, 10%. T_3 not bound to prealbumin[L/]). Approximately 99.8% bound, 0.2% free. Production rate = 30-50 μg/d; at least 50% & probably 85% of this derived from peripheral deiodination of T_4. Half-life = 1 day; volume of distribution = 40 liters. Serum concentration normally 70-200 ng/100 ml.	Thyroid gland & peripheral deiodination of T_4 [Same as for entry 1]	Competitive protein-binding displacement assay Radioimmunoassay	Same as for entry 1	Same as for entry 1	Similar to entry 1, except that in states of low iodine ingestion, T_3 is preferentially synthesized & secreted

Calcitonin ⟨Thyrocalcitonin; CT; TCT⟩ [3,5,6,10,13,14,17,18,20]

3	32 amino acids. Mol wt, ∼3400. N-terminal disulfide ring, positions 1-7. C-terminal prolinamide. Pure peptides soluble in	Ultimobranchial tissue: thyroid parafollicular cells ⟨C-cells⟩ in mammals. Ectopically from several forms of	Bioassay: Decrease in plasma Ca^{2+}, measured 1 hour after i.v. injection into 40-gram rats fasted overnight. Inhibition of re-	Decreases plasma Ca & P. May protect against hypercalcemia under conditions of potential Ca excess (oral Ca intake; lactation):	(−): May increase tendency toward hypercalcemia after Ca loading (+): Used therapeutically (i) transiently to de-	(S): Elevated plasma Ca. GI hormones (gastrin, glucagon, secretin), possibly as part of closed-loop feedback to retard

[L/] Synonyms: Thyroxine-binding prealbumin; TBPA.

continued

Structure & Properties	Source [Targets]	Assay Methods	Principal Actions	Effects of Deficiency (−) & Excess (+)	Control of Secretion: Stimulated by (S), Inhibited by (I)
aqueous solutions at all pH's, optimal stability at pH 4. Inactivated by reduction of disulfide bond or treatment with common proteases. Oxidation of methionine (position 8) inactivates CT. Also inactivated by replacement of C-terminal amide by free carboxyl.	lung malignancy & (rarely) pancreas or mammary gland tissue. [Bone (osteoblasts, osteoclasts), kidney (proximal tubule), GI tract (duodenal & jejunal mucosa)]	lease of ^{45}Ca from incubates of labeled rat bone pretreated with PTH (entry 4). Immunoassay: Guinea pig or rabbit antiserum; ^{125}I-labeled purified CT as tracer. Cross-reactivity among most species very poor, due to sequence differences. Normal human plasma levels, <100 pg/ml.	Bone—inhibits resorption of Ca & P from matrix; retards osteoclastic activity. Kidney—increases clearance of Ca, P, Mg, Na, H_2O; activates renal tubular adenylate cyclase. Gut—inhibits intestinal absorption of Ca & P, increases secretion of Na, K, & Cl into lumen.	crease hypercalcemia due to hyperparathyroidism, malignancy, or immobilization; (ii) to retard excessive bone resorption in certain demineralizing diseases, especially Paget's disease	intestinal Ca absorption after oral Ca intake. Pentagastrin used as provocative test for CT-secreting medullary thyroid carcinoma. (I): Decrease in plasma Ca

Parathyroid Hormone ⟨Parathyrin; Parathormone; PTH⟩ [1-4,8,12,15,16,18]

	Structure & Properties	Source [Targets]	Assay Methods	Principal Actions	Effects of Deficiency (−) & Excess (+)	Control of Secretion: Stimulated by (S), Inhibited by (I)
4	84 amino acid single-chain polypeptide, no disulfide bridges. Mol wt, ∼9500. Soluble & stable in aqueous solvents, optimally at acidic pH. Insoluble in most organic solvents. Inactivated by conventional proteolytic enzymes, acetylation, esterification, or by oxidation of methionine residues. Dilute HCl cleaves peptide chain but yields active fragment (1-29) from N-terminus. Synthetic fragment (1-34) has full biological activity in vivo & in vitro. (Activity detectable in fragment as short as 1-26 of bovine hormone.)	Parathyroid gland (chief cells). Ectopically from malignant tissue, especially lung & kidney. [Bone (osteoblasts, osteoclasts, osteocytes), kidney (proximal, ? distal convoluted tubule), GI tract]	Bioassay: In vivo—hypercalcemia after i.v. injection into parathyroidectomized rats or intact birds (chick, Japanese quail). Phosphaturia & cAMP excretion in parathyroidectomized rats. In vitro—adenylate cyclase activation in renal cortical tissue or isolated bone cells. Release of radioactive Ca from fetal rat bone slices preincubated with ^{45}Ca. Release of Ca, P, or hydroxyproline from postnatal rat calvaria in culture. Immunoassay: Rabbit, guinea pig, or goat antibody, ^{125}I-labeled purified native PTH as tracer. Normal plasma levels <100 to 250 pg/ml, may include	Essential for regulation of normal Ca & P homeostasis: Bone—increases rate of Ca & P resorption from bone, in part by action on osteocytes & osteoclasts. Mediated by cAMP; presence of 1,25-dihydroxy-vitamin D required. Anabolic effect (probably via osteoblasts) stimulates bone formation, with increase in alkaline phosphatase activity. Kidney—promotes phosphate excretion through decrease in tubular resorption. Stimulates resorption of Ca & Mg. Activates renal tubular adenylate cyclase, increasing excretion of cAMP. Stimulates 1-hydroxylation of 25-hydroxy-vitamin D	(−): Hypocalcemia; hyperphosphatemia. Increased neuromuscular irritability, with tetany & seizures. (+): Hypercalcemia; hypophosphatemia. Increased serum alkaline phosphatase. Hypercalciuria (secondary to high filtered Ca load) & phosphaturia (due to decreased tubular resorption), with nephrocalcinosis and/or renal stone formation. Generalized bone demineralization (osteitis fibrosa). Decreased neuromuscular excitability; hypotonicity, stupor or coma.	(S): Decrease in plasma Ca (proportional response over Ca concentrational range of 4-12 mg/100 ml). Decrease in plasma Mg (two- to threefold less sensitive response than to changes in Ca). ? Increased 1,25-dihydroxy-vitamin D. (I): Increase in plasma Ca or (less sensitively) Mg. ? Increase in 24,-25-dihydroxy-vitamin D.

continued

Structure & Properties	Source [Targets]	Assay Methods	Principal Actions	Effects of Deficiency (−) & Excess (+)	Control of Secretion: Stimulated by (S), Inhibited by (I)
		fragments as well as native hormone.	D. GI tract—stimulates intestinal absorption of Ca & P (indirectly through increase in 1,25-dihydroxy-vitamin D)		

Contributors: Ridgway, E. Chester, Daniels, Gilbert H., and Maloof, Farahe; Keutmann, Henry T.

References

1. Arnaud, C. D., ed. 1974. Am. J. Med. 56:743-870.
2. Bayliss, R. I. S., ed. 1974. Clin. Endocrinol. Metab. 3(3).
3. Bondy, P. K., and L. E. Rosenberg, ed. 1974. Duncan's Diseases of Metabolism. Ed. 7. W. B. Saunders, Philadelphia. pp. 951-1679.
4. Buckle, R., ed. 1974. Clin. Endocrinol. Metab. 3(2).
5. Cooper, C. W., et al. 1974. Endocrinology 95:302-307.
6. Copp, D. H., et al. 1962. Ibid. 70:638-645.
7. Gross, J., and R. Pitt-Rivers. 1954. Recent Prog. Horm. Res. 10:109-128.
8. Habener, J. F., and J. T. Potts, Jr. 1976. Handb. Physiol., Sect. 7 Endocrinol. 7:313-342.
9. Ingbar, S. H., and K. A. Woeber. 1974. In R. H. Williams, ed. Textbook of Endocrinology. Ed. 5. W. B. Saunders, Philadelphia. pp. 95-232.
10. Krane, S. M., et al. 1973. Metabolism 22:51-59.
11. Larsen, P. R. 1972. Ibid. 21:1073-1092.
12. Loraine, J. A., and E. T. Bell. 1971. Hormone Assays and Their Clinical Application. Ed. 3. E. and S. Livingstone, Edinburgh.
13. Marx, S. J., and G. D. Aurbach. 1975. In R. V. Talmage, et al., ed. Calcium-Regulating Hormones. Excerpta Medica, Amsterdam. pp. 163-171.
14. Melvin, K. E. W., et al. 1972. Recent Prog. Horm. Res. 28:399-470.
15. Nordin, B. E. C., et al. 1975. (Loc. cit. ref. 13). pp. 239-253.
16. Parsons, J. A., and J. T. Potts, Jr. 1972. Clin. Endocrinol. Metab. 1(1):33-78.
17. Potts, J. R., Jr., et al. 1971. Vitam. Horm. 29:41-93.
18. Rasmussen, H. 1974. (Loc. cit. ref. 9). pp. 660-773.
19. Sterling, K., et al. 1970. J. Am. Med. Assoc. 213:571-575.
20. Tashjian, A. H., et al. 1975. (Loc. cit. ref. 13). pp. 135-148.
21. Tong, W. 1971. In S. C. Werner and S. H. Ingbar, ed. The Thyroid. Ed. 3. Harper and Row, New York. pp. 24-40.

151. DISORDERS OF THYROID FUNCTION

Abbreviations: RAI = radioactive iodine; T_3 = L-triiodothyronine; T_4 = L-thyroxine; TSH = thyrotropin. Figures in heavy brackets are reference numbers.

Principal Signs & Symptoms	Pathophysiology	Diagnosis	Treatment
Hyperthyroidism [6,11,13]			
1 Generalized increase in metabolic rate, tremor, nervousness, anxiety, sweating, heat intolerance, increased appetite, weight loss, hyperdefecation, palpitations, sinus	Most symptoms & signs can be reproduced by excessive circulating levels of T_4 and/or T_3 that result from diffuse hyperplasia (Graves' disease, which can	All causes of hyperthyroidism are associated with elevated serum concentrations of T_4 and/or T_3. Graves' disease may also be associated with	Graves' disease & Plummer's disease are treated with agents which interrupt excessive synthesis or release of thyroid hormones. Antithyroid thiourea drugs (propylthiouracil or methimazole)

continued

Principal Signs & Symptoms	Pathophysiology	Diagnosis	Treatment
tachycardia or atrial fibrillation, gynecomastia, muscle weakness, pretibial myxedema, exophthalmos, variable increase in thyroid size	also include exophthalmos & pretibial myxedema), single or multiple autonomous nodules (Plummer's disease), acute inflammation & release of stored thyroid hormones (subacute thyroiditis or de Quervain's thyroiditis), stimulation & hyperplasia of the thyroid secondary to pituitary hypersecretion of TSH, or ingestion of excessive amounts of thyroid hormones. Only Graves' disease is associated with exophthalmos or pretibial myxedema; these manifestations cannot be reproduced by thyroid hormone excess alone. No thyroid enlargement present during ingestion of exogenous thyroid. "T_3-toxicosis" refers to hyperthyroidism with elevated serum T_3 concentrations, but normal levels of bound & free T_4.	exophthalmos & pretibial myxedema, a high RAI uptake that fails to be suppressed after exogenous T_3 administration for 10 days. Plummer's disease has a nodular enlargement of the thyroid (single or multiple), a normal or high RAI uptake with failure of suppression. Subacute thyroiditis is characterized by exquisitely tender thyroid, low-grade fever, elevated sedimentation rate, & markedly decreased RAI uptake. Hyperthyroidism due to excessive pituitary TSH secretion is associated with inappropriately elevated serum TSH levels. Factitious hyperthyroidism has a reduced RAI uptake, low serum TSH levels, & decreased thyroid size.	block hormone synthesis; RAI (^{131}I) therapy destroys functioning thyroid tissue; surgical resection removes functioning thyroid tissue; exogenous inorganic iodide (^{127}I) in susceptible individuals reduces release of thyroid hormones, causes decreased vascularity and reduction in thyroid size. Subacute thyroiditis is treated symptomatically with salicylates or corticosteroids to reduce pain & inflammation. It is a self-limiting process. Pituitary hypersecretion of TSH is treated with either pituitary irradiation or surgical resection. Factitious hyperthyroidism is treated by withdrawal of thyroid medication.

Hypothyroidism [7,10,12,14]

	Principal Signs & Symptoms	Pathophysiology	Diagnosis	Treatment
2	Decreased metabolic rate, lethargy, fatigue, dry scaly skin, hypodefecation & constipation, weight gain, cold intolerance, sinus bradycardia, carotene deposit in soft tissues, arthralgias; depression; decreased mental function. Thyroid size may be enlarged or small depending on etiology.	Symptoms & signs reproducibly induced by lowering serum concentrations of T_4 & T_3. Decrease in circulating thyroid hormone levels may result from a primary disease in the thyroid caused by iodide deficiency, a congenital enzymatic defect in the biosynthesis of thyroid hormone; blockade of thyroid hormone release by agents, such as iodide or lithium carbonate, in susceptible individuals; by destructive processes in thyroid, such as those occurring after radioactive iodide or surgical therapy of hyper-	Associated with low serum concentrations of T_4 & T_3. Low T_4 is more frequent than low T_3. The characteristic feature of primary thyroid disease is an elevated TSH concentration which results from low serum thyroid hormone levels. Secondary hypothyroidism has low TSH levels, and the pituitary fails to respond to TRH. Tertiary hypothyroidism has low levels of thyroid hormone, TSH, & TRH, but the pituitary can respond to exogenous TRH.	Hypothyroidism from any cause is treated with appropriate replacement with T_4 or T_3. Replacement therapy can be very accurate by following the decline in serum TSH as replacement therapy progresses.

thyroidism, or during the course of autoimmune destruction of the
thyroid gland (Hashimoto's thyroiditis). Secondary or tertiary hypothyroidism due to pituitary disease (TSH deficiency), or hypothalamic disease (thyrotropin-releasing hormone ⟨TRH⟩ deficiency).

continued

	Principal Signs & Symptoms	Pathophysiology	Diagnosis	Treatment
	Subacute Thyroiditis [2,5]			
3	Painful, tender, swollen thyroid gland, pain often radiating to ears. Often follows viral upper respiratory illness. Fever present and may last weeks to months. Initially, mild symptoms of hyperthyroidism may be present; subsequent transient hypothyroidism may occur. Disease is self-limiting; thyroid gland & function almost always return to normal.	Inflammatory nature of the disease process is indicated by an elevated erythrocyte sedimentation rate. Leakage of thyroid hormone from the gland results in transient hyperthyroidism, with suppression of pituitary TSH release. In addition, the extensive nature of thyroid inflammation may render the thyroid gland resistant to exogenous TSH. As the inflammation subsides, pain, swelling, & fever abate and the levels of thyroid hormone fall, often to subnormal levels. As the repair process is completed, thyroid function returns to normal.	Enlarged, often stony-hard, tender thyroid gland, with an elevated sedimentation rate; slightly elevated levels of T_4 & T_3 during very low or absent 24-hour RAI uptake. Rarely, histological proof, showing giant cell granulomas, is necessary, but can be obtained with a percutaneous needle biopsy.	In mild cases, reassurance & salicylates will suffice. With more severe inflammation, glucocorticoids have been employed. T_3 administration, even when mild hyperthyroidism is present, has been reported to be helpful. If hyperthyroid symptoms predominate, β-adrenergic blockade with propranolol should be employed. During hypothyroid phase, which may last for months, T_4 should be administered.
	Multinodular Goiter [1,3,8]			
4	Most patients have asymptomatic enlargement of the thyroid gland. Local symptoms of neck tightness, dysphagia, dyspnea, and/or hoarseness may develop. In areas of the world where iodine deficiency is still prevalent, symptoms of hypothyroidism may coexist. Hyperthyroidism may develop gradually or abruptly in patients with long standing multinodular goiters, cardiac symptoms often predominating.	Most cases are "idiopathic," the pathogenesis being totally obscure. Iodine deficiency, where endemic, & the rare congenital biosynthetic defects in thyroid hormone synthesis can result in multinodular goiter with, or without, hypothyroidism. Euthyroid multinodular goiters may begin to overproduce thyroid hormone if exposed to supraphysiological quantities of inorganic iodide, especially in areas of iodide deficiency.	An asymptomatic enlargement of the thyroid gland, with multiple clinically palpable nodules or visible areas of decreased radioisotope concentration, usually coexists with normal serum concentrations of T_4, T_3, & TSH	Euthyroid, asymptomatic multinodular goiter patients observed clinically, or given suppressive doses of T_4. With significant gland enlargement, local symptoms, or cosmetic disability, surgical removal recommended. In rare situations where hypothyroidism is present, T_4 administration is mandatory. If hyperthyroidism is due to exogenous iodides, they should be withdrawn, and thionamides may be administered concurrently. Spontaneous hyperthyroidism in these conditions is best treated with RAI (^{131}I).
	Thyroid Neoplasms [4,9,15]			
5	Benign neoplasms of the thyroid (including follicular adenomas, microfollicular adenomas, Hürthle cell adenomas, embryonal cell adenomas, & fetal cell adenomas) present with a neck mass and, occasionally, difficulty with swallowing. Well-differentiated thyroid carcinomas (papillary or follicular) may present as a neck mass. Tenderness, dysphagia, dysphonia due to re-	Benign adenomas & well-differentiated carcinomas more likely to develop after radiation exposure, whether it be tonsillar or thymic irradiation in infancy, skin irradiation for acne, or atomic fallout. Medullary carcinoma of the thyroid is a cancer of the parafollicular cells of the thyroid which produce calcitonin; it may occur in conjunction with pheo-	Evaluation of thyroid mass includes careful history & physical examination, thyroid scan (RAI or technetium), thyroid ultrasound, and measurement of the blood levels of thyroid hormones & calcitonin. An isolated nodule that concentrates radioactivity to the exclusion of the remainder of the thyroid gland ("hot" nodule) is almost	Solid, solitary, "cold" nodules should be removed in young children & in most ♂, or if a history of prior neck irradiation was obtained. Presence of vocal cord palsy, suspicous lymph nodes, relentless growth, tracheal obstruction, or difficulty swallowing dictates surgical removal. Suppression of growth for 3-6 mo with the use of exogenous thyroid hormone can be attempted in less suspicious situations. Percutaneous needle biopsy of the

continued

Principal Signs & Symptoms	Pathophysiology	Diagnosis	Treatment
current nerve palsies, or dyspnea may occur. Papillary carcinoma likely to spread locally, with lymph node metastases; follicular carcinoma more likely to spread hematogenously to bone, with osteolytic metastases, & to lungs. Medullary carcinoma of the thyroid often (50%) occurs in conjunction with pheochromocytomas & hyperparathyroidism. Anaplastic carcinoma of the thyroid grows rapidly & relentlessly, with progressive local symptomatology. Benign & malignant neoplasms more common in ♀.	chromocytomas & hyperparathyroidism as part of the dominantly inherited multiple endocrine adenoma (type II) syndrome.	always benign. Most cancers of the thyroid gland concentrate radioactivity less well than the surrounding normal tissue. However, the majority of "cold" nodules are benign. An elevated calcitonin levels suggests diagnosis of medullary carcinoma of the thyroid.	thyroid, where available, allows histological confirmation in almost all cases. Using this technique, thyroid cysts & non-cellular (follicular) adenomas are treated medically; cellular adenomas (microfollicular, embryonal, Hürthle, & fetal cell) & thyroid carcinomas are surgically removed. Before removing a medullary carcinoma of the thyroid, pheochromocytoma should be rigorously excluded. Follicular carcinoma of the thyroid is capable of concentrating RAI (although less well than normal tissue). Local & distant metastatic disease, in this situation, can often be treated with large doses of RAI (^{131}I), after ablation of residual thyroid tissue.

Contributors: Ridgway, E. Chester; Daniels, Gilbert H.

References

1. Astwood, E. B., et al. 1960. J. Am. Med. Assoc. 174: 459-464.
2. Bastenie, P. A., and A. M. Ermans. 1972. Thyroiditis and Thyroid Function. Pergamon Press, Oxford.
3. De Groot, L. J., and J. B. Stanbury. 1975. The Thyroid and Its Diseases. Ed. 4. Wiley-Medimedia, New York. pp. 637-665.
4. De Groot, L. J., and J. B. Stanbury. 1975. (Loc. cit. ref. 3). pp. 666-733.
5. Greene, J. N. 1971. Am. J. Med. 51:97-108.
6. Hamilton, C. R., et al. 1970. N. Engl. J. Med. 283: 1077-1080.
7. Holvey, D. N., et al. 1964. Arch. Intern. Med. 113:89-96.
8. Mortensen, J. D., et al. 1955. J. Clin. Endocrinol. Metab. 15:1270-1280.
9. Refetoff, S., et al. 1975. N. Engl. J. Med. 292:171-175.
10. Ridgway, E. C., et al. 1972. Ann. Intern. Med. 77: 549-555.
11. Ridgway, E. C., et al. 1973. J. Clin. Invest. 52:2783-2792.
12. Ridgway, E. C., et al. 1974. In B. Rothfeld, ed. Nuclear Medicine, In Vitro. J. B. Lippincott, Philadelphia. pp. 205-219.
13. Werner, S. C., and S. H. Ingbar, ed. 1971. The Thyroid. Ed. 3. Harper and Row, New York. pp. 489-711.
14. Werner, S. C., and S. H. Ingbar, ed. 1971. (Loc. cit. ref. 13). pp. 713-845.
15. Woolner, L. B. 1971. Semin. Nucl. Med. 1:481-502.

152. HORMONES OF THE PANCREAS AND GASTROINTESTINAL TRACT

Abbreviations: cAMP = cyclic adenosine 3′,5′-monophosphate; mol wt = molecular wt; GI = gastrointestinal. Figures in heavy brackets are reference numbers. Data in light brackets refer to the column heading in brackets.

	Structure & Properties	Source [Targets]	Assay Methods	Principal Actions	Effects of Deficiency (−) & Excess (+)	Control of Secretion: Stimulated by (S), Inhibited by (I)
			Insulin [1,2,8-10]			
1	Polypeptide, with an A chain of 21	Found in beta cells of islets of	Bioassay: In vivo— mouse convulsion	Carbohydrate: Stimulates glycolytic flux,	(−): Diabetes mellitus (*see* table 153)	(S): Hyperglycemia, metaboliz-

continued

Structure & Properties	Source [Targets]	Assay Methods	Principal Actions	Effects of Deficiency (−) & Excess (+)	Control of Secretion: Stimulated by (S), Inhibited by (I)
amino acids and a B chain of 30 amino acids; chains linked by 2 disulfide bridges. Several crystalline forms can be made as well as various multimers. Heating at low pH produces fibrils or spherites. Soluble in acid ethanol, but insoluble in aqueous solutions, pH 4-7. Relatively resistant to cleavage by proteolytic enzymes.	Langerhans. Equimolar amounts of insulin & C-peptide with small amounts of proinsulins are secreted. [Most tissues are influenced by insulin, but major identifiable effects are upon liver, adipose tissue, & muscle. Insulin effects presumably exerted via receptors on cell membrane. [^{131}I]insulin & [^{125}I]insulin binding to receptors of adipose cells, hepatocytes, & monocytes have been characterized, and receptors are in dynamic flux with changes of receptor number & affinity.]	assay, or measurement of blood glucose in rabbits. In vitro—glucose uptake by rat hemidiaphragm, or oxidation of [1-^{14}C]glucose to $^{14}CO_2$ by rat epididymal adipose tissue. These bioassays measure substances, other than pancreatic insulin, which have insulin-like activity ⟨ILA⟩. Radioimmunoassay: Can detect as little as 50 pg/ml in plasma. Proinsulin contribution to total insulin immunoreactivity, estimated after fractionation, is ∿15% of total. Immunoassay, developed for C-peptide, cross-reacts with proinsulin but gives good estimate of beta cell function	glycogen synthesis, & hexose transport. Gluconeogenesis inhibited. Fat: Stimulates synthesis of fatty acids & triglycerides. Hormone-sensitive lipase & ketogenesis inhibited. Protein: Stimulates protein synthesis, with enhanced amino acid transport & activation of ribosomes. Other: Stimulates or inhibits numerous enzymes, enhances K$^+$ uptake by cells, inhibits glucagon secretion; permissive effects on growth, enhances mucopolysaccharide synthesis. Mechanism of action: Unknown, but can decrease cAMP levels & stimulate phosphodiesterase. Protein phosphorylation can be stimulated or inhibited.	characterized by either relative or absolute insulin deficiency. Resistance to insulin action can lead to glucose intolerance with hyperinsulinism: acromegaly, Cushing's syndrome, obesity, pregnancy, lipoatrophic diabetes, & diseases with decreased receptor number, or antibodies against receptor. (+): Hypoglycemia (see table 153) seen with insulin-producing tumors & in reactive hypoglycemia of early diabetes & alimentary surgery. Possible contribution of hyperinsulinism to idiopathic reactive hypoglycemia is unknown.	able sugars (including D-glyceraldehyde), leucine, sulfonylureas. Stimulation by the following agents probably depends on a permissive effect of glucose: most amino acids, fatty acids, ketones, acetylcholine, isoproterenol, glucagon, prostaglandins, secretin, gastrin, gastric inhibitory peptide ⟨GIP⟩, pancreozymin. Excesses of the following hormones lead to hyperinsulinism secondary to insulin resistance: growth hormone (acromegaly) & hydrocortisone [1]/ (Cushing's syndrome). (I): Hypoglycemia, epinephrine, norepinephrine, somatostatin

Glucagon [2-7,11]

| | Polypeptide of 29 amino acids. Mol wt = 3485. Isoelectric point is ∿ pH 7. Most soluble in acid & alkali. Crystallizes easily in pH 5-8; fibrils form in acid. In dilute aqueous solution, there is little ordered structure. Biosynthesis studies | Primarily found in alpha cells of islets of Langerhans, with smaller amounts in alpha cells of GI tract [Primarily liver & adipose tissue] | Bioassay: In vivo—assays measure hyperglycemic response in cats or rabbits. In vitro—liver slices measuring glucose content of medium, decrease of tissue glycogen, or phosphorylase activation; measurement of cAMP production from particulate fraction of liver; | Pharmacological doses affect most tissues, including heart, hypothalamus, adrenal medulla, GI tract, & gallbladder. Effects caused by physiological concentrations in plasma include stimulation of hepatic glycogenolysis, gluconeogenesis, & ketogenesis; lipolysis in adipose tissues. These effects all op- | (−): No proven examples of isolated glucagon deficiency (+): Hyperglucagonemia of glucagonomas may be associated with abnormal glucose tolerance, weight loss, hypoaminoacidemia, dermatitis (necrolytic migratory erythema), anemia, & stomatitis. In- | (S): Hypoglycemia, amino acids, epinephrine, norepinephrine, acetylcholine, prostaglandins, gastrin, & gastric inhibitory peptide ⟨GIP⟩. Increased plasma glucagon concentrations found in diabetes, stress states (infection, burns, myocardial infarction, |
| 2 | | | | | | |

[1]/ Synonym: Cortisol.

continued

152. HORMONES OF THE PANCREAS AND GASTROINTESTINAL TRACT

Structure & Properties	Source [Targets]	Assay Methods	Principal Actions	Effects of Deficiency (−) & Excess (+)	Control of Secretion: Stimulated by (S), Inhibited by (I)
indicate precursor forms of 12,000 & 9,000 daltons.		use of isolated perfused liver measuring phosphorylase activation or hepatic glucose output. Radioimmunoassay: Detects plasma substances of varying mol wt with glucagon immunoreactivity, approx. weights being 160,000; 9,000 (probable glucagon precursor); 3,500 (glucagon); & 2,000. Non-specific antibodies measure cross-reacting materials from GI tract.	posed by insulin. Physiological role probably is to prevent hypoglycemia after ingestion of protein. May also be important to maintain plasma glucose during fasting & exercise.	creased glucagon secretion in diabetes can contribute to hyperglycemia & ketosis.	trauma), acute pancreatitis, acromegaly, exercise, glucocorticoid excess, renal failure, cirrhosis, & glucagonomas. (I): Hyperglycemia, free fatty acids, secretin, insulin, & somatostatin. Decreased plasma glucagon concentrations seen in hypopituitarism, hyperthyroidism, & chronic pancreatitis.

Gastrin [12]

Structure & Properties	Source [Targets]	Assay Methods	Principal Actions	Effects of Deficiency (−) & Excess (+)	Control of Secretion: Stimulated by (S), Inhibited by (I)
3 Gastrin ⟨G-17⟩ has 17 amino acids; mol wt = 2098. There is also a "big" gastrin of 34 amino acids ⟨G-34⟩, & a "little" gastrin of 13 amino acids ⟨G-13⟩. C-terminus (amino acids 1-5) has same biological actions as larger peptides.	Found in gastric antrum & proximal duodenum. Presence in islets of Langerhans debated. [Gastric parietal cells best known, but effects also found on all portions of GI tract, exocrine pancreas, pancreatic alpha & beta cells, & parafollicular cells[2]]	Bioassay: Stimulation of acid production in dogs, rats, or cats Radioimmunoassay: Synthetic human gastrin I ⟨G-17⟩ usually used as standard. Antisera have variable reactivity with G-34, and G-34 accounts for most of plasma gastrin immunoreactivity.	Stimulation of gastric acid secretion may be major effect at physiological gastrin concentrations. Effect on acid secretion enhanced by acetylcholine & histamine. Pharmacological doses of gastrin can produce many effects, including stimulation of GI tract blood flow & smooth muscle contraction; stimulation of insulin, glucagon, & calcitonin secretion; inhibition of pyloric sphincter.	(−): Seen with antrectomy; may contribute to maldigestion (+): Gastrinoma (associated with Zollinger-Ellison syndrome)—pancreatic gastrin-secreting tumor with multiple peptic ulcers, marked acid secretion, gastric hyperplasia, and associated with multiple endocrine neoplasia type 1. Atrophic gastritis, pernicious anemia—increased gastrin has little effect. Antral G-cell hyperplasia—associated with peptic ulcer.	(S): Digestion products of proteins—peptides & amino acids. Gastric distention, vagal stimulation, calcium, & epinephrine (I): Acid. Pharmacological amounts of secretin, glucagon, vasoactive intestinal peptide ⟨VIP⟩, gastric inhibitory peptide ⟨GIP⟩, & calcitonin.

2/ Synonym: C-cells.

Contributor: Weir, Gordon

continued

References

1. Avruch, J., et al. 1976. J. Biol. Chem. 251:1505-1510.
2. Gerich, J. E., et al. 1976. Annu. Rev. Physiol. 38:353-388.
3. Kuku, S. F., et al. 1976. J. Clin. Endocrinol. Metab. 42:173-176.
4. Lèfèbvre, P. J., and R. H. Unger, ed. 1972. Glucagon; Molecular Physiology, Clinical and Therapeutic Implications. Pergamon Press, New York. pp. 1-370.
5. Mallinson, C. N. 1974. Lancet 2:1-5.
6. Muller, W. A., and G. C. Weir. 1975. In S. C. Sommers, ed. Endocrine Pathology Decennial. Appleton-Century-Crofts, New York. pp. 363-390.
7. Noe, B. D., and G. E. Bauer. 1975. Endocrinology 97:868-877.
8. Roth, J., et al. 1975. Recent Prog. Horm. Res. 31:95-139.
9. Rubenstein, A. H., et al. 1975. In J. Vallence-Owen, ed. Diabetes. Univ. Park Press, Baltimore. pp. 1-30.
10. Steiner, D. F., and N. Freinkel. 1972. Handb. Physiol., Sect. 7 Endocrinol. 1:1-721.
11. Unger, R. H. 1976. Diabetes 25:136-151.
12. Walsh, J. M., and M. I. Grossman. 1975. N. Engl. J. Med. 292:1324-1334, 1377-1384.

153. DISORDERS OF THE PANCREAS

Treatment: i.v. = intravenous.

	Principal Signs & Symptoms	Pathophysiology	Diagnosis	Treatment	Reference
	Diabetes Mellitus				
1	Acute: excessive thirst, appetite, & urination; weight loss; signs of dehydration; blurred vision; pruritus; reactive hypoglycemia	Deficiency of insulin results in decreased glucose disposal & increased gluconeogenesis; consequent hyperglycemia results in following sequence of events: glycosuria, osmotic diuresis, dehydration, & electrolyte depletion (Na^+, K^+, Cl^-, etc.)	Fasting hyperglycemia or glucose tolerance test; glucose intolerance due to the following must be ruled out: starvation, stress, other illnesses (Cushing's syndrome, acromegaly, pheochromocytoma, thyrotoxicosis, renal or hepatic failure, hypokalemia) or drugs (glucocorticoids, diuretics, phenytoin)	Diet: (i) reduction to ideal body weight; (ii) if insulin needed, distribution of calories to match pattern of exercise & time course of insulin action Insulin	1,19, 20, 22
2	Chronic Accelerated atherosclerotic disease (especially cerebrovascular, cardiovascular, & peripheral vascular)	Unknown	Not specific for diabetic patients	Not specific for diabetic patients	11
3	Nephropathy: renal insufficiency, nephrotic syndrome, medullary necrosis	Multifactorial: abnormal quantity (& possibly structure) of glycoprotein of basement membrane, atherosclerosis, autonomic dysfunction of bladder with obstruction, infection	Not specific for diabetic patients. Exception: nodular glomerular lesion (Kimmelstiel-Wilson lesion) on renal biopsy. Nephropathy generally associated with retinopathy.	Not specific for diabetic patients. Dialysis & renal transplantation utilized.	11, 17
4	Retinopathy	Unknown	Ophthalmoscopic examination; fluorescein angiography	Laser photocoagulation in selected cases	5,6, 11
5	Neuropathy: peripheral (distal, symmetrical); mononeuritis multiplex (including peripheral & cranial nerves); autonomic	Peripheral: osmotic effect due to accumulation of sorbitol in peripheral nerves Mononeuritis: occlusion of vasa nervorum Autonomic: unknown	History & physical examination	Efficacy of control of plasma glucose on peripheral neuropathy not known	11

continued

	Principal Signs & Symptoms	Pathophysiology	Diagnosis	Treatment	Reference
6	Pregnancy: Fetal—excessive size, intrauterine death, intrapartum fetal distress, birth trauma, neonatal hypoglycemia, respiratory distress syndrome, congenital abnormalities, neonatal hyperbilirubinemia, neonatal hypocalcemia. Maternal—hydramnios, pre-eclampsia, dystocia, high operative delivery rate.	Fetal hyperinsulinism: glucose crosses placenta, resulting in hyperplasia of fetal islets of Langerhans & hyperresponsiveness to stimuli	Glucose tolerance test	Diet & insulin; frequent medical-obstetrical evaluation	3,4, 15, 18, 21

Diabetic Ketoacidosis

	Principal Signs & Symptoms	Pathophysiology	Diagnosis	Treatment	Reference
7	Same as for entry 1. Also: acetone on breath, Kussmaul breathing, nausea & vomiting, abdominal pain, altered mental status, shock.	Same as for entry 1. Deficiency of insulin also results in accelerated lipolysis in adipose tissue, with release of free fatty acids into circulation; accelerated hepatic ketogenesis; decreased peripheral utilization of ketones.	"Large" ketones in undiluted plasma or serum (nitroprusside test). Blood glucose usually elevated but may be normal.	Insulin, i.v. fluids (normal saline initially, then hypotonic saline), i.v. potassium, i.v. glucose if blood glucose <300 mg/dl	10, 12, 14

Hyperosmolar Non-ketotic Coma

	Principal Signs & Symptoms	Pathophysiology	Diagnosis	Treatment	Reference
8	Same as for entry 1. Profound dehydration; prominent neurologic manifestations, including coma, seizures, focal neurologic signs (often mimicking cerebrovascular accident).	Same as for entry 1, but hyperglycemia more severe (>600 mg/dl), and dehydration more profound. Significant ketosis absent despite advanced degree of insulin deficiency, due to lower rate of adipose tissue lipolysis than in diabetic ketoacidosis (associated in turn with lower plasma levels of growth hormone & hydrocortisone ⟨cortisol⟩ than in diabetic ketoacidosis). Neurologic manifestations correlate with serum osmolality.	Blood glucose, >600 mg/dl; serum osmolality, >350 mosmoles/kg; serum or plasma ketones less than strongly positive in undiluted specimen	Insulin, i.v. fluids (large volume of hypotonic saline), i.v. potassium	2,8,9

Insulinoma

	Principal Signs & Symptoms	Pathophysiology	Diagnosis	Treatment	Reference
9	Symptoms due to sympathetic discharge (e.g., tremor, palpitations, diaphoresis, anxiety). Neuropsychiatric symptoms (e.g., depression; intellectual impairment; seizures; focal abnormalities, such as dysarthria, aphasia, paresis, etc.). Excessive appetite, craving for sweets, weight gain. Exercise intolerance.	Insulin secretion by neoplasm of pancreatic islet beta cell origin; tumors usually benign but may be malignant; tumors may be ectopic or multiple, and may occur as part of the multiple endocrine neoplasia I syndrome	Demonstration of hypoglycemia at time of symptoms, with plasma immunoreactive insulin level inappropriately high for level of blood glucose; or prolonged fast to precipitate symptoms, at which time blood glucose & plasma immunoreactive insulin levels are measured. Provocative tests in selected cases (e.g., tolbutamide test or glucagon test).[1]	Surgical resection; streptozotocin for non-resectable malignant insulinomas; diazoxide, phenytoin, or propranolol may control insulin secretion when streptozotocin not effective	7,16

[1] Other causes of hypoglycemia must be excluded at onset of evaluation. These include the reactive hypoglycemias (e.g., post-gastrectomy, early diabetes mellitus, idiopathic) and other fasting hypoglycemias (e.g., ethanol-induced, primary adrenocortical insufficiency, hypothyroidism, pituitary insufficiency, severe liver disease, non-beta cell tumor-associated hypoglycemia).

continued

Principal Signs & Symptoms	Pathophysiology	Diagnosis	Treatment	Reference
		Glucagonoma		
10 Hyperglycemia, rash (necrolytic migratory erythema), hypo-aminoacidemia, weight loss	Glucagon secretion by neo-plasm of pancreatic alpha cell origin; may be benign or ma-lignant	Elevated plasma immuno-reactive glucagon levels in patient with hyperglyce-mia, characteristic rash & pancreatic mass	Surgical resection; streptozotocin for non-resectable ma-lignant glucagono-mas	13

Contributor: Axelrod, Lloyd

References

1. American Diabetes Association, Committee on Food and Nutrition. 1971. Diabetes 20:633-634.
2. Arieff, A. I., and H. J. Carroll. 1972. Medicine (Baltimore) 51:73-94.
3. British Medical Association. 1974. Br. Med. J. 1:167-168.
4. Brudenell, M., and R. Beard. 1972. Clin. Endocrinol. Metab. 1:673-695.
5. Cheng, H., et al. 1975. Lancet 2:1110-1113.
6. Diabetic Retinopathy Study Research Group. 1976. Am. J. Ophthalmol. 81:383-396.
7. Ensinck, J. W., and R. H. Williams. 1974. In R. H. Williams, ed. Textbook of Endocrinology. Ed. 5. W. B. Saunders, Philadelphia. pp. 627-659.
8. Foster, D. W. 1974. Adv. Intern. Med. 19:159-173.
9. Fulop, M., et al. 1975. Diabetes 24:594-599.
10. Hockaday, T. D. R., and K. G. M. M. Alberti. 1972. Clin. Endocrinol. Metab. 1:751-788.
11. Keen, H., and J. Jarrett, ed. 1975. Complications of Diabetes. E. Arnold, London.
12. Kitabchi, A. E., et al. 1976. Ann. Intern. Med. 84:633-638.
13. Mallinson, C. N., et al. 1974. Lancet 2:1-5.
14. McGarry, J. D., and D. W. Foster. 1976. Am. J. Med. 61:9-13.
15. Persson, B. 1974. Ciba Found. Symp. 27(N.S.)247-273.
16. Service, F. J., et al. 1976. Mayo Clin. Proc. 51:417-429.
17. Shapiro, F. L., et al., ed. 1974. Kidney Int. 6(4: Suppl. 1).
18. Tyson, J. E., and P. Felig. 1971. Med. Clin. North Am. 55:947-959.
19. U.S. National Commission on Diabetes. 1976. U.S. Dep. HEW Publ. (NIH) 76-1021(3).
20. West, K. M. 1973. Ann. Intern. Med. 79:425-434.
21. White, P. 1974. Clin. Perinatol. 1:331-347.
22. Williams, R. H., and D. Porte, Jr. 1974. (Loc. cit. ref. 7). pp. 502-626.

154. ADRENAL HORMONES

Abbreviations & Symbols: absorption max = wavelength of maximum absorbancy; ACTH = adrenocorticotropic hormone; cAMP = cyclic adenosine 3',5'-monophosphate; BMR = basal metabolic rate; CNS = central nervous system; CRH = corticotropin-releasing hormone; DOPA = 3,4-dihydroxyphenylalanine; insol. = insoluble; i.v. = intravenous; mol wt = molecular weight; mp = melting point; sl. = slightly; sol. = soluble; $[\alpha]_D^{20}$, $[\alpha]_D^{25}$ = specific optical rotation based on a sodium light wavelength (D) of 589 nm, at 20°C or 25°C. Figures in heavy brackets are reference numbers. Data in light brackets refer to the column heading in brackets.

Structure & Properties	Source [Targets]	Assay Methods	Principal Actions	Effects of Deficiency (−) & Excess (+)	Control of Secretion: Stimulated by (S), Inhibited by (I)
		Aldosterone [1] [2,4,7-14,16,18,19,27,29,31-35,37-40]			
1 $C_{21}H_{28}O_5$; in equilibrium be-	Zona glomerulosa of adrenal cortex;	Plasma assay: (i) Dou-ble isotope derivative	Participates in reg-ulation of renal	(−): Excessive loss of Na^+ in urine,	(S): Renin-angioten-sin II system (de-

[1] Synonyms: Electrocortin; 11β,21-Dihydroxy-18-oxopregn-4-ene-3,20-dione.

continued

Structure & Properties	Source [Targets]	Assay Methods	Principal Actions	Effects of Deficiency (−) & Excess (+)	Control of Secretion: Stimulated by (S), Inhibited by (I)
tween 11,18-hemiacetal & 18-aldehyde structures when in solution. Mol wt = 360; mp = 164°C; $[\alpha]_D^{20}$ in chloroform = +152.2°; absorption max = 240 nm; fluoresces at 560 nm in alkaline solution	plasma concentration, 5-15 ng/100 ml (35% free); acid-labile metabolite in urine, 5-19 μg/24 h. Synthesized in vivo from cholesterol through pregnenolone, progesterone, deoxycorticosterone, & 18-hydroxycorticosterone [Proximal & distal convoluted tubules of kidney; salivary glands; glands of intestinal tract; sweat glands]	dilution, using [^{14}C]-aldosterone as recovery indicator & [^{3}H]-acetic anhydride as esterifying agent; acetylated derivative quantified after extraction & multiple chromatographic separations. (ii) Radioimmunoassay, with or without preliminary chromatography. Urine assay: Extraction & purification of either acid-labile aldosterone-18-glucuronide or tetrahydro-aldosterone-3-glucuronide, with quantitation by fluorometric or photometric measurement, radioimmunoassay, or double isotope dilution Secretion rate: i.v. injection of [^{3}H]aldosterone followed by quantitation of aldosterone metabolite in a 24-hour urine collection	sodium reabsorption, intravascular volume, & blood pressure	dehydration, hypotension, hyponatremia, hyperkalemia, mild acidosis (+): Increased extracellular volume, increased plasma Na$^+$, hypokalemia (accompanied by glucose intolerance, renal concentrating defect), alkalosis, hypertension, suppression of plasma renin activity (I): Increased intravascular volume (negative feedback on renin-angiotensin system); decreased plasma K$^+$, increased plasma Na$^+$ to a lesser extent	creased renal perfusion leads to renin secretion by juxtoglomerular apparatus, renin cleaves angiotensin I from its substrate; angiotensin I is in turn converted to angiotensin II in the pulmonary vascular bed; angiotensin II stimulates aldosterone secretion and acts as a vasopressor; ACTH; increased plasma K$^+$. Prostaglandins may also stimulate aldosterone production.

Deoxycorticosterone [2]	[3-5,8-13,15,18,19,21,22,24,25,31-35,38-40]				
2	$C_{21}H_{30}O_3$. Mol wt = 330; mp = 141-142°C; $[\alpha]_D^{20}$ in ethanol = +178°; sol. in acetone, benzene, chloroform, other volatile solvents, vegetable oils; insol. in water	Adrenal cortex. Synthesized commercially from cholesterol, diosgenin [Proximal & distal convoluted tubules of kidney; salivary glands; glands of intestinal tract; sweat glands]	Double isotope derivative dilution; competitive protein binding; radioimmunoassay	Mineralocorticoid 1/20 as potent as aldosterone	(−): No syndrome described (+): Excessive plasma concentrations found in some hypertensives of the low-renin type; associated with hypertensive form of adrenal hyperplasia due to steroid 11β-monooxygenase [3] enzymatic defect	....

18-Hydroxy-11-deoxycorticosterone [4]	[20,23,26]				
3	$C_{21}H_{31}O_4$. Mol wt = 346.45; mp = 165-173°C; sol. in most organic solvents; insol. in water; forms aggregates in methylene chloride	Zona fasciculata of adrenal cortex [Proximal & distal convoluted tubules of kidney; salivary glands; glands of intestinal tract; sweat glands]	Gas-liquid chromatography, with electron capture detection; thin-layer chromatography, oxidation to γ-lactone of 18-hydroxy-11-deoxycorticosterone; radioimmunoassay	Has ~60% of mineralocorticoid activity of deoxycorticosterone	(−): No deficiency syndrome described (+): Can result in sodium retention & hypertension of the low-renin type. Associated with Cushing's disease involving bilateral adrenal hyperplasia.	(S): Principally stimulated by ACTH (I): Dexamethasone & other glucocorticoids which suppress ACTH

[2] Synonyms: Cortexone; Δ^4-Pregnen-21-ol-3,20-dione; DOC. [3] Synonym: 11-Hydroxylase. [4] Synonyms: 4-Pregnene-18,21-diol-3,20-dione; 18-OH-DOC.

continued

Structure & Properties	Source [Targets]	Assay Methods	Principal Actions	Effects of Deficiency (−) & Excess (+)	Control of Secretion: Stimulated by (S), Inhibited by (I)
Corticosterone [5] [4,8-10,12,13,18,19,24,28,31-36,38-40]					
4 $C_{21}H_{30}O_4$. Mol wt = 346; mp = 180-182°C; $[\alpha]_D^{20}$ in ethanol = +262°; sol. in organic solvents; sl. sol. in vegetable oils; very sl. sol. in water	Zona fasciculata of adrenal cortex through pregnenolone, progesterone, cholesterol. Synthesized in vitro from deoxycholic acid	Chemical assay of unconjugated steroids: Extraction with organic solvents; purification by paper, column, & gas-liquid chromatography; measurement by acid or alkali fluorescence; Porter-Silber reaction (phenylhydrazine); reduction of tetrazolium salts; double isotope dilution (see entry 1); competitive protein binding Chemical assay of conjugated steroids: Preliminary removal of unconjugated steroids by solvent extraction, followed by hydrolysis of conjugated steroids in aqueous phase by incubation with β-glucuronidase Determination by one of above methods	Action & regulation intermediate between those of the mineralocorticoids (aldosterone & deoxycorticosterone, entries 1 & 2), and those of the glucocorticoids (cortisone & hydrocortisone, entries 5 & 6)		
Cortisone [6] [4,8-10,12,13,15,18,19,21,22,31-35,38-40]					
5 Mol wt = 360; mp = 220-224°C; $[\alpha]_D^{20}$ in ethanol = +209°; sol. in acetone, benzene, chloroform, diethyl ether, vegetable oils; sl. sol. in water	Zona fasciculata of adrenal cortex. Synthesized in vivo from cholesterol through progesterone & hydrocortisone, in equilibrium with hydrocortisone; in vitro from squalene, cholesterol, pregnenolone, progesterone [Most cells, notably liver, striated muscles, kidneys, blood vessels, integument, bone marrow, lymphoid & adipose tissue, reticuloendothelial system, pancreas, & gastrointestinal mucosa]	Double isotope dilution, competitive protein binding Chemical assay: Porter-Silber reaction; m-dinitrobenzene reaction; fluorometric Bioassay (used for comparison of actions, especially for newly synthesized analogues): Life maintenance of adrenalectomized rats on limited salt & water diets; deposition of liver glycogen 1 hour after injection of sample into adrenalectomized, fasting mice or rats; granuloma formation in adrenalectomized rats treated with sample	Antagonistic to insulin Decreases: Nucleotide & protein synthesis in extrahepatic tissues; synthesis of triglycerides & other lipids (lipogenesis); extrahepatic synthesis of sulfated mucopolysaccharide; synthesis & activities of enzymes involved in oxidative catabolism of glucose Increases: Deamination of amino acids to glucose; activities of liver & kidney glucose-6-phosphatase, hexosediphosphatase [7],	(−): Asthenia; hemoconcentration; chronic Addison's disease; decreased blood glucose, liver glycogen, body wt, blood pressure & stress resistance; hyperpigmentation; emaciation; vomiting; diarrhea. In acute deficiency, hypotension, circulatory collapse; hypoglycemia, pyrexia. (+): Cushing's syndrome: abnormal distribution of fat; "buffalo hump"; moon face; truncal obesity, with thin extremities; negative N balance, unless insulin also high; osteoporosis; wasting of muscle; alkalosis; increased gastric acidity; adrenogenital syndrome; hypertension; inhibition of inflammatory repair of wounds & antibody formation	(S): Decreased plasma levels of glucocorticoids; stressful conditions of any kind (mediated by CRH & ACTH release) (I): Increased plasma levels of glucocorticoids—negative feedback through CRH & ACTH

pyruvate decarboxylase, glycogen synthase & arginase, liver pyruvate kinase & alkaline phosphatase, & muscle aminopeptidase; activities of liver tryptophan oxygenase, tyrosine aminotransferase, & other amino acid oxidases & aminotransferases, thereby increasing liver synthesis of protein from amino acids; lipolysis in adipose tissue; fatty acids in plasma; secretion of HCl & pepsinogen by gastric mucosa, and enzymes by pancreas

[5] Synonyms: 11β,21-Dihydroxypregn-4-ene-3,20-dione; Kendall's compound B. [6] Synonyms: Kendall's compound E; 17-Hydroxy-11-dehydrocorticosterone; 17α,21-Dihydroxypregn-4-ene-3,11,20-trione. [7] Synonym: Fructose diphosphatase.

continued

330

Structure & Properties	Source [Targets]	Assay Methods	Principal Actions	Effects of Deficiency (−) & Excess (+)	Control of Secretion: Stimulated by (S), Inhibited by (I)
Hydrocortisone [8] [4,8-10,12,13,15,18,19,21,22,31-35,38-40]					
6 $C_{21}H_{30}O_5$. Mol wt = 362; mp = 217-220°C; $[\alpha]_D^{20}$ in ethanol = +167°; sol. in chloroform, diethyl ether, vegetable oils; sl. sol. in water	Zona fasciculata of adrenal cortex. Synthesized in vivo from cholesterol through pregnenolone, 17α-hydroxyprogesterone, & 11-deoxycortisol. [Same as for entry 5]	Double isotope derivative dilution; competitive protein-binding method accurate & practical Radioimmunoassay methods available, and require smaller sample aliquots	Same as for entry 5	Same as for entry 5	Same as for entry 5
Epinephrine [9] [1,6,9,10,12,17-19,30,32-35,38-40]					
7 Mol wt = 183.2; mp of l-form = 211-212°C; $[\alpha]_D^{20}$ in dilute HCl = −50.72°; sol. in acid, alkali (with decomposition); sl. sol. in water; insol. in chloroform, ethanol, diethyl ether	Adrenal medulla. Synthesized in chromaffin cells or sympathetic neurons (l-form) from l-Tyr through DOPA & norepinephrine; commercially from pyrocatechol. [Sympathetic nervous system; striated, cardiac, & smooth muscle, especially in arterioles; cells producing enzymes involved in glycogenolysis & lipolysis; β-cells of islets of Langerhans. Epinephrine predominantly interacts with catecholamine β-receptors, & to some extent with α-receptors.]	Bioassay: Rise in blood pressure of specially prepared rats; inhibition of contractions in isolated rat uterus; infusion or perfusion of isolated organs, such as guinea pig heart or strips of rat stomach Chemical assay: Extraction & purification by adsorption on aluminum oxide & ion-exchange resins, and by paper chromatography, followed by determination by trihydroxyindole fluorescence, Na ascorbate, Na_2SO_3, K ferricyanide, or ethylenediamine; radioenzymatic assay, utilizing double isotope dilution, most commonly used for clinical purposes	Inhibits intestinal motility; relaxes bladder smooth muscle Stimulates: Catecholamine β-receptors & also α-receptors (cardiac stimulation & lipolysis mediated by β_1-receptors, while bronchodilation & vasodilation are β_2-mediated); CNS; synthesis & activity of adenylate cyclase, thereby increasing level of cAMP which in turn increases concentrations of α-glucan phosphorylase, thus increasing phosphorylation & hydrolysis of liver glycogen to glucose-1-phosphate; release of ACTH Decreases: Insulin secretion (pancreatic β-receptor stimulates insulin secretion, & α-receptor effect inhibits & predominates); activity of glycogen synthase; peripheral resistance; gastrointestinal movement Increases: Cardiac output, heart rate (β-effect), BMR, dilation of bronchi, blood vessels of liver & of striated & cardiac muscle; hyperglycemia following administration; cAMP (when insulin levels low) which activates lipases in adipose tissue, increasing free fatty acids in plasma	(−): No known clinical disease; associated with tuberculous Addison's disease (+): Pheochromocytoma; marked hypertension, pigmentation, tachycardia, headache, nausea, blanching of skin, sweating; increased blood levels of non-esterified fatty acids; α- and β-adrenergic activity	(S): Splanchnic impulses from sympathetic nervous system; stressful stimuli, e.g., trauma, exposure to low temp, hemorrhage, acute hypoxia, severe & prolonged exercise, emotional states such as fear or anger, or hypoglycemia (I): No known inhibitors or feedback mechanism
Norepinephrine ⟨Noradrenaline; L-Arterenol⟩ [1,6,9,10,12,17-19,20,32-35,38-40]					
8 Mol wt = 169.2; mp of l-form =	Adrenal medulla; various nerves, es-	Same as for entry 7 in all tests except	Decreases: Cardiac output	(−): No known clinical disease;	(S): Same as for entry 7

[8] Synonyms: Cortisol; 17-Hydroxycorticosterone; Kendall's compound F; 11β,17α,21-Trihydroxypregn-4-ene-3,20-dione.
[9] Synonyms: Adrenalin; Suprarenine; Adrenine.

continued

Structure & Properties	Source [Targets]	Assay Methods	Principal Actions	Effects of Deficiency (−) & Excess (+)	Control of Secretion: Stimulated by (S), Inhibited by (I)
216.5-218°C (with decomposition), of HCl salt of l-form = 146-147°C; $[\alpha]_D^{25}$ in dilute HCL = −37.3°; solubility same as for entry 7	pecially splanchnic; spleen, heart, & blood vessels [Acts on catecholamine α-receptors]	for pressor & contraction of gravid uterus	Increases: Blood pressure by vasoconstriction; BMR; blood glucose—moderate hyperglycemia following administration	associated with tuberculous Addison's disease (+): Pheochromocytoma; marked hypertension, pigmentation, tachycardia, headache, nausea, blanching of skin, sweating; increased blood levels of non-esterified fatty acids; principally α-adrenergic activity	(I): Unknown

Contributor: Re, Richard

References

1. Axelrod, J., and R. Tomchick. 1958. J. Biol. Chem. 233:702-705.
2. Bayard, F., et al. 1970. J. Clin. Endocrinol. 31:507-510.
3. Biglieri, E. G., et al. 1969. J. Clin. Endocrinol. Metab. 29:1090-1101.
4. Briggs, M. H., ed. 1970. Adv. Steroid Biochem. Pharmacol. 1.
5. Brown, J. J., et al. 1972. Lancet 2:243-246.
6. Coyle, J. T., and D. Henry. 1973. J. Neurochem. 21:61-67.
7. Edelman, I. S., and G. M. Fimognari. 1969. Recent Prog. Horm. Res. 24:1-44.
8. Eliel, L. P., et al. 1971. Pediatrics 47:229-238.
9. Escamilla, R. F., ed. 1971. Laboratory Tests in Diagnosis and Investigation of Endocrine Function. Ed. 2. F. A. Davis, Philadelphia.
10. Frieden, E., and H. Lipner. 1971. Biochemical Endocrinology of the Vertebrates. Prentice-Hall, Englewood Cliffs, NJ.
11. Glaz, E., and P. Vecsei. 1971. Aldosterone. Pergamon Press, New York.
12. Gray, C. H., and A. L. Bacharach, ed. 1967. Hormones in Blood. Ed. 2. Academic Press, New York. v. 2.
13. Heftmann, E. 1970. Steroid Biochemistry. Academic Press, New York.
14. Ito, T., et al. 1971. J. Clin. Endocrinol. 34:106-112.
15. James, V. H. T., ed. 1968. Recent Adv. Endocrinol. Ed. 8.
16. Kliman, B. 1965. Adv. Tracer Methodol. 2:213-220.
17. Levine, R. J., and L. Landsberg. 1974. In P. K. Bondy and L. E. Rosenberg, ed. Duncan's Diseases of Metabolism. Ed. 7. W. B. Saunders, Philadelphia. v. 2, pp. 1181-1224.
18. Litwack, G., ed. 1972. Biochemical Actions of Hormones. Ed. 2. Academic Press, New York. v. 1.
19. Loraine, J. A., and E. T. Bell. 1971. Hormone Assays and Their Clinical Application. Ed. 3. Williams and Wilkins, Baltimore.
20. Mason, P. A., and R. Fraser. 1975. J. Endocrinol. 64:277-288.
21. McKerns, K. W., ed. 1968. Functions of the Adrenal Cortex. Appleton-Century-Crofts, New York. v. 1 and 2.
22. McKerns, K. W. 1969. Steroid Hormones and Metabolism. Appleton-Century-Crofts, New York.
23. Melby, J. C., et al. 1971. Circ. Res. 28(Suppl. 2):143-152.
24. Murphy, B. E. P. 1970. Acta Endocrinol., Suppl. 147:37-60.
25. Oddie, C. J., et al. 1972. J. Clin. Endocrinol. Metab. 34:1039-1054.
26. Oliver, J. T., et al. 1973. Science 182:1249-1251.
27. Poulsen, K., et al. 1974. Clin. Immunol. Immunopathol. 2:373-380.
28. Prunty, F. T. G., and H. Gardiner-Hill, ed. 1972. Mod. Trends Endocrinol. 4.
29. St. Cyr, M. J., et al. 1972. Clin. Chem. 18:1395-1402.
30. Sawin, C. T. 1969. The Hormones: Endocrine Physiology. Little, Brown; Boston.
31. Schwartz, T. B., ed. 1968. Yearb. Endocrinol. 1967/1968.
32. Schwartz, T. B., ed. 1969. Ibid. 1969.
33. Schwartz, T. B., ed. 1970. Ibid. 1970.
34. Schwartz, T. B., ed. 1971. Ibid. 1971.
35. Schwartz, T. B., ed. 1972. Ibid. 1972.
36. Smellie, R. M. S., ed. 1971. The Biochemistry of Steroid Hormone Action. Academic Press, London.
37. Speckart, P., et al. 1975. Program Endocr. Soc. 57th Annu. Meet., p. 184(A).
38. Sunderman, F. W., and F. W. Sunderman, Jr. 1971. Laboratory Diagnosis of Endocrine Diseases. W. H. Green, St. Louis.
39. Turner, C. D., and J. T. Bagnara. 1976. General Endocrinology. Text ed. W. B. Saunders, Philadelphia.
40. Williams, R. H., ed. 1974. Textbook of Endocrinology. Ed. 5. W. B. Saunders, Philadelphia.

Abbreviations: ACTH = adrenocorticotropic hormone. Figures in heavy brackets are reference numbers.

Principal Signs & Symptoms	Pathophysiology	Diagnosis	Treatment
Cushing's Syndrome [1,3,4,8,9,13]			
1 Central obesity, "buffalo hump," "moon facies"; thin skin, oily, easy bruisability, purple striae, plethora, acne, hirsutism; hypertension, myopathy, osteoporosis, glucose intolerance	Results from excessive levels of circulating hydrocortisone [L/] (or other glucocorticoid) which in turn result from (i) hypersecretion of ACTH by the pituitary (Cushing's disease), leading to bilateral adrenal hyperplasia; (ii) adrenal cortical adenoma; (iii) nodular hyperplasia of adrenal glands; (iv) adrenal carcinoma; (v) ectopic secretion of ACTH by neoplasm; or (vi) ingestion of glucocorticoids. Excessive hydrocortisone [L/] produces all signs & symptoms; in addition, hypertension can result from high circulating concentrations of hydrocortisone [L/], and from mineralocorticoids released by the adrenal under stimulation by ACTH.	Characterized by failure to suppress plasma hydrocortisone [L/], urinary 17-hydroxysteroids, or urinary free hydrocortisone [L/] by administration of dexamethasone. Suppression after high- but not low-dose dexamethasone seen with Cushing's disease. Other forms of Cushing's syndrome generally not suppressed with high- or low-dose dexamethasone. Plasma ACTH elevated in Cushing's disease & ectopic ACTH production. Other forms of Cushing's syndrome can be distinguished by history, physical examinations, intravenous pyelogram, & adrenal vein catheterization. Responses to ACTH or metyrapone administration can be of value. A good outpatient screening test to exclude Cushing's syndrome is 1 mg dexamethasone at midnight followed by plasma hydrocortisone [L/] determination at 0800 (normal level: <5 μg/dl).	(i) Pituitary hypersecretion of ACTH can be treated with pituitary irradiation (X ray, proton beam), radioactive implants, or pituitary surgery. If adrenalectomy is performed for therapy of Cushing's disease, Nelson's syndrome (pituitary tumor & hyperpigmentation) can occur in some cases as a late result. (ii) Adrenal adenomas, adrenal carcinoma, bilateral nodular hyperplasia can be treated with adrenal surgery. Bilateral nodular hyperplasia may also require therapy directed toward the pituitary. Adrenal carcinoma may require additional therapy with inhibitors of adrenal steroidogenesis or with the adrenal toxin 1,1-dichloro-2-(o-chlorophenyl)-2-(p-chlorophenyl)-ethane ⟨o-p'-DDD⟩.
Addison's Disease [2,9]			
2 Weakness, weight loss, hyperpigmentation, salt craving, hypotension, hyponatremia, hyperkalemia, hypoglycemia, pyrexia, abdominal cramps	Destruction of adrenal glands by autoimmune mechanisms, tuberculosis, hemorrhage, granulomatous disease, or surgery leads to deficiency of hydrocortisone [L/] (glucocorticoid activity), aldosterone (mineralocorticoid activity), & adrenal medullary epinephrine	Low plasma hydrocortisone [L/] during stress is suggestive, but diagnosis must be confirmed by demonstrating subnormal responsiveness of plasma hydrocortisone [L/] & urinary steroids to exogenous ACTH infusion	Administration of glucocorticoid (usually cortisone); large dose in A.M., smaller in P.M. Often fludrocortisone ⟨Florinef⟩ must be administered to provide mineralocorticoid activity.
Hyperaldosteronism [5,6]			
3 Hypertension, alkalosis, high normal serum sodium, hypokalemia. Hypokalemia may be associated with glucose intolerance, renal con-	Hypersecretion of aldosterone by adrenal adenoma (very rarely a carcinoma), or by bilaterally hyperplastic adrenal glands, results in renal sodium retention, kaliuresis, & hydro-	(i) Hypernatremia, hypokalemia, alkalosis, urinary potassium wasting; (ii) elevated plasma aldosterone, aldosterone excretory rate, or aldosterone secretory rate which is	Adrenal adenoma best treated by surgical removal of adenoma. Bilateral hyperplasia best treated with the aldosterone antagonist spironolactone, diuretics, & antihyper-

[L/] Synonym: Cortisol.

continued

	Principal Signs & Symptoms	Pathophysiology	Diagnosis	Treatment
	centrating defects & polyuria, weakness, cardiac arrhythmias. Low salivary Na$^+$/K$^+$ ratios are also seen.	gen ion loss. Sodium retention results in hypertension.	not suppressed by sodium loading; (iii) suppressed & poorly stimulatable plasma renin activity	tensive agents, since surgery can correct electrolyte abnormalities but often does not benefit hypertension.
	Isolated Hypoaldosteronism [10,12,14]			
4	Hypotension, hyperkalemia	Deficient production of aldosterone leads to urinary sodium loss, dehydration, hyperkalemia, & postural hypotension. Isolated deficiency of aldosterone can result from enzymatic defect in aldosterone production (usually in infancy), or from hyposecretion of renin (usually in older patients with some abnormality of renal function).	....	Fludrocortisone
	Pheochromocytoma [7,11]			
5	Hypertension, fixed or paroxysmal; headache; excessive sweating; orthostatic hypotension; palpitation; tremor; elevated hematocrit; hyperglycemia; fever	Hypersecretion of epinephrine & norepinephrine by adrenal medullary tumors (usually benign) or by extra-adrenal chromaffin tissue. Can be sporadic or familial; can be associated with multiple endocrine neoplasia syndrome type II, with the mucosal neuroma syndrome, & with phakomatosis.	Elevated concentrations of catecholamines or their metabolites (4-hydroxy-3-methoxymandelic acid[2]; metanephrine) in urine. Provocative tests (e.g., tyramine infusion) or blocking tests (phentolamine) are not much used.	Adrenergic blockade (phenoxybenzamine and, if needed, propranolol) followed by surgical removal of tumor

[2] Synonyms: Vanillyl-mandelic acid; VMA.

Contributor: Re, Richard

References

1. Besser, G. M., and T. London. 1968. Br. Med. J. 4: 552-554.
2. Christy, N. P., ed. 1971. The Human Adrenal Cortex. Harper and Row, New York.
3. Connolly, C. K., et al. 1968. Br. Med. J. 2:665-667.
4. Federman, D. D. 1967. Hosp. Pract. 2(4):60-65.
5. Horton, R. 1973. Metabolism 22:1525-1545.
6. Kaplan, N. M. 1973. Clinical Hypertension. Medcom Press, New York. pp. 243-271.
7. Levine, R. J., and L. Landsberg. 1974. In P. K. Bondy and L. E. Rosenberg, ed. Duncan's Diseases of Metabolism. Ed. 7. W. B. Saunders, Philadelphia. v. 2, pp. 1203-1224.
8. Liddle, G. W. 1960. J. Clin. Endocrinol. 20:1539-1560.
9. Liddle, G. W. 1974. In R. H. Williams, ed. Textbook of Endocrinology. Ed. 5. W. B. Saunders, Philadelphia. pp. 233-283.
10. Michelis, M. F., and H. V. Murdaugh. 1975. Am. J. Med. 59:1-5.
11. Ross, E. J., et al. 1967. Br. Med. J. 1:191-198.
12. Schambelan, M., et al. 1972. N. Engl. J. Med. 287: 573-578.
13. Tyler, F., and C. D. West. 1972. Am. J. Med. 53:664-672.
14. Ulick, S. 1976. J. Clin. Endocrinol. Metab. 43:92-96.

Abbreviations: Absorption max = wavelength of maximal absorbancy; BMR = basal metabolic rate; cAMP = cyclic adenosine 3′,5′-monophosphate; DNA = deoxyribonucleic acid; insol. = insoluble; mol wt = molecular weight; mp = melting point; mRNA = messenger ribonucleic acid; sl. = slightly; sol. = soluble; $[\alpha]_D$ = specific optical rotation based on a sodium light wavelength (D) of 589 nm. Data in light brackets refer to the column heading in brackets.

Testosterone ⟨Δ⁴-Androsten-17β-ol-3-one⟩					
Structure & Properties	Source [Targets]	Assay Methods	Principal Actions	Effects of Deficiency (−) & Excess (+)	Control of Secretion: Stimulated by (S), Inhibited by (I)
$C_{19}H_{28}O_2$. Mol wt = 288; mp = 155-156°C; $[\alpha]_D$ in ethanol = +109°; absorption max = 238 nm; sol. in ethanol, diethyl ether, volatile solvents; sl. sol. in vegetable oils; insol. in water	Leydig ⟨interstitial⟩ cells of testis; plasma Main pathway for peripheral conversion— from acetate through cholesterol, pregnenolone, progesterone, & androstenedione— from adrenal cortex (dehydroepiandrosterone is main cortical C_{19}-steroid) [All ♂ sex organs; anterior pituitary; muscle; hair follicles; epiphyses of long bones; vocal cords]	Bioassay: Increase in comb size of castrated cock (capon); blackening of bill of English sparrow (Pfeiffer's test); increase in weight in seminal vesicles of castrated ♂ rat (Mathieson & Hays test) Chemical assay (plasma): [³⁵S]thiosemicarbazide; thin-layer chromatographic purification of doubly labeled (¹⁴C-ring & [³H]acetate ester) testosterone; measurement of [³H]testosterone chloroacetate by gas-liquid chromatography & electron capture Chemical assay (urine): Extraction with diethyl ether & measurement by gas-liquid chromatography; scintillation counting of [³H, ¹⁴C]testosterone Radioimmunoassay (plasma): Antibodies raised to testosterone conjugates are reactive to testosterone, with limited 30% cross-reactivity to stanolone ⟨5α-dihydrotestosterone⟩; extraction with diethyl ether or methylene chloride; dried residue combined with antibody & [³H]testosterone tracer; liquid scintillation counting of ³H with comparison to standard assay curve, expressed as ng/dl Radioimmunoassay (urine): Glucuronidase hydrolysis, extraction of released testosterone. Assay as for plasma, with results expressed as μg/24 hours.	Androgenic; little effect on weight of heart, urinary bladder; produces positive balances of Ca, N, P, K, & S Inhibits: Growth of thymus, adrenals Decreases: Folliculoid & luteoid activity in immature ♀; amino acid catabolism; creatinuria; Na⁺ & Cl⁻ excretion; kidney alkaline phosphatase Increases: Development of ♂ secondary sex organs & sex characteristics; libido; BMR; protein anabolism by DNA-based stimulation of mRNA synthesis; amino acid transport in striated muscle; amino acid incorporation & activities of D-amino acid oxidase, arginase, acid phosphatase, & β-glucuronidase in kidney cortex; renal transport of Na⁺ & K⁺; rate of synthesis of fatty acids, citrate, & fructose in seminal vesicles; respiration rate in seminal vesicles & prostate	(−): Immaturity or atrophy of accessory sex organs; lack of secondary sex characteristics & ♂ behavior patterns; poor muscle development & function; delayed closure of epiphyses; decreased excretion of 17-ketosteroids in urine; functional decrease with age; deficiency effects more pronounced before puberty than after (+): Precocious sex development; hypertrophy of ♂ accessory sex organs; increased muscle mass; increased skeletal growth until epiphyseal closure; increased excretion of 17-ketosteroids in urine; decreased scalp hair; increased hirsutism. Effects mediated via testosterone in kidney & muscle, & via stanolone in other tissues	(S): Luteinizing hormone ⟨LH⟩, mediated through activation of Leydig cell membrane receptors & stimulation of adenylate cyclase system, resulting in cAMP formation & subsequent stimulation of steroid biosynthesis (I): High levels of testosterone—negative feedback through LH

continued

156. MALE REPRODUCTIVE HORMONE

Contributor: Kliman, Bernard

General References

1. Briggs, M. H., ed. 1970. Adv. Steroid Biochem. Pharmacol. 1.
2. Chen, J. C., et al. 1971. Clin. Chem. 17:581-584.
3. Eik-Nes, K. B. 1971. Recent Prog. Horm. Res. 27: 517-535.
4. Escamilla, R. F., ed. 1971. Laboratory Tests in Diagnosis and Investigation of Endocrine Function. Ed. 2. F. A. Davis, Philadelphia.
5. Frieden, E., and H. Lipner. 1971. Biochemical Endocrinology of the Vertebrates. Prentice-Hall, Englewood Cliffs, NJ.
6. Gray, C. H., and A. L. Bacharach, ed. 1967. Hormones in Blood. Ed. 2. Academic Press, New York. v. 2.
7. Heftmann, E. 1970. Steroid Biochemistry. Academic Press, New York.
8. Judd, H. L., et al. 1974. J. Clin. Endocrinol. Metab. 38:134-141.
9. Litwack, G., ed. 1972. Biochemical Actions of Hormones. Ed. 2. Academic Press, New York. v. 1.
10. Loraine, J. A., and E. T. Bell. 1971. Hormone Assays and Their Clinical Application. Ed. 3. Williams and Wilkins, Baltimore.
11. McKerns, K. W. 1969. Steroid Hormones and Metabolism. Appleton-Century-Crofts, New York.
12. McKerns, K. W. 1971. The Sex Steroids: Molecular Mechanism. Appleton-Century-Crofts, New York.
13. Prunty, F. T. G., and H. Gardiner-Hill, ed. 1972. Mod. Trends Endocrinol. 4.
14. Sawin, C. T. 1969. The Hormones: Endocrine Physiology. Little, Brown; Boston.
15. Schwartz, T. B., ed. 1969. Yearb. Endocrinol. 1969.
16. Schwartz, T. B., ed. 1970. Ibid. 1970.
17. Schwartz, T. B., ed. 1971. Ibid. 1971.
18. Schwartz, T. B., ed. 1972. Ibid. 1972.
19. Stollerman, G. H., ed. 1970. Adv. Intern. Med. 16.
20. Sunderman, F. W., and F. W. Sunderman, Jr. 1971. Laboratory Diagnosis of Endocrine Diseases. W. H. Green, St. Louis.
21. Turner, C. D., and J. T. Bagnara. 1976. General Endocrinology. Text ed. W. B. Saunders, Philadelphia.
22. Williams, R. H., ed. 1974. Textbook of Endocrinology. Ed. 5. W. B. Saunders, Philadelphia.
23. Wilson, J. D. 1972. N. Engl. J. Med. 287:1284-1291.

157. DISORDERS OF MALE REPRODUCTIVE SYSTEM

Figures in heavy brackets are reference numbers.

Part I. Defects of the Hypothalamus

	Principal Signs & Symptoms	Pathophysiology	Genetics	Treatment
	Kallmann's Syndrome [3,4,9-11]			
1	Hypogonadotropic hypogonadism with anosmia	Partial or complete deficiency of gonadotropin-releasing hormone	Unclear; most compatible with autosomal dominant pattern	Clomiphene if defect is partial; gonadotropin-releasing hormone or one of its analogues; testosterone for androgenization; gonadotropins for fertility
	Familial Gonadotropin Deficiency [1/] [1,2,9,10,12]			
2	Hypogonadotropic hypogonadism	Partial or complete deficiency of gonadotropin-releasing hormone	Autosomal recessive	Gonadotropin-releasing hormone or an analogue [7]; testosterone for androgenization; gonadotropins for fertility
	Prader-Labhart-Willi Syndrome [6,10]			
3	Hypogonadotropic hypogonadism; obesity; mental retardation; diabetes; short stature	Partial or complete deficiency of gonadotropin-releasing hormone	Sporadic (rare condition which may or may not be due to a genetic inheritance, e.g., autosomal recessive; most likely a single, random mutation)	Dependent somewhat on degree of mental retardation. Clomiphene and/or luteinizing hormone—releasing hormone or its analogues; testosterone for androgenization; gonadotropins for fertility.

1/ *See also* entry 1, **Part II.**

continued

157. DISORDERS OF MALE REPRODUCTIVE SYSTEM

Part I. Defects of the Hypothalamus

Principal Signs & Symptoms	Pathophysiology	Genetics	Treatment
Laurence-Moon-Biedl Syndrome [5,8,10]			
4 Hypogonadotropic hypogonadism; retinitis pigmentosa; obesity; mental retardation; polydactyly	Partial or complete deficiency of gonadotropin-releasing hormone	Autosomal recessive	Dependent somewhat on degree of retardation

Contributor: Crowley, William F., Jr.

References
1. Biben, R. L., and G. S. Gordan. 1955. J. Clin. Endocrinol. Metab. 15:931-942.
2. Ewer, R. W. 1968. J. Clin. Endocrinol. Metab. 28: 783-788.
3. Hamilton, C. R., et al. 1973. Ann. Int. Med. 78:47-55.
4. Kallmann, F. J., et al. 1944. Am. J. Ment. Defic. 48: 203-236.
5. Laurence, J. Z., and R. C. Moon. 1866. Ophthal. Rev. 2:32-52.
6. McGuffin, W. L., and A. D. Rogol. 1975. J. Clin. Endocrinol. Metab. 41:325-331.
7. Mortimer, C. H., et al. 1974. Br. Med. J. 4:617-621.
8. Reinfrank, R. F., and F. L. Nichols. 1964. J. Clin. Endocrinol. Metab. 24:48-53.
9. Reitano, J. F., et al. 1975. J. Clin. Endocrinol. Metab. 41:1035-1042.
10. Rimoin, D. L., and R. N. Schimke. 1971. Genetic Disorders of the Endocrine Glands. C. V. Mosby, St. Louis.
11. Santen, R. J., and C. A. Paulsen. 1973. J. Clin. Endocrinol. Metab. 36:47-54.
12. Spitz, I. M., et al. 1974. N. Engl. J. Med. 290:10-15.

Part II. Pituitary Defects

Abbreviations: LH = luteinizing hormone; FSH = follicle-stimulating hormone.

Principal Signs & Symptoms	Pathophysiology	Genetics	Treatment
Familial Gonadotropin Deficiencies[1/] [1,2,4,5]			
1 Hypogonadotropic hypogonadism	Deficiency of LH & FSH	Autosomal recessive	Exogenous gonadotropins if fertility desired; testosterone replacement for virilization
Isolated LH Deficiency[2/] [3]			
2 Eunuchoidism in presence of spermatogenesis	Deficiency of LH resulting in defective virilization	Sporadic (rare condition which may or may not be due to a genetic inheritance, e.g., autosomal recessive. Most likely a single, random mutation.)	Human chorionic gonadotropin administration or testosterone replacement
Panhypopituitarism [4]			
3 Hypogonadotropic hypogonadism	Deficiency of LH & FSH, with either isolated growth hormone deficiency, or with defects in all other anterior pituitary functions	Autosomal recessive; sporadic (rare condition which may or may not be due to a genetic inheritance. Most likely a single, random mutation.)	Exogenous gonadotropins if fertility desired; testosterone therapy for virilization

[1/] *See also* entry 2, **Part I.** [2/] Synonym: "Fertile eunuch syndrome."

continued

157. DISORDERS OF MALE REPRODUCTIVE SYSTEM

Part II. Pituitary Defects

Contributor: Crowley, William F., Jr.

References

1. Biben, R. L., and G. S. Gordan. 1955. J. Clin. Endocrinol. Metab. 15:931-942.
2. Ewer, R. W. 1968. Ibid. 28:783-788.
3. Faiman, C., et al. 1968. Mayo Clin. Proc. 43:661-667.
4. Rimoin, D. L., and R. N. Schimke. 1971. Genetic Disorders of the Endocrine Glands. C. V. Mosby, St. Louis.
5. Spitz, I. M., et al. 1974. N. Engl. J. Med. 290:10-15.

Part III. Defects of Androgen Metabolism

	Principal Signs & Symptoms	Pathophysiology	Genetics	Treatment
	Congenital Adrenal Lipoid Hyperplasia [7,10]			
1	Phenotypic ♀, Addisonian crises in neonatal period	Defects of cholesterol side-chain cleavage enzyme (adrenal gland & testes)	Autosomal recessive	Glucocorticoid & mineralocorticoid replacement
	Cholesterol 17,20-Lyase Deficiency [14]			
2	Ambiguous external genitalia (usually ♀ escutcheon); inguinal or intra-abdominal testes; hypospadias	Partial deficiency of cholesterol 17,20-lyase (adrenal gland & testes)	♂-limited autosomal dominant or X-linked recessive	Surgery of external genitals after decision as to sexual assignment; glucocorticoid replacement if evidence of hydrocortisone[1/] deficiency
	3β-Hydroxysteroid Dehydrogenase Deficiency [1,9]			
3	Incomplete virilization; hypospadias, mild to severe (perineoscrotal); Addisonian crises (usually, but not invariably); gynecomastia at puberty	Partial deficiency of 3β-hydroxysteroid dehydrogenase (adrenal gland & testes)	Autosomal recessive	Glucocorticoid & mineralocorticoid replacement therapy; surgical correction of external genitals after decision as to sexual assignment
	17-Ketosteroid Reductase Deficiency [3,4,11,12]			
4	Ambiguous external genitalia; ♀ body habitus; gynecomastia (usually); virilization at puberty	Partial deficiency of 17-ketosteroid reductase (in testes only)	Autosomal recessive	Surgical correction of external genitals after decision as to sexual assignment
	Steroid 17α-Hydroxylase Deficiency [2]			
5	Incomplete virilization (usually ♀ escutcheon)	Deficiency of steroid 17α-hydroxylase (adrenal gland & testes); hypokalemic alkalosis; hypertension	Autosomal recessive	Glucocorticoid replacement
	Male Pseudohermaphroditism Type II[2/] [5,6,8,13]			
6	Ambiguous external genitalia; pubertal virilization; no gynecomastia	Steroid 5α-reductase deficiency	Autosomal recessive	Genital surgery depending on sexual assignment

[1/] Synonym: Cortisol. [2/] Synonym: Pseudovaginal perineoscrotal hypospadias.

Contributor: Crowley, William F., Jr.

References

1. Bongiovanni, E. M. 1964. J. Clin. Invest. 41:2086-2192.
2. Bricaire, H., et al. 1972. J. Clin. Endocrinol. Metab. 35:67-72.

continued

Part III. Defects of Androgen Metabolism

3. Givens, J. R., et al. 1974. N. Engl. J. Med. 291:938-944.
4. Goebelsmann, U., et al. 1972. J. Clin. Endocrinol. Metab. 36:867-879.
5. Imperato-McGinley, J., and R. E. Peterson. 1976. Am. J. Med. 61:251-272.
6. Imperato-McGinley, J., et al. 1974. Science 186:1213-1215.
7. Kirkland, R. T., et al. 1973. J. Clin. Endocrinol. Metab. 36:488-496.
8. Opitz, J. M., et al. 1971. Clin. Genet. 3:1-26.
9. Parks, E. S., et al. 1971. J. Clin. Endocrinol. Metab. 33:269-278.
10. Rimoin, D. L., and R. N. Schimke. 1971. Genetic Disorders of the Endocrine Glands. C. V. Mosby, St. Louis.
11. Saez, J. M., et al. 1971. J. Clin. Endocrinol. Metab. 32:604-610.
12. Saez, J. M., et al. 1972. Ibid. 34:598-600.
13. Walsh, P. C., et al. 1974. N. Engl. J. Med. 291:944-949.
14. Zachman, M., et al. 1972. Clin. Endocrinol. 1:369-385.

Part IV. Peripheral Target Organ Defects

Principal Signs & Symptoms	Pathophysiology	Genetics	Treatment
Complete Testicular Feminization [1,3,4,8]			
1 ♀ body habitus; scant axillary & pubic hair; no Müllerian structures; intra-abdominal testes; gonadoblastomas	Defect of androgen binding to its cytosol receptor, or failure of testosterone receptor complex to effect protein synthesis	X-linked recessive	Castration; estrogen replacement
Incomplete Testicular Feminization [3,5,7]			
2 ♀ body habitus with some degree of virilization; absent Müllerian structures; variable degree of axillary & pubic hair; intra-abdominal testes; gonadoblastomas	Partial defect of androgen effect upon peripheral target organs (see entry 1)	Sporadic (rare condition which may or may not be due to a genetic inheritance, e.g., autosomal recessive. Most likely a single, random mutation)	Castration; estrogen replacement
Male Pseudohermaphroditism Type I [1/] [2,5-7,9-12]			
3 Variable degree of virilization from Lubs syndrome (♀ escutcheon) to Rosewater's syndrome (familial gynecomastia in otherwise normal ♂); infertility; gynecomastia	Partial defect of androgen effect upon peripheral target organs (see entry 1)	X-linked recessive	Genital surgery depending on sexual assignment

1/ Includes: Lubs syndrome, Gilbert-Dreyfus syndrome, Reifenstein syndrome, and Rosewater's syndrome.

Contributor: Crowley, William F., Jr.

References
1. Amrhein, J. A., et al. 1976. Proc. Natl. Acad. Sci. USA 73:891-894.
2. Bowen, P., et al. 1965. Ann. Intern. Med. 62:252-270.
3. Crawford, J. D. 1970. Clin. Pediatr. 9:167-170.
4. Faiman, C., and J. S. D. Winter. 1974. J. Clin. Endocrinol. Metab. 39:631-639.
5. Federman, D. D. 1968. Abnormal Sexual Development. W. B. Saunders, Philadelphia.
6. Gilbert-Dreyfus, S., et al. 1957. Ann. Endocrinol. (Paris) 18:93-101.
7. Imperato-McGinley, J., and R. E. Peterson. 1976. Am. J. Med. 61:251-272.
8. Judd, H. L., et al. 1972. J. Clin. Endocrinol. Metab. 34:229-237.
9. Lubs, H. A., et al. 1959. Ibid. 19:1110-1120.
10. Reifenstein, E. C., Jr. 1947. Proc. Am. Fed. Clin. Res. 3:86.
11. Rosewater, S., et al. 1965. Ann. Intern. Med. 63:377-385.
12. Wilson, J. D., et al. 1974. N. Engl. J. Med. 290:1097-1103.

Abbreviations & Symbols: $[\alpha]_D$ = specific optical rotation based on a sodium light (D) wavelength of 589 nm; BSA = bovine serum albumin; CHO = carbohydrate; FSH = follicle-stimulating hormone; GH = growth hormone; GI = gastro-intestinal; insol. = insoluble; LH = luteinizing hormone; LH-RH = luteinizing hormone—releasing hormone; λ_{max} = wavelength of maximal absorbancy; mp = melting point; pI = isoelectric point; sl. = slightly; sol. = soluble; TRH = thyrotropin-releasing hormone; TSH = thyrotropin; UV = ultraviolet. Data in light brackets refer to the column heading in brackets. Figures in heavy brackets are reference numbers.

Structure & Properties	Sources [Targets]	Assay Methods	Principal Actions	Effects of Deficiency (−) & Excess (+)	Control of Secretion: Stimulated by (S), Inhibited by (I)
			Estradiol[1] [1]		
1 $C_{18}H_{24}O_2$. Mol wt = 272; mp = 174-176°C; $[\alpha]_D$ in dioxane = +76°; λ_{max} = 281 nm; sol. in alkali, volatile solvents; sl. sol. in vegetable oils; insol. in water. [18]	Ovaries; placenta; adrenal cortex (♂♀); testes; blood & urine (♂♀). Synthesized in vivo from acetate through cholesterol, pregnenolone, testosterone, & intermediates; synthesized in vitro from cholesterol. [44,47-49, 61] [All ♀ sex organs; mammary glands; mucous membranes; hypothalamus; anterior pituitary; osteoblasts; tumors of breast & endometrium; spermatozoa [8,9]]	Bioassay: Cornified epithelial cells in vaginal smear from castrated ♀ rats & mice. Increase in uterine wt in immature rats or mice. Vaginal opening of intact immature animals. Enlargement of oviduct in chickens. Increased mitotic figures in vaginal smear from castrated ♀ mice. [40] Chemical assay: Splitting of protein bond by boiling with dilute HCl or heating with 0.1 N NaOH over steam bath. Hydrolysis of conjugates by concentrated HCl or enzymes (sulfatases, glucuronidases). Extraction with diethyl ether, drying, and partition between aqueous NaOH & organic solvent phases. Chromatographic separation by paper partition, column adsorption, thin layer, ion-exchange, countercurrent distribution, column, or gas-liquid chromatography. Colorimetric estimation (quinol-sulfuric acid). Fluorometric estimation (phosphoric acid, sulfuric acid). Enzy-	Estrogenic; antagonizes androgen effects. Development & maintenance of ♀ sex organs & secondary sex characteristics. Maintenance of menstrual cycle & pregnancy. Mild vasodilator. Slows growth of skeleton. Affects: Maturation of hypothalamus; hypothalamic releasing hormones (LH-RH, TRH); pituitary secretion of hormones (LH, FSH, GH). Plasma proteins (transcortin, thyroxine-binding globulin, steroid-binding β-globulin[2]). Cholesterol levels (decreases). Growth & development of breast & uterus. Endometrial proliferation & vaginal mucosa. Promotes: Epiphyseal closure Stimulates: Enzymes (isocitrate dehydrogenase, monophenol monooxygenase[3], peroxidase, transhydrogenases) in placenta. Calcification of bones (moderately). Peripheral circulation. Decreases: Erythrocyte P uptake. Plasma	(−): Immaturity or atrophy of accessory sex organs. Lack of secondary ♀ sex characteristics & behavior patterns. Decreased mammary gland development. Delayed epiphyseal closure and continued growth of long bones. Osteoporosis. Hot flashes; increased emotionality. (+): Precocious maturity. Hypertrophy of secondary ♀ sex organs & mammary glands. Cystic hyperplasia of endometrium. Blocking of ovulation. Skeletal growth deceleration; excessive calcification of tissues if parathyroids are normal.	(S): Combined FSH & LH; cyclic changes in blood levels with menstrual periods (I): Increased level of estradiol, which inhibits FSH & LH production

[1] Synonyms: Estradiol-17β; Estra-1,3,5(10)-triene-3,17β-diol; Dihydroestrone. [2] Synonym: Sex-steroid-binding globulin. [3] Synonym: Phenolase.

continued

	Structure & Properties	Sources [Targets]	Assay Methods	Principal Actions	Effects of Deficiency (−) & Excess (+)	Control of Secretion: Stimulated by (S), Inhibited by (I)
			mic estimation (hydroxysteroid dehydrogenase). [40] Isotope dilution: Using [^{3}H]estrogen or [^{14}C]estrogen standards, or formation of radioactive derivatives with [^{14}C]acetic anhydride or [^{3}H]acetic anhydride. [40] Radioimmunoassay: Plasma extracted with fresh diethyl ether and separated with column chromatography; fraction containing estradiol incubated with anti-estradiol antibodies (generated in sheep to estradiol hemisuccinate coupled to BSA & polymerized using ethyl chloroformate) & [^{3}H]estradiol [2,33,40]	cholesterol; β-lipoproteins. Increases: Mammary gland duct development; uterine motility; growth of uterine (fallopian) tubes, axillary & pubic hair (♀), & all secondary ♀ sex organs. Tissue growth & cell division. Uterine uptake of Na^+, K^+, glucose, & water; endometrial alkaline phosphatase & glycogen; vaginal glycogen; protein anabolism in uterus by stimulation of RNA nucleotidyltransferase [4] & serine hydroxymethyltransferase synthesis. Retention of Ca^{2+}, Na^+, & water. Phospholipid, RNA, & protein synthesis. [14, 15,53]		

Estrone [5] [3,5,16]

	Structure & Properties	Sources [Targets]	Assay Methods	Principal Actions	Effects of Deficiency (−) & Excess (+)	Control of Secretion: Stimulated by (S), Inhibited by (I)
2	$C_{18}H_{22}O_2$. Mol wt = 270; mp = 260°C; $[\alpha]_D$ in chloroform or dioxane = +160°; sol. in alkali, volatile solvents; sl. sol. in vegetable oils; very sl. sol. in water. [18, 40,44]	Adrenal cortex; ovary; urine. Synthesized in vivo from cholesterol. [47-49, 51,61] [Same as for entry 1]	Same as for entry 1	Same as for entry 1	Same as for entry 1	Same as for entry 1

Estriol [6] [1]

	Structure & Properties	Sources [Targets]	Assay Methods	Principal Actions	Effects of Deficiency (−) & Excess (+)	Control of Secretion: Stimulated by (S), Inhibited by (I)
3	$C_{18}H_{24}O_3$. Mol wt = 288; mp = 282°C; $[\alpha]_D$ in dioxane = +53° to +63°; sol. in alkali, volatile solvents; sl. sol. in vegetable oils; insol. in water. [18]	Post-menopausal ovary; menstruating, early luteal phase ovary; human placenta; urine of pregnant women. Synthesized from estrone & estradiol. [29, 32,46,51,61] [Same as for entry 1, but estriol is a weaker es-	Bioassay, chemical assay, & isotope dilution, all same as for entry 1 Radioimmunoassay: Plasma extracted with diethyl ether, and incubated with radio-labeled estriol & rabbit antiserum (against estriol-3-O-carboxymethyl ether complexed to BSA). Separation of bound & free	Causes greater elasticity of vaginal structures and improvement in epithelial texture. Does not cause endometrial proliferation & bleeding. Stimulates: Cervical, vaginal, & vulvar cornification; mitotic activity; ovarian growth; body wt. Phospholipid, RNA, & protein synthesis. Imbibition	(−): None known in non-pregnant human. During pregnancy when urinary or plasma concentrations decrease, fetal distress is suspected. Fetal adrenal gland provides estriol conjugates which are converted to free es-	(S): FSH & LH during menstrual cycles & pregnancy (I): During gestation, decreased fetal adrenal function, decreased LH & FSH or degeneration of corpora lutea in menstrual cycles

---

[4] Synonym: RNA polymerase. [5] Synonyms: Ketohydroxyestrin; $\Delta^{1,3,5:10}$-Estratrien-3-ol-17-one. [6] Synonyms: Trihydroxyestrin; $\Delta^{1,3,5:10}$-Estratriene-3,16α,17β-triol.

continued

Structure & Properties	Sources [Targets]	Assay Methods	Principal Actions	Effects of Deficiency (−) & Excess (+)	Control of Secretion: Stimulated by (S), Inhibited by (I)
	trogen in terms of cellular growth & replication promotion. Mainly cervix, vagina & vulva. [15,32]]	by means of dextran-coated charcoal. [8]	of uterine fluid. Phagocytosis of carbon by reticuloendothelial cells. [8] Decreases: Post-menopausal symptoms, dysmenorrhea; NADH oxidase [7] activity in uterus; uterine motility	triol by placenta. [24] (+): None known in non-pregnant or pregnant women [24]	

Progesterone [8] [1]

4	$C_{21}H_{30}O_2$. Mol wt = 314; mp of α-form = 128°C, of β-form = 121°C; $[\alpha]_D$ in dioxane = +172° to +182°; λ_{max} = 240 nm; sol. in volatile solvents; sl. sol. in vegetable oils; insol. in water. [18]	Follicle, corpus luteum, stromal tissue of ovary; placenta; adrenal cortex; testes. Synthesized in vivo from cholesterol through pregnenolone; in vitro from acetate. [3,17,23, 44,48,49] [Uterus (endometrium & myometrium); uterine ⟨fallopian⟩ tubes; lobules & alveoli of mammary gland; kidney tubules; anterior pituitary; hypothalamus; spermatozoa [30]]	Bioassay: Proliferation of endometrium after injection of unknown extract into isolated segment of uterine horn of immature female rabbits [31]. Hypertrophy of stromal nuclei of endometrium of ovariectomized mice after intra-uterine injection [25]. Increase in endometrial carbonate dehydratase [9] in immature female rabbits [42]. Maintenance of pregnancy in spayed rats & mice [58]. Implantation in ovariectomized rabbits [43]. Physicochemical assays: UV absorption by progesterone at 240 nm. Dinitrophenylhydrazone, isonicotinic acid hydrazide, or thiosemicarbazide derivative formation and spectrophotometric measurements with Allen's procedure to correct for interference. KOH-H_2SO_4 fluorescence.	Negative feedback on hypothalamus suppresses LH-RH stimulation of LH at pituitary. Luteinizing effect—affecting preparation of endometrium for implantation of zygote; proliferation of decidual tissue or placenta. Antagonistic to aldosterone, promoting excretion of Na^+, Cl^-, & water. Stimulates: Protein catabolism, galactose oxidation Decreases: Myometrial contractility; alkaline phosphatase in uterus; cytoplasmic estrogen receptors in endometrium Increases: Growth of lining epithelial cells in estrogen-primed endometrium, with increased glycogen, mucin, & fat. Lobule development in mammary glands. Basal metabolic rate; body temperature.	(−): Lack of normal cyclic changes of endometrial development for implantation & gestation; functional uterine bleeding (+): Progestational changes. Pregnancy prolongation. Na^+, K^+, excretion & catabolism.	(S): FSH & LH. Small doses of estrogens induce cytoplasmic progesterone receptors. (I): Decreased LH & FSH secretion. Degeneration of corpora lutea in menstrual cycles.

Conversion of progesterone to 20β-hydroxypregn-4-en-3-one and measurement in H_2SO_4-ethanol reagent by fluorescence. Gas-liquid chromatography. [34]

Isotope-derivative technique: Progesterone is reacted with sodium [³H]bo-

[7] Synonym: Diphosphopyridine nucleotide oxidase. [8] Synonyms: Δ⁴-Pregnene-3,20-dione; Pregn-4-ene-3,20-dione. [9] Synonym: Carbonic anhydrase.

continued

Structure & Properties	Sources [Targets]	Assay Methods	Principal Actions	Effects of Deficiency (−) & Excess (+)	Control of Secretion: Stimulated by (S), Inhibited by (I)
		rohydride, [^{35}S]thiosemicarbazide, or [^{3}H]acetic anhydride to form progesterone derivatives which are purified, and the amount of radioactivity in the final residue is proportional to the amount of progesterone or its derivative. In double isotope dilution derivative assay, a known amount of tracer of ^{3}H- or ^{14}C-labeled progesterone is added to the starting material to correct for losses; ratio of labeled steroid added to labeled derivative is determined. [34] Competitive protein-binding analysis: Progesterone, extracted with petroleum benzin [10] and separated by chromatography (thin layer, paper, or column), is incubated with transcortin and radio-labeled progesterone. Separation of bound & free achieved with inert materials such as activated magnesium silicate [11] or Fuller's earth. [37,38] Radioimmunoassay: Progesterone, extracted with diethyl ether and separated by microcolumn chromatography, is incubated with anti-progesterone antibody (made to 11-deoxycortisol 21-hemisuccinate in sheep) and radio-labeled progesterone. Separation of bound & free by dextran-coated charcoal. [4] Spin immunoassay: Spin-labeled derivative (3-(progesterone-11α-hemisuccinyl)-3-methylamino-2,2,5,5-tetramethylpyrrolidine-1-oxyl) is produced and antibodies to this made. Then an electron spin resonance spectrum is obtained. [56]		

Relaxin [1]

Structure & Properties	Sources [Targets]	Assay Methods	Principal Actions	Effects of Deficiency (−) & Excess (+)	Control of Secretion: Stimulated by (S), Inhibited by (I)
5 Polypeptide. Mol wt = 9000; pI = 5.5; sol. in water, 95% ethanol.	Endometrium, corpus luteum & blood of pregnant women; placenta [Pubic ligaments, uterus, cervix]	Bioassay: Degree of relaxation of guinea pig pubic ligament Radioimmunoassay: Double antibody radioimmunoassay, with porcine relaxin (NIH-R-P$_1$) used as standard and anti-porcine relaxin antibody generated in rabbits [10]	Effects relaxation of pubic ligament and separation of symphysis pubis during last stages of pregnancy. After presensitization with estrogen, connective tissues of symphysis become more vascular, collagen fibers are dissolved, and mucopolysaccharides are depolymerized, rendering ligament more flexible. Effects softening & relaxation of uterine cervix after pretreatment with estrogen. Inhibits uterine motility. [59]	(−): Not definitely known; may prolong labor (+): Not definitely known	(S): Not definitely known; probably increased levels of progesterone during pregnancy (I): Not definitely known; possibly changes in balances of estrogen & progesterone during parturition (levels in blood peak during terminal stages of pregnancy and decline rapidly just prior to, during, & 1 day after delivery)

Human Chorionic Gonadotropin ⟨HCG⟩ [6,7,11-13,21,22,27,35,36,41,45,50,52,54,55,59]

Structure & Properties	Sources [Targets]	Assay Methods	Principal Actions	Effects of Deficiency (−) & Excess (+)	Control of Secretion: Stimulated by (S), Inhibited by (I)
6 Glycopeptide. Mol wt = 37,000. Resembles pituitary glycoprotein hormones in	Syncytiotrophoblastic cells of placenta. Ectopically from certain malignancies (of lung, ovary, liver, GI	Bioassays & bioreceptor assays employ same systems as LH (see entry 4 in table 145) Radioimmunoassay: Rabbit, guinea pig,	Maintains corpus luteum & progesterone [12] production through first trimester of pregnancy, hence sustaining pregnancy until onset of fetal hormon-	(−): Absence of HCG incompatible with continuation of pregnancy beyond 1-2 mo. No known instances	(S): HCG production & secretion correlate directly with trophoblastic tissue mass during first 2 mo of pregnancy. Levels

[10] Synonym: Petroleum ether. [11] Synonym: Florisil. [12] Synonym: Progestin.

continued

Structure & Properties	Sources [Targets]	Assay Methods	Principal Actions	Effects of Deficiency (−) & Excess (+)	Control of Secretion: Stimulated by (S), Inhibited by (I)
chemical structure & properties. Two dissimilar subunits, non-covalently associated: alpha (common) subunit, identical to LH-, FSH-, & TSH-alpha; beta (hormone-specific) subunit, with 145	tract). Normal placenta also secretes free alpha subunit. Free alpha and/or beta subunit found in trophoblastic neoplasms (hydatidiform mole; choriocarcinoma) & ectopic tumors. [Corpus luteum of ovary]	goat, or sheep antisera; ^{125}I- or ^{131}I-labeled purified HCG as tracer. Specific assays for separate subunits as well as intact HCG. Antisera to HCG or its subunits usually cross-react with LH; specific sera for HCG may be prepared using peptide fragment from C-terminus of beta subunit, where sequence is unique to HCG.	al autonomy. ? Immunosuppressive action on lymphocytes, perhaps protecting fetus against immunologic rejection. ? Weak thyroid-stimulating activity, of uncertain physiological significance. When given exogenously in absence of pregnancy, exerts same actions on reproductive system as LH.	of isolated HCG deficiency in otherwise normal pregnancy. (+): Exogenously or from certain tumors, yields elevated plasma testosterone, estrogen, & progesterone (see entry 4 in table 145)	reach maximum at 60-80 days, then diminish. No specific feedback or other control mechanism known. (I): None known

amino acids, closely similar to LH with extra 30-residue sequence at carboxyl terminus. Contains 30% CHO linked to asparagine residues, and to serine residues within HCG-specific C-terminal portion of beta subunit. Separate subunits biologically inactive.

Human Placental Lactogen [13]/ [7,19,20-22,26,28,39,57,59,60]

Structure & Properties	Sources [Targets]	Assay Methods	Principal Actions	Effects of Deficiency (−) & Excess (+)	Control of Secretion: Stimulated by (S), Inhibited by (I)
7 Polypeptide, 191 amino acids. Mol wt = 22,000; two disulfide bridges. Chemical properties & amino acid sequence closely resemble GH (entry 3, table 145).	Syncytiotrophoblastic cells of placenta. Ectopically, in ♂♀, by trophoblastic & occasionally non-trophoblastic tumors. [Mammary gland]	Bioassay & immunoassay procedures employ same systems as those for prolactin (see entry 5 of table 145). Immunological cross-reactivity generally stronger with GH than with prolactin.	Along with prolactin, stimulates mammary gland growth & milk production during pregnancy. Exhibits most of the general anabolic effects of GH, at potency intermediate between prolactin and GH itself (may be of physiological significance during pregnancy).	(−): None known (+): From ectopic or exogenous sources in ♂ or non-puerperal ♀, may produce gynecomastia & galactorrhea	(S): Production & secretion increase steadily throughout pregnancy. ? Augmented by period of fasting or hypoglycemia. No specific feedback or other control mechanism known. (I): None known

[13]/ Synonyms: Human chorionic somatomammotropin; HPL; HCS.

Contributors: Beitins, Inese Z.; Keutmann, Henry T.

References

1. Altman, P. L., and D. S. Dittmer, ed. 1973. Biology Data Book. Ed. 2. Federation of American Societies for Experimental Biology, Bethesda, MD. v. 2, pp. 652-655.

2. Abraham, G. E. 1969. J. Clin. Endocrinol. Metab. 29:866-870.

3. Abraham, G. E., and A. D. Tait. 1971. Res. Reprod. 3(5).

continued

4. Abraham, G. E., et al. 1971. J. Clin. Endocrinol. Metab. 32:619-624.

5. Ball, P., et al. 1975. Ibid. 40:406-408.

6. Bayliss, R. I. S., ed. 1974. Clinics in Endocrinology and Metabolism. W. B. Saunders, Philadelphia. v. 3, pt. 3.

7. Bondy, P. K., and L. E. Rosenberg, ed. 1974. Duncan's Diseases of Metabolism. Ed. 7. W. B. Saunders, Philadelphia. v. 2, pp. 951-1679.

8. Brecher, P. I., and H. H. Wotiz. 1967. Steroids 9:431-442.

9. Briggs, M. 1974. Acta Endocrinol. (Copenhagen) 75:785-792.

10. Bryant, G. D., and T. Stelmasiak. 1974. Endocrinol. Res. Commun. 1(5-6):415-433.

11. Canfield, R. E., et al. 1971. Recent Prog. Horm. Res. 27:121-164.

12. Canfield, R. E., et al. 1976. In J. A. Parsons, ed. Peptide Hormones. Macmillan, London. pp. 299-315.

13. Carlsen, R. B., et al. 1973. J. Biol. Chem. 248:6810-6827.

14. Chan, L., and B. W. O'Malley. 1976. N. Engl. J. Med. 294:1322-1328.

15. Chan, L., and B. W. O'Malley. 1976. Ibid. 294:1430-1437.

16. De Hertogh, R., et al. 1975. J. Clin. Endocrinol. Metab. 40:93-101.

17. Eik-Nes, K. B. 1971. Recent Prog. Horm. Res. 27:517-535.

18. Fasman, G. D., ed. 1975. Handbook of Biochemistry and Molecular Biology. Ed. 3. CRC Press, Cleveland. v. 3, pp. 539-540, 542.

19. Frantz, A. G. 1976. (Loc. cit. ref. 12). pp. 199-230.

20. Frantz, A. G., et al. 1972. Recent Prog. Horm. Res. 28:527-590.

21. Frieden, E. H. 1976. Chemical Endocrinology. Academic Press, London.

22. Friesen, H. G. 1973. Handb. Physiol., Sect. 7 Endocrinol. 2(2):295-309.

23. Garren, L. D., et al. 1971. Recent Prog. Horm. Res. 27:433-478.

24. Goebelsmann, U., et al. 1975. J. Steroid Biochem. 6:703-709.

25. Hooker, C. W., and T. R. Forbes. 1947. Endocrinology 41:158-169.

26. Horrobin, D. F. 1973. Prolactin: Physiology and Clinical Significance. Medical and Technical, Lancaster, England.

27. James, V. H. T., and L. Martin, ed. 1974. Curr. Top. Exp. Endocrinol. 2.

28. Josimovich, J. B., et al., ed. 1974. Lactogenic Hormones, Fetal Nutrition, and Lactation. J. Wiley, New York.

29. Kao, M., et al. 1975. J. Lab. Clin. Med. 86:513-520.

30. MacLaughlin, D. T., and G. S. Richardson. 1976. J. Clin. Endocrinol. Metab. 42:667-678.

31. McGinty, D. A., et al. 1939. Endocrinology 24:829-832.

32. Merrill, R. C. 1958. Physiol. Rev. 38:463-480.

33. Mikhail, G., et al. 1970. Steroids 15:333-352.

34. Molen, H. J. van der, and A. Aakvaag. 1967. In C. H. Gray and A. L. Bacharach, ed. Hormones in Blood. Ed. 2. Academic Press, New York. v. 2, pp. 221-303.

35. Morgan, F. J., et al. 1975. J. Biol. Chem. 50:5247-5258.

36. Moudgal, N. R., ed. 1974. Gonadotropins and Gonadal Functions. Academic Press, New York.

37. Murphy, B. E. P. 1964. Nature (London) 201:679-682.

38. Murphy, B. E. P. 1967. J. Clin. Endocrinol. Metab. 27:973-990.

39. Niall, H. D., et al. 1973. Recent Prog. Horm. Res. 29:387-416.

40. O'Donnell, V. J., and J. R. K. Preedy. 1967. (Loc. cit. ref. 34). v. 2, pp. 109-186.

41. O'Malley, B. W., and A. R. Means, ed. 1973. Receptors for Reproductive Hormones. Plenum Press, New York.

42. Pincus, G., et al. 1957. Endocrinology 61:528-533.

43. Rennie, P., and J. Davies. 1965. Ibid. 76:535-537.

44. Richardson, G. S. 1967. Ovarian Physiology. Little, Brown; Boston. pp. 55-88.

45. Rosemberg, E., ed. 1968. Gonadotropins 1968. Geron-X, Los Altos, CA.

46. Rotti, K., et al. 1975. Steroids 25:807-816.

47. Ryan, K. J. 1963. Monogr. Pathol. 3:69-83.

48. Ryan, K. J., and O. W. Smith. 1965. Recent Prog. Horm. Res. 21:367-409.

49. Savard, K., et al. 1965. Ibid. 21:285-365.

50. Saxena, B. B., et al., ed. 1972. Gonadotropins. Wiley-Interscience, New York.

51. Smith, O. W. 1960. Endocrinology 67:698-707.

52. Sussman, H. H., et al. 1974. Cancer (Philadelphia) 33:820-827.

53. Taylor, R. W. 1974. J. Obstet. Gynaecol. Br. Commonw. 81:856-866.

54. Vaitukaitis, J. L. 1973. J. Clin. Endocrinol. Metab. 37:505-514.

55. Vaitukaitis, J. L., et al. 1976. Recent Prog. Horm. Res. 32:289-331.

56. Wei, R., and R. Almirez. 1975. Biochem. Biophys. Res. Commun. 62:510-516.

57. Weintraub, B. D., and S. W. Rosen. 1971. J. Clin. Endocrinol. Metab. 32:94-101.

58. Wiest, W. G., and T. R. Forbes. 1964. Endocrinology 74:149-150.

59. Williams, R. H., ed. 1974. Textbook of Endocrinology. Ed. 5. W. B. Saunders, Philadelphia.

60. Wolstenholme, G. E. W., and J. Knight, ed. 1972. Lactogenic Hormones. Churchill-Livingstone, Edinburgh.

61. Wotiz, H. H., et al. 1956. J. Biol. Chem. 222:487-495.

Part I. Ovarian Hypofunction

Abbreviations: ACTH = adrenocorticotropic hormone; DHT = dihydrotestosterone; FSH = follicle-stimulating hormone; GH = growth hormone; LH = luteinizing hormone; LH-RH = luteinizing hormone—releasing hormone; TRH = thyrotropin-releasing hormone; TSH = thyrotropin.

	Disorder	Principal Signs & Symptoms	Pathophysiology	Diagnosis	Treatment	Reference
				Primary		
1	General Constitutional delay	Delayed menarche beyond age 16; early signs of thelarche & pubarche; short stature	Familial traits; delay in maturation of hypothalamic-pituitary-gonadal axis	Family history. Short stature; delayed bone age. Normal outflow tract: hymen, cervix; uterus palpable. No evidence of systemic disorder: obesity, cachexia, thyroid, or adrenal disease. Normal buccal smear.	Assurance until age 18. If condition persists beyond that time, investigation for primary amenorrhea.	19, 20, 30
2	Agonadism	Normal stature; pubarche, but no thelarche or menarche; blind vagina & no uterus	Karyotype 46 XY, with early destruction of gonad	Buccal smear negative; karyotype 46 XY. Serum & urinary LH & FSH increased; serum & urinary estrogens & progesterone low.	Replacement with estrogens	12, 27
3	Gonadal agenesis	Normal stature; pubarche, but no thelarche or menarche; normal vagina & infantile uterus	Karyotype 46 XY, with absent gonads but normal Müllerian duct development	Buccal smear negative; karyotype 46 XY. Serum & urinary LH & FSH increased; serum & urinary estrogens & progesterone low.	Cyclic replacement with estrogens & progesterone	12, 27
4	Resistant ovary syndrome	Normal stature; normal thelarche & pubarche; primary or secondary amenorrhea	Resistance of primordial follicles to respond to high concentrations of circulating gonadotropins	Serum & urinary LH & FSH increased; maturation index midzone; serum & urinary estrogens & progesterone low. Ovarian pathology reveals: "fat streak ovaries"; numerous primordial follicles without corpora albicans formation.	If desirous of fertility, clomiphene citrate or exogenous gonadotropin therapy	17, 31
	Gonadal dysgenesis					
5	Turner's syndrome	Short stature; early signs of pubarche, but none of thelarche or menarche; clitoris normal or slightly enlarged; normal vagina; infantile uterus. Other signs which may or may not be present: triangular facies; prominent ears & otitis; short, broad neck with webbing; low posterior hairline; multiple pigmented nevi; broad, shield-like chest, with widely spaced nipples; lymphedema of hands & feet; clinodactyly; cubitus valgus; congenital heart disease; hypertension.	Chromosomal abnormality: karyotype 45 XO or 46 XX-, resulting in streak ovaries	Abnormal physical signs; short stature; delayed bone age. Buccal smear negative or with abnormal Barr body; karyotype 45 XO or 46 XX-, or with abnormal X chromosome: isochromosome, deletion of short arm of X, deletion of long arm of X or ring X chromosome; mosaic XO/XX. Increased serum & urinary LH & FSH; no cornification on vaginal smear. Renal anomalies on intravenous pyelogram.	Androgenic steroid therapy for short stature. 1.5-2.0 mg estradiol 17β-cypionate ⟨estradiol 17β-cyclopentylpropionate⟩ in oil, intramuscularly at monthly intervals, then cyclic replacement with estrogens ⟨estrone sulfate 1.25 or 2.5 mg for 3 wk out of 4⟩. When bleeding starts, add medroxyprogesterone acetate, 5-10 mg during last week.	12, 16, 19, 20, 27- 30, 35

continued

Part I. Ovarian Hypofunction

	Disorder	Principal Signs & Symptoms	Pathophysiology	Diagnosis	Treatment	Reference
6	Pure gonadal dysgenesis	Normal stature; early signs of pubarche, but none of thelarche or menarche; normal clitoris & vagina, infantile uterus; eunuchoid habitus; no somatic signs of Turner's syndrome; occasionally slight virilization	Chromosomal abnormalities, leading to streak gonads	Family history. Buccal smear positive or negative; karyotype: 46 XX, 46 XY, 45 XO/46 XY, 45 XO/46 XX. Delayed bone age. Plasma & urinary LH & FSH increased; plasma & urinary estrogens decreased; no vaginal cornification; occasionally increased plasma testosterone.	If Y chromosome present, surgical removal of gonads at time of puberty (because of increased predisposition to gonadal tumors); cyclic replacement with estrogens & progesterone	3,5, 11, 13
7	True hermaphrodite or mixed gonadal dysgenesis	Normal or short stature; pubarche, but no signs of thelarche or menarche; normal clitoris, vagina & uterus; may have signs of virilization	Presence of both ovarian & testicular tissue (separately or combined as ovotestis)	Family history. Buccal smear positive or negative; karyotype: 46 XX, 46 XY or mosaic. Serum & urinary LH & FSH normal or increased; at surgery, both testis & ovary, or ovotestis, found.	Gonadectomy (because of increased predisposition to gonadal tumors); cyclic replacement with estrogens & progesterone	12, 27
8	Testicular feminization syndrome	Tall, eunuchoid proportions; good breast development; deficient pubic & axillary hair; no menarche; inguinal masses; normal clitoris, short vagina, no cervix or uterus	Lack of cytosolic & nuclear receptor for DHT in androgen-sensitive tissues	Family history. Buccal smear negative; karyotype 46 XY. Serum & urinary LH & FSH, normal; serum & urinary estrogens, normal adult range; plasma testosterone, normal ♂ adult range.	Gonadectomy at time of puberty (because of increased predisposition to gonadal tumors); replacement with estrogens	1,2, 12, 22, 24, 27
9	Menopause, premature	Cessation of menses before age 40; hypogonadism	Unknown; possibilities: (i) late manifestation of gonadal dysgenesis; (ii) associated with autoimmune disease	Karyotype: mosaic. Presence of other autoimmune conditions. Serum & urinary LH & FSH increased; serum & urinary estrogens low; poor cornification on vaginal smear.	Cyclic replacement with estrogens & progesterone; trial with exogenous gonadotropins	4,10, 15, 19, 20, 30
			Secondary			
	General Hypothalamic					
10	Kallmann's syndrome	Tall stature; eunuchoid proportions; pubarche, but no thelarche or menarche. Hyposmia or anosmia; may have midline defects.	Unknown; possibilities: (i) developmental abnormality of hypothalamus, with decreased synthesis and/or release of LH-RH; (ii) agenesis of olfactory lobes of brain	Family history. Hyposmia or anosmia. Delayed bone age. Serum & urinary LH & FSH decreased; serum & urinary estrogens decreased; no cornification on vaginal smear; variable response to LH-RH stimulation.	Cyclic replacement therapy with estrogens & progesterone; when desirous of fertility, clomiphene citrate or LH-RH therapy	18- 20, 27, 30, 32
11	Laurence-Moon-Biedl syndrome	Retinitis pigmentosa; polydactyly; obesity; mental retardation; pubarche, but some delay in thelarche	Unknown; perhaps hypothalamic defect responsible for obesity & hypogonadism	Signs & symptoms as listed. Serum & urinary LH & FSH decreased; serum & urinary estrogens decreased; no cornification on vaginal smear; variable response to LH-RH stimulation.	Same as for entry 10	6,19, 20, 26, 27, 30

continued

Part I. Ovarian Hypofunction

	Disorder	Principal Signs & Symptoms	Pathophysiology	Diagnosis	Treatment	Reference
12	Hypothalamic destructive lesions	Obesity; emotional lability; hypogonadism; amenorrhea; galactorrhea	Surgical stalk section, basilar meningitis, granulomas, craniopharyngiomas, & hypothalamic tumors lead to hypophysiotropic hormone deficiency	Past history. Increased serum prolactin; serum & urinary LH & FSH decreased; poor vaginal cornification; abnormal responses to TRH & LH-RH stimulation.	Same as for entry 10	19, 20, 25, 27, 30, 34
13	Weight loss	Recent weight loss due to dieting; amenorrhea	Unknown; possible decrease in synthesis and/or release of LH-RH from hypothalamus	Weight below expected for height. Serum & urine LH decreased, whereas FSH normal; poor cornification on vaginal smear; prepubertal or pubertal response to LH-RH stimulation.	Increase in food consumption. If desirous of pregnancy, clomiphene citrate, LH-RH therapy.	7,14, 19-21, 23, 30, 36
14	Emotional strain	Depression, agitation, recent change in occupation or environment	Unknown; possible decrease in synthesis and/or release of LH-RH from hypothalamus	History & signs of emotional problems. Serum & urine LH low, FSH normal; poor cornification on vaginal smear.	Psychotherapy. If desirous of pregnancy, same as for entry 13.	19, 20, 30
15	Hypopituitarism	Short stature; infantile facies & proportions. Sexual infantilism, with no pubarche, thelarche or menarche; secondary amenorrhea if onset later. Headache; visual disturbances; decreased visual fields.	Craniopharyngioma; chromophobe or eosinophilic adenoma of pituitary; necrosis of pituitary due to postpartum hemorrhage (Sheehan's syndrome); granulomatous disease, causing partial or complete destruction of pituitary gland	X-ray visualization of sella turcica & suprasellar region. Decreased upper lateral visual fields. Early: Decreased serum & urinary LH & FSH; decreased serum & urinary estrogens; poorly cornified vaginal smear. Later: May have GH, TSH, ACTH deficiencies, prolactin increase; variable response to LH-RH stimulation.	Definitive treatment of primary lesion by surgery, proton beam therapy, or radiation. Cyclic replacement therapy with estrogens & progesterone; exogenous gonadotropin therapy for fertility.	8,9, 19, 20, 30, 33
	Compartmental					
16	Anovulatory bleeding	Normal sexual development & height. Painless menorrhagia, interspersed with periods of amenorrhea; occasionally follicle cyst palpable on bimanual examination.	Absence of midcycle LH surge, & sluggish waxing & waning of ovarian follicles, leading to prolonged estrogen secretion	Monophasic basal body temperature chart; no midcycle LH surge in serum or urine; no luteal estrogen or progesterone increase in serum. Negative search for vaginal or endometrial malignancy.	Younger patient: 2.5-10 mg of norethynodrel, with mestranol ⟨Enovid⟩ for 3 wk, and then withdrawn for "medical curettage"; if ovulation does not resume, clomiphene citrate. Older patient; dilation & curettage.	19, 20, 30
17	Inadequate luteal phase	Normal height & sexual development. Abbreviated menstrual cycles; infertility; tendency to early abortion.	Relative deficiency of FSH during follicular phase or impaired follicle development, leading to impaired corpus luteum formation & function	Basal body temperature chart shows slow rise & abbreviated luteal plateau; low plasma progesterone during luteal phase; endometrial biopsy abnormal for luteal stage	Clomiphene citrate	19, 20, 30

continued

159. FEMALE REPRODUCTIVE DISORDERS

Part I. Ovarian Hypofunction

Contributor: Beitins, Inese Z.

References
1. Addison, W. A., et al. 1976. Obstet. Gynecol. 47: 331-336.
2. Amrhein, J. A., et al. 1976. Proc. Natl. Acad. Sci. USA 73:891-894.
3. Bardin, C. W., et al. 1969. J. Clin. Endocrinol. Metab. 29:1429-1437.
4. Blizzard, R. M., et al. 1966. Clin. Exp. Immunol. 1: 119-128.
5. Boczkowski, K. 1970. Am. J. Obstet. Gynecol. 106: 626-628.
6. Bowen, P., et al. 1965. Arch. Intern. Med. 116:598-604.
7. Boyar, R. M., et al. 1974. N. Engl. J. Med. 291:861-865.
8. Chaussain, J. L., et al. 1974. J. Clin. Endocrinol. Metab. 38:58-63.
9. Coscia, A. M., et al. 1974. Ibid. 38:83-88.
10. de Moraes-Ruehsen, M., and G. E. S. Jones. 1967. Fertil. Steril. 18:440-461.
11. Elliott, G. A., et al. 1959. J. Clin. Endocrinol. Metab. 19:995-1003.
12. Federman, D. D. 1967. Abnormal Sexual Development. W. B. Saunders, Philadelphia.
13. Ferguson-Smith, M. A. 1965. J. Med. Genet. 2:142-155.
14. Frisch, R. E., and J. W. McArthur. 1974. Science 185:949-951.
15. Irvine, W. J., et al. 1968. Lancet 2:883-887.
16. Johanson, A. J., et al. 1969. J. Pediatr. 75:1015-1021.
17. Jones, G. S., and M. de Moreas-Reuhsen. 1969. Am. J. Obstet. Gynecol. 104:597-600.
18. Kallmann, F. J., et al. 1944. Am. J. Ment. Defic. 48: 203-236.
19. Kase, N. G., and L. Speroff. 1974. In P. K. Bondy and L. E. Rosenberg, ed. Duncan's Diseases of Metabolism. Ed. 7. W. B. Saunders, Philadelphia. v. 2, pp. 1585-1628.
20. McArthur, J. W. 1974. In M. M. Wintrobe, et al., ed. Harrison's Principles of Internal Medicine. Ed. 7. McGraw-Hill, New York. pp. 570-582.
21. McArthur, J. W., et al. 1976. Mayo Clin. Proc. 51: 607-616.
22. Morris, J. M. 1953. Am. J. Obstet. Gynecol. 65:1192-1211.
23. Nillius, S. J., and L. Wide. 1975. Br. Med. J. 3:405-408.
24. Polani, P. E. 1970. Phil. Trans. R. Soc. London B259: 187-204.
25. Reichlin, S., et al. 1976. Annu. Rev. Physiol. 38:389-424.
26. Reinfrank, R. F., and R. L. Nichols. 1964. J. Clin. Endocrinol. Metab. 24:48-53.
27. Rimoin, D. L., and R. N. Schimke. 1971. Genetic Disorders of the Endocrine Glands. C. V. Mosby, St. Louis. pp. 285-356.
28. Rosenbloom, A. L., and J. L. Frias. 1973. Am. J. Dis. Child. 125:385-387.
29. Rosenfield, R. L., et al. 1973. J. Clin. Endocrinol. Metab. 37:574-580.
30. Ross, G. T., and R. L. Vande Wiele. 1974. In R. H. Williams, ed. Textbook of Endocrinology. Ed. 5. W. B. Saunders, Philadelphia. pp. 368-422.
31. Starup, J., et al. 1971. Acta Endocrinol. 66:248-256.
32. Tagatz, G., et al. 1970. N. Engl. J. Med. 283:1326-1329.
33. Taymor, M. L., et al. 1974. Am. J. Obstet. Gynecol. 120:721-732.
34. Tolis, G., et al. 1973. J. Clin. Invest. 52:783-788.
35. Turner, H. H. 1938. Endocrinology 23:566-574.
36. Warren, M. P., and R. L. Vande Wiele. 1973. Am. J. Obstet. Gynecol. 117:435-449.

Part II. Ovarian Hyperfunction

Abbreviations: FSH = follicle-stimulating hormone; LH = luteinizing hormone; LH-RH = luteinizing hormone—releasing hormone; TSH = thyrotropin; T_4 = thyroxine.

	Disorder	Principal Signs & Symptoms	Pathophysiology	Diagnosis	Treatment	Reference
			Primary			
1	Feminizing tumors: Granulosa-theca cell tumor	Prepubertal girl: thelarche, menarche. Sexually mature woman: intermittent uterine bleeding; may have hirsutism; clitoromegaly, increased libido.	Tumors excrete estrogens leading to pseudopuberty in girls & menstrual disturbances in women	80% of tumors palpable on bimanual examination. High proportion of cornifield cells on vaginal smear. Plasma & urinary estrogens increased; serum & urinary LH & FSH suppressed for age; decreased response to LH-RH stimulation.	Surgical removal of tumor	3,7, 10, 14, 16

continued

Part II. Ovarian Hyperfunction

	Disorder	Principal Signs & Symptoms	Pathophysiology	Diagnosis	Treatment	Reference
2	Masculinizing tumors: Arrhenoblastoma; hilus cell tumor	Prepubertal girl: tall stature, acne, pubarche, clitoromegaly. Older women: virilism & amenorrhea.	Tumors secrete androgens	Tall stature, advanced bone age. Abdominal mass. Serum & urinary testosterone increased; 17-ketosteroids in urine elevated in 50% and are not suppressed with dexamethasone.	Surgical removal of tumor	7,10, 14
			Secondary			
3	General True precocious puberty	Pubertal growth spurt, tall stature, thelarche, pubarche, & menarche before age 8	Early maturation of hypothalamus (escapes inhibition from small amounts of estrogens secreted by ovary)	Tall stature; advanced bone age. Serum & urinary LH & FSH increased; serum & urinary estrogens increased; cornification on vaginal smear; pubertal LH & FSH secretion pattern on LH-RH stimulation.	School acceleration. Medroxyprogesterone acetate, 100-200 mg, i.m., biweekly.	2,6-8, 10, 11, 14, 15
4	Albright's syndrome	Precocious puberty, with bone lesions & skin pigmentation	Unknown; some investigators suggest overproduction of releasing hormones from hypothalamus	Same as for entry 3. In addition, osteitis fibrosa disseminata, & brown, nonelongated, pigmented areas on skin	Same as for entry 3	1,5, 7, 10, 14
5	Hypothyroidism	Short stature; signs of hypothyroidism; thelarche & menarche	Unknown; possible that excessive TSH secretion leads to increased LH & FSH secretion	Bone age delayed. Low T_4, high TSH in serum; serum & urinary LH & FSH increased.	Thyroxine	7,9, 10, 14, 17
6	Compartmental Persistent follicle cyst	Prepubertal girl: tall stature; thelarche, menarche. Sexually mature woman: intermenstrual bleeding or post-menopausal bleeding.	Persistent follicle cyst secretes estrogens	Prepubertal girl: advanced bone age. All ages: cornified vaginal epithelium; urinary estrogens increased; serum & urinary FSH & LH depressed	Surgical removal	7,10, 12, 14
7	Stein-Leventhal syndrome & hyperthecosis	Oligomenorrhea or amenorrhea; anovulatory infertility & hirsutism in 50%; obesity in 30%	Arrested ovarian follicle maturation associated with noncyclic "dampening" of pituitary-ovarian axis	Ovaries may be enlarged, with multiple follicle cysts under capsule. Pathology: hyperplastic fibrosis of cortical stroma; luteinization of theca cells; endometrium hyperplastic. Plasma testosterone, androstenedione, & dehydroepiandrosterone high; serum & urinary LH high, FSH normal; LH hyperresponds to LH-RH stimulation; urinary 17-ketosteroids elevated.	For ovulation induction, clomiphene citrate, 25-50 mg daily for 3-5 d; wedge resection; oral contraceptives	4,7, 10, 13, 14

Contributor: Beitins, Inese Z.

continued

Part II. Ovarian Hyperfunction

References

1. Albright, F., et al. 1937. N. Engl. J. Med. 216:727-746.
2. Boyar, R. M., et al. 1973. Ibid. 289:282-286.
3. Diddle, A. W. 1952. Cancer (Philadelphia) 5:215-228.
4. Givens, J. R., et al. 1976. Am. J. Obstet. Gynecol. 124:333-339.
5. Hall, R., and C. Warrick. 1972. Lancet 1:1313-1316.
6. Job, J. C., et al. 1972. J. Clin. Endocrinol. Metab. 35:473-476.
7. Kase, N. G., and L. Speroff. 1974. In P. K. Bondy and L. E. Rosenberg, ed. Duncan's Diseases of Metabolism. Ed. 7. W. B. Saunders, Philadelphia. v. 2, pp. 1585-1628.
8. Kupperman, H. S., and J. A. Epstein. 1962. J. Clin. Endocrinol. Metab. 22:456-458.
9. Lee, P. A., and R. M. Blizzard. 1974. Johns Hopkins. Med. J. 135:55-60.
10. McArthur, J. W. 1974. In M. M. Wintrobe, et al., ed. Harrison's Principles of Internal Medicine. Ed. 7. McGraw-Hill, New York. pp. 570-582.
11. Money, J., and J. Neill. 1967. Clin. Pediatr. 6:277-280.
12. Monteleone, J. A. 1973. J. Pediatr. Surg. 8:949-950.
13. Rebar, R., et al. 1976. J. Clin. Invest. 57:1320-1329.
14. Ross, G. T., and R. L. Vande Wiele. 1974. In R. H. Williams, ed. Textbook of Endocrinology. Ed. 5. W. B. Saunders, Philadelphia. pp. 368-422.
15. Sadeghi-Nejad, A., et al. 1970. Clin. Res. 18:202.
16. Serment, H., et al. 1970. Rev. Fr. Endocrinol. Clin. 11:489-514.
17. Van Wyk, J. J., and M. M. Grumbach. 1960. J. Pediatr. 57:416-435.

160. MISCELLANEOUS HORMONES

Abbreviations: cAMP = cyclic adenosine 3',5'-monophosphate; CNS = central nervous system; GI = gastrointestinal; insol. = insoluble; mol wt = molecular weight; PNS = peripheral nervous system; sol. = soluble. Figures in heavy brackets are reference numbers. Data in light brackets refer to the column heading in brackets.

Structure & Properties	Source [Targets]	Assay Methods	Principal Actions	Effects of Deficiency (−) & Excess (+)	Control of Secretion: Stimulated by (S), Inhibited by (I)
Prostaglandins ⟨PG's⟩ [1-13]					
1 C_{20} fatty acids with cyclopentane ring; derivatives of prostanoic acid; class of compound defined by structure of ring (PGA, PGE, PGF, etc.); subscript determined by degree of unsaturation of fatty acid, e.g., PGE_1 versus PGE_2.	Reproductive organs: accessory genital glands in ♂, semen, testis; uterus, endometrium, menstrual fluid, & ovary; umbilical cord, placenta, amniotic fluid. Other endocrine glands: thyroid, adrenal cortex. Adipose tissue. Platelets. Lung. Cardiac muscle. Gastric mucosa, gastric fluid, & other parts of GI tract. Kidney (especially medulla). Thymus. Iris. Ner-	Bioassay: Contraction of smooth muscle in preparations such as trachea, stomach, jejunum, ileum, colon, or uterus, from a variety of species. Vasodepressor activity. Inhibition of norepinephrine-induced lipolysis in isolated rat fat cells[1]. Gas-liquid chromatography: Detection by (i) flame ionization detector, (ii) electron capture detector, or (iii) mass spectrometer	Numerous physiological functions suggested, but actual roles not yet clearly delineated in most situations Reproduction: Multiple effects on normal menstrual cycle, fertilization, labor, & delivery; induction of ovulation by $PGF_{2\alpha}$; effect on rate of tubal transport & implantation; effects on rate of sperm transport & fertilization, and on uterine contractility & duration of labor. Can induce abortion or parturi-	(−): Not definitely known (+): PGE's cause bone resorption & mediate hypercalcemia of some patients whose hypercalcemia is associated with malignant tumors. PGE_2 produced by synovial membrane of patients with rheumatoid arthritis. May mediate inflammation & bone	(S): Catecholamines (in fat cells[1]) (I): Acetylsalicylic acid[2], indomethacin, phenylbutazone, *p*-hydroxyphenylbutazone[3], fenoprofen, ibuprofen, ketoprofen, naproxen, meclofenamic acid, mefenamic acid, glucocorticoids, & others

[1] Synonym: Adipocytes. [2] Synonym: Aspirin. [3] Synonym: Oxyphenylbutazone.

continued

Structure & Properties	Source [Targets]	Assay Methods	Principal Actions	Effects of Deficiency (−) & Excess (+)	Control of Secretion: Stimulated by (S), Inhibited by (I)
Mol wt of PGE$_1$ = 354. Sol. in alkaline solution, fat & fat solvents; insol. in water; destroyed by concentrated alkali.	vous system (CNS & PNS). [Virtually all cells & tissues]	Ultraviolet spectrophotometry Enzymatic analysis Radioimmunoassay: Usually after extraction in organic solvent & chromatographic separation	tion. Adipose tissue: Regulation of rate of lipolysis; PGE$_2$, an antilipolytic substance, is released by lipolytic stimuli such as norepinephrine Cardiovascular system: PGA's & PGE's reduce blood pressure by vasodilatation, & possibly also by inhibition of sympathetic nervous system activity and by diuresis of NaCl & H$_2$O Renal: PGE's (& perhaps PGA's) synthesized in renal medulla, and carried to cortex by either vasa recta or loop of Henle. PG's modulate renal blood flow, promote diuresis of NaCl & H$_2$O, and may be "medullin," postulated renal vasodepressor substance(s). GI system: Decreases gastric acid secretion. Alters motility. Regulates synthesis of cAMP in numerous tissues. Stimulates cAMP release in numerous tissues, decreases cAMP release in tissues in which PG's inhibit responses induced by hormones (e.g., fat cells[1]). Produces inflammation in joints & other tissues	resorption of rheumatoid joints.	
Thromboxanes [10]					
2 C$_{20}$ fatty acids with oxane ring; derivatives of prostanoic acid. Thromboxane A$_2$ has a bicyclic oxane-oxetane ring system, and a half-life of 32 s under physiological conditions.	Platelets, lung [Platelets]	Gas-liquid chromatography, with detection by mass spectrometry Radioimmunoassay of thromboxane B$_2$, a metabolite of thromboxane A$_2$	Thromboxane A$_2$ is a potent inducer of platelet aggregation	(−): Deficiency of the platelet cyclooxygenase that catalyzes formation of PGG$_2$[4] is associated with a defect in hemostasis (+): Not definitely known	(S): Not definitely known (I): Inhibitors of fatty acid cyclooxygenase, e.g., acetylsalicylic acid[2] & indomethacin

[1] Synonym: Adipocytes. [2] Synonym: Aspirin. [4] The cyclic endoperoxide which is the precursor of thromboxane A$_2$.

Contributor: Axelrod, Lloyd

References

1. Anderson, R. J., et al. 1976. Kidney Int. 10:205-215.
2. Hansen, H. S. 1976. Prostaglandins 12:647-679.
3. Jaffe, B. M., and H. R. Behrman. 1974. In B. M. Jaffe and H. R. Behrman, ed. Methods of Hormone Radioimmunoassay. Academic Press, New York. pp. 19-34.
4. Karim, S. M. M., ed. 1976. Prostaglandins: Chemical and Biochemical Aspects. Univ. Park Press, Baltimore.
5. Karim, S. M. M., ed. 1976. Prostaglandins: Physiological, Pharmacological and Pathological Aspects. Univ. Park Press, Baltimore.
6. Kelly, R. W. 1973. Clin. Endocrinol. Metab. 2:375-392.
7. Lee, J. B. 1974. In R. H. Williams, ed. Textbook of Endocrinology. Ed. 5. W. B. Saunders, Philadelphia. pp. 854-868.
8. Robinson, D. R., et al. 1975. J. Clin. Invest. 56:1181-1188.
9. Samuelsson, B., et al. 1975. Annu. Rev. Biochem. 44:669-695.
10. Samuelsson, B., and R. Paoletti, ed. 1976. Advances in Prostaglandin and Thromboxane Research. Raven Press, New York. v. 1 and 2.
11. Seyberth, H. W., et al. 1975. N. Engl. J. Med. 293:1278-1283.
12. Shaw, J., et al. 1971. Ann. N.Y. Acad. Sci. 180:241-260.
13. Zins, G. R. 1975. Am. J. Med. 58:14-24.

161. RELATIVE RADIOTOXICITY OF NUCLIDES PER UNIT ACTIVITY

The relative radiotoxicity of each nuclide in the table is based on its average rank from the classification schemes in references 1-4. Although the classification criteria of the quoted references are not identical, all present similar radio-activity ranks for most nuclides. Toxicity: Med-A = medium toxicity, upper sub-group A; Med-B = medium toxicity, lower sub-group B.

	Element	Mass No.	Toxicity		Element	Mass No.	Toxicity		Element	Mass No.	Toxicity
1	$_1$H	3	Low	45		72	Med-B	89		105	Med-B
2	$_4$Be	7	Med-B	46	$_{32}$Ge	71	Low	90	$_{46}$Pd	103	Med-B
3	$_6$C	14	Med-B	47	$_{33}$As	73	Med-B	91		109	Med-B
4	$_8$O	15	Low	48		74	Med-B	92	$_{47}$Ag	105	Med-B
5	$_9$F	18	Med-B	49		76	Med-B	93		110m	Med-A
6	$_{11}$Na	22	Med-A	50		77	Med-B	94		111	Med-B
7		24	Med-B	51	$_{34}$Se	75	Med-B	95	$_{48}$Cd	109	Med-B
8	$_{14}$Si	31	Med-B	52	$_{35}$Br	82	Med-B	96		115m	Med-A
9	$_{15}$P	32	Med-B	53	$_{36}$Kr	85m	Med-B	97		115	Med-B
10		33	Med-B	54		85	Med-B	98	$_{49}$In	113m	Low
11	$_{16}$S	35	Med-B	55		87	Med-B	99		114m	Med-A
12	$_{17}$Cl	36	Med-A	56	$_{37}$Rb	84	Med-B	100		115m	Med-B
13		38	Med-B	57		86	Med-B	101		115	Med-B
14	$_{18}$Ar	37	Low	58		87	Low	102	$_{50}$Sn	113	Med-B
15		41	Med-B	59	$_{38}$Sr	85m	Low	103		125	Med-B
16	$_{19}$K	42	Med-B	60		85	Med-B	104	$_{51}$Sb	122	Med-B
17		43	Med-B	61		89	Med-A	105		124	Med-A
18	$_{20}$Ca	45	Med-A	62		90	High	106		125	Med-A
19		47	Med-B	63		91	Med-B	107	$_{52}$Te	125m	Med-B
20	$_{21}$Sc	46	Med-A	64		92	Med-B	108		127m	Med-A
21		47	Med-B	65	$_{39}$Y	90	Med-B	109		127	Med-B
22		48	Med-B	66		91m	Low	110		129m	Med-A
23	$_{23}$V	48	Med-B	67		91	Med-A	111		129	Med-B
24	$_{24}$Cr	51	Med-B	68		92	Med-B	112		131m	Med-B
25	$_{25}$Mn	52	Med-B	69		93	Med-B	113		132	Med-B
26		54	Med-A	70	$_{40}$Zr	93	Low	114	$_{53}$I	124	Med-A
27		56	Med-B	71		95	Med-A	115		125	Med-A
28	$_{26}$Fe	52	Med-B	72		97	Med-B	116		126	Med-A
29		55	Med-B	73	$_{41}$Nb	93m	Med-B	117		129	Low
30		59	Med-B	74		95	Med-B	118		130	Med-B
31	$_{27}$Co	56	Med-A	75		97	Low	119		131	Med-A
32		57	Med-B	76	$_{42}$Mo	99	Med-B	120		133	Med-A
33		58m	Med-B	77	$_{43}$Tc	96m	Low	121		134	Med-B
34		58	Med-B	78		96	Med-B	122		135	Med-B
35		60	Med-A	79		97m	Med-B	123	$_{54}$Xe	131m	Low
36	$_{28}$Ni	59	Med-B	80		97	Med-B	124		133	Med-B
37		63	Med-B	81		98	Med-B	125		135	Med-B
38		65	Med-B	82		99m	Low	126	$_{55}$Cs	131	Med-B
39	$_{29}$Cu	64	Med-B	83		99	Med-B	127		134m	Low
40		67	Med-B	84	$_{44}$Ru	97	Med-B	128		134	Med-A
41	$_{30}$Zn	65	Med-B	85		103	Med-B	129		135	Low
42		69m	Med-B	86		105	Med-B	130		136	Med-B
43		69	Low	87		106	Med-A	131		137	Med-A
44	$_{31}$Ga	67	Med-B	88	$_{45}$Rh	103m	Low	132	$_{56}$Ba	131	Med-B

continued

161. RELATIVE RADIOTOXICITY OF NUCLIDES PER UNIT ACTIVITY

	Element	Mass No.	Toxicity		Element	Mass No.	Toxicity		Element	Mass No.	Toxicity
133		140	Med-A	177		194	Med-B	221		232	High
134	$_{57}$La	140	Med-B	178	$_{78}$Pt	191	Med-B	222		233	Med-A
135	$_{58}$Ce	141	Med-B	179		193m	Low	223		234	Med-A
136		143	Med-B	180		193	Med-B	224		235	Low
137		144	Med-A	181		197m	Low	225		236	Med-A
138	$_{59}$Pr	142	Med-B	182		197	Med-B	226		238	Low
139		143	Med-B	183	$_{79}$Au	196	Med-B	227		240	Med-B
140	$_{60}$Nd	147	Med-B	184		198	Med-B	228	U-nat	235 + 238	Low
141		149	Med-B	185		199	Med-B	229	$_{93}$Np	237	High
142	$_{61}$Pm	147	Med-B	186	$_{80}$Hg	197m	Med-B	230		239	Med-B
143		149	Med-B	187		197	Med-B	231	$_{94}$Pu	238	High
144	$_{62}$Sm	147	Low	188		203	Med-B	232		239	High
145		151	Med-B	189	$_{81}$Tl	200	Med-B	233		240	High
146		153	Med-B	190		201	Med-B	234		241	High
147	$_{63}$Eu	152	Med-A	191		202	Med-B	235		242	High
148		154	Med-A	192		204	Med-A	236		243	Med-B
149		155	Med-B	193	$_{82}$Pb	203	Med-B	237		244	Med-B
150	$_{64}$Gd	153	Med-B	194		210	High	238	$_{95}$Am	241	High
151		159	Med-B	195		212	Med-A	239		242m	High
152	$_{65}$Tb	160	Med-A	196	$_{83}$Bi	206	Med-B	240		242	Med-B
153	$_{66}$Dy	165	Med-B	197		207	Med-A	241		243	High
154		166	Med-B	198		210	Med-A	242		244	Med-B
155	$_{67}$Ho	166	Med-B	199		212	Med-B	243	$_{96}$Cm	242	High
156	$_{68}$Er	169	Med-B	200	$_{84}$Po	210	High	244		243	High
157		171	Med-B	201	$_{85}$At	211	Med-A	245		244	High
158	$_{69}$Tm	170	Med-A	202	$_{86}$Rn	220	Med-B	246		245	High
159		171	Med-B	203		222	Med-B	247		246	High
160	$_{70}$Yb	175	Med-B	204	$_{88}$Ra	223	High	248		248	High
161	$_{71}$Lu	177	Med-B	205		224	Med-A	249		249	Med-B
162	$_{72}$Hf	181	Med-A	206		226	High	250	$_{97}$Bk	249	Med-A
163	$_{73}$Ta	182	Med-A	207		228	High	251		250	Med-B
164	$_{74}$W	181	Med-B	208	$_{89}$Ac	227	High	252	$_{98}$Cf	249	High
165		185	Med-B	209		228	Med-A	253		250	High
166		187	Med-B	210	$_{90}$Th	227	High	254		251	High
167	$_{75}$Re	183	Med-B	211		228	High	255		252	High
168		186	Med-B	212		230	High	256		253	High
169		187	Low	213		231	Med-B	257		254	High
170		188	Med-B	214		232	Low	258	$_{99}$Es	253	High
171	$_{76}$Os	185	Med-B	215		234	Med-A	259		254m	Med-A
172		191m	Low	216	Th-nat	228 + 232	Low	260		254	High
173		191	Med-B	217	$_{91}$Pa	230	Med-A	261		255	High
174		193	Med-B	218		231	High	262	$_{100}$Fm	254	Med-B
175	$_{77}$Ir	190	Med-B	219		233	Med-B	263		255	Med-A
176		192	Med-A	220	$_{92}$U	230	High	264		256	High

Contributor: Aamodt, Roger L.

General References

1. International Atomic Energy Agency. 1963. Int. At. Energy Agency Tech. Rep. Ser. 15.
2. International Commission on Radiological Protection. 1964. ICRP Publ. 5.
3. Morgan, K. A., et al. 1964. Health Phys. 10:151-169.
4. National Institutes of Health. 1972. U.S. Dep. HEW (NIH) Publ. 73-18.

162. MAMMALIAN CELL TYPES RANKED ACCORDING TO RADIOSENSITIVITY

Group represents a generalization of observations [ref. 2].

	Cell Type	Group	Properties	Examples	Radio-sensitivity
1	Vegetative intermitotic cells	I	Divide regularly; no differentiation	Erythroblasts; intestinal crypt cells; germinal cells of epidermis; lymphocytes[1]	High ↑
2	Differentiating intermitotic cells	II	Divide regularly; some differentiation between divisions	Myelocytes	
3	Connective tissue cells[2]	...	....	....	
4	Reverting post-mitotic cells	III	Do not divide regularly; variably differentiated	Liver	
5	Fixed post-mitotic cells	IV	Do not divide; highly differentiated	Nerve cells; muscle cells	Low ↓

[1] The small lymphocyte is one of the most radiosensitive cells, and is believed to die an intermitotic death after irradiation (most sensitive cells are considered to die a mitotic death). [2] Supporting structures, such as connective tissue and endothelial cells of small blood vessels, are regarded as intermediate in sensitivity between groups II and III of the parenchymal cells.

Contributor: Broseus, Roger W.

References

1. Casarett, G. W. 1963. In R. J. C. Harris, ed. Cellular Basis and Aetiology of Late Somatic Effects of Ionizing Radiations. Academic Press, New York. pp. 189-205.

2. Hall, E. J. 1973. Radiobiology for the Radiologist. Harper and Row, Hagerstown, MD. p. 193.
3. Rubin, P., and G. W. Casarett. 1968. Clinical Radiation Pathology. W. B. Saunders, Philadelphia. v. 1.

163. ANNUAL AVERAGE RADIATION DOSES TO INDIVIDUALS IN THE UNITED STATES

Data are averages based on estimates, weighted by appropriate factors to account for differences in geographic location, living habits, diet, etc. **Remarks:** Figures in heavy brackets are reference numbers.

	Source	Body Area Exposed	Dose mrem/yr	Remarks
				Natural Background Radiation[1]
1	Cosmic radiation	GI tract	28	Estimates include 10% reduction to account for structural shielding. Dose is mildly dependent on geomagnetic latitude (within the USA) & on altitude. Dose ranges from 50 mrem/yr in Denver (altitude, 1600 m) & 125 mrem/yr at Leadville, Colorado (altitude, 3200 m) [2], to as low as 30 mrem/yr in Puerto Rico [4] (uncorrected for shielding).
2		Lung	28	
3		Bone surfaces	28	
4		Bone marrow	28	
5		Gonads	28	
6	Cosmogenic radionuclides	GI tract	0.7	Cosmogenic radionuclides are produced by cosmic ray bombardment of nuclei, primarily in the atmosphere, e.g., carbon-14 produced by the $n[^{14}N,p]^{14}C$ reaction. Carbon-14 is responsible for virtually all of the dose from this source.
7		Lung	0.7	
8		Bone surfaces	0.8	
9		Bone marrow	0.7	
10		Gonads	0.7	
11	External terrestrial radiation	GI tract	26	Estimate includes a 20% reduction for shielding by housing, & a 20% reduction for self-shielding by the body
12		Lung	26	
13		Bone surfaces	26	
14		Bone marrow	26	
15		Gonads	26	

[1] Adapted from reference 2, Table 44.

continued

163. ANNUAL AVERAGE RADIATION DOSES TO INDIVIDUALS IN THE UNITED STATES

	Source	Body Area Exposed	Dose mrem/yr	Remarks
16	Inhaled radionuclides	Lung	100	Due primarily to α-ray emitters present in air, yielding dose to the bronchial epithelium; local dose to segmental bronchioles is 450 mrem/yr. The dose to small areas of bifurcations in the bronchial epithelium has been calculated to be as high as 10 rem/yr from ^{210}Pb & ^{210}Po present in cigarette smoke, for smokers of 2 packs/d [1].
17	Radionuclides in the body	GI tract	24[2/]	Estimate excludes cosmogenic contribution shown separately. Most of dose from this source is due to ^{40}K (19 mrem/yr), a naturally occurring isotope of potassium.
18		Lung	24	
19		Bone surfaces	60	
20		Bone marrow	24	
21		Gonads	27	
22	Total radiation from natu-	GI tract	80	Dose totals were rounded
23	ral sources, including cos-	Lung	180	
24	mic	Bone surfaces	120	
25		Bone marrow	80	
26		Gonads	80	
	Other Sources			
27	Medical uses of radiation	Whole body	20	Radiographic examinations. Value is the "genetically significant dose," a composite index based on actual doses received, weighted for the reproductive potential of the individual receiving the dose [3].
28	Fallout from nuclear-weapons testing	Whole body	4	Dose from this source is decreasing due to cessation of large-scale testing of nuclear weapons [4]
29	Miscellaneous sources	Whole body	3	Examples of miscellaneous sources are air transport & consumer products [4]
30	Nuclear power generation & reactor fuel reprocessing	Whole body	<1	Estimated average dose to individuals living within 100 km of a processing plant is 0.2-0.5 mrem/yr per 100 metric tons of fuel processed [4]
31	Total radiation from all sources	Whole body	∿107	Estimated average

2/ Does not include any contribution from radionuclides in the gut contents.

Contributor: Broseus, Roger W.

References

1. Little, J. B., et al. 1965. N. Engl. J. Med. 273:1343-1351.
2. National Council on Radiation Protection and Measurements. 1975. NCRP Rep. 45.
3. U.S. Department of Health Education and Welfare, Bureau of Radiological Health. 1976. U.S. Dep. HEW (FDA) Publ. 76-8034.
4. U.S. Environmental Protection Agency. 1972. U.S. EPA Publ. ORP/CSD 72-1.

164. RADIATION SYNDROME AFTER ACUTE WHOLE-BODY EXPOSURE

	Exposure [Midline Absorbed Dose]	Time After Exposure	Effects
1	Asymptomatic range, 100 R or less [65 rads or less]	Months	No symptoms, except very mild hematopoietic effects in upper range of doses

continued

	Exposure [Midline Absorbed Dose]	Time After Exposure	Effects
2	Sublethal range, 100-200 R [65-130 rads]	Weeks to months	Chills, fever, headache, exertional dyspnea, sore throat. General deterioration. Mucosal reddening, tonsillar swelling; bleeding gums; hematuria, melena, & mild purpura. Weight loss. Secondary infection. Complete recovery within 6 mo.
3	Median-lethal range, 400-500 R [270-330 rads]	Weeks	Fever & sore throat. Pharyngitis with ulceration, hyperemia, bleeding gums, & loosening of teeth. Nausea & vomiting on 1st day for doses above 300 R. Partial epilation above 300 R, complete epilation above 600 R. Purpura of skin & mouth. Blood in stool. Pancytopenia, acellular marrow. Prostration & lethargy, intermittent disorientation. Diarrhea, severe abdominal pain. Shock, coma. Death (25-40 d) in half of exposed cases, slow recovery in half of exposed cases.
4	Supralethal range, 1,000-10,000 R [670-6700 rads]	Hours to days	Nausea, vomiting, diarrhea, high fever, & pancytopenia. Blood in stool & vomitus. Extreme prostration with shock & cyanosis. Death (5-30 d).
5	Acute CNS range, above 10,000 R [above 6700 rads]	Immediate	Disorientation, ataxia & mental incapacitation; rapid progression to semiconsciousness & severe prostration.
6		Minutes	Cardiovascular shock. Patient appears almost moribund, may be incoherent, retching, vomiting, hyperventilating. Skin dusky reddish violet and may be cold. Mucous membranes cyanotic, conjunctivae hyperemic.
7		Hours	Watery diarrhea, vomiting. Temperature high, then falling. Lymphopenia & destruction of marrow.
8		Days	Death (minutes to a few days) preceded by severe restlessness, incoherence, abdominal pain, sweating, collapse, & coma

Contributor: Aamodt, Roger L.

General References

1. Alexander, P. 1965. Atomic Radiation and Life. Penguin, Baltimore. pp. 132-151.
2. Bond, V. P., et al. 1969. In C. F. Behrens, et al., ed. Atomic Medicine. Ed. 5. Williams and Wilkins, Baltimore. pp. 221-228.
3. Hemplemann, L. 1961. Diagnosis and Treatment of Acute Radiation Injury. IAEA/WHO International Documents Service, New York. pp. 49-65.
4. National Council on Radiation Protection and Measurements. 1971. NCRP Rep. 39.
5. National Research Council, Committee on Pathologic Effects of Atomic Radiation. 1963. NAS-NRC Publ. 1134:3-7.
6. Saenger, E. L., ed. 1963. Medical Aspects of Radiation Accidents. U.S. Government Printing Office, Washington, D.C. pp. 63-73.
7. Upton, A. C., and R. F. Kimball. 1967. In K. Z. Morgan and J. E. Turner, ed. Principles of Radiation Protection. J. Wiley, New York. pp. 398-447.
8. Wald, N. 1967. (Loc. cit. ref. 7). pp. 457-465.

165. DOSE RESPONSE TO TOTAL BODY IRRADIATION

Data are derived from radiation therapy and a few nuclear industry accident cases, and are applicable to adults only since the very young (especially the fetus) are more susceptible to radiation effects. **Dose:** Entries are representative compromises of variable ranges of values, in part because whole body irradiation—representative absorbed dose of whole body penetrating (X or gamma) radiation—is not a uniquely definable entity.

	Dose	Response
		Acute Exposure
1	5-25 rads	Minimum dose detectable by chromosomal aberration analysis or other specialized analysis

continued

165. DOSE RESPONSE TO TOTAL BODY IRRADIATION

	Dose	Response
2	50-75 rads	Minimum acute dose readily detectable in a specific individual, e.g., one who presents himself as a possible exposure case
3	75-125 rads	Minimum acute dose likely to produce vomiting in about 10% of individuals exposed
4	150-200 rads	Acute dose likely to produce transient disability and clear hematological changes in a majority of individuals exposed
5	300 rads	Median lethal dose for single short exposure [1]
6	1,000 rads	Necrosis of progenitive tissues (hematopoietic, gastrointestinal); 100% death in 30-60 d [1]
7	10,000 rads	Disruption of central nervous system and cardiovascular function; death within minutes to hours
8	100,000 rads	Spastic seizures; death within seconds
		Chronic Exposure
9	0.001 rad/d	No effect; ∿ natural radiation levels
10	0.01 rad/d	No effect [2]; within recommended occupational exposure limit of 5 rads/yr
11	0.1 rad/d	No effect [2]; within recommended occupation exposure limit in effect during the period 1930-1950
12	1 rad/d	Debilitation in 3-6 mo; death in 3-6 yr, as projected from animal data
13	10 rads/d	Debilitation in 3-6 wk; death in 3-6 mo, as projected from animal data

[1] Prognosis may be significantly altered by intensive medical care, especially at somewhat lower doses. [2] Chronic effects possible, e.g., malignancy, with increasing probability at increased accumulated doses and at increasing dose rates.

Contributor: Broseus, Roger W.

General References

1. Claus, W. D., ed. 1958. Radiation Biology and Medicine. Addison-Wesley, Reading, MA. p. 336.

2. National Council on Radiation Protection and Measurements. 1971. NCRP Rep. 39:46.

166. ESTIMATED DOSE-RESPONSE RELATIONSHIPS FOR GENERAL LIFE-SHORTENING AND INCREASED INCIDENCE OF LEUKEMIA

Site of dose estimation is 5-cm depth, whole body exposure. Data adapted from reference 1.

	Radiation Dose	Response	
		Life-Shortening	Leukemia
1	High-intensity exposure, >50 rads/d	∿10 d/rad	2-4 cases per 10^6 man-yr per rad
2	Low-intensity exposure, <1 rad/d	∿3 d/rad	1-2 cases per 10^6 man-yr per rad [1]

[1] Considered to be an upper limit for increased leukemic incidence in adults at low dose rates [ref. 2]. *See also* reference 3.

Contributor: Broseus, Roger W.

References

1. Langham, W. H., ed. 1967. NAS-NRC Publ. 1487: 263.
2. National Council on Radiation Protection and Measurements. 1975. NCRP Rep. 43.
3. National Research Council, Advisory Committee on the Biological Effects of Ionizing Radiations. 1972. The Effects on Populations of Exposure to Low Levels of Ionizing Radiation. National Academy of Sciences, Washington, D.C.

167. EFFECTS OF RADIATION DOSE ON EARLY LETHALITY

Radiation Dose: Effects from exposure to <100 rems have not been detected. **Tissue Primarily Affected** is the one most sensitive at the indicated dose. Data in brackets refer to the column heading in brackets.

	Radiation Dose [Time After Exposure]	Tissue Primarily Affected	General Symptoms	Critical Post-Exposure Period	Convalescent Period	Mortality
1	100-200 rems [3 h]	Hematopoietic	Moderate leukopenia. Incidence of vomiting: 100 rems, 5%; 200 rems, 50%.	....	Several wk	None
2	200-600 rems [2 h]	Hematopoietic	Severe leukopenia; purpura; hemorrhage; infection. Epilation at >300 rems. Incidence of vomiting: 300 rems, 100%.	4-6 wk	1-12 mo	Death within 2 mo from hemorrhage and/or infection in 0-80% of cases (variable)
3	600-1000 rems [1 h]	Hematopoietic	Severe leukopenia; purpura; hemorrhage; infection. Epilation at >300 rems. Incidence of vomiting: 100%.	4-6 wk	Long	Death within 2 mo from hemorrhage and/or infection in 80-100% of cases (variable)
4	1000-5000 rems [30 min]	Gastrointestinal tract	Diarrhea; fever; disturbance of electrolyte balance. Incidence of vomiting: 100%.	5-14 d	....	Death within 2 wk from circulatory collapse in 90-100% of cases
5	>5000 rems [30 min]	Central nervous system	Convulsions; tremor; ataxia; lethargy. Incidence of vomiting: 100%.	1-48 h	....	Death within 2 d from respiratory failure and/or brain edema in 90-100% of cases

Contributor: Wagner, William M.

Reference: Glasstone, S., ed. 1962. The Effects of Nuclear Weapons. U.S. Government Printing Office, Washington, D.C. p. 591.

168. RADIATION TOLERANCE DOSES FOR VARIOUS ORGANS

Organs are grouped in classes based on life-threatening potential: Class I = organs in which radiation lesions are fatal or result in severe morbidity; Class II = organs in which radiation lesions result in moderate to mild morbidity (in exceptional circumstances a fatality may occur, but permanent sequelae are generally compatible with survival); Class III = organs in which radiation lesions result in mild, transient, reversible effects, or in no morbidity. **Whole or Part** = field size or length of organ irradiated. $TD_{5/5}$ = the minimal tissue tolerance dose associated with a 5% rate of complications occurring within five years of treatment. $TD_{50/5}$ = the maximal tissue tolerance dose associated with a 50% complication rate over the same time span. The reason for defining the terms "minimal" and "maximal" as 5% and 50% respectively, relates to clinical decision-making, as expressed in "operating characteristics" of the radiation oncologist.

	Organs		$TD_{5/5}$	$TD_{50/5}$	Injury
	Class	Whole or Part	rad	rad	
	Class I				
1	Fetus	Whole	200	400	Death
2	Brain	Whole	6000	7000	Infarction, necrosis
3		25%	7000	8000	
4	Spinal cord	10 cm	4500	5500	Infarction, necrosis
5	Stomach	100 cm²	4500	5500	Perforation, ulcer, hemorrhage
6	Intestine	400 cm²	4500	5500	Ulcer, perforation, hemorrhage
7		100 cm²	5000	6500	

continued

	Organs		TD$_{5/5}$	TD$_{50/5}$	Injury
	Class	Whole or Part	rad	rad	
8	Liver	Whole	2500	4000	Acute & chronic hepatitis
9		Whole strip	1500	2000	
10	Lung	Whole	1500	2500	Acute & chronic pneumonitis
11		100 cm²	3000	3500	
12	Heart	60%	4500	5500	Pericarditis & pancarditis
13	Bone marrow	Whole	250	450	Aplasia, pancytopenia
14		Segmental	3000	4000	
15	Kidney	Whole	2000	2500	Acute & chronic nephrosclerosis
16		Whole strip	1500	2000	
	Class II				
17	Skin	100 cm²	5500	7000	Acute & chronic dermatitis
18	Peripheral nerves	10 cm	6000	10,000	Neuritis
	Eye				....
19	Retina	Whole	5500	7000	
20	Cornea	Whole	5000	>6000	
21	Lens	Whole or part	500	1200	
	Ear				
22	Middle	Whole	5000	7000	Serous otitis
23	Vestibule	Whole	6000	7000	Meniere's syndrome
24	Oral cavity & pharynx	50 cm²	6000	7500	Ulceration, mucositis
25	Salivary glands	50 cm²	5000	7000	Xerostomia
26	Esophagus	75 cm²	6000	7500	Esophagitis, ulceration
27	Rectum	100 cm²	6000	8000	Ulcer, stricture
28	Bladder	Whole	6000	8000	Contracture
29	Ureter	5-10 cm	7500	10,000	Stricture
30	Testis	Whole	100	200	Sterilization
31	Ovary	Whole	200-300	625-1200	Sterilization
	Endocrine glands				
32	Adrenal	Whole	>6000	....	Hypoadrenalism
33	Pituitary	Whole	4500	20,000-30,000	Hypopituitarism
34	Thyroid	Whole	4500	15,000	Hypothyroidism
35	Growing cartilage, bone[1]	Whole or 10 cm²	1000	3000	Growth arrest, dwarfing
36	Mature cartilage, bone[2]	Whole or 10 cm²	6000	10,000	Necrosis, fracture, sclerosis
	Class III				
37	Large arteries & veins	10 cm²	>8000	>10,000	Sclerosis
38	Lymph nodes & lymphatics	Whole node	5000	>7000	Atrophy, sclerosis
39	Breast[1]	Whole	1000	1500	No development
40	Breast[2]	Whole	>5000	>10,000	Atrophy, necrosis
41	Uterus	Whole	>10,000	>20,000	Necrosis, perforation
42	Vagina	Whole	9000	>10,000	Ulcer, fistula
43	Muscle[1]	Whole	2000-3000	4000-5000	Atrophy
44	Muscle[2]	Whole	6000	8000	Fibrosis
45	Articular cartilage	Joint surface, mm²	>50,000	>500,000	None

[1] Child. [2] Adult.

Contributor: Swain, Robert W.

Reference: Rubin, P., and R. A. Cooper, Jr., ed. 1975. Radiation Biology and Radiation Pathology Syllabus. American College of Radiology, Chicago. pp. 2-7.

169. TIME-DOSE RELATIONSHIP FOR CATARACT PRODUCTION

Graph is based on data from 233 clinical cases, 128 with cataracts and 105 without. The X- and γ-radiation employed varied from 100 to 1200 kV, and total doses from approximately 20 to 4300 rads. Exposures ranged from single doses to doses fractionated over periods up to approximately 10 years. Data for single treatments were plotted at 4 hours (0.16 day). For those individuals treated with radon seeds, the data were plotted at 13 days, the time at which 90% of the treatment was administered. Points for non-cataract patients were plotted and a line drawn at the upper limit of the points. Points for cataract cases were plotted and a line drawn along the lower limits. Below the lower line are the non-cataract cases, and above the upper line are those with cataracts. In the zone between are both cataract and non-cataract cases. A combination of dose and overall treatment time which falls above the shaded area would usually produce a progressive opacity with visual loss. Time-dose combinations falling below the shaded area would not be expected to produce injury to the lens. Those combinations falling within the shaded area may or may not produce a cataract; within this zone, the probability of a progressive cataract increases with increasing dose.

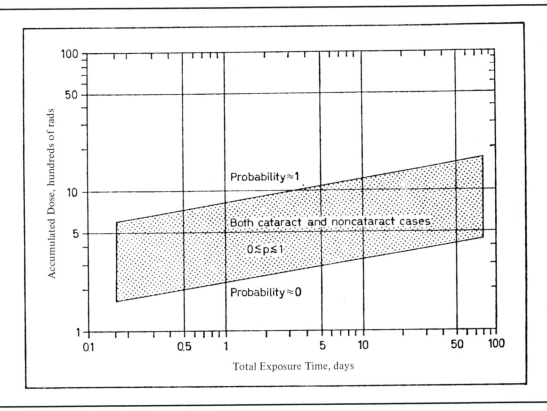

Contributors: Swain, Robert W.; Broseus, Roger B.

Reference: Merriam, G. R., et al. 1972. Front. Radiat. Ther. Oncol. 6:346-385.

170. LENS OPACITIES FROM LOW LET RADIATION

LET = linear energy transfer—the rate of energy release along an ionization track. **Minimum Dose** is the minimum dose at which lens change was detected.

	Type of Radiation	Duration of Exposure	Minimum Dose rad	Grade of Change at Minimum Dose	Reference
			Infants & Children		
1	X rays	3 wk-3 mo	560	Just visible by use of ophthalmoscope or slit lamp	3
2	Radium	>3 mo	550		

continued

170. LENS OPACITIES FROM LOW LET RADIATION

	Type of Radiation	Duration of Exposure	Minimum Dose rad	Grade of Change at Minimum Dose	Reference
3	Radium	>3 mo	1380	Just visible by use of ophthalmoscope or slit lamp	4
			Adults[1]		
4	X rays	Single exposure	600	Just visible by use of ophthalmoscope or slit lamp	2
5		3 wk-3 mo	800		
6	Radium	Single exposure	200	Just visible by use of ophthalmoscope or slit lamp	3
7		3 wk-3 mo	400		
8		>3 mo	550		
9	Radon gold seeds	3 wk-3 mo	1600	Minor—not noticed by patient	1
10		>3 mo	3100	Major—vision impaired	

[1] Includes children 10 years and older.

Contributor: Wagner, William M.

References

1. Britten, M. J. A., et al. 1966. Br. J. Radiol. 39:612-617.
2. Cogan, D. G., and K. K. Dreisler. 1953. Arch. Ophthalmol. 50:30-34.
3. Merriam, G. R., and E. F. Focht. 1957. Am. J. Roentgenol. Radium Ther. Nucl. Med. 77:759-785.
4. Qvist, C. F., and B. Zachau-Christiansen. 1959. Acta Radiol. 51:207-216.

171. RADIATION EFFECTS ON THE SKIN

The skin is tissue that has been studied extensively, and the observed chronic and late effects exemplify what may happen in other tissues. **Effects** are for acute dose. **Doses** cited for each effect are representative rather than precise. The exposures were given in roentgen (R) in the reference, but an exposure in air of 1 R ≈ 1 rad in tissue. Data are adapted from reference 1.

	Dose rad	Effects	
		Early	Chronic
1	50	Chromosomal changes only	None. (Possible slight risk of neoplastic alterations.)
2	500	Transitory erythema[1]. Transitory epilation[2]	Usually none. Risk of altered function increased.
3	2500	Temporary ulceration. Permanent epilation.	Atrophy; telangiectasis. Altered pigmentation.
4	5000	Permanent ulceration (unless area very small)	Chronic ulcer; substantial risk of carcinogenesis
5	50,000	Ordinarily necrotizing, but recovery possible when radiation has extremely low penetration	Permanent destruction to a depth dependent on radiation energy

[1] Degree of erythema is dependent on dose and penetrating power of radiation, as well as the dose rate, complexion, and area exposed [ref. 2]. Erythema may appear within hours after 1000-rad dose, to 1-3 wk after lower doses (200-400 rad) of X- or γ-radiation of energy <150 KeV.
[2] Complete epilation at >450 rad in 16-18 d [ref. 2].

Contributors: Broseus, Roger B.; Swain, Robert W.

References

1. National Council on Radiation Protection and Measurements. 1971. NCRP Rep. 39:49.
2. Parker, J. F., Jr., and V. R. West, ed. 1973. NASA SP-3006:444.

172. ESTIMATED ABSORBED DOSES OF RADIATION FOR PRODUCTION OF ERYTHEMA, DESQUAMATION, AND LATE NECROSIS OF SKIN

	Response	Dose Specification	Absorbed Dose, rad, for Response Probability of		
			10%	50%	90%
1	Erythema	High intensity; estimated at 0.1-mm depth over 35-100 cm² exposed area	400	575	750
2	Desquamation	High intensity; estimated at 0.1-mm depth over 35-100 cm² exposed area	1400	2000	2600
3	Late necrosis	High intensity 1-d dose; estimated at 0.1 mm depth over <150 cm² exposed area	2000	2800	3600
4		Fractionated or protracted over 7 wk or longer; estimated at 0.1 mm depth over <150 cm² exposed area	4600	6400	8200

Contributor: Broseus, Roger W.

Reference: Langham, W. H., ed. 1967. NAS-NRC Publ. 1487:247, 262.

173. RELATIONSHIP OF SKIN ERYTHEMA DOSE AND RELATIVE BIOLOGICAL EFFECTIVENESS TO HALF-VALUE LAYER

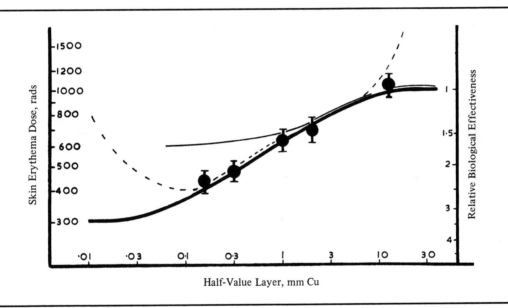

Half-Value Layer, mm Cu

⬦ : estimated median erythema doses and their associated confidence limits.

▬ : observed relation of skin erythema dose, a reciprocal function of relative biological effectiveness, to quality (half-value layer in copper).

── : same function corrected for absorbed dose.

--- : demonstrates skin-sparing effects of various energies.

Contributor: Wagner, William M.

Reference: Cohen, L. 1966. In E. E. Schwartz, ed. The Biological Basis of Radiation Therapy. J. B. Lippincott, Philadelphia. p. 260.

174. RELATIVE BIOLOGICAL EFFECTIVENESS FOR SKIN REACTION FOR VARIOUS ENERGY PHOTONS

Cesium-137 is used as the standard for relative-biological-effectiveness comparison. **KVP** = kilovolt peak; **HVL** = half-value layer; **RBE** = relative biological effectiveness.

	Energy		HVL	RBE		Energy		HVL	RBE
	KVP	Filtration	mm Cu			KVP	Filtration	mm Cu	
1	140	1 mm Al	0.09	1.71	9	230	1 mm Al plus 0.22 mm Cu	1	1.50
2		2 mm Al	0.15	1.66	10		1 mm Al plus 0.68 mm Cu	1.5	1.40
3		3 mm Al	0.21	1.63	11		1 mm Al plus 1.18 mm Cu	2	1.33
4		1 mm Al plus ¼ mm Cu	0.38	1.58	12		1 mm Al plus 0.81 mm Cu plus 0.65 mm Sn	3	1.24
5	200	0.08 mm Cu	0.52	1.55	13	400	1 mm Cu plus 0.5 mm Sn	4	1.19
6		0.5 mm Cu	0.955	1.50		^{137}Cs		10.8	1.00
7		1 mm Cu	1.4	1.47					
8		2 mm Cu	1.8	1.45					

Contributor: Wagner, William M.

Reference: Cohen, L. 1966. In E. E. Schwartz, ed. The Biological Basis of Radiation Therapy. J. B. Lippincott, Philadelphia. pp. 208-348.

175. ESTIMATED GONADAL TOLERANCE TO RADIATION

Dose = amount of radiation necessary to produce the specified effect on 50% of the subjects, unless otherwise indicated; R = roentgens. Data in brackets refer to the column heading in brackets.

	Organ or Cell Type	Effect	Dose, rads[1] [Dose Rate]	Reference
1	Testis	Temporary sterility or reduced fertility	15-30 [20 rads/min]	7
2			250	6
3			416	7
4		Permanent sterility	500-600	3
5			600	10
6			950	1
7	Spermatogonia B	Cell death	∿15	7
8	Spermatocytes, preleptotene	Cell death	∿200	7
9	Ovary	Temporary sterility or reduced fertility	170	6
10			400[2]	13
11			640	8
12			1200 [300 rads/d]	11
13			1740 [3 series over 2½ yr]	4
14		Permanent sterility	320 R	6
15			400[3]	11
16			625	12
17			800-1000 R	9
18			2000 R [3 series over 2 yr]	8
19			[2000 mg radium/h[4]]	5
20	Ovary or uterus	Carcinogenesis	360-720[5,6]	2
21			[1200-1800 mg radium/h[7]]	14

[1] Unless otherwise indicated. [2] Women >40 years old but not of menopausal age. [3] Women <40 years old. [4] Intrauterine. [5] Estimated ovarian dose. [6] >5 years after irradiation, carcinogenesis in 33 of 2068 patients. [7] Carcinogenesis in 3 of 958 patients, with mean time of 6.7 years for induction, and in 17 of 590 patients, with mean time of 9.5 years for induction.

continued

175. ESTIMATED GONADAL TOLERANCE TO RADIATION

Contributor: Wagner, William M.

References

1. Callaway, J. L., et al. 1947. Arch. Dermatol. Syphilol. 56:471-479.
2. Doll, R., and P. G. Smith. 1968. Br. J. Radiol. 41: 362-368.
3. Fabrikaut, J. I. 1970. At. Energy Comm. Rep. NYO-39740-41.
4. Gans, B., et al. 1963. Obstet. Gynecol. 22:596-600.
5. Ganzoni, M., and H. Widmer. 1930. Strahlentherapie 38:754-761.
6. Glucksmann, A. 1947. Br. J. Radiol. (Suppl. 1):101-108.
7. Heller, C. G. 1967. NAS-NRC Publ. 1487:133.
8. Jacox, H. W. 1939. Radiology 32:538-545.
9. LaCassagne, A., et al. 1962. In S. Zucherman, ed. The Ovary. Academic Press, New York. v. 2, pp. 498-501.
10. Lushbaugh, C. C., and R. C. Ricks. 1972. Front. Radiat. Ther. Oncol. 6:228-248.
11. Paterson, R. 1963. The Treatment of Malignant Disease by Radiotherapy. Ed. 2. Williams and Wilkins, Baltimore.
12. Peck, W. S., et al. 1940. Radiology 34:176-186.
13. Ricks, R. C., and E. W. Hupp. 1964. Tex. J. Sci. 16: 491-492.
14. Speert, H. 1952. Cancer (Philadelphia) 5:478-484.

176. ESTIMATES OF GONADAL DOSE PER EXAMINATION

Films: Average number of films per examination.

	Examination	Films	Dose, millirads Testis	Ovary		Examination	Films	Dose, millirads Testis	Ovary
1	Skull	3.7	<1	4	12	Total[3]	...	137	558
2	Cervical spine	3.1	8	2		Barium enema			
3	Upper extremity[1]	2.3	2	1	13	Radiography	3.5	1535	439
4	Lower extremity[2]	2.4	96	<1	14	Fluoroscopy	...	50	366
	Chest				15	Total[3]	...	1585	805
5	Radiography	1.4	5	8	16	Cholecystography	3.7	2	193
6	Photofluorography	...	<1	8	17	Intravenous or retrograde pyelography	5.0	2091	407
7	Fluoroscopy	...	1	71					
8	Thoracic spine	2.1	196	9	18	Abdomen	1.7	254	289
9	Shoulder	1.8	<1	<1	19	Lumbar spine	2.5	2268	275
	Upper gastrointestinal series				20	Pelvis	1.5	717	41
10	Radiography	4.4	130	360	21	Hip	2.3	1064	309
11	Fluoroscopy	...	7	198					

[1] Excluding shoulder. [2] Excluding hip. [3] Totals derived by adding radiography and fluoroscopy.

Contributor: Wagner, William M.

Reference: Penfil, R. L., and M. L. Brown. 1968. Radiology 90:209-216.

177. EFFECT OF RADIATION ON SPERMATOGENESIS

Dose = 190 kilovolt peak X rays, 1-3 mA, 20 rads/min.

	Dose, rad	Observed Effect on Sperm Count		Dose, rad	Observed Effect on Sperm Count
1	15-20	Moderate oligospermia	3	100	Marked oligospermia & azoospermia
2	50	Pronounced oligospermia	4	200-600	Azoospermia

Contributor: Wagner, William M.

Reference: Heller, C. G. 1967. NAS-NRC Publ. 1487:133.

178. EFFECT OF RADIATION ON PROGENITIVE TISSUE

The congenital anomalies were produced by irradiating the mouse embryo and fetus with X rays during each of the 20 gestation days. The black spot indicates the gestation age at which the anomaly can most easily be produced by radiation; the solid, black line shows the gestation spread during which the anomaly can be produced, usually by a higher level of radiation. The comparable human gestation days (with embryonic measurement, in millimeters) are shown at the bottom of the chart.

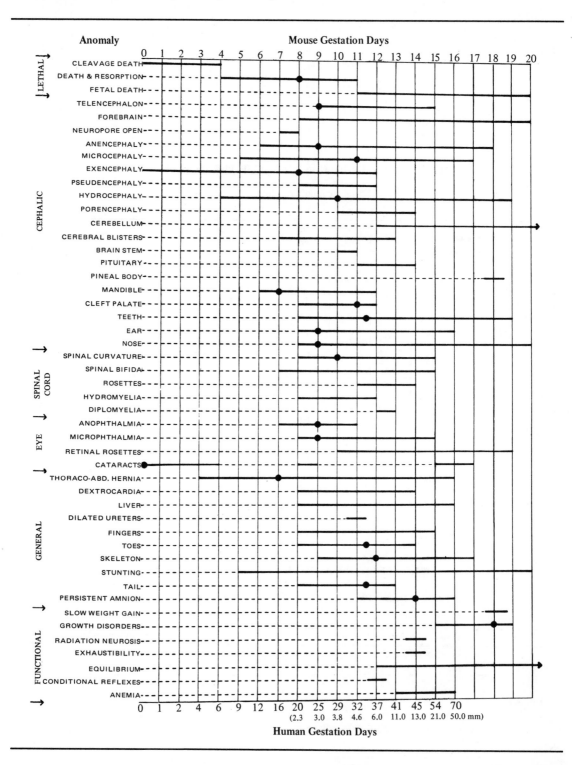

continued

178. EFFECT OF RADIATION ON PROGENITIVE TISSUE

Contributor: Wagner, William M.

Reference: Rugh, R. 1964. Radiology 82:917-920.

179. IDEALIZED RESPONSE OF VARIOUS CIRCULATING ELEMENTS TO RADIATION EXPOSURE

The time-course of changes in most of the peripheral blood elements is fairly well correlated with the dose of radiation to the bone marrow. FIGURES 1-3 indicate roughly the smoothed average time-course (based on human cases of accidental exposure) for neutrophils, lymphocytes, and platelets. The changes are represented as percentages of normal counts (the average levels for the population), and the curves portray generally the time-course of changes as a function of radiation dose. FIGURE 4 shows the idealized average dose-response relationship for neutrophils, lymphocytes, and platelets, in which the minimum value for each blood element has been plotted against the dose.

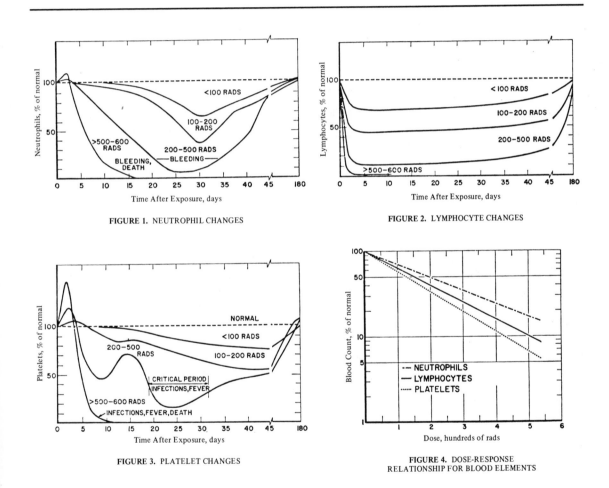

FIGURE 1. NEUTROPHIL CHANGES

FIGURE 2. LYMPHOCYTE CHANGES

FIGURE 3. PLATELET CHANGES

FIGURE 4. DOSE-RESPONSE RELATIONSHIP FOR BLOOD ELEMENTS

Contributor: Broseus, Roger W.

Reference: Langham, W. H., ed. 1967. NAS-NRC Publ. 1487:94-95.

180. DEGREE OF HEMATOLOGICAL DEPRESSION EXPECTED AFTER HIGH DOSES OF RADIATION

The time after the dose at which a given degree of reduction would be expected decreases with increasing dose.

	Circulating Blood Elements	Absorbed Dose, rads, for Reduction of		
		25%	50%	75%
1	Neutrophils	80	190	390
2	Lymphocytes	60	150	300
3	Platelets	50	120	250

Contributor: Broseus, Roger W.

Reference: Langham, W. H., ed. 1967. NAS-NRC Publ. 1487-249.

181. RADIATION EFFECTIVENESS IN PRODUCING FETAL CHROMOSOME MUTATION

Estimated Dose or Exposure: R = roentgen.

	Fetal Age at Exposure	Estimated Dose or Exposure	Type of X ray Examination	Age at Chromosome Analysis	Tissue Studied	Chromosome Mutations	Reference
1	1 wk	2.5 R	Radiopelvimetry	25 mo	Lymphocytes, fibroblasts	Mosaic for 1-3 markers (extra)	2
2	6 wk	3.0 R	....	6 wk[1]	Skin, lung	Translocations, monosomics, trisomics	4
3		3.9 rads	Digestive tract roentgenography[2]	6 wk[1]	Chorionic fragments	Deletions, dicentrics	3
4	10 & 11 wk	0.19 rad	Abdominal hysterosalpingograph	12 wk[1]	....	None	3
5	20-30 wk	....	Radiation therapy	1, 2, 3, & 4 yr	Lymphocytes	All types	1

[1] Induced abortuses. [2] Barium meal and enema.

Contributor: Wagner, William M.

References
1. Kucerova, M. 1970. Acta Radiol. Ther. Phys. Biol. 9: 353-361.
2. Lejeune, L., et al. 1964. C. R. Acad. Sci. 259(D):485-488.
3. Sato, H. 1966. Lancet 11:551.
4. Thiede, H. A., and S. B. Salm. 1964. Am. J. Obstet. Gynecol. 90:205-215.

182. GENETIC RISK AFTER IRRADIATION

Data were adapted from reference 1. **Doubling Dose** = the dose of radiation required to induce a mutation rate equal to the spontaneous rate. Doses include ranges from the following sources: 10-30 rads [ref. 1]; 10-100 rads [ref. 6]; 30-80 rads [ref. 2, 4]; and 30-100 [ref. 5]. **Additional Risk** = risk to the child resulting from one rad to a parent.

continued

Type of Determinant	Current Frequencies		Doubling Dose, rads	Additional Risk	Risk Formulas
	All Cases	New Cases			
1 Autosomal domi- nant gene traits (births)	8×10^{-3}	3×10^{-4}	10	1.6×10^{-5}	Birth frequency of all dominant gene traits of any social importance is 0.8%; estimated proportion of mutants is 4%. Therefore, mutants are $\frac{4}{100} \times \frac{8}{1000} = 3.2 \times 10^{-4}$. This represents effects of mutation in *both* parents. If doubling dose is 20 rads, then number of induced mutations per rad to *one* parent is $$\frac{1}{2} \times \frac{1}{20} \times \frac{32}{100,000} = 0.000008 = 8 \times 10^{-6}.$$
2			20	8×10^{-6}	
3			30	5×10^{-6}	
4			50	3×10^{-6}	
5			80	2×10^{-6}	
6			100	1.6×10^{-6}	
7 Sex-linked gene traits (births)	5×4^{-4}	$<1.7 \times 10^{-4}$	10	$<1.7 \times 10^{-5}$	The birth frequency of all sex-linked gene traits which are almost all recessive is $\sim 10^{-4}$. Of these (equilibrium distributions assumed), a maximum of $\frac{1}{3}$ will have arisen de novo, all on maternal X chromosomes (i.e., the frequency of mutants is 1.7×10^{-4}). If the doubling dose is 20 rads, a dose of 1 rad to mothers would be expected to determine $$\frac{1}{20} \times \frac{17}{100,000} = 8.5 \times 10^{-6} \text{ new mutants.}$$
8			20	$<8.5 \times 10^{-6}$	
9			30	$<5.7 \times 10^{-6}$	
10			50	$<3.4 \times 10^{-6}$	
11			80	$<2.1 \times 10^{-6}$	
12			100	$<1.7 \times 10^{-6}$	
13 Chromosomal aberrations (births)	7×10^{-3}	7×10^{-3}	....	Unknown	No predictions are made, but current frequencies are shown to draw attention to their magnitudes.
14 Abortion associated with chromosomal aberrations (recognized pregnancies)	3×10^{-2}	3×10^{-2}	....	Unknown	No predictions are made, but current frequencies are shown to draw attention to their magnitudes.
15 "Genetic death" (zygotes)	2×10^{-1}	5×10^{-3}	....	9×10^{-5}	If each individual carries 8 small dominant genes and each has a 2.5% independent chance of elimination in a generation, then the total risk is $0.025 \times 8 = 2 \times 10^{-1}$. If a total mutation rate per gamete of 0.1 on an average is assumed, each individual would receive 0.2 freshly arisen mutations; the risk of elimination by 0.2 mutations each conferring an independent risk of 2.5% is $0.025 \times 0.2 = 5 \times 10^{-3}$. If, as Muller [ref. 3] suggests, 140 rad induces 0.5 mutations/gamete, then 1 rad induces 0.0036 such mutations, and 0.025 are eliminated in the first generation; thus, the risk of a "genetic death" in the first generation from 1 rad is $0.0036 \times 0.025 = 9 \times 10^{-5}$.

Contributor: Aamodt, Roger L.

References

1. International Commission on Radiological Protection. 1966. ICRP Publ. 8:45.
2. Medical Research Council. 1956. Hazards to Man of Nuclear and Allied Radiation. H. M. Stationery Office, London.
3. Muller, H. J. 1964. Am. J. Public Health 54(2):42-50.
4. National Academy of Sciences. 1956. The Biological Effects of Atomic Radiation: Summary Reports. Washington, D.C. pp. 23-27.
5. Purdom, C. E. 1963. Genetic Effects of Radiation. G. Newnes, London. p. 162.
6. United Nations Scientific Committee on the Effects of Atomic Radiation. 1962. U.N. Gen. Assem. 17th Sess. Off. Rec. Suppl. 16:101.

183. LOW-LEVEL IONIZING RADIATION AND INCIDENCE OF DISEASE

This table has been only slightly modified from the original BEIR 1972 report. Values are for the estimated effect of 5 rem per generation on a population of one million live births. This includes conditions for which there is some evidence of a genetic component. The doubling dose of radiation required to induce a disease rate equal to the spontaneous rate is 20-200 rem.

Disease Classification		Current Incidence	Effect of 5 rem/generation no. of cases/10^6 live born	
			First Generation	Equilibrium
1	Dominant diseases	10,000	50-500	250-2500
2	Chromosomal & X-linked recessive diseases	10,000	65-80	90-180
3	Congenital anomalies	15,000	5-500	50-5000
4	Anomalies expressed later	10,000		
5	Constitutional & degenerative diseases	15,000		
	Totals	60,000	120-1100	400-7700
	Geometric mean	....	360	1760

Contributor: Abrahamson, Seymour

Reference: National Research Council, Advisory Committee on the Biological Effects of Ionizing Radiations. 1972. The Effects on Populations of Exposure to Low Levels of Ionizing Radiation. National Academy of Sciences, Washington, D.C. p. 57.

184. CANCER RISK PER RAD

ESSENTIAL FACTS RELATED TO RADIATION CARCINOGENESIS

1. Radiation-induced cancer is essentially identical to that arising from other causes.
2. Most human data related to radiation carcinogenesis come from limited studies on populations irradiated with widely-varying, crudely-known doses.
3. Many studies relate to populations subjected to partial body irradiation. The choice of dose values and extent of the body area at risk is necessarily somewhat subjective.
4. Empirical risk estimates are valid only for the population studied under the conditions which applied to that population.
5. Although risk estimates in the following tables are expressed as cases of cancer per million persons exposed per rad of exposure, no evidence exists that risk is in fact a linear function of dose, and serious errors are possible if these data are applied to cases of low-dose exposure.
6. These data are intended primarily as an indication of the current state of knowledge of radiation carcinogenesis in humans and provide an index of risk to various organs.

	Type of Cancer	Cases per 10^6 Persons per Rad	Reference
1	Leukemia	10-50	3
2		14-40	4
3		20	2
4	Lung	10-200	3
5		12-40	4
6		20	2
7	Breast	6-20	4
8		10-100	3

	Type of Cancer	Cases per 10^6 Persons per Rad	Reference
9	Thyroid	10-20	2
10		20-40[1]	4
11		40-80[2]	4
12		30-200	3
13	All cancers	40	1
14		100-200	4
15		100-500	3

[1] Males. [2] Females.

continued

184. CANCER RISK PER RAD

Contributor: Aamodt, Roger L.

References

1. International Commission on Radiological Protection. 1966. ICRP Publ. 8.
2. Ibid. 14, 1969.
3. National Research Council, Advisory Committee on the Biological Effects of Ionizing Radiations. 1972. The Effects on Populations of Exposure to Low Levels of Ionizing Radiation. National Academy of Sciences, Washington, D.C. pp. 93-211.
4. United Nations Scientific Committee on the Effects of Atomic Radiation. 1972. Ionizing Radiation: Levels and Effects. United Nations, New York. v. 2, pp. 402-447.

185. CANCER MORTALITY AS A FUNCTION OF ESTIMATED RADIATION DOSE

See ESSENTIAL FACTS RELATED TO RADIATION CARCINOGENESIS, page 370.

The following data are from the Japanese population exposed to radiation from atomic bombs [ref. 2]. Excess Cases: Calculated from mortality of specified dose group minus mortality of 0-9 rad group (the control population). Rad Dose: Values were based on the theoretical calculations of Auxier, et al., and are designated as tentative 1965 (T65) values [ref. 1]; doses in parentheses are ranges. NV = negative value.

	Type of Cancer	Excess Cases per 10^6 Exposed Persons per Rad Dose of				
		3.0 (0-9)	21.7 (10-49)	70.2 (50-99)	141.6 (100-199)	434 (200+)
1	Leukemia	0	503	981	3657	14,346
2	All except leukemia	0	2846	6514	382	9754
3	Digestive organs & peritoneum	0	NV	2942	NV	3998
4	Respiratory system	0	1216	1047	900	1842
5	Breast (♀ only)	0	671	1037	3424	1159
6	Cervix & uterus	0	1566	NV	NV	NV
7	Other	0	400	1771	NV	3914
8	All cancers	0	3349	7495	4039	24,100

Contributor: Aamodt, Roger L.

References

1. Auxier, J. A., et al. 1966. Health Phys. 12:425-429.
2. Jablon, S., and H. Kato. 1972. Radiat. Res. 50:649-698.

186. ORGAN SENSITIVITY TO THE INDUCTION OF FATAL MALIGNANCY

See ESSENTIAL FACTS RELATED TO RADIATION CARCINOGENESIS, page 370.

Average Radiation Dose: Dosimetry values were taken from referenced papers when possible. No corrections were made for partial body exposure. Atomic Bomb Casualty Commission doses used were based on the theoretical calculations of Auxier, et al., and are designated as tentative 1965 (T65) values in all cases [ref. 3]. Biological Effects of Ionizing Radiation (BEIR) data include their modifications as referenced.

continued

Population at Risk: Groups of individuals exposed to ionizing radiation, and includes patients irradiated to treat various conditions.

Excess Cases per 10^6 Persons per Rem: BEIR data were converted from cases per 10^6 persons per rem per year to cases per 10^6 persons per rem by multiplying by elapsed time calculated from person-years per number in population at risk. Crude estimates of the lower and upper limits of the 90% range (in parentheses) were made by the method detailed in Appendix IV of reference 15.

	Type of Cancer	Average Radiation Dose rad	Population at Risk	Average Duration of Study yr	No. of Persons Exposed	No. of Cases	Expected Cases	Excess Cases per 10^6 Persons per Rem	Reference
1	Leukemia	30[1,2]	Tinea capitis	15	2043	4	0.9	51(13.5-115.5)	1,2,15, 18
2		65[1,3]	Thymic enlargement (Series I)	18	1451	6	0.96	53(23-101)	10,15
3		86[4,5,6]	Japanese A-bomb survivors[7]	25	19,472	62	16.8	27(21-33)	11,15
4		135	Metropathia haemorrhagica	13.6	2068	6	1.31	17(3.7-26.2)	7
5		136	Metropathia haemorrhagica	13.6	2068	6	1.3	17(6.8-32.6)	7,15
6		275[1]	Thymic enlargement	16.4	2878	6	2	5(0-10)	10
7		300[1,2]	Tinea capitis	15	2043	4	0.9	5(0-8)	1,2,18
8		335[5,6]	Japanese A-bomb survivors	25	2770	42	2.3	43(38-48)	11
9		372[8]	Ankylosing spondylitis	9.7	14,554	52	5.48	9(6.9-10.7)	5,6,15
10		724	Polycythemia vera patients given ^{32}P	13	228	25	1.7	141(115-162)	14
11		757[1,2]	Head irradiation	12.9	971	1	0.33	1(0-2)	9
12		879[8]	Ankylosing spondylitis	13	14,554	60	6.75	4(3.6-4.7)	5,6
13	Salivary	275	Thymic enlargement	25	2878	3	0.07	4(2-4)	10
14		757	Head irradiation	12.9	971	2	0.04	3(1-3)	9
15	Digestive[9]	82[4,5,6]	Japanese A-bomb survivors[7]	25	23,979	378	363	8(0-26)	11,15
16		250[8]	Ankylosing spondylitis	11	14,554	58	33.7	7(3-10)	5,6,15
17		335[5,6]	Japanese A-bomb survivors	25	2770	79	68	12(0-30)	11
18		500[8]	Ankylosing spondylitis	11	14,554	58	33.7	3(1-5)	5,6,15
19	Lung	50	Thorotrast injection	20	921	5	1.12	8(3-18)[10]	15
20		86[4,5,6]	Japanese A-bomb survivors[7]	25	19,472	71	56.3	9(1-16)	11,15
21		172	Metal miners	30	1759	45	16.1	10(7-13)[10]	15
22		277	Fluorspar miners	26	800	51	2.8	22(18-36)[10]	15
23		335[5,6]	Japanese A-bomb survivors	25	2770	15	10	5(0-13)	11
24		400[8]	Ankylosing spondylitis	11	14,554	96	54.2	7(5-10)	5,6,15
25		468	Uranium miners	17	4146	135	16	6(5-7)[10]	15
26		879[8]	Ankylosing spondylitis	13	14,554	96	54.2	3(2-5)	5,6
27	Breast	81[4,5,6]	Japanese A-bomb survivors[7]	25	11,968	26	12.9	14(6-21)	11,15
28		200	Mastitis patients	19	606	11	4.23	56(23-102)	15
29		335[5,6]	Japanese A-bomb survivors	25	1503	4	2.3	3(0-12)	11
30		1215	Pulmonary tuberculosis	20	243	22	2.5	128	15

[1] Air dose to head and thymus of these patients may not reflect the biologically effective dose. [2] The BEIR Committee reduced the tinea capitis dose to 10% to compensate for the small amount of red bone marrow irradiated. [3] BEIR data for leukemia for Hempelmann's thymic enlargement patients include only the heavily exposed cases of Series I; dose is based on 20% of the air dose to the thymus as estimated by Marinelli. [4] BEIR data for the Japanese atomic bomb-exposed population include 10->200 rad exposures. [5] Data used from reference 11 is only for exposure of >200 rads. [6] Relative biological effectiveness (RBE) for neutrons was taken as 1 by Jablon and Kato [ref. 11] for the Japanese atomic bomb-exposed population.

A recent paper by Rossi and Mays [ref. 16] indicates that neutrons may be much more biologically effective in inducing cancer than has been thought previously; they estimate 800 leukemias per 10^6 persons per rad for the period 1945-1972 in the Japanese A-bomb survivors who received a biologically significant neutron dose in Hiroshima. [7] Age at exposure, >10 years. [8] The dose to ankylosing spondylitis patients is that to the spinal marrow in all cases since values were not available for individual organs. [9] Data for stomach cancer and gastrointestinal cancer have been combined, except for stomach cancer from the BEIR report [ref. 15]. [10] BEIR data include a quality factor of 10 for alpha-emitting radionuclides.

continued

	Type of Cancer	Average Radiation Dose rad	Population at Risk	Average Duration of Study yr	No. of Persons Exposed	No. of Cases	Expected Cases	Excess Cases per 10⁶ Persons per Rem	Refer- ence
31	Thyroid[11]	143[4,5,6]	Japanese A-bomb survivors[12]	24	811	6	1.6	38(2-61)	11,15
32		220	Thymic enlargement	19.7	867	1	0.059	5(0-5)	13
33		229	Thymic enlargement	16	2878	19	0.14	29(21-39)	10,15
34		275	Thymic enlargement	16.4	2878	19	0.14	24(21-24)	10
35		329	Thymic enlargement	24	223	14	0.06	190(122-261)	10,15
36		330	Thymic enlargement	18.4	1644	11	0.12	20(16-20)	17
37		335	Rongelap Islanders[7]	15	34	2	0.030	173(47-178)	4
38		400	Thymic irradiation	30.1	466	2	0.061	10(2-11)	12
39		585	Head irradiation (Subgroup I)	10.7	170	3	0.014	30(17-30)	9
40		757	Head irradiation (all)	12.9	971	3	0.08	4(2-4)	9
41		836	Tuberculous adenitis	17	162	7	0.051	52(40-52)	8
42		1125	Rongelap Islanders[12]	15	19	1	0.017	46(0-48)	4
43	Bone	204	²²⁴Ra-exposed adults	18	708	10	0.088	7(4-11)[10]	15
44		372[8]	Ankylosing spondylitis	11	14,554	4	0.63	1(0.2-1.4)	15
45		1103	²²⁴Ra-exposed juveniles	21	217	35	0.033	15(11-18)[10]	15
46		1700	²²⁶Ra-exposed persons	49	775	48	0.39	4(3-4.4)[10]	15

[4] BEIR data for the Japanese atomic bomb-exposed population include 10->200 rad exposures. [5] Data used from reference 11 is only for exposure of >200 rads. [6] Relative biological effectiveness (RBE) for neutrons was taken as 1 by Jablon and Kato [ref. 11] for the Japanese atomic bomb-exposed population. A recent paper by Rossi and Mays [ref. 16] indicates that neutrons may be much more biologically effective in inducing cancer than has been thought previously; they estimate 800 leukemias per 10⁶ persons per rad for the period 1945-1972 in the Japanese A-bomb survivors who received a biologically significant neutron dose in Hiroshima. [7] Age at exposure, >10 years. [8] The dose to ankylosing spondylitis patients is that to the spinal marrow in all cases since values were not available for individual organs. [10] BEIR data include a quality factor of 10 for alpha-emitting radionuclides. [11] Data are based on morbidity rather than mortality since thyroid carcinoma is rarely fatal. [12] Age at exposure, <10 years.

Contributor: Aamodt, Roger L.

References

1. Albert, R. E., and A. R. Omran. 1968. Arch. Environ. Health 17:899-918.
2. Albert, R. E., et al. 1966. Am. J. Public Health 56: 2114-2120.
3. Auxier, J. A., et al. 1966. Health Phys. 12:425-429.
4. Conrad, R. A., et al. 1970. J. Am. Med. Assoc. 214: 316-324.
5. Court-Brown, W. M., and R. Doll. 1957. Med. Res. Counc. (GB) Spec. Rep. Ser. 295.
6. Court-Brown, W. M., and R. Doll. 1965. Br. Med. J. 2:1327-1332.
7. Doll, R., and P. G. Smith. 1968. Br. J. Radiol. 41: 362-368.
8. Hanford, J. M., et al. 1962. J. Am. Med. Assoc. 181: 404-410.
9. Hazen, R. W., et al. 1966. Cancer Res. 26:304-311.
10. Hempelmann, L. H., et al. 1967. J. Natl. Cancer Inst. 38:317-341.

11. Jablon, S., and H. Kato. 1972. Radiat. Res. 50:649-698.
12. Janower, M. L., and O. S. Miettinen. 1971. J. Am. Med. Assoc. 215:753-756.
13. Latourette, H., and F. J. Hodges. 1959. Am. J. Roentgenol. 82:667-677.
14. Modan, B., and A. M. Lilienfeld. 1965. Medicine (Baltimore) 44:304-341.
15. National Research Council, Advisory Committee on the Biological Effects of Ionizing Radiations. 1972. The Effects on Populations of Exposure to Low Levels of Ionizing Radiation. National Academy of Sciences, Washington, D.C. pp. 93-211.
16. Rossi, H. H., and C. W. Mays. Unpublished. Radiobiological Research Laboratory, Columbia Univ., New York, 1976.
17. Saenger, E. L., et al. 1960. Radiology 74:889-904.
18. Schulz, R., and R. E. Albert. 1968. Arch. Environ. Health 17:935-950.

INDEX

* indicates diagram or graph
fn indicates footnote material
hn indicates headnote material

Aldolase, 110, 113, 118, 154
Aldosterone, 328-329, 333-334, 342
Alexander's disease, 248
Alexia, 292
Alimentary surgery: insulin, 324
Alimentary transmission: viruses, 3-4
Alkaline phosphatase
    blood assay, 116-117
    cortisone, 330
    graft-versus-host disease, 70
    inherited disorders, 102, 111
    liver diagnostic test, 211
    parathyroid hormone, 319
    reproductive hormones, 335, 341-342
Alkaline ribonuclease, 119
Alkalosis, 279, 329-330, 333, 338
Alkaptonuria: tests, 109
Alleles, 103-104, 126-127
Allergic diseases & disorders, 52-53, 55-56, 246-247
Allergic reactions: anaphylactic hypersensitivity, 82
                hearing loss, 262
                immunoprophylaxis, 49
                vaccines, 42, 44
Allescheria boydii, 234, 236
Allogeneic cells, 65, 80
Allogeneic skin graft, 65
Allograft rejection, 83, 88
Alloisoleucine, 98
Al(OH)$_3$ (*see* Aluminum hydroxide)
Alopecia, 71, 80
Alpha cells, 315, 317, 328 (*see also* Acidophils)
Alpha-particle therapy, 310
Alphaviruses, 2-3
Alpha waves, electroencephalographic, 297 hn, 297-298, 298 fn
Altitude: sickle cell trait, 158
Altitudinal hemianopia, 292
Aluminum hydroxide [Al(OH)$_3$], 121 hn
Alveolar basement membrane antigens, 83
Alveolar gases, 183
Alveolar macrophages, 64
Alveoli, mammary gland, 342
Alzheimer astrocytes, 248
Amantadine, 8, 45
Amaurosis, Leber's, 291
Amaurosis fugax, 291
Amaurotic cat's eye, 292
Ambient temperature, 2-3, 23, 183-184, 186-187, 308-309, 331
Amblyopia, 259-260, 292
Ameloblastoma, melanotic, 221
Amenorrhea: acromegaly, 310
             follicle-stimulating hormone, 305
             ovarian dysfunction, 346, 348, 350
Americium [Am], 354
Amikacin, 19
Amine oxidases, 117, 251 fn
Amine:oxygen oxidoreductase, 117
Amino-acid aminotransferase, branched-chain, 99
Aminoacidemias, sulfur, 99
Amino acid oxidases, 330, 335
Amino acids (*see also* specific amino acid)
    anterior pituitary hormones, 305-308
    digestion, 203 hn, 203*, 203 fn
    disorders, 91, 97-109

gastrin, 325
human placental lactogen, 344
iron absorption, 207 hn
keto acid production, 139 hn-140 hn, 140
luteinizing hormone—releasing hormone, 315
normal blood concentrations, 105-106
normal urine concentrations, 200
oxidation, 139 hn
pancreas hormones, 323-324
parathyroid hormone, 319
renal clearance, 97 hn, 103 hn, 106-107
testosterone, 335
thyroid hormones, 318
trauma, 149
Aminoacidurias, 103, 105, 109
Aminoacyl-histidine dipeptidase, 102
α-Aminoacylpeptide hydrolase, 117-118
α-Aminoadipic aciduria, 100
p-Aminobenzoic acid, 31
Aminoglycosides, 36, 37 hn, 38, 40
p-Aminohippuric acid, 194 hn, 195-196, 197 hn, 197-198
p-Aminohippuric acid tubular maxima, 194 hn, 195-196
β-Aminoisobutyric aciduria, 102
δ-Aminolevulinate synthase, 274
2-Amino-2-methyl-1-propanol buffer, 116
Aminopeptidases, 117, 203 hn, 203*
Aminoquinolines, 31
p-Aminosalicylic acid, 24
Amino sugars, 200
Aminotransferases, 330
β-Amino transport system, 102
Ammonia [NH$_3$], 99-100, 104, 213, 303
Ammonia nitrogen, 100, 116
Ammonium chloride, 197 hn
Ammonium sulfate [(NH$_4$)$_2$SO$_4$], 121 hn
Amnesia, retrograde, 229
Amnestic confabulatory syndrome, 239
Amnion: radiation, 366*
Amniotic fluid, 96-97, 308, 351
Amodiaquin, 31, 145
Amoeba, enteric, 234
Amoxicillin, 38 fn, 40
AMP, 113, 119 (*see also* Adenosine 5'-monophosphate)
cAMP (*see also* Adenosine 3',5'-monophosphate, cyclic)
    allergic diseases, 54-56
    amino acid disorder, 104
    anterior pituitary hormones, 305 hn, 305-307, 309
    epinephrine, 328 hn, 331
    insulin, 323 hn, 324
    parathyroid hormone, 317 hn, 319
    prostaglandins, 351 hn, 352
    testosterone, 335 hn, 335
    vasopressin, 311 hn, 312
cAMP phosphodiesterases, 55
Amphoric breathing, 14
Amphotericin B, 36, 40
Ampicillin, 16, 19-20, 36, 37 hn, 37-40
Amputation: bacterial infection, 17
Amylase, 117, 202 hn, 202, 209
Amylo-1,6-glucosidase, 92, 110
Amyloid, 26, 273
Amyloidosis, 261, 273, 282
Amylopectin, 202*, 202 fn
Amylose, 202*
Amylo-(1,4→1,6)transglucosidase, 92

Amylphenol, 147
Amyotrophy, 275
Anabolism, protein: estradiol, 341
Anaerobe infections, 16, 20, 233
Anaerobes, 37-38, 206 fn
Analbuminemia, 125, 130
Analphalipoproteinemia, 126 fn
Anaphylactic shock, 82
Anaphylactoid purpura, 89, 284
Anaphylatoxin, 82, 88
Anaphylaxis, 51, 54 hn, 55-56
Anaplasia, 222-223
Anaplastic carcinoma, 323
Ancylostoma duodenale, 32*, 33
Andrade type amyloidosis, 273
Androgen-binding protein, 305
Androgenic steroid therapy, 346
Androgens, 338-339, 350
Androgen-sensitive tissues, 347
Androstenedione, 335, 350
Δ^4-Androsten-17β-ol-3-one, 335
Anemia, 169, 324, 366*
    aplastic, 76, 284
    Cooley's, 157-159
    hemolytic
        cytomegalic inclusion disease, 244
        hemoglobinopathies, 158-159
        hereditary, 110, 113-115, 154-155
        plasma proteins, 127-128
        serum complement level, 88
    iron deficiency, 157-158
    megaloblastic, 128, 157-158
    nutritional macrocytic, 113
    pernicious: enzyme assay, 113
        gastrin, 325
        hemorrhages, 284
        immunofluorescence test, 87
        immunopathologic mechanism, 84
        vitamin B_{12} absorption, 206 fn
    sickle cell, 96, 158-159, 284-285
Anemic anoxia, 248
Anencephaly, 97, 252, 366*
Anesthesia: bacterial infections, 20, 26
        blunt-force contusion, 230
        cranial nerve disorder, 264
        electroencephalographic changes, 300 hn
Aneurysmal bone cyst, 256
Aneurysms: central nervous system, 282
        cranial nerve disorders, 261, 263-264
        hemorrhages, 284-285
        neuro-ophthalmic disorders, 289, 292
        trauma, 228-229
Anger: epinephrine, 331
Angiitis, 261, 282-284
Angioblastic meningioma, 224, 283 fn
Angioblastoma, 283
Angiogram, 53, 258
Angiography, fluorescein, 326
Angiokeratoma corporis diffusum, 274
Angioma, 224, 283
Angioneurotic edema, 89, 110, 127, 130
Angiopathies, 282-283
Angiosarcoma, 221, 224
Angiostrongylus cantonensis, 283
Angiotensin, 329

Anhidrosis, 272, 288
Animal (*see also* specific animal)
    bite, 3, 9, 242
    dander, 82
    disease hosts, 233
Anisocoria, 288
Anisocytosis, 159
Ankle: skeletal fusion, 217
Ankylosing spondylitis, 69, 372-373
Anomalies, 254 hn, 254-255, 366 hn, 366*, 370
Anophthalmia, 366*
Anosmia, 258, 336, 347
Anovulatory bleeding, 348
Anovulatory infertility, 350
Anoxia: myelin disorders, 248
Anterior commissure, 249
Anterior fontanelle, 243
Anterior horn cells, 251
Anterior horns, spinal cord, 240
Anterior midbrain (paratectal), 290
Anterior pituitary gland
    disorders, 310-311
        hypothalamic hormones, 314-316
        reproductive hormones, 335, 340, 342
Anterior pituitary hormones, 305-309
Anterior sacral roots, 281
Anterior temporal area: encephalographic spikes, 302
Anterior temporal lobectomy, 259-260
Anterior tibial nerve, 269 fn
Anterior uveitis, 69
Anthrax, 14, 17, 49
Anti-A isohemagglutinin, 66
Antibiotic-resistant strains, 18 hn, 18-19
Antibiotics, 1, 15-19, 30-31, 211
Anti-B isohemagglutinin, 66
Anti-blood-group sera, 86
Antibodies (*see also* specific antibody)
    autoimmune diseases, 85-86
    bacterial infections, 18, 29
    hormones, 324, 330
    IgE anti-penicillin, 55
    IgE assay, 51-52
    immune-complex reaction, 82
    immunodeficiency diagnosis, 65 hn, 66, 66 fn
    leukocyte function, 64
    plasma proteins, 128-129
    tests, 25, 29
    transplants, 73 fn, 80
    viral infections, 238 hn, 238-245
Antibody-mediated reactions, 83
Anti brain T-cell, 57
Anti chronic lymphatic leukemia, 57
α_1-Antichymotrypsin, 126
Anticoagulant therapy, 284
Anticonvulsants, 144-145
Antidepressants, 277 hn
Antidiuretic, 197 hn
Antidiuretic hormone, 311-312
Antidiuretic hormone syndrome, 314
Anti-DNase B, 25
Antigens (*see also* specific antigen)
    autoimmune diseases, 85-87
    bacterial infections, 26, 29
    immunodeficiency diagnosis, 65 hn, 65-66, 66 fn
    immunopathologic mechanisms, 82-84

Craniosynostosis, 101
Cranio-vertebral anomalies, 254
Cranium: circulatory disorders, 283
C-reactive protein, 18, 128
Creatine kinase, 110, 117
Creatine phosphate, 117
Creatine phosphokinase, 110
Creatinine, 148, 200
Creatinine clearance, 36 hn, 39 hn, 40, 194 hn, 195, 198 fn
Creatinuria, 335
Crepitation, 15
Crest, iliac, 257
Cretinism, 109
Creutzfeldt-Jakob disease, 245-246
Crigler-Najjar syndrome, 209 hn
Crohn's disease, 83 fn
Cromolyn sodium, 55
Croup, 4
Cryoproteinemia, 26
Cryptococcus neoformans, 234, 236
Cryptogenic cirrhosis: immunofluorescence test, 87, 212
Crypts, intestinal, 72
Cubitus valgus: Turner's syndrome, 346
Culex, 10 fn-11 fn
Cultures: bacterial infections, 14-16
Curettage, 348
Curium [Cm], 353
Curvature of the spine, 255
Cushing's disease, 137, 329, 333
Cushing's syndrome: adrenocorticotropic hormone, 305
    cortisone, 330
    diagnosis & treatment, 333
    glucose intolerance, 326
    insulin, 324
    pigment metabolism, 143
Cusp, mitral valve, 175 hn, 177*-178*
Cutaneous albinism, 291
Cutaneous anaphylaxis, 51
Cutaneous angiitis, 261
Cutaneous nerves, 272, 272 fn
Cutaneous viral infections, 46, 242
Cyanosis, 8, 19, 357
Cyclic AMP (*see* Adenosine 3',5'-monophosphate, cyclic)
Cyclizine, 54
Cyclooxygenase, 352
Cyclophosphamide, 74-76, 145
Cycloserine, 24
Cyproheptadine, 54
Cyst, aneurysmal bone, 256
Cyst: helminth infections, 237
    nervous system, 225-226, 259
    ovarian follicle, 348, 350
    post-hemorrhage, 229 fn
    thyroid gland, 323
Cystathionine, 99, 108
Cystathionine γ-lyase, 99
Cystathioninemia, 108
Cystathionine β-synthase deficiency, 94, 99, 108, 143
Cystathioninuria, 99
Cysteine, 103, 117
Cystic cerebellar tumors, 222
Cystic cerebral ependymoma, 223
Cystic degeneration: birth trauma, 231
Cysticercus cellulosae, 234, 237
Cystic fibrosis, 53, 110, 182

Cystic hyperplasia, 340
Cystine, 103-106, 108-109
Cystinelysinuria, neonatal, 103
Cystinosis, 91, 104
Cystinuria, 91, 103, 109, 203 fn
Cystitis, 14, 22
Cystometrogram, 281
Cystyl-aminopeptidase, 117-118
Cytidine intermediates: digestion, 204*
Cytochalasin B, 63
Cytochrome oxidase system, 104
Cytochrome b_5 reductase, 111, 155
Cytokaryorrhexis, 72
Cytolysis, 82, 123
Cytomegalic inclusion disease, 244, 252
Cytomegalovirus, 2-3
Cytomegalovirus infections
    associated immunodeficiency, 68
    central nervous system, 244, 252
    characteristics & therapy, 8
    therapeutic agent, 45
Cytoplasm: graft-versus-host reactions, 71 fn
    Negri bodies, 242
    peripheral nerve pathology, 274
    respiratory viruses, 5*
    virus particles, 244
Cytoplasm antigens, 84, 244
Cytoplasmic basophilia, 251
Cytoplasmic hormone receptors, 342
Cytoplasmic RNA, 251 fn
Cytoplasmic vacuoles, 245-246
Cytosine arabinoside, 75 fn-76 fn
Cytosol, 339
Cytosolic receptor, 347
Cytosol peptidases, 203 hn, 203*
Cytotoxic antibodies, 73 fn
Cytotoxicity, target cell, 61
Cytoxan, 145

Dactinomycin: abnormal pigmentation, 145
Dander: hypersensitivity, 82
Dandy-Walker syndrome, 243
Dark adaptation, 291
Daunomycin, 76
Dead space, lung: formula, 179 hn
Deafness: CNS viral infections, 238, 242-243
    nerve disorders, 248, 262-263
    retinitis pigmentosa, 291
    trauma, 227
Death: drug inhalation, 54
    fetal, 252, 327, 366*
    infections, 21-22, 244-246
    myelin disorders, 247
    radiation, 357-359, 364, 366*-367*
    sudden infant, 67-68
    transplants, 74-80
    trauma, 149-150, 231
Debrancher enzyme, 110
Decompression sickness, 285
Decubitus ulcers, 230
Deer, 21
Deerflies, 21
Degeneration, pigmentary retinal, 288
Degenerative diseases, 255, 257, 370 (*see also* specific degenerative disease)

Dihydroxyacetone phosphate, 115, 156
p-Dihydroxybenzene, 147
3,4-Dihydroxyphenylalanine, 142 hn, 143, 328 hn, 331
1,25-Dihydroxy-vitamin D, 319-320
24,25-Dihydroxy-vitamin D, 319
1α,25-Dihydroxy-vitamin D_3, 206 hn, 207*
Diisopropyl fluorophosphate, 163 hn, 163
Dilantin, 260, 290 fn
1,4-Di(methanesulfonoxyl)butane, 145
Dimethyl sulfoxide, 45 hn, 46
Dimorphic fungi, 234
Dinitrofluorobenzene, 65 fn
Dinitrophenylhydrazine, 107 hn, 108
Diodone clearance, 194 hn
Diosgenin, 329
Dipeptidases, 203 hn, 203*
Dipeptides, 203 hn, 203*
Diphenhydramine, 54
p-Diphenylenediamine, 118
Diphenylhydantoin, 205 fn, 260, 290 (see also Phenytoin)
Diphenylhydantoin sodium, 144
1,3-Diphosphoglycerate, 113-115
2,3-Diphosphoglycerate, 113, 156
Diphosphoglyceromutase, 110, 154
Diphosphopyridine nucleotide oxidase, 342 fn
Diphtheria, 48-49, 81
Diphtheria-tetanus toxoid, 65
Diphtheritic neuropathy, 247, 270
Diphyllobothrium latum, 22, 32*, 33
Diplococcus pneumoniae, 233, 235
Diploid cell strains, human, 42 fn
Diplomyelia, 366*
Diplopia, 288-290
Dipylidium caninum, 34
Disaccharidases, 124-125
Disaccharides: digestion, 202*
Discoid lupus erythematosus, 85-86, 129
Disks, spinal, 255, 257
Dislocation, spinal, 254, 258
Disorientation: radiation exposure, 357
Distal tubules, 329
Disulfide bridges: anterior pituitary hormones, 306-307
        calcitonin, 319
        corticotropin-releasing hormone, 314
        human placental lactogen, 344
        insulin, 324
Diuresis, 326, 352
Diuretics, 277 hn, 313, 326, 333
Diurnal rhythm: hormones, 305-306, 308
Diurnal temperature reversal, 19
Dizziness, 257 hn, 258, 262
DNA (see Deoxyribonucleic acid)
DNA antigen, double-stranded, 85
DNA nucleotidyltransferase, 45-46
Dog: antirabies prophylaxis, 9
    cardiac cycle, 167 hn, 168*
    disease transmission, 27, 233-234, 242
    parasite host, 21-22
Dominant gene traits (see Autosomal dominant inheritance pattern)
DOPA, 142 hn, 143, 328 hn, 331
Dopamine, 308, 315
Dopamine β-hydroxylase, 118
Dopamine β-monooxygenase, 118

DOPA quinone, 143
Dorsal columns, 241, 271, 275
Dorsal funiculi, 230
Dorsal horn neurons, 241-242
Dorsal pedal vein, 173
Dorsal root ganglia, 240-241, 270-271, 279
Dorsal spinal root lesions, 242
Doxorubicin hydrochloride, 145
Doxycycline, 37 hn, 40
DPNH methemoglobin reductase, 111
Dracunculus medinensis, 22
Drug-induced angiopathy, 283
Drug-induced hemolytic anemia, 154
Drugs, 14, 285-286, 290, 300 hn (see also specific drug)
Drusen, optic nerve, 260
Dubin-Johnson syndrome, 209 hn
Duchenne's muscular dystrophy, 110
Duck, 21
Duck embryo vaccine, 9 hn, 9, 45
Ducts, 213, 278, 312, 341
Dumb-bell neurilemoma, 263
Duodenal IgA, 43*
Duodenal ulcer, 201
Duodenum, 207 hn, 317, 319, 325
Dura, 254
Dural hematoma, 228
Dural shunt, 289
Dural thrombosis, traumatic, 228
Dural veins, 231
Dust, 53, 82
Dwarfing: radiation, 360
Dwarfism, 255, 306, 311
Dysarthria, 242-246, 289, 327
Dysautonomia, familial, 272
Dyscrasias, 228, 273 fn, 284-285
Dysentery, 236-237
Dysfibrinogenemia, 121 fn
Dysgammaglobulinemic states, 88
Dysgenesis, gonadal, 346-347
Dysgerminoma, 225
Dysglobulinemia, 137-138, 273-274
Dyskeratosis, 70
Dyskinesia, 289
Dysmenorrhea, 342
Dysmetria, 289
Dysmyelinogenetic leukodystrophy, 248
Dysostosis, cleidocranial, 254
Dysphagia: bacterial infection, 14
    nerve disorders, 242, 245, 263-264
    spine fractures, 229
    thyroid disorders, 322
Dysphonia, 322
Dysplasia, 255, 259, 283
Dyspnea, 8, 52-53, 322-323, 357
Dysprosium [Dy], 354
Dysrhaphia, 252, 254
Dysrhythmias, cardiac, 287
Dysthyroid orbitopathy, 288
Dystocia, 327
Dystonia, 252
Dystrophy: muscular, 110, 264
    myotonic, 96, 260
    neuroaxonal, 275 fn
    neuro-ophthalmic disorders, 288

primary optic, 259
Dysuria, 14

Eagle tests: syphilis, 29
Ear (*see also* Auditory)
    audiometry, 293 hn-294 hn, 294 fn
    bacterial infection, 14
    operations, 37
    radiation, 360, 366*
    skin thickening, 26
    thyroiditis, 322
    trauma, 227
    Turner's syndrome, 346
    vesicles, 241
    vestibular function tests, 295 hn, 295
Early normoblast counts, 164
Eastern equine encephalitis, 10, 21, 239, 239 fn
EB virus, 3 hn, 3, 57
Ecchymoses, mastoid, 227
Echinococcus granulosus, 234, 237
Echinostoma, 32*
Echocardiograms, 168 hn, 168*, 175 hn, 176*-178*
Echoviruses, 2-4, 5*, 6-7, 238-240, 252
Eclampsia, 285-286
Eczema, 81, 82 fn
Eczema vaccinatum, 43, 46
Edema
    complement system deficiencies, 89, 110, 127, 130
    graft-versus-host reaction, 71
    heart failure, 53
    immunoprophylaxis reaction, 49
    lepromatous leprosy, 26
    myelin disorder, 248
    nasal: adrenergic agents, 55
    optic nerve disorder, 259
    radiation, 359
    trauma: brain, 228-229, 229 fn
        central nervous system, 249, 286-287
        spinal cord, 230, 232
Edinger-Westphal nucleus, 277
Edmonston vaccine, 42
Edrophonium, neuro-ophthalmic response, 288
Efferent pathways, 278-281
Effusion: bacterial infection, 15
Egg allergy, 44, 48-49
Eggs, helminth, 33-35, 234
Egg white lysozyme, 119
Ehlers-Danlos syndrome: prenatal diagnosis, 91
Einsteinium [Es], 354
Ejaculation, 281
Elastase, 203 hn, 203*
Elbow, 145, 217
Electrocardiogram
    pulmonary embolism, 52 hn, 53
    related cardiovascular events, 168*, 178*
    rheumatic fever, 18
Electrocortin, 328 fn
Electroencephalogram
    CNS viral infections, 238 hn, 238-239, 243-245
    patterns: abnormal, 300*-303*
        normal, 296 hn, 296*-299*
    transplacental infection, 252 hn, 252
Electrolytes (*see also* specific electrolyte)
    cystic fibrosis, 53
    diabetes mellitus, 326

    hyperaldosteronism, 334
    lethal radiation, 359
    surgery, 140
Electromechanical systole, 175
Electrophoresis: autonomic responses, 278
        genetic disorders, 107 hn, 109-110
        plasma proteins, 131, 212
Electrophoretic mobility, 122-123, 137 fn
Electroretinogram, 291
Emaciation: cortisone, 330
Embolic lesions, 14
Embolism, 53, 285
Embolus, 291
Embryo, helminth, 33-35
Embryonal tumors, 225, 323
Emesis: graft-versus-host reaction, 70
Emotional disturbances, 340, 348
Emphysema, 53, 171, 182, 212
Empyema, 18-19
Encephalitis infections
    drug toxicity, 46
    electroencephalographic abnormalities, 300 hn
    laboratory findings, 10-11, 239, 242, 243 fn, 244
    non-viral, 235 fn-237 fn
    occurrence: United States, 10-11, 239 fn
    virus types, 7
Encephalitis viruses
    California, 11, 21
    eastern equine, 10, 21, 239, 239 fn
    equine, 2 (*see also* specific equine encephalitis)
    Japanese B, 21, 239 fn
    Murray Valley, 21, 239 fn
    Russian spring-summer, 21
    St. Louis, 11, 21
    tick-borne, 21
    Venezuelan equine, 11, 21, 239 fn
    western equine, 10, 21, 252
Encephalomalacia, 228-229, 231, 286
Encephalomyelitis: acute disseminated, 247
        allergic, 42
        congenital rubella, 243
        encephalitis viruses, 21, 252
        immunopathologic mechanism, 84
        intrauterine pathogens, 252
Encephalopathy: hypoxic, 248
        lead, 286
        liver diagnostic test, 213
        spongiform, 245, 286
        thymus transplants, 78
        trauma, 23 1
Endarterectomy, carotid, 263
Endocardial deformities, 7
Endocarditis: chemoprophylaxis, 37
        diagnosis, 14
        nerve disorders, 235, 272
        pneumonia complication, 19
        serum complement level, 88
        therapy, 16
Endocervical culture, 16
Endochondral ossification, 254 hn
Endocrine adenoma syndrome, 323
Endocrine disorders, 69, 109, 323 (*see also* specific disorder or disease)
Endocrine glands, 351, 360 (*see also* specific gland)
Endocrine neoplasia, 325, 327, 334

Fibrous gliosis, 245
Fibula, 217
Filtration rate, glomerular, 305 hn, 306
Filum terminale, 223
Finger: deformity, 310
    ossification, 217
    radiation, 366*
    sensory loss, 257
    ulcer, 14
Firearm injuries, 227
Fish, 22, 27
Fission, binary, 1
Fissure, interlobar, 18-19
Fistula, 228-229, 263-264, 360
Fitzgerald coagulation factor, 121 hn
Flaccid paralysis, 240, 242
Flaccid paraparesis, 248
Flaujeac trait, 121 hn
Flavin-adenine dinucleotide [FAD], 114, 155
Flaviviruses, 2-3
Fleas, 14, 21, 27
Fletcher coagulation factor, 121 hn
Flocculation tests, 29
Florinef, 333
Flucytosine, 30 fn, 36 fn
Fludrocortisone, 333-334
Fluids: amniotic, 351
    bloody spinal, 229
    gastric, 351
    intravenous, 327
    menstrual, 351
    synovial, 83 fn, 88 fn, 218-220
Flukes, 32*, 234 (see also Trematodes)
Fluorescein angiography, 326
Fluorescein-conjugated concanavalin A capping: poly-
   morphonuclear leukocytes, 63
Fluorescent rabies antibodies, 242
Fluorescent treponemal antibody tests, 29
Fluorine [F], 353
5-Fluorocytosine, 36, 40
Fluorodinitrobenzene, 65
Fluorometric assay, 107 hn, 107-108
Fluoroscopy, 365
Foam cells, 271, 274
Focusing: neuro-ophthalmic disorders, 288
Foix-Alajouanine disease, 224
Folate, 165 hn, 165
Folic acid, 97, 205*, 209 hn
Follicle: hair, 335
    ovarian, 305-306, 342, 346, 348, 350
Follicle-stimulating hormone
   biochemistry, 305-307
   female reproductive disorders, 346 hn, 346-348,
    349 hn, 349-350
   female reproductive hormones, 340 hn, 340-342
   luteinizing hormone—releasing hormone, 315
   pituitary disorders, 337 hn, 337
Follicular cells, thyroid gland, 309
Follicular tumors, 322-323
Follitropin, 305
Fontanelle, anterior, 221, 243
Foods, 27, 82, 202*-203*, 205*-206*, 207 hn, 207
Food vacuole, 31
Foot: acromegaly, 310
    edema, 26

    motor loss, 257
    ossification centers, 216 hn
    skeletal fusion, 217
    Turner's syndrome, 346
Foramen magnum, 263, 290
Forced expiratory flow rate, 181 hn, 181-182
Forced expiratory volume, 52 hn, 52-53, 181 hn, 181-182
Forced vital capacity, 52 hn, 52-53, 181 hn, 181
Forceps delivery, 231
Forearm, 141-142, 145, 171, 257 (see also Arm)
Forebrain, 366*
Forehead, 146
Formalin-ethylene oxide, 48
[^{14}C]Formate oxidation, 62
Formazan, 63
Formic acid oxidation, 62
Formiminoglutamic aciduria, 109
Fornix of eye, inferior, 278
Foshay's test, 14, 17
Fossa: tumors, 224, 261, 289, 310
Fowl, 2-3 (see also Poultry)
Fowler's solution, 145
Fox, 9, 21, 242
Fractures, 227-229, 258, 264, 360
Francisella tularensis, 17, 21, 49
Free cholesterol: plasma concentrations, 134
Free fatty acids (see Fatty acids, free)
Free water clearance, 197 hn, 197-198
Friedlander's bacillus, 18
Frontal gyrus, superior, 250
Frontal lobe, 229, 239, 281
β-Fructofuranosidase, 202 hn, 202*
Fructose, 104, 202*, 213, 335
Fructose 1,6-bisphosphate, 113, 115, 118, 155-156
Fructose-bisphosphate aldolase: blood assay, 113, 118
               disorders, 104, 110, 154
Fructose 6-phosphate, 114-115, 156
Fructose-1-phosphate aldolase, 104
Fruits: botulism incidence, 27
Fucose, 200
α-L-Fucosidase, 91
Fucosidosis, 91
Functional residual capacity, 179-180, 182 hn, 182
Fundus oculi, 260
Fungal infections, 234, 236, 285 (see also Mycoses; specific
   fungal infection)
Fungi: hypersensitivity, 83 (see also Molds)
Funiculi, dorsal, 230
Furosemide, 262
Fusiform aneurysms, 282
Fusiform cavitation, 230
Fusion, skeletal, 216-217, 254
Fusobacterium, 38
F. necrophorum, 233, 235

Gadolinium [Gd], 354
Galactocerebroside-β-galactosidase, 248
Galactokinase, 104, 109-110, 113, 154
Galactorrhea, 308, 310, 344, 348
Galactose: digestion, 202*, 202 fn
    enzyme assay, 113
    inherited disorders, 104, 109
    progesterone, 342
Galactosemia, 91, 104, 109-110, 154
Galactose 1-phosphate, 113

Hemoptysis, 8
Hemorrhage: Addison's disease, 333
  bacterial infection, 21
  central nervous system, 284-285, 287, 287 fn
  cranial nerve disorder, 261
  epinephrine, 331
  growth hormone deficiency, 311
  hemoglobinopathies, 159
  hypopituitarism, 348
  intrauterine pathogen, 252
  myelin disorders, 247
  neuro-ophthalmic disorders, 289
  poliomyelitis, 240
  radiation, 359
  trauma, 149-150, 228-229, 231-232
  tumors, 224
  vasopressin, 314
Hemorrhagic diathesis, 231
Hemorrhagic encephalitis, 236 fn
Hemorrhagic encephalopathy, 247
Hemorrhagic fever viruses, South American, 2
Hemorrhagic lesions, 247
Hemorrhagic necrosis, 241
Hemorrhagic retinopathy, 292
Hemosiderin pigment, 228, 231
Hemostasis, 121 hn, 121-122, 352
Henderson-Hasselbalch equation, 194 hn
Henle, loop of, 352
Heparan N-sulfatase, 94
Hepatic (see also Liver)
Hepatic bilirubin, 209 hn, 210*
Hepatic cirrhosis, 98, 104
Hepatic excretion: antimicrobial agents, 40
Hepatic failure, 237, 271, 287, 326
Hepatic glycogenolysis, 324
Hepatic heme turnover, 209 hn
Hepatic insufficiency, 303*
Hepatic ketogenesis, 327
Hepatic necrosis, 213
Hepatic neoplasia, 212
Hepatic schizonticides, 30 hn, 31
Hepatic toxicity: antituberculous drugs, 24
Hepatic venous pressure, wedged, 173
Hepatitis: blood product hazards, 13
  cardiac output, 169
  congenital rubella encephalomyelitis, 243
  epidemiologic features, 4, 12
  histocompatibility leukocyte antigens, 69
  immunodeficiency, 68
  immunofluorescence tests, 85, 87
  immunoglobulin M, 129
  immunoprophylaxis, 47
  Leptospira, 21, 235
  liver diagnostic tests, 211
  lymphoid replacement therapy, 81
  plasma amino acids, 101
  radiation, 360
  Schistosoma, 22
  serum complement level, 88
Hepatitis surface antigens, 12, 87 hn, 87
Hepatitis viruses, 2 hn, 3, 7, 42, 82
Hepatobiliary disorders, 209 hn-210 hn, 211, 213
Hepatocellular disease, 211-213
Hepatocytes, 72, 211-212, 324

Hepatolenticular degeneration, 104, 127, 131 (see also Wilson's disease)
Hepatomegaly, 100, 236
Hepatosplenomegaly, 157, 159, 236, 244
Hering, canals of, 72
Hermaphrodite, 347
Herniation, 254, 290, 366*
Heroin addiction: pneumonia, 20
Herpangina, 6
Herpes simplex (see also Herpesviruses)
  CNS infections, 238-240, 252, 282
  epidemiological features, 4
  facial nerve, 261
  therapy, 10, 45 fn-46 fn
  transmission, 3
Herpes simplex encephalitis, 239, 239 fn
Herpes stomatitis, 81
Herpesviruses (see also specific herpes infection)
  CNS infections, 238, 238 fn, 239, 239 fn, 244, 252
  DNA core, 5*
  facial nerve, 261
  physical characteristics, 2
  respiratory illnesses, 4
  therapy, 10, 45-46
Herpesvirus hominis, 2
Herpesvirus varicellae, 241-242
Herpes zoster infections, 241-242, 259 (see also specific infection)
Herpes zoster ophthalmicus, 259
Herpes zoster oticus, 261
Herpetic gingival stomatitis, 261
Herpetic keratitis, 45-46
Herpetic kerato-uveitis, 45
Hetacillin, 38 fn
Heterodera marioni, 32*
Heterophyes heterophyes, 32*, 34
Heterotopia, nasal glial, 226
Heterozygotes, 91-95, 103 hn, 103-104, 212
Hexachlorophene, 248
Hexamidase A, 116
n-Hexane, 271
Hexokinase, 110, 114, 155
Hexosamine, 200
Hexosaminidases, 91-92, 111
Hexosediphosphatase, 330
Hexose monophosphate shunt, 62
Hexose-1-phosphate uridylyltransferase, 91
Hexoses, 200, 324
Hilus cell tumor, 350
Hindbrain: age-related change, 251
Hinton test: syphilis, 29
Hip, 217, 257, 365
Hippocampus, 229, 242
Hirsutism, 310, 333, 335, 349-350
Histamine: allergic disorders, 54-55, 82
  anaphylactic importance, 51
  enzyme assay, 117
  gastrin secretion, 325
Histamine methyltransferase, 251
Histamine phosphate, 201 hn, 279
Histamine release, leukocyte, 51-52
Histamine test, intradermal, 279
Histidine, 98, 103, 105-106, 108
L-Histidine ammonia-lyase, 98, 143

Hyperdibasic aminoaciduria, 103, 109
Hyperemia, 357
Hyperfunctioning thyroid nodule, 318
Hypergammaglobulinemia, 26, 88
Hyperglucagonemia, 324
Hyperglycemia: adrenal hormones, 330-332
liver diagnostic test, 213
pancreas disorders, 326-328
pancreas hormones, 323, 325
pheochromocytoma, 334
Hyperglycinemias, 99, 108, 111
Hyperglycinuria, 103
Hyperhistidinemias, 98, 108
Hyperimmune serum globulin, 13
Hyperimmunoglobulinemias, 59-60, 271, 273
Hyperinflation, chest, 53
Hyperinsulinism, 324, 327
Hyperkalemia, 329, 333-334
Hyperkeratosis, 71
Hyperleucinemia, 99, 108
Hyperlipidemia, 136 hn, 137-138, 212
Hyperlipoproteinemias, 136-138
Hyperlysinemia, 92, 100, 102, 108
Hypermelanosis, 143
Hypermethioninemia, 98
Hypermotility, 231
Hypermyelination, 231
Hypernatremia, 284-285, 333
Hyperornithinemia, 100
Hyperosmolality, blood, 313
Hyperosmolar non-ketotic coma, 327
Hyperostosis, 230
Hyperparathyroidism, 254, 319, 323
Hyperphenylalaninemia, 92, 97-98, 107-108
Hyperphosphatemia, 319
Hyperpigmentation
    adrenal disorders, 333
    chemical agents, 145-146
    congenital rubella encephalomyelitis, 243
    cortisone, 330
    Fanconi's syndrome, 143, 143 fn
Hyperplasia: adrenal, 329, 333
    congenital adrenal lipoid, 338
    cystic, 340
    endometrial, 350
    endoneural, 270
    gastric, 325
    hyperthyroidism, 320-321
    islets of Langerhans, 327
    Kupffer cell, 72
    nodular, 333
    peripheral nerves, 275
    Schwann cell, 271, 274-275
Hyperplastic fibrosis, 350
Hyperplastic myelinopathy, 272
Hyperprolinemia, 92, 100, 102, 108
Hyperpyrexia, 242 (see also Fever)
Hyperreflexia, autonomic, 230, 281
Hypersensitivity, 53, 65 hn, 65, 82-83, 278, 288 (see also
    Allergic reactions)
Hypertension: acromegaly, 310
    adrenal disorders, 333-334
    adrenal hormones, 329-330, 332
    adrenocorticotropic hormone, 305
    blood flow, 171

cardiac output, 169
CNS disorders, 287
female reproductive disorder, 346
heart failure, 53
spinal cord contusion, 230
steroid 17α-hydroxylase deficiency, 338
vasopressin, 312
viral infections, 7
Hyperthecosis, 350
Hyperthyroidism, 143, 288, 320-322, 325
Hypertonicity, blood, 312
Hypertriglyceridemia, familial, 137 fn, 138
Hypertrophy: bony & soft tissues, 306
    interstitial cells, 307
    Kupffer cell, 72
    ovary, 306
    peripheral nerves, 248, 271, 275, 275 fn
    right ventricle, 105
Hypertropia, 290
Hypertyrosinemias, 98, 108
Hyperuricemia, 24
Hypervalinemia, 99, 108, 111
Hyperventilation, 277 hn, 279, 357
Hyperviscosity, 292
Hypervolemia, 312
Hypoadrenalism, 292, 360
Hypoalbuminemia, 212
Hypoaldosteronism, 334
Hypoaminoacidemia, 324, 328
Hypobetalipoproteinemia, 139
Hypocalcemia, 104, 319, 327
Hypochromia, 157-159
Hypodefecation, 321
Hypoesthesia, facial, 289
Hypofibrinogenemia, 121
Hypogammaglobulinemia, 59-60, 131
Hypoglossal nerve disorders, 263
Hypoglycemia
    Addison's disease, 333
    adrenal hormones, 330-331
    amino acid disorders, 101, 103
    anterior pituitary hormones, 305-306, 308
    electroencephalographic abnormalities, 300 hn
    growth hormone deficiency, 311
    human placental lactogen, 344
    liver diagnostic test, 213
    pancreas disorders, 326-327, 327 fn
    pancreas hormones, 324-325
Hypogonadism, 258, 336-337, 347-348
Hypokalemia, 326, 329, 333
Hypokalemic alkalosis, 338
Hypolipoproteinemias, 138-139
Hypomyelination, 248
Hyponatremia: Addison's disease, 333
    aldosterone, 329
    autonomic nervous system, 277 hn
    edema, 287
    peripheral nerve pathology, 270
    vasopressin, 312, 314
Hypoosmolality, blood, 312
Hypophosphatasia, 101, 109, 111
Hypophosphatemia, 319
Hypophysiotropic hormone, 348
Hypopigmentation, 146
Hypopituitarism: abnormal pigmentation, 143

Indium [In], 353
Indocyanine green, 213
Indomethacin, 351-352
Infant death, sudden, 67-68
Infant disorders, 126, 290
Infantile uterus, 346-347
Infantilism, sexual, 348
Infarction: glucagon, 324
   hemoglobinopathies, 158
   intrauterine pathogen, 253
   nerves, 260, 272, 275
   radiation, 359
Infectious angiitis, 282-283
Inferior olive, 250-251
Inferior salivatory nucleus, 278
Infertility, 310, 339, 348, 350 (see also Fertility; Sterility)
Influenza infections (see also Influenzaviruses)
 central nervous system, 239
 diagnosis, 8
 pneumonia complication, 18
 therapy, 8, 44-45, 48
 transmission, 4
Influenza vaccines, 42, 44, 44 fn, 263
Influenzaviruses, 2-4, 5*, 6, 239
Infundiboloma, 226
Inhalation: disease transmission, 28
Inheritance patterns (see also autosomal & sex-linked inheritance patterns)
 amino acid disorders, 97 hn, 98-105
 coagulation factor deficiencies, 121 hn, 121-122
 hyperlipoproteinemias, 136 hn, 137-138
 inborn errors of metabolism, 91-95
 nerve disorders, 248, 269 hn, 271, 273
Inhibitory concentration correlates: antimicrobial agents, 38-39
Injection: virus transmission, 3
Inoculation: viral disease transmission, 4
Inorganic iodide: goiter, 322
Inorganic iron: absorption, 207 hn, 207*
Inorganic orthophosphate: enzyme assay, 112 hn, 116
Inorganic phosphorus: urine, 200
Inorganic sulfur: urine, 200
Inorganic toxins: peripheral nerves, 270
Insomnia, 229
Insulin: adrenal hormones, 330-331
  biochemistry, 323-324
  central nervous system, 281, 284
  gastrin, 325
  glucagon, 325
  growth hormone, 306, 311
  hemorrhage, 284
  keto acid production, 139 hn, 140
  obesity, 101
  pancreas disorders, 84, 326-327
  somatostatin, 316
  trauma, 148 hn, 149
Insulin-dependent diabetes, 87
Insulinoma, 87, 327
Integument, 254 hn, 330
Intellectual impairment, 243-244, 248, 327 (see also Mental retardation)
Intercellular bridge antigens, epithelial, 83
Intercellular edema, 71
Intercostal nerve, 242
Interferon, 1, 46, 61

Interlobar fissure, 18-19
Intermediate normoblast count, 164
Intermitotic cells: radiosensitivity, 355
Intermittent porphyria: diagnosis, 94, 111
    hyperlipoproteinemia, 137
    uroporphyrinogen I synthase, 155
    vasopressin, 314
Internal jugular vein, 264
Internode length: peripheral nerves, 268 hn, 268-269
Interpeduncular fossa, 289
Interstitial cells: testis, 307, 335
Interstitial-cell-stimulating hormone, 307
Interstitial edema, 53
Interstitial fibrosis, 53, 182
Interstitial fluid, 191, 191 fn
Interstitial infiltrates, 8
Interstitial nephritis, methicillin-induced, 87
Inter-α-trypsin inhibitor, 126
Interventricular septum, 175 hn-176 hn, 176*, 178*
Intestinal bacteria, 209 hn, 210* (see also specific genus)
Intestinal crypts, 72, 355
Intestinal glands, 72
Intestinal helminths, 32*, 33-35
Intestinal lumen, 72, 202*-207*, 319
Intestinal lymphangiectasis, 68
Intestinal mucosa, 72, 202*, 202 fn, 203*-207*
Intestinal peptide, vasoactive, 325
Intestinal tract, 33-34, 310, 329 (see also specific tissue)
Intestines: amino acid disorders, 103-104
   calcium absorption, 206 hn, 319
   disaccharidases, 124-125
   immunopathologic mechanisms, 82-83
   lesions, 72
   motility, 331
   radiation tolerance doses, 359
   tumor, 307
Intoxication, water, 287
Intrauterine death, 327
Intrauterine infection, 244
Intrauterine pathogens, 252-253
Inulin clearance, 194 hn, 195-196
Iodide, 62, 318, 321
Iodide, inorganic: goiter, 322
Iodination: ingested particles, 62
Iodine [I], 308, 320 hn, 321-323
Iodochlorhydroxyquin, 259
Iododeoxyuridine, 46
Ionic composition: body compartments, 191-192
Ionizing radiation, low-level, 370
Ipsilateral pupil response, 277
Ir gene defect, 67 fn
Iridium [Ir], 354
Iridocyclitis, 26
Iridoviridae, 2 hn
Iris, 143-144, 278, 351 (see also Eye; Pupil)
Iron [Fe]: absorption, 207 hn, 207*
   deficiency, 68
   hemoglobinopathies, 157, 159
   radiotoxicity, 353
   serum concentrations, 165 hn, 165
   transferrin, 128
Iron-binding capacity: serum, 165 hn, 165
Iron-binding globulins, 207 hn, 207*
Iron deficiency anemia, 157-158
Iron (II):oxygen oxidoreductase, 118

Kwashiorkor, 124, 143
Kyphosis, 229, 255

Labor (birth), 37, 343, 351
Labyrinthine disorders, 238, 262, 290
Lacerations, 228, 229 hn, 230, 232
Lacrimal gland, 278
Lacrimal nucleus, 278
Lacrimation test, 272, 278
β-Lactamases, 37 hn
Lactase, 124 hn, 124-125, 202 hn, 202 fn (*see also* Galactosidases)
Lactate, 119, 141-142, 148, 150, 156
Lactate dehydrogenase, 114, 119, 212
L-Lactate:NAD⁺ oxidoreductase, 114, 119
Lactation, 316, 318
Lactic acid, 109
Lactic acidosis, 101, 139 hn, 140, 142
Lactobacillus, 165
Lactogen, human placental, 306, 308, 344
Lactose, 202*, 202 fn
Lactoyl-glutathione lyase, 114
Lacunae, intraepithelial, 71
Lamina, vertebral, 258
Lamina propria, 65, 72
Laminar necrosis, 248
Lanthanum [La], 354
Large intestine, 72
Larvae, 32*, 33
Larval migrans, visceral, 237
Laryngotracheitis, 7
Larynx, 82
Laser photocoagulation, 326
Lassa virus, 3
Lateral columns of spinal cord, 281
Lateral femoral cutaneous nerve, 272
Lateral horns, 241
Lateral mass of atlas, 258
Lateral popliteal nerve, 272 fn
Laurence-Moon-Biedl syndrome, 337, 347
Lead [Pb], 270, 354
Lead encephalopathies, 286
Lead poisoning, 155, 209 hn
Leber's disease, 259, 260, 291
Lecithin, 133
Left atrium, 167 hn, 168*, 174, 175 hn, 176*, 177 hn, 177*-178*, 178 fn
Left ventricle, 150, 167 hn, 168*, 174, 175 hn, 175, 176*, 177 hn, 177*-178*, 178 fn
Leg: ataxia, 245
    blood lactate & pyruvate levels, 141-142
    degenerative disk disease, 257
    paralysis, 242
    ulcers, 158-159
Leiner's disease, 89
Leishmania, 22
Lemon juice: autonomic responses, 278
Lens, 288, 290 fn, 360-362
Lenticular degeneration, progressive, 143
Lenticular deposits, 291
Leprosy, 26, 236, 270
Leptomeningeal infections, 285
Leptomeninges, spinal, 224
Leptomeningitis, 235 hn, 235-237, 243
Leptospira, 21, 233, 235, 253 fn

Lesch-Nyhan syndrome, 92, 111, 114, 155
Lesions: autonomic nervous system, 277 hn, 278, 280-281
    bacterial infection, 14
    central nervous system, 221, 223, 226, 239-242, 252
    cranial nerves, 259-260, 263
    diabetes mellitus, 326
    graft-versus-host reactions, 71-72
    growth hormone deficiency, 311
    intrauterine pathogens, 252
    liver diagnostic tests, 211-213
    myelin disorders, 246-249
    neuro-ophthalmic disorders, 288-290
    ovarian dysfunction, 348, 350
    protozoan infection, 22
    small blood vessels, 285
    spinal neoplasms, 256
    trauma, 229, 231-232
    viral infections, 239-242, 244-245
Lesser multangular bone, 217
Lesser petrosal nerve, 278
Lethargy, 243, 314, 321, 357, 359
Leucine: insulin, 324
    metabolic disorders, 98-99, 101, 108
    normal blood concentrations, 105
    renal clearance, 106
    trauma, 149
Leucine aminopeptidase, 117, 203 hn, 212 fn
Leucine aminotransferase, 99
L-Leucine-*p*-nitroanilide, 117
Leukemia: fungal infection, 236
    graft survival, 74-76
    hemorrhages, 284
    lymphocyte surface marker system, 57
    ocular involvement, 259
    peripheral nerve pathology, 270
    plasma proteins, 128-129
    pneumonia, 19
    radiation, 358, 370-372
Leukocyte antigens, histocompatibility (*see* Histocompatibility leukocyte antigens)
Leukocyte count, 14 hn
Leukocyte function tests, 62-64
Leukocyte inhibitory factor, 61
Leukocytes (*see also* specific leukocyte; WBC)
    function, 62 hn, 62-64
    IgE antibody detection, 51-52
    immunodeficiency diagnosis, 65
    immunopathologic mechanisms, 82 hn, 82-84
    inherited disease diagnosis, 111
    migration, 61, 66
    peripheral blood, 161
    synovial fluid, 218-220
    transplants, 72, 74 hn
    viral infections, 10, 238 hn, 238-242, 244
Leukocytorrhexis, 72
Leukocytosis, peripheral, 242
Leukocytosis, polymorphonuclear, 240
Leukodystrophy, 93, 111, 247-248, 274
Leukoencephalopathy, 245, 247, 292
Leukopenia, 20, 161 fn, 359
Leydig cells, 307 fn, 335
Lhermitte-Duclos disease, 223
Libido, 307, 335, 349
Life span: red cells, 163

Ligaments: congenital spinal anomalies, 254-255
    ossification, 263
    relaxin, 343
    trauma, 229, 257 hn, 257-258
Ligandin, 210*
Limbic system, 281
α-Limit dextrins, 202*, 202 fn
Lincomycin, 16, 18-19, 36, 38, 40
Linea alba, 143
Linoleic acid, 132-134
Lip: abnormal pigmentation, 146
Lipase, 119, 324, 331
Lipexal, 64 fn
Lipids (*see also* Fatty acids; Triglycerides)
    anaphylactic importance, 51
    brain content, 251
    cortisone, 330
    digestion & absorption, 204*, 204 fn
    lipoproteinemias, 137-139
    normal blood concentrations, 132-135, 162
    normal urine concentrations, 200
    plasma proteins, 126-127
Lipoamide dehydrogenase, 94
Lipoate acetyltransferase, 94
Lipoatrophic diabetes, 324
Lipofuscin, 251
Lipofuscinosis, ceroid, 291
Lipogenesis, 330
Lipoid hyperplasia, congenital adrenal, 338
Lipolysis: adrenal hormones, 330-331
    glucagon, 324
    growth hormone, 306
    pancreas disorders, 327
    prostaglandins, 352
    trauma, 148 hn
Lipopolysaccharide, 63
Lipoproteinemias, 135-139 (*see also* specific disease)
Lipoproteins: disorders, 136 hn, 137, 138 hn, 138-139
    estradiol, 341
    liver diagnostic test, 212
    method of definition, 135-136
    properties & function, 126-127
    Tangier disease, 131, 274
    variation in disease, 131
Liquid petrolatum, 63
Listeria, 22, 233, 236, 253, 253 fn
Lithium, 318
Lithium carbonate, 321
Livedo reticularis, 143
Liver (*see also* Hepatic)
    abnormal pigmentation, 143
    adrenal hormones, 330-331
    amino acid disorders, 98 fn, 101, 103
    anterior pituitary disorders, 310-311
    bilirubin, 209 hn, 210*
    calcium absorption, 206 hn
    cell differentiation failure, 67
    diagnostic tests, 211-213
    fetal transplants, 79-80
    glucagon, 324
    graft-versus-host reactions, 71-72
    keto acids, 139 hn
    metabolic activity, 318
    plasma coagulation factors, 121-122
    pneumonia, 19

    posterior pituitary hormones, 312
    radiation, 355, 360, 366*
Liver abscesses, 236
Liver cell carcinoma, 212-213
Liver cell plates, 72
Liver disease (*see also* specific disease)
    alcoholic: diagnostic test, 211
    central pontine myelinolysis, 249
    galactose-1-phosphate uridylyltransferase, 154
    hyperlipoproteinemias, 137-138
    hypoglycemia, 327 fn
    plasma proteins, 125-128
    serum complement level, 88
Liver flukes, 32*
Liver lesions, 71-72, 211-213
Liver malignancy, 343
Liver membrane, 87
Live vaccines, 42, 43*, 43-45, 48-49 (*see also* specific vaccine)
Lobar pneumonia, 14, 18-20, 182
Lobectomy, anterior temporal, 259-260
α-Lobeline hydrochloride, 279
Lobes: frontal, 229, 281
    occipital, 292-293
    parietal, 292-293
    temporal, 221, 229, 310
Lobules: mammary gland, 342
Lobules, paracentral, 281
Lochia, foul, 14
Locus coeruleus, 250
Loop of Henle, 352
Lordosis, 229
Louse, 27-28, 233
Lowe's oculocerebrorenal syndrome, 104
Lubs syndrome, 339, 339 fn
Lucio phenomenon, 26
Luder-Sheldon syndrome, 105
Lumbar agenesis, 255
Lumbar disks, 257 hn, 257
Lumbar nerve root, 257 hn, 257
Lumbar sensory ganglia, 242
Lumbar spine radiation, 365
Lumbar stenosis, 255
Lumbar tap, 14
Lumbar trauma, 258
Lumbar vertebra, 254 hn, 254
Lumen, 72, 202*-207*, 319
Luminal membrane, 103
Lung (*see also* Pulmonary)
    diffusing CO capacity, 52 hn, 52-53, 181 hn, 182
    echocardiogram, 176 hn, 178*
    hormones, 351-352
    IgE antibody detection, 51
    immunopathologic mechanisms, 82-84
    radiation, 355-356, 360, 368
    spinal neoplasms, 256 hn
Lung abscesses, 14, 16, 236
Lung cancer, 323, 370, 372
Lung capacity, total, 179-180, 182 hn, 182
Lung compliance, static, 181 hn, 182
Lung diseases, 8, 14, 19-20, 84 (*see also* specific disease)
Lung flukes, 32*, 234
Lung malignancies, 306, 319, 343 (*see also* Lung cancer)
Lung tumors, 305, 307, 314
Lung volumes, 179 hn, 179-180, 182 hn, 182

liver diagnostic test, 213
myelin disorders, 247-248
ovarian hypofunction, 348
radiation, 358-360, 362-363
sensory ganglia, 241
trauma, 229-230
Necrotizing lesions, 285
Negative free water clearance, 197 hn, 197-198
Negri bodies, eosinophilic, 242
Neisseria, 15-17, 233, 235
Nelson's syndrome, 143, 333
Nematodes, 33, 234, 283
Neodymium [Nd], 354
Neomycin, 37-38, 262
Neonatal cholestasis, 212
Neonatal cystinelysinuria, 103
Neonatal hyperbilirubinemia, 327
Neonatal hyperphenylalaninemia, 97
Neonatal hypocalcemia, 327
Neonatal iminoglycinuria, 103
Neonatal meningitis, 252-253
Neonatal tyrosinemia, 98, 108
Neonate, 129
Neoplasms: circulatory system, 283-285, 287
cranial nerves, 258-263
Cushing's syndrome, 333
gastrin, 325
glucagonoma, 328
human chorionic gonadotropin, 344
islets of Langerhans, 327
liver diagnostic test, 212
nervous system, 221-226, 291-293
non-viral infections, 236
plasma proteins, 126
pneumonias, 19
radiation, 362
spine, 256
thyroid, 322-323
Nephritic factor, 88, 122
Nephritis, 21, 80, 82-83, 87, 100
Nephritogenic serotypes, 24-25
Nephrocalcinosis, 319
Nephrolithiasis, 230
Nephron permeability, 312
Nephropathy, 104, 262, 273, 326
Nephrosclerosis, 360
Nephrosis, 68, 125, 127-128, 137
Nephrotic syndrome: diabetes mellitus, 326
fetal liver transplants, 80
hyperlipoproteinemias, 138
liver diagnostic test, 212
α_1-macroglobulin, 127
Nephrotoxic serum nephritis, 83
Neptunium [Np], 354
Nerve cells, 239-240, 242, 247-248, 355
Nerve endings, 278
Nerve fibers, 231-232, 268-275, 291
Nerve palsies, 260-261, 323
Nerve plaques, 247
Nerve root, 254, 257 hn, 272-273 (*see also* specific nerve)
Nerves (*see also* specific nerve)
atrophy, 230, 259-260, 263
lepromatous leprosy, 26
norepinephrine, 331
tumor, 256

Nerve surgery, facial, 262
Nervousness: hyperthyroidism, 320
Nervous system, 233-237
autonomic, 277 hn, 277-281
central (*see also* Central nervous system)
asthma, 56
circulatory disorders, 282
hormone secretion, 314 hn, 314-316
intrauterine pathogens, 252-253
prostaglandins, 351 hn, 352
untreated syphilis, 29*
peripheral, 246 hn, 247-249, 351 hn, 352
sympathetic, 331, 352
Neuralgia, 242, 261, 263
Neural tube, 97, 254 hn, 254
Neuraminidase antigens, 6 hn, 6 fn
Neurapraxia, 230
Neurilemoma, 225, 261-263
Neuritis, 243 fn, 259, 360
Neuroaxonal dystrophy, 275 fn
Neuroblastomas, 221, 225, 258, 289
Neurocutaneous melanosis syndrome, 224
Neurodeficit: spinal neoplasms, 256
Neuroepithelial tumors, 221-223, 225
Neurofibrillary tangles, 251
Neurofibril regeneration, 230
Neurofibromas, 225, 256, 262-263
Neurofibromatosis, 224, 259, 292
Neurofibrosis, 275
Neurofilaments, 271, 275
Neuroglia, 226, 250
Neurohypophyseal tumors, 226
Neurohypophysis, 314-315
Neurologic disorders
antituberculous drugs, 24
associated enzymes, 110 fn, 154-155
CNS viral infections, 238-239, 244
congenital spinal anomalies, 254 hn, 254-255
intrauterine pathogens, 252-253
rubella, 243
Trypanosoma cruzi infection, 22
viral disease immunization, 43-45
Neuroma, 230, 262, 334
Neuromuscular disorders, 69, 258-264, 319
Neuromyelitis, 247, 259
Neuronophagia, 239-242
Neurons, 239-245, 250, 280, 331
Neuro-ophthalmic disorders, 288-293
Neuropathy: cranial nerves, 259-263
diabetes mellitus, 326
hypolipoproteinemias, 139
Mycobacterium leprae infection, 236 fn
myelin, 247-249
ocular motor system, 289
peripheral nerves, 270-275, 275 fn
Neurophysin, 312
Neuropore, 366*
Neurosecretory cells, 314
Neurosis, 366*
Neurosyphilis, 30, 288
Neurotmesis, 230
Neurovascular cross-compression, 262
Neutralization antibodies, 238 hn, 238, 241-244
Neutropenia, 99
Neutrophilic cell counts, 164

Oleic acid, 132-134
Olfactory (see also Nose)
Olfactory bulb glomeruli, 250
Olfactory genetics, 258
Olfactory lobes, 347
Olfactory nerve disorders, 258-259
Oligodendrocytes, 244-246
Oligodendroglia, 239
Oligodendrogliomas, 221, 223
Oligo-1,6-glucosidase, 202 hn, 202*
Oligomenorrhea, 350
Oligopeptidases, 203 hn, 203*
Oligopeptides, 203 hn, 203*
Oligosaccharides, 200, 202 fn
Oligospermia, 365
Oliguria, 36
Olivary nuclei, 250
Olive oil emulsion, 119
Olives: botulism incidence, 27
Olives (brain), 231, 250
Olivopontocerebellar degeneration, 259
Oocytes: hormones, 305, 307
Opacification, retinal, 291
Open-heart surgery, 285
Operations: chemoprophylaxis, 37
Ophthalmia, gonococcal, 37
Ophthalmic nerve, 241-242
Ophthalmic zoster, 241
Ophthalmoplegia, 14, 260-261, 288-292
Opisthorchis, 35
Opisthotonus, 243
Opossum, 21-22
Opsonification, 63
Optic (see also Eye; Ocular; Orbital)
Optical density: leukocytes, 62 hn, 63
Optical rotation: hormones, 328 hn, 329-332, 335 hn,
    335, 340 hn, 340-342
Optic atrophy, 244, 259-260, 291-292
Optic chiasma, 259-260, 292, 310
Optic-chiasmatic arachnitis, 259
Optic disk, 259, 291-292
Optic dystrophy, 259
Optic foramen, 259
Optic nerve: autonomic pathways, 277
            disorders, 222, 247, 259-260, 291-292
Optic neuritis, 24, 245 fn, 259
Optic neuropathy, 259-260
Optokinetic nystagmus, 292-293
Oral cavity, 360
Oral contraceptives, 146, 350
Oral mucosa, 145
Oral pharynx, 82
Oral ulcerations, 111, 154
Orbital (see also Eye; Ocular; Optic)
Orbital apex lesions, 289
Orbital fissure syndrome, superior, 260
Orbital pain, 289
Orbital plate fractures, 227
Orbitopathy, dysthyroid, 288
Orbiviruses, 2-3
Orchitis, 7
Orf virus, 2-3
Organic acid metabolism, 109
Organic phosphorus, 200
Organic toxins, 270-271

Organophosphate, 270
Oriboca virus, 2
Ornithine, 100, 102-103, 105-106, 108-109
Ornithine carbamoyltransferase, 100, 108, 119
Ornithine decarboxylase, 100
Ornithinemia, 108
Ornithine—oxoacid aminotransferase, 94
Ornithine transcarbamylase, 100, 108
Ornithosis chlamydias, 21
Oropharyngeal operations, 37
Orotate phosphoribosyltransferase, 94
Orotic aciduria, 94, 110-111
Orotidine 5'-phosphate decarboxylase, 94, 110-111
Orthomyxoviruses, 3, 5*, 6 hn
Orthopedic operations: chemoprophylaxis, 37
Orthophosphate, 162
Orthophosphate, inorganic, [P_i], 116
Orthostatic hypotension, 281
Oscillations, head, 290
Osmium [Os], 354
Osmolality, 197 hn, 197-198, 314, 327
Osmoreceptors, hypothalamic, 311-312
Osmoregulation: albumin, 125
Osmotic diuresis, 326
Os odontoideum, 254
Osseous necrosis, 230
Osseous spicule, 254
Ossification, 216-217, 254 hn, 255, 263
Osteitis fibrosa, 319, 350
Osteoarthritis, 218, 310
Osteoblastic lesions, 256
Osteoblastoma, 256
Osteoblasts, 211, 319, 340
Osteochondroma, 256, 285
Osteoclasts, 319
Osteocytes, 319
Osteodystrophy, renal, 254
Osteogenic sarcoma, 256
Osteoid osteoma, 256
Osteolytic metastases, 323
Osteoma, osteoid, 256
Osteomalacia, 254
Osteomyelitis, 15, 17, 236
Osteoporosis, 230, 306, 330, 333, 340
Otic ganglion, 278
Otitis, 261, 263, 346, 360
Otitis media, 18-19, 235
Otolithic function, 295
Otorrhea, 227
Ototoxicity: neomycin, 262
Ova: intestinal helminths, 32*
Ovarian cortical stroma, 350
Ovarian follicles, 305, 307, 346, 348, 350
Ovary: anterior pituitary hormones, 305-307
        mosaicism, 258
        post-menopausal, 341
        prostaglandins, 351
        radiation, 364-365
        reproductive disorders, 346-350
        reproductive hormones, 340-344
Ovary syndrome, resistant, 346
Ovotestis, 347
Ovulation, 305-307, 315, 340, 348, 350-351
Oxacillin, 36-37, 39-40
Oxaloacetate, 113, 117, 119

420

Renal transplants, 326
Renal tubular acidosis, 104
Renal tubular adenylate cyclase, 319
Renal tubular brush border, 82
Renal tubular defects, 128
Renal tubular failure, 98
Renin, plasma, 280, 329, 334
Renin-angiotensin II system, 328
Reoviruses, 2-3, 5*
Reproductive disorders, 336-339, 346-350
Reproductive hormones: biochemistry, 335, 340-344
Reproductive organs, 351 (see also specific organ)
Reserpine, 308
Residual volume, 52 hn, 52-53, 182 hn, 182
Resistant ovary syndrome, 346
Respiratory diseases (see also specific respiratory disease)
    bacterial, 14, 19
    viral, 4, 37, 322
Respiratory failure: radiation, 359
Respiratory insufficiency, 240
Respiratory muscle weakness, 182
Respiratory syncytial virus vaccine, 42
Respiratory syndromes, 6, 182, 238, 327
Respiratory system cancer, 371
Respiratory viruses, 2-4, 5* (see also specific virus)
Reticular cells, 84, 164, 256
Reticular dysgenesis, 67
Reticular formation: brain, 250
Reticulin antigen, 87
Reticulocyte count, 157-159
Reticuloendothelial cells, 121, 342
Reticuloendothelial system: bilirubin excretion, 210*
    cortisone, 330
    nerve disorders, 247
    Tangier disease, 139, 274
Reticulum, 72
Retina: radiation, 360, 366*
Retinal anlage tumor, 221
Retinal opacification, 291
Retinal pigmentation, 243, 288, 291
Retinal receptors, 277
Retinal vessel occlusion, 291-292
Retinitis, 237
Retinitis pigmentosa, 139, 291, 337, 347
Retinoblastoma, 221, 292
Retinol-binding protein, 126
Retinopathies, 289, 291-292, 326
Retrobulbar neuritis, 259, 292
Retrograde pyelography, 365
Retro-orbital infection, 236
Retroperitoneum, 221
Rhabditiform larvae, 32*
Rhabdoviruses, 2-3, 242
Rh blood group: erythroblastosis fetalis, 82
Rhenium [Re], 354
Rhesus monkey erythrocyte, 57
Rheumatic fever, 18, 37, 283-284
Rheumatic heart disease, 18, 170-171
Rheumatoid arteritis, 283
Rheumatoid arthritis: HLA association, 69
    immunofluorescence test, 85
    immunopathologic mechanism, 83
    peripheral nerves, 272
    plasma proteins, 126-127
    prostaglandins, 351

serum complement level, 88
    synovial fluid, 218-219
Rheumatoid factor, 26, 83
Rhinitis, 4, 6, 18, 54-55, 236
Rhinorrhea, 227
Rhinoviruses, 2-4, 5*, 46
Rhizopus, 234, 236
Rhodium [Rh], 353
Rhomboencephalitis, 236 fn
Rhonchi, 8, 14
Rib cage, expanded, 310
Riboflavin, 110 fn
Ribonuclease I, 85-86, 119
Ribonucleic acid: antiviral agents, 46
    central nervous system, 251
    enzyme assay, 119
    microorganisms, 1
    sclerosing panencephalitis, 244
    synthesis: hormones, 306
Ribonucleic acid, messenger, 335
Ribonucleoprotein, 85, 244
Ribonucleotide reductase, 45
Ribosomes, 1, 324
Ribs: spinal trauma, 258
Ribulose 5-phosphate, 115
Richner-Hanhart syndrome, 98
Rickets, 101-102, 104, 254
Rickettsia, 21, 27-28, 49, 233, 235
Rickettsial diseases, 27-28, 49, 233, 235, 283
Rickettsias, 1, 21
Rickettsiosis, North Asian tick-borne, 27
Rifampin, 24, 36-37, 40
Rift Valley fever virus, 2
Rimantidine HCl, 45
Right atrium, 174, 175 hn, 176*
Right ventricle, 105, 167 hn, 168*, 174, 175 hn-177 hn,
    176*-178*, 178 fn
RNA (see Ribonucleic acid)
RNA nucleotidyltransferase, 46, 341
RNA viruses, 1-2, 5*, 242 fn-244 fn (see also specific virus)
Rochalimaea quintana, 28
Rocky Mountain spotted fever, 21, 27-28, 49, 283
Rodents, 11, 21-22, 27-28, 233-234
Roentgenography, 53, 368 (see also Radiography)
Romberg's disease, 264
Rosenthal fibers, 248
Rose spots: bacterial infection, 14
Rosettes, 57, 366* (see also E-rosettes)
Rosewater's syndrome, 339, 339 fn
Rotaviruses, 2-3
Rotor syndrome, 209 hn
Rowley-Rosenberg syndrome, 105
Rubella: CNS infection, 282
    epidemiological features, 4
    immunodeficiency mechanism, 68
    immunoprophylaxis, 44, 47-48
Rubella encephalomyelitis, congenital, 243
Rubella panencephalitis, chronic progressive, 243
Rubella syndrome, congenital, 44 fn
Rubella vaccine, 42, 44
Rubella virus, 2-3, 243, 252
Rubidium [Rb], 353
Ruminants, 21 (see also specific animal)
Runyon groups: Mycobacterium, 23
Rupture: trauma, 228-229

Ruptured arterial aneurysms, 284-285
Russian spring-summer encephalitis virus, 21
Russian tick-borne virus, 2
Ruthenium [Ru], 353

Sabin vaccine, 42
Sac, conjunctival, 278
Saccades, 289
Saccharopine, 100, 108
Saccharopine dehydrogenase, 92, 100
Saccharopine oxidoreductase, 92
Saccharopinuria, 93, 100, 108
Saccular aneurysms, 263-264, 282
Sacral disks, 257 hn, 257
Sacral nerve roots, 257, 281
Sacral parasympathetic nerves, 280-281
Sacral segments, 277 hn, 281
Sacral vertebra, first, 254 hn, 254
Sacrococcygeal agenesis, 255
St. Louis encephalitis, 11
St. Louis encephalitis virus, 21, 239 fn
Salbutamol, 55
Salicylates, 321
Saline, hypotonic, 327
Saliva: autonomic responses, 281
    CNS viral infections, 238, 242, 244
    immunoglobulin concentrations, 58
    viral encephalitis, 10
Salivary α-amylase, 202 hn, 202*
Salivary glands, 310, 329, 360, 372 (see also Parotid gland)
Salivation, 278, 310
Salivatory nucleus, inferior, 278
Salk neutralizing antibodies, 66
Salk vaccine, 42
Salmonella, 64, 69 fn, 233, 235
S. typhi, 16, 49, 80, 253 fn
Salt craving, 333
Salt intake, 313
Samarium [Sm], 354
Sandfly, 22
Sandhoff's disease, 92, 111, 260
Sanfilippo syndrome, 94
Sarcoidosis, 263
Sarcomas, 221, 224, 256
Sarcomatosis, primary meningeal, 224
Sarcosinemia, 99, 108
Sarcosine oxidase, 99
Sausage-body neuropathy, 273
Scalp hair, 146-147, 310, 335
Scalp tenderness, 292
Scandium [Sc], 353
Scaphoid bone, 217
Scapula, 257
SCARI regimen, 76
Scarlet fever, 18
Scarring, 48-49
Scars, glial, 231
Schilder's disease, 231 fn, 292
Schistosoma, 22, 32*, 35, 234, 237
Schizogyria, sclerotic, 231
Schizonticides, 30 hn, 31
Schwann cells
    hyperplasia, 271, 274-275
    lepromatous leprosy, 26
    myelin disorders, 247-248

    nuclei, 269, 273, 275
    peripheral nerve pathology, 270-271, 273-275
Schwannoma, 225 (see also Neurilemoma)
Sciatic nerve, 230, 242, 272
Scleroderma, 283
Sclerosing panencephalitis, 10 fn, 244
Sclerosis: CNS neoplasm, 222
    cranial nerve disorders, 258-262, 264
    immunofluorescence test, 86
    myelin disorder, 246-247
    neuro-ophthalmic disorders, 289-290
    radiation, 360
    trauma, 231
Sclerotic atrophy, cerebellar, 243
Sclerotic platygyria, 231
Sclerotic polymicrogyria, 231
Sclerotic schizogyria, 231
Scoliosis, 229, 255
Scopoletin fluorescence, 62
Scotoma, 291-292
Scrapie, 245 fn
Scrotum, 281
Scrub typhus, 27, 283
Sea level: alveolar O_2 pressure, 183
Secondary sex characteristics, 207, 335, 340
Secretin, 316, 318, 324-325
Secretin-producing cells, 317
Secretin test: pancreatic function, 208-209
Secretions, body, 58, 128, 281
Secretory component synthesis, 67
Secretory IgA, 128
Sedatives: asthma, 56
Sedimentation rate: erythrocytes, 18, 292, 321
Segmental demyelination, 269 hn, 270-275
Segmental infarction, 272
Segmentation: congenital spinal anomalies, 254 hn, 254-255
Segmented cells, 161, 161 fn, 163 hn, 164
Seizures: amino acid disorders, 102
    antituberculous drugs, 24
    electroencephalogram, 301*-302*
    growth hormone deficiency, 311
    intrauterine pathogens, 252
    nerve disorders, 242-245, 247-248, 263, 289
    pancreas disorders, 327
    parathyroid hormone, 319
    vasopressin, 314
    viral encephalitis, 10-11, 239
    whole-body radiation exposure, 358
Selenium [Se], 353
Sella turcica, 292, 310, 348
Semen, 351
Semicircular canal function, 295 hn, 295
Semimydriasis, 288
Seminal vesicles, 335
Seminiferous tubules, 305
Semliki Forest virus, 2
Semple vaccine, 42
Senile macular degeneration, 291
Senile plaques, 251
Sensorimotor neuropathy, 270-275
Sensorineural hearing loss, 294 hn, 294, 294 fn
Sensory deficit: trauma, 228
Sensory ganglia, 241-242
Sensory loss, 249, 257 hn, 257

Toes, 217, 257, 366*
Togaviruses, 2-3
Tolbutamide test, 327
Toluene, 271
Tomogram, 257-258
Tone decay, 293 hn, 294
Tongue, 71, 310
Tonsillitis, 14, 16
Tonsils: hyperlipoproteinemia, 139
    immunodeficiency diagnosis, 65
    radiation, 322, 357
    viral encephalitis, 10
Tonsils, cerebellar, 229
Topographic agnosia, 293
Tourniquet injury, 249
Toxic amblyopia, 292
Toxicosis, T$_3$-, 321
Toxins, exogenous: peripheral nerves, 270-271
Toxocara canis, 234, 237
Toxoplasma gondii, 234, 237, 253
Toxoplasmosis, 231 fn
Tracheal obstruction, 322
Tracheal secretions, 244
Tracheal shift, ipsilateral, 18, 20
Tracheal stenosis, 53
Tracheobronchial secretions, 58
Tracheobronchitis, 4
Tracheostomy, 53
Traction: spinal trauma, 258
Transcobalamin, 126, 128, 206 hn, 206*, 206 fn
Transcortin, 126, 340
Transferrin: deficiency, 131
    iron absorption, 207 hn
    properties, 128
    serum concentrations, 165
    synovial fluid, 218
Transfusion, 3, 73 (*see also* Blood products)
Transhydrogenases, 340
Transient hypogammaglobulinemia, 59-60
Transplacental infections, 3, 252 hn, 252, 252 fn, 253,
    253 fn
Transplants, 72-78, 245
Transport, amino acid, 102-103, 109, 203*, 203 fn
Transverse atlantal ligament, 254
Transverse myelitis, 292
Transverse process: spinal trauma, 258
Trapezium bone, 217
Trapezius muscle, 257
Trapezoid bone, 217
Trauma: bacterial infection, 236
    birth, 230-232, 327
    central nervous system, 148 hn, 284-285, 287
    cranial nerves, 227-229, 231, 258, 260-264
    cranio-cerebral, 227-231
    diabetes mellitus, 327
    electroencephalographic abnormalities, 300 hn
    epinephrine, 331
    glucagon, 325
    growth hormone deficiency, 311
    hemodynamic function & blood, 149-150
    metabolic constituents, 148-149
    myelin, 249
    neuro-ophthalmic disorders, 289, 291-293
    peripheral nerves, 230, 232
    pigment metabolism, 144

    spine & spinal cord, 229-230, 232, 257-258
    synovial fluid, 220
    vasopressin, 313-314
Traumatic aneurysms, 229, 282
Traumatic apoplexy, 229
Traumatic dural thrombosis, 228
Traumatic hematomyelia, 230
Traumatic neuroma, 230
Traumatic porencephalia, 231
Trematodes, 34-35, 234 (*see also* Flukes)
Tremor: hyperthyroidism, 320
    insulinoma, 327
    nerve disorders, 240, 245, 289
    pheochromocytoma, 334
    radiation, 359
Trench fever, 28
Treponemal antibody tests, fluorescent, 29
Treponema pallidum, 29*, 29, 233, 235, 252
Triacetyloleandomycin, 56
Triacylglycerol lipase, 119, 204 hn, 204*
Triangular bone: ossification, 216
Triatomids, 22
Triceps muscle, 257
Trichinella spiralis, 22, 234, 237
Trichorrhexis nodosa, 100
Trichostrongylus, 32*
Trichuris trichiura, 32*, 33
Tricuspid valve, 167 hn
Trigeminal afferents, 278
Trigeminal facial vascular malformation, 225
Trigeminal ganglion, 241, 261
Trigeminal herpes, 241-242
Trigeminal neuralgia, paroxysmal, 261
Trigeminal neurilemomas, 261
Trigeminal sensory neuropathy, 261-262
Triglycerides: digestion & absorption, 204*, 204 fn
    hormones, 324, 330
    lipoproteinemias, 136 hn, 137-139
    plasma concentrations, 132
Trigone, 223, 281
L-Triiodothyronine, 308, 318, 320 hn, 320-322
Trimethoprim, 16
Trimethoprim-sulfamethoxazole, 8, 39
Triosephosphate isomerase, 110, 113, 115, 155
Trioxsalen, 146
Triparanol, 147
Tripeptidases, 203 hn, 203*
Triple response of Lewis, 279
Tritium, 188 hn, 189
Trochlear nerve, 260, 289
Trochlear nucleus, 250
Trombiculid mite, 28
Trophic disturbances: birth trauma, 232
Trophoblastic neoplasms, 344
Trophoblastic tissue, 343
Tropical sprue, 124
Trunk, body (*see* Body trunk)
Trypanosoma, 22, 234, 236
Trypsin, 126, 203 hn, 203*, 206 hn, 206*, 305-307
Tryptic proteolysis, 314
Tryptophan, 101, 106, 306
Tryptophan oxygenase, 330
Tsetse fly, 22, 234
Tuberal nuclei, 242
Tuberculin-purified protein derivative, 61